P9-EKS-152

03210309

Phobic and Anxiety Disorders in Children and Adolescents

OKANAGAN UNIVERSITY COLLEGE
LIBRARY
BRITISH COLUMBIA

PHOBIC AND ANXIETY DISORDERS IN CHILDREN AND ADOLESCENTS

A Clinician's Guide
to Effective Psychosocial
and Pharmacological Interventions

Edited by
THOMAS H. OLLENDICK
JOHN S. MARCH

OXFORD
UNIVERSITY PRESS
2004

OXFORD
UNIVERSITY PRESS

Oxford   New York
Auckland   Bangkok   Buenos Aires   Cape Town   Chennai
Dar es Salaam   Delhi   Hong Kong   Istanbul   Karachi   Kolkata
Kuala Lumpur   Madrid   Melbourne   Mexico City   Mumbai   Nairobi
São Paulo   Shanghai   Taipei   Tokyo   Toronto

Copyright © 2004 by Oxford University Press, Inc.

Published by Oxford University Press, Inc.
198 Madison Avenue, New York, New York 10016

www.oup.com

Oxford is a registered trademark of Oxford University Press

All rights reserved. No part of this publication may be reproduced,
stored in a retrieval system, or transmitted, in any form or by any means,
electronic, mechanical, photocopying, recording, or otherwise,
without the prior permission of Oxford University Press.

Library of Congress Cataloging-in-Publication Data
Phobic and anxiety disorders in children and adolescents : a clinician's
guide to effective psychosocial and pharmacological interventions /
[edited by] Thomas H. Ollendick, John S. March.
p. cm.
Includes bibliographical references and index.
ISBN 0-19-513594-6
1. Anxiety in children.   2. Phobias in children.   I. Ollendick,
Thomas H.   II. March, John S., MD.
RJ506.A58   P48   2003
618.92'85223—dc21   2002156296

1 3 5 7 9 8 6 4 2

Printed in the United States of America
on acid-free paper

To the real giants in the field—Albert Bandura,
B. F. Skinner, and Joseph Wolpe. They have greatly
influenced not only my professional development but
my personal development as well.

—THO

To John Greist, Edna Foa, and Keith Conners,
mentors and friends extraordinaire.

—JSM

PREFACE

Anxiety disorders are common, cause considerable morbidity and perhaps mortality, and (most important) are now treatable with evidence-based treatment procedures. This book is designed to help clinicians from a variety of disciplines learn about the etiology, developmental course, assessment, and treatment of children and adolescents with anxiety disorders. Thus, clinicians and their patients are the primary targets for this book.

In the past, psychology and psychiatry have been at odds over these issues—sometimes for scientific reasons and at other times because stakeholder issues were paramount. The editors and chapter authors of this book believe strongly that it is not possible to practice competent and ethical psychopharmacology without the availability of empirically supported psychotherapy. Similarly, it is not possible to practice competent and ethical psychotherapy without the availability of empirically supported psychopharmacology. We believe that physicians (who typically write prescriptions) and psychologists (who, for the most part, have developed and are better versed in psychological treatments) must join hands in the care of individual patients, if for no other reason than that the complexity of modern mental health care is beyond the capacity of any one individual to master.

In this context, this book intentionally models both the benefits and the difficulties of multidisciplinary practice in which practitioners of both disciplines become stakeholders for the experiment (the research question) or the benefit of the individual patient (the clinical question). Without this commitment to multidisciplinary practice, we shortchange our patients.

ORGANIZATION OF THE BOOK

In writing this book, we married as authors an outstanding group of psychologists and psychiatrists who are expert in their respective areas. The book is organized in three parts.

In part I, "Foundational Issues," we lay the foundation for the chapters on specific phobic and anxiety disorders that follow by providing a broad and integrative view of issues that affect the psychopathology, assessment, and treatment of the various childhood anxiety disorders. Specific chapters cover diagnostic issues, etiology, epidemiology development, and comorbidity.

In part II, "Assessment and Treatment of Specific Disorders," we focus on the *DSM-IV* anxiety disorders. Each chapter includes sections on clinical manifestation or phenomenology of the disorder, diagnosis and classification (including differential diagnosis and comorbidity), and developmental course of the disorder, with the bulk of the chapter focused on assessment and treatment. With respect to assessment, the authors focus on best assessment practices—using an assessment tree—to arrive at a correct diagnosis and to assist in treatment planning and evaluation of treatment outcome. In this way, assessment serves treatment (i.e., it should possess clinical or treatment utility). In turn, treatment is discussed in a stages-of-treatment model, illustrating the decision-making process in determining which treatments to use and the order in which the treatments should be selected or tried. As such, the best treatment practices will be illustrated. Selected treatments must have some empirical support for their use and (ideally) have been subject to randomized clinical trials for their consideration.

In part III, "Future Directions for Research and Practice," we highlight issues that will continue to characterize the field in the new millennium, in an attempt to set the stage for future research and practice. In particular, we focus on prevention and early intervention, the need to move from efficacy to effectiveness research, translating research to practice, and services research to see if our treatments are actually implemented and working.

ACKNOWLEDGMENTS

It has been our good fortune to participate in the development and dissemination of empirically supported medication and psychosocial treatments for youth with anxiety disorders, but many others also deserve credit. The authors of the chapters in this volume are truly pioneers. Much, if not most, of what is known in this area devolves from these individuals and their students. We are grateful to them for conveying their accumulated wisdom, which highlights the extraordinary progress made in pediatric anxiety disorders over the past 10 to 15 years.

Most of all, we owe a special debt of gratitude to the many patients and their families who have taught us so much about anxiety disorders in young people. With so much of mental health care still driven by ineffective relationship-oriented psychotherapies and poorly implemented drug treatments, it often seems to us that our patients and their parents are ahead of the field in their understanding of mental illness and its treatment. Their thoughtful observations, cheerfulness in the face of anxiety, and willingness to wonder along with us as we endeavor to find answers to their conditions have been and remain professionally rewarding and personally inspiring. Without them, this book would not have been written.

There is, of course, much more to life than academic pursuits, and I (THO) want to thank my wife, Mary; my now-grown children, Laurie and Katie; and my grandchildren, Braden and Ethan. And I (JSM) want to thank my wife, Kathleen, and my children, Matthew and Maggie, for their patience as we put this volume together. Their love and support make all other things, including the varied tasks of academic life, possible. Because research is a collaborative endeavor, we also wish to thank the members of our research groups, without whom our own small scientific contributions would soon founder.

Finally, as in most areas of psychiatry and psychology, controversy abounds. This book, though rich in information and recommendations, will in some instances not do justice to the edge of the field, and the reader may not agree with everything we say. The errors of fact are ours; the controversies will eventually lead to good science. Our goal in producing this volume is to help children and adolescents with anxiety disorders lead more normal, happy, and productive lives. We hope we have achieved this goal, even if only modestly.

CONTENTS

CONTRIBUTORS

ANNE MARIE ALBANO, New York University Child Studies Center, New York University Medical Center

ALETA ANGELOSANTE, Department of Psychology, Temple University, Philadelphia, Pennsylvania

ADRIAN ANGOLD, Duke University Medical Center, Durham, North Carolina

PAULA M. BARRETT, Department of Psychology, Griffith University, Queensland, Australia

GAIL A. BERNSTEIN, Division of Child and Adolescent Psychiatry, University of Minnesota Medical School, Minneapolis

BORIS BIRMAHER, Department of Psychiatry, Western Psychiatric Institute and Clinic, University of Pittsburgh Medical School, Pittsburgh, Pennsylvania

BARBARA J. BURNS, Department of Psychiatry and Behavioral Sciences, Duke University Medical Center, Durham, North Carolina

JUDITH A. COHEN, Department of Psychiatry, MCP Hahnemann University School of Medicine, Allegheny General Hospital, Pittsburgh, Pennsylvania

E. JANE COSTELLO, Duke University Medical Center, Durham, North Carolina

JOHN F. CURRY, Department of Psychiatry, Duke University Medical Center, Durham, North Carolina

MARK R. DADDS, Department of Psychology, Griffith University, Queensland, Australia

HELEN L. EGGER, Department of Psychiatry and Behavioral Sciences, Duke University Medical Center, Durham, North Carolina

ROBERT F. FERDINAND, Department of Child and Adolescent Psychiatry, Sophia Children's Hospital, Erasmus University, Rotterdam, the Netherlands

GRETA FRANCIS, Brown University School of Medicine and the Bradley School, East Providence, Rhode Island

MARTIN E. FRANKLIN, Department of Psychiatry, University of Pennsylvania School of Medicine, Philadelphia, Pennsylvania

JENNIFER B. FREEMAN, Brown University School of Medicine, East Providence, Rhode Island

EDNA B. FOA, Department of Psychiatry, University of Pennsylvania School of Medicine, Philadelphia, Pennsylvania

ABBE M. GARCIA, Child and Family Psychiatry, Rhode Island Hospital, Providence, Rhode Island

GOLDA S. GINSBURG, Division of Child and Adolescent Psychiatry, Johns Hopkins University School of Medicine, Baltimore, Maryland

POLLY GIPSON, Center for the Advancement of Children's Mental Health, Department of Child Psychiatry, New York State Psychiatric Institute/Columbia University, New York

CHRIS HAYWARD, Department of Psychiatry, Stanford University Medical Center, Stanford, California

AARON S. HERVEY, Department of Psychology: Social and Health Sciences, Duke University, Durham, North Carolina

DAVID HEYNE, Department of Medicine, Dentistry, and Heath Sciences, University of Melbourne, Victoria, Australia

RACHAEL C. JAMES, Department of Psychology, Griffith University, Queensland, Australia

PETER JENSEN, Center for the Advancement of Children's Mental Health, Department of Child Psychiatry, New York State Psychiatric Institute/Columbia University, New York

PHILIP C. KENDALL, Department of Psychology, Temple University, Philadelphia, Pennsylvania

NEVILLE J. KING, Department of Education, Monash University, Clayton, Victoria, Australia

HENRIETTA L. LEONARD, Brown University School of Medicine, East Providence, Rhode Island

ANTHONY P. MANNARINO, Department of Psychiatry, MCP Hahnemann University School of Medicine, Allegheny General Hospital, Pittsburgh, Pennsylvania

JOHN S. MARCH, Department of Psychiatry, Child and Family Study Center, and Department of Psychology: Social and Health Sciences, Duke University Medical Center, Durham, North Carolina

LAUREN M. MILLER, Child and Family Psychiatry, Rhode Island University, Providence, Rhode Island

ROBIN NEMEROFF, Center for the Advancement of Children's Mental Health, Department of Child Psychiatry, New York State Psychiatric Institute/ Columbia University

THOMAS H. OLLENDICK, Child Study Center, Department of Psychology, Virginia Polytechnic Institute and State University, Blacksburg, Virginia

AMY R. PERWIEN, Department of Clinical and Health Psychology, University of Florida Medical School, Gainesville, Florida

SANDRA PIMENTEL, Department of Psychology, Temple University, Philadelphia, Pennsylvania

DANNY PINE, Department of Psychiatry, Columbia University, New York

MOIRA A. RYNN, Department of Psychiatry, University of Pennsylvania School of Medicine, Philadelphia, Pennsylvania

WENDY K. SILVERMAN, Child and Family Psychosocial Research Center, Department of Psychology, Florida International University, Miami, Florida

L. ALAN SROUFE, Institute of Child Development, Minneapolis, Minnesota

MICHAEL SWEENEY, Department of Child and Adolescent Psychiatry, Columbia University, New York

BRUCE TONGE, Centre for Developmental Psychiatry and Psychology, Monash Medical Centre, Clayton, Victoria, Australia

PHILIP D. A. TREFFERS, Academic Centre for Child and Adolescent Psychiatry Curium, Leiden University Medical Center, Leiden, The Netherlands

FRANK C. VERHULST, Department of Child and Adolescent Psychology, Erasmus University, Rotterdam, The Netherlands

JOHN T. WALKUP, Division of Child and Adolescent Psychiatry, Johns Hopkins University School of Medicine, Baltimore, Maryland

SUSAN L. WARREN, Center for Family Research, George Washington University, Washington, DC

ALICIA WEBB, Department of Psychology, Temple University, Philadelphia, Pennsylvania

I

FOUNDATIONAL ISSUES

1

DIAGNOSTIC ISSUES

Mark R. Dadds, Rachael C. James,
Paula M. Barrett, & Frank C. Verhulst

Diagnostic issues lie at the heart of contemporary scientific approaches to psychopathology. The medical/categorical approach is currently the most frequently used and influential model of diagnosis, with the *Diagnostic and Statistical Manual of Mental Disorders: DSM-IV* (American Psychiatric Association [APA], 1994) and *ICD-10: International Statistical Classification of Diseases and Related Health Problems* (World Health Organization [WHO], 1992–1994) being the most popular contemporary diagnostic systems in this model. In its purest form, the categorical approach has an explicit acceptance of the idea that the normal differs from the pathological by kind rather than by degree and that there are clear distinctions between qualitatively different types of disorder. It sees childhood disorders as discrete entities that are displayed in clusters of interrelated clinical symptoms. Each disorder can be distinguished from other disorders by the way the symptoms cluster and by the extent to which these clusters have specific sets of associations with other clinically significant factors. This type of model also identifies common features of people that are placed in the same category, for instance, a distinctive set of symptoms, pathological features, epidemiology, course, and response to treatment (Werry, 1994). Categorical systems are developed by panels of experts who negotiate categories and criteria on the basis of empirical evidence and clinical experience.

DEVELOPMENT OF THE CURRENT SYSTEMS:
DSM AND *ICD*

The *DSM* system has undergone many revisions in the last few decades, facilitating a common vocabulary and improved communication between clinicians and researchers. Most salient progress occurred with the publication of the *DSM-III* (APA, 1980). It differed from existing classification schemes in several ways—multiaxiality; explicit criteria for each disorder; exclusionary criteria; hierarchical organization in which particular disorders are held to be mutually exclusive, with emphasis on phenomenological criteria rather than etiological criteria; anchored points for the axes; supporting manual; and attempts to empirically establish reliability.

The *DSM-III-R* (APA, 1987) anxiety disorders consisted of adult anxiety disorders (panic disorder, agoraphobia, social phobia, simple phobia, obsessive-compulsive disorder, posttraumatic stress disorder, generalized anxiety disorder, and anxiety disorder not otherwise specified) and anxiety disorders with onset usually in childhood or adolescence. Children were given adult diagnoses using adult-derived criteria when they had symptoms of disorders, unless specifically excluded in the definition. Childhood anxiety disorders included separation anxiety disorder, overanxious disorder, and avoidant disorder. Due to problems with reliability, stability of diagnoses, comorbidity, and poor discriminant validity, criteria in *DSM-IV* were tightened to remove overlap with other disorders and to improve compatibility with adult anxiety disorders. Avoidant disorder, which was semantically identical with social phobia, was removed from the *DSM-IV*, and it was assumed that avoidant personality disorder would take its place. Overanxious disorder was also removed, due to lack of discriminant validity; it was subsumed under the diagnosis of generalized anxiety disorder. Therefore, the only specific childhood anxiety disorder that remained in the *DSM-IV* was separation anxiety disorder.

The *DSM* employs a phenomenological approach in that disorders are diagnosed on the basis of observable symptoms. The theories of the cause behind the disorder are of little consequence, and hence the *DSM* may be considered atheoretical, based on an empirical process of continually updating categories in response to new research (Sonuga-Barke, 1998). Although the *DSM* may be atheoretical with regard to specific disorders, it inherently promotes the theory that disorders are discrete entities with a categorical rather than a dimensional structure, that these result from organismic dysfunction, and that these are endogenous and thus situated within the child (Dawson, 1994; Sonuga-Barke, 1998).

The *International Classification of Disorders* (*ICD*) is the official diagnostic system that members of the United Nations use in preparing their national health statistics. Notable similarities were introduced in the *DSM-III* and the *ICD-9* (WHO, 1975) systems. The two diagnostic systems both had separate sections for childhood disorders, the *ICD-9* could be used as a multiaxial system, and they both adopted an atheoretical approach to

diagnosis (Sonuga-Barke, 1998). However, there were also several significant differences. First, the *ICD* contains no operational diagnostic criteria,
just general descriptions. Second, the *ICD-9* contained fewer subcategories,
with the anxiety disorders being divided into four categories: (1) neurotic
disorders (those that were similar to adult anxiety disorders, such as phobias),
(2) disturbances of emotions specific to childhood, (3) mixed disturbance of
emotion and conduct (comorbidity), and (4) adjustment reactions, which
included stress-related disorders. Third, the axes were different, as well as being
optional (I—Clinical psychiatric syndrome, II—Developmental delays, III—
Intellectual level, IV—Physical disorders, V— Abnormal psychosocial situations). Fourth, comorbidity in the *ICD* was dealt with by "mixed disorders"
rather than multiple diagnoses. Finally, the *ICD* manual was very brief (Werry,
1994). Subsequently, research into the *ICD-9* was more limited than that
conducted for *DSM-III*. Reliability was inconsistent but low for emotional
and neurotic disorders, but it improved when these disorders were combined
(Gould, Shaffer, Rutter, & Sturge, 1988). When attempts were made to more
finely discriminate the anxiety disorders, reliability was diminished.

   ICD-10 was published in 1992, in two versions: one for clinicians and
one for researchers, detailing the operational criteria. The fact that *ICD*
does not view it as important for clinicians to have access to the operational
criteria reduces its credibility as a scientific classification system (Werry,
1994). In the *ICD-10*, as in *DSM*, all the childhood anxiety disorders are
aggregated in a single category, with a number of subcategories: *separation anxiety disorder, phobic disorder*, and *social phobic disorder* (with these
disorders differing from the adult anxiety disorders by being only exaggera-
tions of normal developmental fears); *other* (which includes overanxious
disorder); and a new disorder, *sibling rivalry disorder*.

   The list of disorders that follows is based on the current *Diagnostic and
Statistical Manual of Mental Disorders* (fourth edition), or *DSM-IV*. There
are several disorders—such as posttraumatic stress disorder, acute stress
disorder, and adjustment disorder—that can include anxious symptoms;
however, only categories in which anxiety is the primary problem are discussed in this chapter. Readers are referred to the subsequent chapters in
this book for substantive reviews of these specific disorders. It should be
noted that little developmental sophistication is to be found in the current categorization of anxiety disorders. Thus, the presentation, epidemiology, and correlates of the following disorders differ across age groups.
For older adolescents, use of the adult anxiety disorder literature is increasingly appropriate.

Separation Anxiety Disorder (SAD)

SAD is defined as undue anxiety regarding separation from significant figures in the child's life. The child must meet three of the following criteria:
recurrent, excessive distress when separation from home or attachment figures occurs or is anticipated; persistent and excessive worry about harm

happening to attachment figures; persistent and excessive worry that some event will lead to separation from an attachment figure; persistent reluctance or refusal to attend school due to fear of separation; persistent and excessive fear or reluctance to be alone or without attachment figures at home; persistent reluctance to go to sleep without being near an attachment figure; repeated nightmares about separation; and repeated complaints of physical symptoms when separation from attachment figures occurs or is anticipated. To be diagnosed with the disorder, a child must have symptoms lasting for more than four weeks, and the child must be younger than 18.

Generalized Anxiety Disorder (GAD)

GAD is characterized by excessive and uncontrollable anxiety and worry, occurring more days than not for at least 6 months. The anxiety must be about several areas of life functioning and must be associated with at least three psychophysiological or somatic complaints. This disorder subsumes the category of overanxious disorder, which was a childhood anxiety disorder in the *DSM-III-R* but was discontinued for the *DSM-IV*.

Social Phobia

Social phobia is identified by a persistent and excessive fear of social situations in which the child is exposed to unfamiliar people or to possible evaluation by others. The child fears that he or she will act in a way that will be humiliating or embarrassing. *DSM-IV* also specifies that exposure to the feared social situation will almost always provoke anxiety, which in children may be expressed by crying, tantrums, freezing, or shrinking from social situations. To be diagnosed with this disorder, adults must recognize that their fear is irrational, but this criterion is not essential for children. Children with social phobia will avoid the social situation or endure it with extreme distress. The avoidance or anxiety must significantly interfere with the child's functioning, and the symptoms must last for at least 6 months.

Specific Phobia

A specific phobia is characterized by a marked and persistent fear, that is excessive and unreasonable, of a specific object or situation. The presence of the feared object or situation or the anticipation of it can bring on an almost immediate anxiety response. In children, this anxiety may be expressed by crying, tantrums, freezing, or clinging. For adults to be diagnosed with this disorder, they must recognize that the fear is irrational, but this criterion is not essential for children. Children with a specific phobia will avoid the situation or endure it with extreme distress. The avoidance or anxiety must significantly interfere with the child's functioning, and the symptoms must be of at least a 6-month duration. Common phobias in children center on the dark, animals, blood, heights, and medical/dental procedures.

Obsessive-Compulsive Disorder (OCD)

OCD is characterized by obsessions, compulsions, or both. Obsessions are defined as recurrent and persistent thoughts, images, or impulses that are intrusive and distressing (e.g., relating to germs/contamination, harm/danger); they are not simply excessive worries about ordinary problems. The person attempts to ignore or suppress the obsessions and acknowledges that the obsessions are products of the mind. Compulsions are defined as repetitive behaviors or mental acts that a person feels that he or she must perform in response to an obsession, to prevent or reduce distress or prevent some dreaded event or situation from occurring (e.g., washing, checking, touching). The compulsions are performed according to rigid rules and are not realistically connected with what they are designed to prevent, or they are clearly excessive. For adults to be diagnosed with the disorder, they must recognize that their obsessions or compulsions are irrational. Children do not necessarily have to meet this criterion. The obsessions or compulsions also must significantly interfere with the child's functioning.

Panic Disorder

Panic disorder is identified by the presence of recurrent and unexpected panic attacks and subsequent worry for at least one month about future attacks. Agoraphobia, which is characterized by avoidance of certain situations due to anxiety about not being able to escape from these situations if a panic attack occurs, often coincides with panic disorder. Therefore, children can either be diagnosed with panic disorder with agoraphobia or panic disorder without agoraphobia. Cognitive factors are central to contemporary models of adult panic attacks (adults often report a fear that they are going crazy or about to die), and onset of panic disorder is usually in early adulthood or late adolescence, concurrent with the development of more sophisticated cognitive representations of the self. Thus, there has been much discussion about whether panic disorder actually occurs in children and younger adolescents (see Schniering, Hudson, & Rapee, 2000). Speculation also exists about whether SAD is an early form of panic disorder (see Silove & Manicavasagar, 2001).

POSITIVE ASPECTS AND PROBLEMS
OF DIAGNOSTIC SYSTEMS

Diagnostic classification has been defined as "the assumption that experience can be captured, that it will be repeated, and that subgroups of human beings share certain behaviors, emotions, foibles, challenges, and stresses that differentiate them from others" (Werry, 1994, p. 22). Classification facilitates communication in an efficient manner and, used effectively, can benefit all stakeholders by guiding resources and priorities in treatment and prevention. A good classification system not only tells what is absolutely necessary to make the diagnosis, but also alerts the examiner as to the other features of the disorder (Werry, 1994). Poland, Von Eckardt, and Spalding (1994) described diagnostic systems as providing clinical and scientific disciplines with a common set of ideas about the nature of disorders, which therefore inform practice in the clinic and laboratory. Categorization can also be a useful aid to clinical practice, potentially increasing the efficiency of therapeutic decisions and relieving uncertainty in clients. Assigning a diagnostic label to describe what is wrong with a child often brings great relief to the worried parent. An accurate diagnosis presented with clinical acumen can greatly enhance knowledge; can empower children, their families, and all those who deal with them; and can reduce distress and isolation (Werry, 1994).

But diagnostic systems can be problematic (Poland et al., 1994; Sonuga-Barke, 1998; Werry, 1994). The reliability and validity of many diagnostic categories remain questionable. The extent to which current categorical systems adequately fit and cover the varied structure of symptoms displayed by referred clients is also questionable. Increasing recognition of the high levels of comorbidity typically found between and within disorders has presented a major challenge to the usefulness of the categorical approach. The widespread use of diagnostic categories as the criteria to form groups for research may actually be hampering the precision of research findings on etiology and treatment. When a disorder represents a state that is clearly abnormal, characterized by qualitatively different symptoms, then the categorical model can be adequate. However, with many disorders such as anxiety, the abnormality is not one of a qualitative combination of abnormal symptoms (e.g., hallucinations) but is one of extreme degrees of characteristics found in all people (e.g., anxiety). A challenge thus becomes defining an appropriate cutoff score based on predictive power for poor functioning.

Clinically, the use of diagnostic classification can and has been criticized. First, applying a ready-made diagnosis may deter clinicians from undertaking more extensive assessment and conceptualization of a client's problems. Clinical practice in which a packaged treatment is selected to match a given diagnosis (e.g., cognitive-behavioral therapy, or CBT, for depression) is on the rise due to economic pressures and may be efficient where diagnosis is accurate, the client is typical, and the treatment is efficacious. On the other hand, however, such facile matching may be grossly inefficient when a more careful consideration of the client's problems may indicate different and nonstandard therapeutic strategies. Furthermore, serious doubts have been raised about the actual relevance of many diagnostic categories to treatment planning. In the area of child anxiety, few differences in response to standardized CBT treatments have been noted for the different subgroups of disorders (Dadds & Barrett, in press). The use of diagnoses has also been criticized for the potential social stigma associated with use of psychiatric labels, and it is important that clinicians handle labels with sensitivity. An accurate diagnosis presented in a way that empowers children and their caregivers can relieve uncertainty in clients and bring relief to a worried child or parent, enhance knowledge, normalize distress, and reduce isolation (Werry, 1994). But the insensitive use of labels (such as attention-deficit/hyperactivity disorder or social phobia) with a child and his or her caregivers can facilitate negative cycles in the child's life that perpetuate problems.

With regard to diagnosis and treatment matching, it should be noted that there is considerable controversy about the relative advantages of individually tailored treatments versus standardized interventions designed for specific diagnostic categories. Many writers in the behavioral tradition have argued that tailored treatment is optimal (e.g., Hickling & Blanchard, 1997). However, it is rarely found that specific interventions have precise impact on the targets they are designed to alter. Furthermore, evidence that tailored treatments produce superior benefits is almost nonexistent. Thus, much evidence is available to support the public health benefits of standardized and empirically validated interventions for designated diagnostic categories.

COMPLEMENTARY APPROACHES TO CATEGORIZATION

A dimensional model is based on the assumption that psychopathology is a quantitative rather than qualitative deviation from normality and asserts that there are a number of dimensions on which all individuals vary. Examples of dimensional systems that have been extensively researched are the Child Behavior Checklist (CBCL; Achenbach, 1991) and the Conners Scales (Conners & Barkley, 1985). All such systems are derived from symptom rating scales and developed by empirical multivariate statistical methods. A dimensional approach encourages the focus on common factors (that cut across the anxiety disorders) and how they vary with development, for example, the content of fears (Anxiety Disorders Association of America, 1998). For disorders with early onset, the content of the anxiety is often safety and security issues (SAD, simple phobia). For disorders with a later onset (overanxious disorder, social phobia), though, the anxiety is more likely to be about performance evaluation and social/evaluative concerns. Therefore, there is some support for the notion that the content of the anxiety disorders changes with age or development and is a unifying factor of several anxiety disorders.

An advantage of dimensional models is that most have been established statistically and empirically through the use of factor analysis (Werry, 1994) and thus have the potential to reduce large number of categories to a smaller number of dimensions of behavioral and emotional dysfunction. They are more sensitive to the range of severity of problems, from mild to severe rather than disordered versus healthy. Thus, they are useful for screening risk and early signs of a problem and are often used in large early intervention programs (e.g., Dadds, Spence, Holland, Barrett, & Laurens, 1997). Finally, they partially sidestep the issue of comorbidity, in that various dimensions can be considered side by side (Werry, 1994).

Werry (1994) also noted that dimensional systems have several limitations and suggested that these systems should not be used for individual diagnosis and treatment, but should be used instead in conjunction with categorical systems. Sonuga-Barke (1998) acknowledged that the dimensional system is probably a better model than the categorical approach for science, but there are concerns about its clinical utility due to problems about the transparency and communicability. He asserted that, by adopting this system, we run the risk of dismantling the bridge of meaning that provides a common understanding of disorders that enables communication between clinician and researcher. Also, the categorical and dimensional models share certain structural features, namely that dimensions derived in the psychometric approach can be roughly equivalent to categories in the diagnostic approach. For the child anxiety disorders, a recently developed child and parent report measure (Spence, 1998) was designed to reflect *DSM* categories and does in fact show good convergence with these.

It should be noted that the distinction between categorical and dimensional systems is somewhat arbitrary. Many contemporary categorical systems utilize dimensional criteria. For example, the *DSM* specifies that patients must show certain levels of impairment, as judged on a healthy-impaired continuum. Similarly, dimensional measures such as the CBCL incorporate cutoffs that are derived from normative studies and specify when a person's problems can be considered to be in the clinical range.

Another alternative to the categorical or symptom-oriented dimensional models that classifies on the basis of presenting symptoms is the functional model, largely derived from behavioral analytic theory. It classifies on the basis of the functional meaning and consequences of behavior rather than its simple presence or absence. The great advantage of functional systems of diagnosis is that they are highly relevant for treatment. An excellent example of functional criteria incorporated in a diagnostic system is that of Kearney and Silverman's (1996) diagnostic system for school-refusal behavior. Their system is empirically and clinically grounded and creates a template for classification of other diagnoses. Functional criteria are applied on the basis of children's reasons for refusal: (a) to avoid specific (e.g., classrooms, teachers, buses) or general stimuli-provoking negative affectivity, (b) to escape from aversive social/evaluative situations (e.g., public speaking, interacting with peers), (c) to gain verbal/physical attention (e.g., via tantrums, clinging, noncompliance), or (d) to pursue positive tangible reinforcement (e.g., watching television, visiting with friends).

Kearney and Silverman (1993) developed the School Refusal Assessment Scale, designed specifically for this type of behavior. It has demonstrated reliability and validity and consists of 16 items for parents and children. The scale provides categorical and dimensional as well as functional analyses. Treatment strategies may be informed by the functional criteria of the diagnosis. However, clinician judgments show questionable reliability when rating the reinforcement functions of children's school refusal behavior, with years of training and experience being the only variables found that related to the reliability of judgments (Daleiden, Chorpita, Kollins, & Drabman, 1999).

CRITERIA FOR EVALUATING DIAGNOSTIC SYSTEMS

Reliability refers to the replicability of the diagnosis (Blashfield & Draguns, 1976), that is, whether a specific diagnostic method produces the same information at different administrations. There are various types of reliability: (a) interrater reliability, which means that two clinicians or researchers assessing the same child will agree on the diagnosis they give to the child; (b) test-retest reliability, which means the stability of the diagnostic procedure across time; and (c) across-samples reliability, in which the same child would receive the same diagnosis in different clinics, cities, and countries. However, this type of reliability is really only another type of interrater reliability. Schniering et al. (2000) identified the importance of interrater reliability and test-retest reliability but also included parent-child reliability. To conduct a comprehensive assessment of children and adolescents, it is important to obtain information from the child or adolescent, as well as information from significant others in the child's life.

Validity refers to the ability of the diagnostic and measurement system to represent reality and includes predictive, concurrent, and discriminative validity. Both reliability and validity are affected by the particular system used, the methods of eliciting the data used to make the diagnosis, and the disorder itself, and it is important to separate these. Most studies have assessed a combination of reliability and validity indices, so the following review considers them together. Although self-reports, parent reports, and other behavioral and physiological measures are often used to test diagnostic hypotheses, the main method for reaching a diagnosis is structured interviews. Structured or semistructured interviews have several advantages over unstructured interviews, and the reliability of unstructured interviews has been found to be quite poor. Silverman and Saavedra (1998) argued that the almost universal usage of diagnostic interview procedures in research studies has greatly enhanced interrater reliability of diagnoses. Thus, the review focuses mainly on these interview strategies.

Several structured interviews have been developed for assessing children with anxiety disorders. These include the Diagnostic Interview Schedule for Children (DISC; Shaffer et al., 1993), the Kiddie Schedule for Affective Disorders and Schizophrenia: Present and Lifetime Version (K-SADS-PL; Kaufman, Birmaher, Brent, Rao, & Ryan, 1997), the Anxiety Disorders Interview Schedule for *DSM-IV*, Child Version (ADIS-IV-C; Silverman & Albano, 1996), and the Diagnostic Interview for Children and Adolescents

(DICA; Welner, Reich, Herjanic, Jung, & Amado, 1987). To improve diagnostic reliability or to parallel changes in the diagnostic systems, most of these interviews have been revised in recent years. The ADIS is the only structured interview that focuses primarily on the assessment of anxiety disorders.

Interrater Reliability and Concurrent and Discriminative Validity

In terms of interrater reliability, Schniering et al.'s (2000) review concluded that studies have generally reported moderate to high independent-interrater agreement in the assessment of anxiety in children using structured interviews. For instance, Rapee, Barrett, Dadds, and Evans (1994) found moderate to strong interrater reliability for most of the childhood anxiety disorders when interviewing parents and low to moderate reliability when interviewing children using the ADIS-C.

It should be noted, though, that the methods used in these studies result in an artificially inflated level of agreement between two raters. Typically, one rater interviews the child, and another rater observes the interview either live or later, via videotape, and makes an independent diagnosis based on the observed interview. This type of procedure only estimates reliability on the basis of observing the same interview. The clinician conducting the interview takes the interview in the desired direction on the basis of hypotheses being entertained about the diagnosis. The rater observing will have no choice but to base his or her diagnosis on the information yielded in the interview, even if his or her hypotheses would have taken the interview in a different direction. Based on this method, it is more likely that the two raters will reach the same diagnosis. A possibly more reliable method of measuring interrater reliability would be to have one rater interview the child and then to have another rater, some time later, interview the child again. This is expensive and redundant for the family and child, but the advantage of this method would be that both interviewers would be able to independently ask the questions that they felt were pertinent in making a certain diagnosis. Although superior to the previous method, it still has flaws, in that it is likely that the way the interviewee responds to the second interviewer will be influenced by his or her experiences in the first interview. Thus, a rigorous method for assessing interrater reliability of diagnoses does not exist, and it must be concluded that current estimates of agreement reflect upper limits to the real levels and do not apply to unstructured interviews.

Concurrent validity has also been assessed by examining the level of agreement between structured interviews and clinicians' ratings. Moderate levels of agreement have been reported between the DISC-R (Piacentini et al., 1993) and the DICA and clinician-generated diagnoses (Welner et al., 1987). Good concordance has been found between the K-SADS and other structured interviews for children when assessing most childhood disorders (Hodges, McKnew, Burbach, & Roebuck, 1987). In general, it has been found that concordance has been weaker for the anxiety disorders than other disorders, particularly when the diagnosis has been solely based on child interviews. In summary, Schniering et al. (2000) concluded that structured interviews provide a reasonably accurate picture of the primary features of anxiety in children and adolescents.

Discriminant validity refers to the ability of the diagnosis to differentiate children with a specific anxiety disorder from children with another anxiety disorder or children with other disorders of childhood. If the childhood anxiety disorders do not demonstrate discriminant validity, there is little point in having distinct disorders. Silverman and Saavedra (1998) described discriminant validity as being concerned with whether there was enough evidence to support the distinctiveness of each disorder. Sonuga-Barke (1998) asserted, "A system of classification is valid if it helps clinicians to distinguish between children who differ in clinically significant ways" (p. 117). Preliminary research has indicated that the DISC is able to discriminate psychiatric from pediatric referrals for children with severe psychopathology, but not in children with milder symptoms (Costello, Edelbrock, & Costello, 1985). Fisher et al. (1993) found the DISC to be adequately sensitive in the diagnosis of specific childhood disorders, including the anxiety disorders. It also appears that the DICA is able to differentiate clinical from nonclinical children, from 7 years of age (Sylvester, Hyde, & Reichler, 1987). These results provide some evidence that the structured interviews are moderately able to differentiate between different diagnostic categories.

Schniering et al. (2000) reviewed the research on the discriminant validity of childhood anxiety disorders. They examined the four areas of research that have addressed the extent to which children and adolescents with anxiety disorders can be differentiated from children (a) without psychiatric disorders, (b) with other anxiety disorders, (c) with depressive disorders, and (d) with behavior disorders. These areas of research are discussed in subsequent sections, followed by a discussion of the ability of specific factors such as family history to discriminate anxiety disorders.

Differentiating Children With Anxiety Disorders From Children Without Psychiatric Disorders

Little research has compared children with anxiety disorders with non-clinically anxious children; however, the results are generally promising. For example, Beidel (1991) compared three groups of children: children with overanxious disorder, children with social phobia, and children who were not clinically anxious. Children with social phobia could be differentiated from the nonanxious children, in that children with social phobia reported more anxiety-provoking situations over a 2-week period, more distress, and lower levels of perceived cognitive competence than the nonanxious children. But the overanxious children could not be differentiated from the control group on these variables. In response to these results, Beidel argued that overanxious disorder did not demonstrate adequate discriminant validity to be deemed a clinical diagnosis. Instead, she thought that overanxious disorder may represent a prodromal condition preceding the development of other anxiety disorders.

Tracey, Chorpita, Douban, and Barlow (1997) examined the discriminant validity of the childhood GAD diagnosis. They compared children diagnosed with GAD and children without anxiety disorders. They found that these two groups of children could be significantly differentiated on the basis of the number of worries, the number of GAD symptoms, and scores on the worry/oversensitivity factor on the Revised Children's Manifest Anxiety Scale (Reynolds & Richmond, 1978). Therefore, it appears that the diagnosis of childhood GAD has better discriminant validity than the diagnosis of overanxious disorder. In summary, when structured diagnostic interviews and self-report measures of anxiety are used, children with anxiety disorders can quite reliably be differentiated from children without anxiety disorders.

Differentiating Between Disorders: The Problem of Comorbidity

Werry (1994) argued that the lack of discriminant validity of the childhood anxiety disorders has been swept under the carpet by use of the term *comorbidity*. Comorbidity exists when a person is diagnosed with more than one disorder. Very high rates of comorbid anxiety disorders or consistent patterns of comorbidity tend to indicate that the diagnostic system is not differentiating between anxiety disorders, but rather depicts a single category. Alternatively, lower comorbidity rates tend to indicate that the anxiety disorders are deserving of separation into several different types. Anxiety disorders most commonly share comorbidity with other anxiety disorders, affective disorders, and externalizing disorders (Silverman & Saavedra, 1998). There also appears to be a basic pattern of development when a child has several disorders. The chronology is anxiety, externalizing disorder, dysthymia, major depression, and substance use (Silverman & Saavedra, 1998).

Silverman and Saavedra (1998) have also suggested that different comorbid patterns appear for different anxiety disorders, which may be indicative of discriminant validity. For instance, Last, Perrin, Hersen, and Kazdin (1992) found that children with a primary diagnosis of SAD were more likely to have comorbid anxiety disorders than those with a primary diagnosis of overanxious disorder. Children with a primary diagnosis of overanxious disorder were more likely to be diagnosed with social phobia.

Jensen, Martin, and Cantwell (1997) examined the comorbid rates for attention-deficit/hyperactivity disorder (ADHD) and other anxiety disorders, with the primary purpose being to determine whether comorbid patterns that exist are distinctive from what exists when the disorder appears alone. They concluded that "it is the interaction of the two or more conditions that conveys unique information that should set the standard for determining whether the comorbid pattern should be regarded as a unique syndrome; that is, what appears as a comorbid condition should be atypical from what is observed with the primary disorder" (p. 1067). Very few studies have examined whether anxiety plus an additional disorder is significantly different from anxiety alone. Some research has investigated the differences between anxiety alone and anxiety plus depression. There was some preliminary evidence that there might be some distinguishing features, indicating the possibly of a distinct syndrome (Jensen et al., 1997).

In clinic samples, it has been found that the majority of children had been diagnosed with more than one anxiety disorder (Last, Hersen, Kazdin, Finkelstein, & Strauss, 1987). Of those children with SAD, 42% were diagnosed with an additional anxiety disorder. In children with overanxious disorder, 55% had been diagnosed with an additional anxiety disorder, and 64% of children with social phobia had been diagnosed with an additional anxiety disorder. Alessi and Magen (1988) found comorbid SAD in six out of seven children diagnosed with panic disorder. However, Last and Strauss (1989) reported that only 35% of adolescents with panic disorder had been diagnosed with an additional anxiety disorder.

The rates of comorbid anxiety and other internalizing disorders in clinic samples ranges from 24 to 79% (e.g., Last, Strauss, & Francis, 1987). The rates of comorbid anxiety and other externalizing disorders in clinic samples ranges from 8 to 61% (e.g., Last, Strauss, et al., 1987).

Comorbidity rates in community samples are much lower than those found in clinic samples. Lewinsohn, Zinbarg, Seeley, Lewinsohn, and Sack (1997) found an overall anxiety comorbidity rate of 18.7% in a sample of adolescents identified in the community who had experienced an anxiety disorder. 81.3% of the sample had only met criteria for one anxiety disorder, 15.7% had been diagnosed with two disorders, and only 3% had been diagnosed with three anxiety disorders. In contrast to this low community comorbidity rate, Valleni-Basile et al. (1994) found high comorbidity in a community sample of adolescents with OCD. 34% met criteria for an additional diagnosis of SAD and 29% met criteria for a phobic disorder. The rates of comorbid anxiety and other internalizing disorders in community samples ranges from 13 to 72% (e.g., Anderson, Williams, McGee, & Silva, 1987; McGee, Feehan, & Williams, 1990). The rates of comorbid anxiety and externalizing disorders in community samples ranges from 7 to 39% (e.g., Bird et al., 1988; McGee et al., 1990).

It tends to be assumed that comorbidity is genuine, but it is possible that it is actually due to errors in the diagnostic methods used or lack of discriminant validity in the diagnostic system used. Silverman and Saavedra (1998) have discussed some of the methodological issues that complicate research investigating comorbidity. First, they concluded that comorbidity is not simply a product of measurement overlap and thus artifactual. For instance, even when items in measures that overlap are removed, there still remains a relationship between the disorders (e.g., depression and anxiety). With regard to comorbidity rates being higher in clinic samples than in community samples, they reason that if children have more than one disorder, they are likely to be more impaired, and therefore more likely to be seeking treatment. In addition, in many studies using children in the community, comprehensive assessments are not always conducted of all the possible anxiety disorders. Therefore, comorbidity may often be missed.

Differentiating Between Childhood Anxiety Disorders

Research in this area has primarily focused on differentiating the diagnoses of SAD, overanxious disorder, and social phobia. Silverman and Saavedra (1998) discussed the discriminant validity of the different childhood anxiety disorders, in terms of how well they were able to distinguish children with different disorders, on the basis of demographic variables, psychometrics, patterns of comorbidity, and family history. They asserted that there were significant differences between the anxiety disorders on the basis of demographic variables.

As in the previous section, evidence supporting the discriminant validity of (the previous *DSM* category) of overanxious disorder is less solid. However, preliminary studies provide better support for the discriminant validity of GAD. For instance, Last, Hersen, et al. (1987) compared children with overanxious disorder and SAD. They found that children with SAD were younger, came from poorer families, and were less likely to have a comorbid anxiety disorder than overanxious children. Silverman and Saavedra (1998) also reported that SAD is more prevalent in girls than in boys, and that children with SAD are of lower socioeconomic status than children with overanxious disorder or phobic disorders. But Pruis, Lahey, Thyer, and Christ (1990) were not able to find these significant differences between the two groups.

In terms of the differences between social phobia and simple phobias, it has been found that children with social phobia were referred at an older age and had an older age of onset (Silverman & Saavedra, 1998), reported more distress in the form of fearfulness, loneliness and depression, and were more likely to have additional anxiety disorders than those with simple phobias (Strauss & Last, 1993). Therefore, there appears to be sufficient evidence for the discriminant validity of social phobia and simple phobias.

Gender ratios in both clinic and community samples have not been of much assistance in differentiating between the anxiety disorders due to inconsistent findings (Schniering et al., 2000). No differences have been found in the gender ratios between children from clinic samples with SAD, overanxious disorder, and social phobia (Last, Strauss, et al., 1987; cf. Silverman & Saavedra, 1998). Similarly, no differences in gender ratios were identified between children from clinic samples with social phobia or simple phobias (Strauss & Last, 1993). However, Swedo, Rapoport, Leonard, Lenane, and Cheslow (1989) found a greater proportion of males to females had OCD using a clinic sample. When community samples have been used, some gender differences in the anxiety disorders have been identified. For all anxiety disorders, except overanxious disorder, there was found to be a greater proportion of females to males (Anderson et al., 1987). In a community sample of adolescents with OCD, equal gender ratios were observed (Valleni-Basile et al., 1994). The general finding is that when clinic samples are used, there are no significant differences in the gender ratios, but when community samples are used, there appears to be a greater proportion of females with anxiety disorders. Schniering et al. (2000) suggest that this finding might be a reflection of societal values, where an anxious boy is more unacceptable than an anxious girl, and therefore a greater proportion of boys are referred for treatment.

A recent study looked at the discriminant validity between two anxiety problems with the strongest construct validity. Compton, Nelson, and March (2000) examined the progression and pattern of self-reported symptoms of social phobia (SP) and separation anxiety (SA) using the Multidimensional Anxiety Scale for Children (March et al., 1997) in large community and clinical samples of children and adolescents. In general, SP and SA dimensions were readily discriminable by age, gender, and racial/cultural background.

Silverman and Saavedra (1998) concluded that on the basis of demographic variables and psychological variables that there is mixed evidence for the discriminant validity of the different childhood anxiety disorders. Some support has been demonstrated for the discriminant validity of social phobia, SAD, and preliminary evidence is tentatively supportive of GAD.

Differentiating Between Anxiety and Depression

Much argument has occurred as to whether anxiety and depression are actually different constructs, or whether they are best considered as the same construct. Some researchers have proposed that anxiety and depression lie on the same continuum, where anxiety leads into depression (Dobson, 1985), whereas others have argued that they form part of a larger construct of negative affectivity (King, Ollendick, & Gullone, 1991). Comorbidity rates of anxiety and depression vary considerably, from 15.9% to 61.9% (Brady & Kendall, 1992). There is considerable overlap between anxiety and depression symptoms, particularly in relation to somatic symptoms (Schniering et al., 2000). For instance, for both sets of disorders the criteria include symptoms such as irritability, restlessness, concentration difficulty, sleep disturbance and fatigue. This overlap of symptoms better enables a child to meet criteria for two rather than one diagnosis, possibly elevating comorbidity rates.

Some factors have been identified that differentiate anxiety from depression. Schniering et al. (2000) suggested that the child's current age and age of onset are some factors that can enable separation of the disorders. For instance, children with anxiety alone tended to be younger than children with depression alone (Strauss, Last, Hersen, & Kazdin, 1988). In addition, the evidence suggested that as an anxious child grows older, they may be more likely to develop depression (Cole, Peeke, Martin, Truglio, & Seroczynski, 1998).

Differentiating Between Anxiety Disorders and Behavior Disorders

Comorbidity rates of anxiety and behavior disorders are generally much lower than those reported for anxiety and depression (Schniering et al., 2000). But some research has reported surprisingly high rates of comorbidity. Anderson et al. (1987) reported that 39% of children diagnosed with an anxiety disorder had an additional diagnosis of ADHD, oppositional defiant disorder, or conduct disorder. Last, Hersen, et al. (1987) also found that 16.7% of children with SAD also met criteria for an additional diagnosis of ADHD and 16.7% met criteria for oppositional defiant disorder. 36.4% of children diagnosed with overanxious disorder met criteria for oppositional defiant disorder and 18.2% met criteria for ADHD. Children with social phobia were less likely to have an additional diagnosis of a behavior disorder. Weissman et al. (1999) assessed 44 children with anxiety disorders, before puberty and 10 to 15 years later. They found that compared with normal controls, those children with anxiety were more likely to develop conduct disorder and were more at risk of substance abuse.

Even though anxiety disorders appear very different from behavior disorders, there has been limited evidence to support the clear differentiation of these disorders. For example, Perrin and Last (1992) found that the Fear Survey Schedule for Children-Revised (FSSC-R), Revised Children's Manifest Anxiety Scale (RCMAS), and the Modified State-Trait Anxiety Inventory for Children (STAIC-M) could not significantly discriminate between boys with anxiety disorders and those with ADHD. In comparison, a recent study showed that the Multidimensional Anxiety Scale for Children (MASC; March et al., 1997) can discriminate between anxiety and ADHD at a reasonable level of accuracy. This indicates that many problems of discrimination may be primarily due to problems with specific anxiety measures rather than the constructs of anxiety versus ADHD.

Some studies have examined the differentiating factors. Werry, Reeves, and Elkind (1987) identified three factors that differentiated children with anxiety disorders from children with attention-deficit, oppositional defiant, or conduct disorders. First, children with behavior disorders were more likely to be boys, whereas children with anxiety disorders were more likely to be girls. Second, anxious children were more likely to have a parent with an anxiety disorder. Third, even though both anxious children and children with behavior disorders were significantly more likely than nonclinical children to interpret ambiguous scenarios as indicating threat, differences were found, in that anxious children were more likely than oppositional children and nonclinical children to avoid situations they interpreted as threatening (Barrett, Rapee, Dadds & Ryan, 1996).

Similar to the difficulty in differentiating children with anxiety disorders from children with depression is that of differentiating between anxiety and behavior disorders, which also share common symptoms. Children with GAD often experience concentration difficulties at school and home as a consequence of excessive worry. This could be mistakenly identified as ADHD. Children with anxiety disorders also tend to avoid situations that cause them anxiety. This could be mistakenly identified as oppositional behavior.

Discriminant Validity Based on Family History

Silverman and Saavedra (1998) discussed the discriminant validity of the anxiety disorders by examining whether the family histories of children who develop anxiety disorders are significantly different than those of other children. Kovacs and Devlin (1998) reported that children with parents with internalizing disorders are much more likely to develop internalizing disorders. This is especially the case with depression but less so with anxiety. Turner, Beidel, and Costello (1987) reported that anxious parents were significantly more likely than nonanxious parents to have children with anxiety disorders; however, there was no significant difference in the anxiety disorder rates of children who had anxious parents as compared with anxiety disorder rates of children who had parents with dysthymia. Therefore, parental history was used successfully to discriminate children with anxiety disorders from normal controls, but not from children with other psychiatric disorders. Last, Hersen, Kazdin, & Orvaschel (1991) reported that there were significantly more anxiety disorders in the first-degree relatives of children with anxiety disorders than in the first-degree relatives of children with ADHD or those of normal controls. Some specificity was noted; it was found that children with SAD were more likely to have first-degree relatives with panic disorders. Some nonspecificity was also found: there was a tendency for female first-degree relatives of children with ADHD to show an increased rate of anxiety disorders as compared with the first-degree relatives of children without psychiatric disorders. Biederman, Milberger, Faraone, and Kiely (1995) also reported a family relationship between ADHD and childhood anxiety disorders (see also Biederman et al., 1992).

Silverman and Saavedra (1998) summarized the family studies by concluding that children with relatives with anxiety disorders are more likely to have anxiety disorders themselves but that this may not be a specific relation. For instance, people with anxiety disorders have also been shown to be more likely to have relatives with ADHD and depression.

Age-of-Onset Studies

Silverman and Saavedra (1998) suggested that age-of-onset studies are another way of examining the progression and stability of the anxiety disorders. These studies indicated that there is some tendency for different disorders to have different ages of onset. For instance, SAD tends to have an early onset, specific phobias have an early onset, overanxious disorder has a broader age range but also has a younger age of onset, social phobia tends to begin in middle adolescence, and panic disorder with or without agoraphobia tends to have an onset in adolescence or early adulthood. Beiderman et al. (1995) documented the average age of onset of anxiety disorders among children with panic disorder and agoraphobia. It was found that the earliest anxiety disorder was simple phobia, followed by avoidant and separation disorders, followed by agoraphobia. Social phobia, over-anxious disorder, and OCD tended to occur later than agoraphobia. Children with panic disorders showed a similar course but had an older age of onset. In summary, there appear to be multiple developmental progressions whereby anxiety disorders change into different anxiety and other disorders, especially depressive disorders.

Stability, Test-Retest Reliability, and Predictive Validity

With regard to the stability of disorders and their measurement, three related elements can be identified. First is the stability of the disorder itself. Second is the test-retest reliability of the measurement system, and third is the validity of the disorder to predict processes and outcomes external to the diagnosis per se. With respect to test-retest reliability, it is essential to note the important distinction between the disorder's actually changing and the unreliability of the diagnostic methods. In other words, if a child is assessed 2 weeks after the first interview and the assessment indicates that the child no longer meets criteria for a specific anxiety disorder, the question is "Did the child get better in those 2 weeks, or is the interview an unreliable measure of the anxiety disorder?" Researchers have tended to assume that the symptoms are stable and that, if there is a discrepancy, it is a consequence of the measure's not being reliable. When this is the case, the studies may be underestimating the reliability of the measure. Thus, a study in which the test-retest reliability of a diagnostic procedure is assessed needs to consider both the stability of the method of diagnosis and the stability of the disorder. Ideally, the test-retest reliability of a diagnostic procedure is its reliability assuming that the disorder has remained present. Thus, the chosen time period must not be too long, given the expected duration of the disorder

It has been found that test-retest reliability of diagnoses of anxiety disorders based on children's self-reports, using time intervals of 10 to 21 days, range from moderate (Jensen et al., 1995) to excellent (Silverman & Eisen, 1992). When only the symptoms are considered, the test-retest reliability of children's self-reports has varied considerably, from having poor to fair stability (Boyle et al., 1993) to having satisfactory to high stability (March et al., 1997; March & Sullivan, 1999; Silverman & Rabian, 1995).

Schniering et al. (2000) discussed some variables that seem to correlate with poor test-retest reliability. Reliability with younger children, those with more limited cognitive ability, and boys has tended to be less consistent, with the finding that such children tend to report more symptoms of anxiety in the first interview than in subsequent interviews (Fallon & Schwab-Stone, 1994). Estimates of test-retest reliability of parents' reports of their children's anxiety have ranged from moderate to high for both diagnoses and individual symptoms (Silverman & Eisen, 1992).

With regard to stability, there is conflicting evidence that a diagnosis of any of the childhood anxiety disorders is stable over time. Caspi, Henry, McGee, Moffit, and Silva (1995), using a longitudinal design, examined children through childhood and adolescence. They found that shy 5-year-olds were more likely to be shy in childhood or adolescence. In adulthood, they were more likely to take longer to marry, have children, and establish stable careers. Pollack, Otto, Sabatino, and Majcher (1996) interviewed a sample of adults with anxiety disorders, and 50% of them retrospectively reported that they had anxiety disorders as children.

Cantwell and Baker (1987) studied a group of children for 3 years. Some 10 to 15% received treatment. They found that 71% of children initially diagnosed with avoidant disorder no longer met criteria for the disorder after three years, 89% of children initially diagnosed with SAD no longer met criteria for the disorder after three years, and 75% of children diagnosed with overanxious disorder did not meet criteria for the disorder after 3 years. However, almost a third of the children initially diagnosed with anxiety disorders received different anxiety diagnoses at the 3-year follow-up, and 25% of the children received new behavior disorder diagnoses. These results tended to indicate that the anxiety disorders were much more changeable. Last, Perrin, Hersen, and Kazdin (1996) found similar results. They found that after a period of 4 years, 82% of children no longer met criteria for the anxiety disorders they had been diagnosed with, but 15% were diagnosed with new and different anxiety disorders. An additional 13% of children shifted to depressive diagnoses, and 7% developed behavior disorders. However, these results may be questionable, because during the 4 years, 73% of the children received treatment. The results do indicate that although one anxiety diagnosis may dissipate, another may develop.

Beidel, Flink, and Turner (1996) examined children diagnosed with anxiety disorders before and after a 6-month period. They found that two thirds of the children initially diagnosed with either social phobia or overanxious disorder still met criteria for one of these disorders at follow-up. Also, even those children who were initially diagnosed with anxiety disorders and who did not meet criteria for the same disorders at follow-up were still reporting anxiety symptoms, but at subthreshold levels. Only a very small percentage of children no longer met criteria for any diagnosis.

Beitchman, Wekerle, and Hood (1987) examined the stability of four groups of children over 5 years: those with conduct disorder, ADHD, developmental delay, and emotional disorder. They found that the group of children with emotional disorders (which consisted of overanxious disorder, avoidant disorder, dysphoria, adjustment problems, and selective mutism) were the most unlikely to receive the same diagnosis at follow-up. In other words, the emotional disorders demonstrated the lowest predictive validity, with children receiving the same diagnosis only 29% of the time.

Therefore, research indicates that a significant percentage of children who have been diagnosed with anxiety disorders do not retain their anxiety disorder diagnosis but are later diagnosed with different disorders, such as another anxiety disorder, depression, or behavior disorder. Silverman and Saavedra (1998) suggested that the low stability may indicate that environmental or social factors are important contributors to the diverse diagnostic outcomes. But they also suggest that much of the variance over time could be due to comorbidity that was present but not adequately measured at initial diagnosis.

Predictive validity is the ability of a diagnosis to predict, with an accuracy greater than chance, a range of variables external to the diagnosis itself, such as treatment outcome, and specific areas and global functioning in the present and the future. The predictive validity of diagnostic systems as applied to childhood anxiety disorders has not been well researched. However, those studies done have produced little evidence that the different anxiety disorders evident in childhood predict different outcomes. Apart from differences in sociodemographic profiles and presenting symptoms, few differences in etiology and treatment outcomes have been noted for the different subgroups of disorders (see Dadds & Barrett, 2001; Vasey & Dadds, 2001).

Agreement Between Child and Adult Reports

Agreement between adults and children is not a form of reliability in the purest sense, because they have access to and report on different samples of behavior and experience. This form of agreement is often used as an index of reliability, though, for pragmatic reasons. Results have been inconsistent, but low agreement tends to be the rule. Schniering et al. (2000) suggested that there is a trend for parents to report more symptoms than their children, and as would be expected, parents appear to be more reliable in reporting complex details. Possible explanations for the inconsistent agreement between parents and children includes the assessment methods' not being developmentally relevant to the children, resulting in their failing to comprehend the questions; the children's wanting to present in a socially desirable manner; and, in some cases, the parents' not having an accurate understanding of their children's difficulties, or the inflation of their perceptions of their children's anxiety (as a consequence of their own anxiety). Rapee et al. (1994) suggested that, when there is a significant discrepancy between the child's and parent's reports, it is best to base the diagnosis on the information provided by the parent. Of course, each case is different, and the therapist needs to be aware of the interpersonal dynamics between the child and parent and of issues such as the associated gains for the parent or child in receiving such a diagnosis.

COVERAGE

Coverage refers to the ability of the diagnostic system to cover most of the children judged to have a psychological disorder. One of the central issues in the area of childhood anxiety disorders is the number of diagnostic categories. Blashfield and Draguns (1976) noted that, due to economic, legal, and administrative pressures, the *DSM* was required to have 100% coverage. Therefore, when *DSM-III* and *DSM-III-R* were published, the number of diagnostic classes increased from 182 to almost 300. Many investigators thought that a majority of the new categories were overrefined, untested, and excessive in number. When *DSM-IV* was published, anxiety disorders of childhood and adolescence and its two subcategories, overanxious and avoidant disorder, were eliminated. The only anxiety disorder specific to childhood that was retained in the *DSM-IV* was SAD.

Silverman and Saavedra (1998) suggested that the reason avoidant disorder was eliminated from the *DSM* was because there was insufficient evidence to discriminate avoidant disorder from social phobia, generalized type. The reason that overanxious disorder was eliminated from the *DSM* was because there was insufficient evidence to discriminate overanxious disorder from GAD. In addition, inconsistent reliabilities were found for overanxious disorder. It also had a very high prevalence, which suggested that the threshold for the diagnosis was too low. Beidel, Silverman, and Hammond-Laurence (1996) reported more similarities than differences between overanxious children in community and clinic samples. Ginsburg, La Greca, and Silverman (1998) also reported that, even though it was normal for children to worry, it was possible to derive thresholds for pathological worry. Therefore, they suggested that if the thresholds had been altered somewhat, there might have remained some justification to retain the overanxious disorder diagnosis. The symptoms were not very specific, which often resulted in artifactual comorbidity. Another reason that these two disorders were eliminated from the *DSM-IV* was because the approach of having separate childhood and adult disorders for similar constructs was inconsistent with the way in which the other disorders that both children and adults experienced was handled (e.g., depression).

Silverman and Saavedra (1998) raised the question of whether there was sufficient evidence for these two disorders to be removed from the *DSM*. Last and Perrin (1992) reported that avoidant disorder was the least diagnosed of the childhood disorders. They also found that children with avoidant disorder and children with social phobia were not significantly different on any sociodemographic or clinical variables. Instead, avoidant disorder and social phobia tended to have the same age of onset, or the two disorders overlapped quite significantly.

Last et al. (1992) did not find convincing evidence for the removal of overanxious disorder. Instead, they noted that many children who qualified for a diagnosis of overanxious disorder did not also meet criteria for

GAD. The main reason was that the diagnosis of GAD required the presence of multiple somatic complaints. When the *DSM-IV* was published, the number of physical symptoms for GAD was reduced. Kendall and Warman (1996) reported a very high consistency between *DSM-III-R* overanxious disorder and *DSM-IV* GAD. However, this study only consisted of a small sample of 8- to 13-year-olds.

Silverman and Saavedra (1998) concluded that the coverage of the anxiety disorders was satisfactory and that it made sense to subsume avoidant disorder under social phobia. But they remained unconvinced that the spectrum of children presenting with problematic worry and anxiety were sufficiently covered by subsuming overanxious disorder under GAD.

Using Self-Report and Other Measures in Diagnosis

Several self-report measures are designed to measure anxiety in children and adolescents. These measures are quick and easy to administer, are helpful in assessing treatment outcome, and provide useful normative data (Schniering et al., 2000). In general, test-retest reliability for the self-report measures has been reported to be moderate to high. However, one of their major disadvantages is their limited ability to discriminate between diagnostic groups and, as with the structured interviews, there is poor concordance between the parent's report and the child's report across most self-report measures (Engel, Rodrigue, & Geffken, 1994).

In terms of discriminant validity, there is some evidence that self-report questionnaires can differentiate between clinically anxious children and children without anxiety disorders (Schniering et al., 2000). But there is inconsistent evidence about the ability of the self-report measures to discriminate children with anxious disorders from those with other psychiatric disorders (Hoehn-Saric, Maisami, & Wiegand, 1987; Perrin & Last, 1992; Strauss et al., 1988). Exceptions include Beidel (1996), who found that the Social Phobia and Anxiety Inventory for Children (SPAI-C) could be used to distinguish between anxious children and those with behavior disorders, and March et al. (1997) who were able to discriminate between anxiety disorders and ADHD using the MASC.

Little research has examined the ability of self-report measures to differentiate between the different anxiety disorders. However, the Screen for Child Anxiety Related Emotional Disorders (SCARED) has been shown to demonstrate good discriminant validity within the childhood anxiety disorders (Birmaher et al., 1997). In addition, Ginsburg et al. (1998) found that the Social Anxiety Scale for Children–Revised could differentiate between children with social phobia and anxious children without the diagnosis. Similarly, Ginsburg et al. found that they could differentiate between the different phobias using the FSSC-R. Preliminary evidence also indicates that the Spence Children's Anxiety Scale (SCAS) has also been able to discriminate between the different childhood anxiety disorders (Spence, 1998).

Silverman and Saavedra (1998) concluded that, when more specific measures are used, there tends to be better discrimination than when more general measures are used. Schniering et al. (2000) pointed out that the general poor ability of the self-report measures to discriminate between the different types of anxiety disorders needs to be interpreted in the context of the high rates of comorbidity among the anxiety disorders. That is, many of the self-report measures contain items that are relevant to all of the anxiety disorders and do not contain subcategories to assess the different types of anxiety disorders. Therefore, it would be expected that the self-report questionnaires would show poor discriminant validity in differentiating between the anxiety disorders.

A range of other behavioral and physiological measures has been used effectively to measure associated aspects of anxiety problems in young people, and reviews can be found elsewhere in this and other books. Many of these reliably discriminate between anxious and nonanxious children, but none has been shown to reliably discriminate between the individual categories of anxious disorders. As noted, this is due both to characteristics within these measures and to unresolved problems with overlap between the diagnostic categories of anxiety disorders.

CONCLUSIONS

Major unresolved issues in the diagnosis of child anxiety disorders include (a) the high levels of comorbidity in the anxiety disorders and with other behavioral and emotional problems; (b) the lack of adequate reliability in children's self-reports across some measures and the low level of agreement between parent and child reports, to the point that children's reports may be contributing little to diagnostic decisions; and (c) the lack of discriminant and predictive validity across specific diagnostic categories.

It is interesting to note that diverse authors are concluding that progress with these problems will be best made by adopting a more developmental focus and taking into account the child's level of cognitive development, language skills, and understanding of emotions; concept of self and self-awareness; perception of others; and need to appear socially desirable (Schniering et al., 2000). Similarly, Silverman and Saavedra (1998) asserted that, in order to develop our understanding of anxiety disorders in children, future research needs to examine developmental changes in terms of cognitive development, emotional development, and social cognitive development.

A child's ability to reason, form concepts, and communicate and comprehend develops at a rapid rate (Bee & Mitchell, 1980). It is thought that the accuracy of information obtained during an assessment is strongly influenced by the sensitivity of the particular assessment measure to these cognitive developmental abilities. However, most self-report measures of children's anxiety are simply modified versions of adult measures. For instance, the RCMAS is based on the adult Manifest Anxiety Scale (Taylor,

1953). Therefore, it is unclear whether assessment measures of child anxiety are actually assessing the constructs they are designed to measure, given that it has been assumed that children think and respond just like adults. Campbell, Rapee, and Spence (1996) found that adults equated the term *worry* with frequency of thought and viewed the aversiveness of feared outcomes as a different construct. However, children under 10 years of age interpreted worry as meaning the same thing as aversiveness and interpreted frequency of thought as a different construct. In other words, younger children interpreted worry in terms of how bad they would find an event, rather than how often they thought about the event. Clearly, children and adults have a different understanding of the language used in self-report measures.

McCathie and Spence (1991) found that children and adolescents reported a high level of fearful thoughts and avoidance behavior concerning events (on the FSSC-R) that are highly unlikely to occur. That is, they rated fears of death, illness, injury, and danger as most fearful, even though they were unlikely to encounter these events in daily life. In a very similar study, King and Gullone (1990) added to the FSSC-R the stimulus item of getting AIDS. They stated that 65.9% of children and adolescents reported the highest level of fear towards AIDS, even though it was extremely unlikely that this would occur. The results of these two studies indicated that, when self-report measures such as the FSSC-R are administered to children, they may not measure the same constructs as they measure when given to adults. That is, adults are likely to respond by checking the items that elicit a fearful response in daily life, not the aversiveness to the thought of the occurrence of specific events.

In order to report on internal states, children must have developed a concept of the self, have an understanding of emotion, and have some insight into processes within themselves. However, research indicates that distinct changes occur in children's understanding of themselves (Damon & Hart, 1982). Harter (1990) found that children have little interest in observing, understanding, and evaluating internal processes (and little ability to do so) until adolescence. Stone and Lemanek (1990) asserted that children are not able to provide accurate reports of their emotions until they are 8 to 9 years old, when their understanding of emotions becomes based on internal mental cues. Therefore, even if they are experiencing anxiety disorders, they may be unable to give a name to their experiences (Quay & La Greca, 1986).

Schniering et al. (2000) recognized that social desirability is an important factor in assessing children. It is particularly likely that children with anxiety disorders will behave in this way, because they are especially concerned about being evaluated negatively and criticized. In line with this, children with social phobia would be especially expected to respond is socially desirable ways (Schniering et al., 2000). Hagborg (1991) examined the effect of social desirability on RCMAS scores in adolescents. It was found that social desirability was significantly related to a lower level of anxiety's being reported by the males, but not the females. Dadds, Perrin, and Yule (1999) showed similar results, and Dadds et al. (1997) showed that high social desirability may influence treatment success. Schniering et al. (2000) suggested that it is necessary to make efforts to minimize and perhaps monitor the effect of social desirability in the assessment process.

Another important issue that needs to be considered when assessing children for anxiety disorders is understanding what constitutes normal fears and anxiety during development. Clear changes in the content of children's fears have been found to occur throughout development. Vasey (1993) found that the content of worry in children follows a progression, from physical threats to psychological and abstract threats. Vasey also reported that, as young people develop more advanced cognitive skills, they are more capable of mediating severe and generalized anxiety through worry. Therefore, Schniering et al. (2000) suggested that it is very important for examiners to take into account normal developmental fears and the changes that occur in anxiety over the course of development.

Finally, the lack of stability of anxiety problems in children led Silverman and Saavedra (1998) to argue that more emphasis needs to be placed on the idea that many children will naturally recover from anxiety problems. Understanding the developmental progression of normal anxiety will shed light on this.

The following suggestions for clinical practice are noted. Categorical systems such as the *DSM* have much to recommend their use but also have inherent problems. A cautious approach to their use is recommended, with attention to the following issues:

1. The use of multiple informants to ensure that diagnosis is based on comprehensive data.
2. Sensitivity to the cognitive developmental aspects of the child and his or her competence with identifying and reporting internal states, the child's existing vocabulary to describe emotions, and his or her need for social approval.
3. Use of a combination of categorical, dimensional, and functional models in diagnosing a child.
4. Awareness of the complex patterns of comorbidity that are common in the anxiety disorders.
5. Awareness that disorders are in flux over time and that anxiety problems may be transient, may persist, and often change form or into other disorders such as depression.
6. Sensitivity to the interpersonal context of the diagnosis, such that the provision of such a label can be a blessing or a burden to the child and family.

REFERENCES

Achenbach, T. M. (1991). *Manual for the Child Behavior Checklist: 4–18 and 1991 profile.* Burlington: University of Vermont Department of Psychiatry.

Alessi, N. E., and Magen, J. (1988). Panic disorder in psychiatrically hospitalized children. *American Journal of Psychiatry, 145,* 1450–1452.

American Psychiatric Association. (1980). *Diagnostic and statistical manual of mental disorders* (3rd ed.). Washington, DC: Author.

American Psychiatric Association. (1987). *Diagnostic and statistical manual of mental disorders: DSM-III-R* (3rd ed., rev.). Washington, DC: Author.

American Psychiatric Association. (1994). *Diagnostic and statistical manual of mental disorders: DSM-IV* (4th ed.). Washington, DC: Author.

Anderson, J. C., Williams, S., McGee, R., & Silva, P. A. (1987). *DSM-III* disorders in preadolescent children: Prevalence in a large sample from the general population. *Archives of General Psychiatry, 44,* 69–76.

Anxiety Disorders Association of America. (1998, October). Paper presented at the symposium, *Treating anxiety disorders in youth: Current problems and future solutions.* Alexandria, VA.

Barrett, P. M., Rapee, R. M., Dadds, M. R., & Ryan, S. (1996). Family enhancement of cognitive style in anxious and aggressive children. *Journal of Abnormal Child Psychology, 24,* 187–203.

Bee, J. L., & Mitchell, S. K. (1980). *The developing person: A life-span approach.* New York: Harper & Row.

Beidel, D. C. (1991). Social phobia and overanxious disorder in school-age children. *Journal of the American Academy of Child and Adolescent Psychiatry, 30,* 545–552.

Beidel, D. C. (1996). Assessment of childhood social phobia: Construct, convergent, and discriminative validity of the Social Phobia and Anxiety Inventory for Children (SPAI-C). *Psychological Assessment, 8,* 235–340.

Beidel, D. C., Flink, C. M., & Turner, S. M. (1996). Stability of anxious symptomatology in children. *Journal of Abnormal Child Psychology, 24,* 257–269.

Beidel, D., Silverman, W., & Hammond-Laurence, K. (1996). Overanxious disorder: Subsyndromal state or specific disorder? A comparison of clinic and community samples. *Journal of Clinical Child Psychology, 25,* 25–32.

Beitchman, J., Wekerle, C., & Hood, J. (1987). Diagnostic continuity from preschool to middle childhood. *Journal of the American Academy of Child and Adolescent Psychiatry, 26,* 694–699.

Biederman, J., Faraone, S. V., Keenan, K., Benjamin, J., Krifcher, B., Moore, C., Sprich, S., et al. (1992). Further evidence for family-genetic risk factors in attention deficit hyperactivity disorder. Patterns of comorbidity in probands and relatives psychiatrically and pediatrically referred samples. *Archives of General Psychiatry, 49,* 728–738.

Biederman, J., Milberger, S., Faraone, S., & Kiely, K. (1995). Impact of adversity on functioning and comorbidity in children with attention-deficit hyperactivity disorder. *Journal of the American Academy of Child and Adolescent Psychiatry, 34,* 1495–1503.

Bird, H. R., Canino, G., Rubio-Stipec, M., Gould, M. S., Ribera, J., Sesman, M., Woodbury, M., et al. (1988). Estimates of the prevalence of childhood maladjustment in a community survey in Puerto Rico. *Archives of General Psychiatry, 45,* 1120–1126.

Birmaher, B., Khetarpal, S., Brent, D., Cully, M., Balach, L., Kaufman, J., & McKenzie Neer, S. (1997). The Screen for Child Anxiety Related Emotional Disorders (SCARED): Scale construction and psychometric characteristics. *Journal of the American Academy of Child and Adolescent Psychiatry, 36,* 545–553.

Blashfield, R. K., & Draguns, J. G. (1976). Evaluative criteria for psychiatric classification. *Journal of Abnormal Psychology, 85*(2), 140–150.

Boyle, M. H., Offord, D. R., Racine, Y., Sanford, M., Szatmari, P., Fleming, J. E., & Price-Munn, N. (1993). Evaluation of the Diagnostic Interview for Children and Adolescents for use in general population samples. *Journal of Abnormal Child Psychology, 21,* 663–681.

Brady, E. U., & Kendall, P.C. (1992). Comorbidity of anxiety and depression in children and adolescents. *Psychological Bulletin, 111,* 244–255.

Campbell, M. A., Rapee, R. M., & Spence, S. (1996). Developmental changes in the interpretation of instructions on a questionnaire measure of worry. Manuscript in preparation.

Cantwell, D. P., & Baker, L. (1987). The prevalence of anxiety in children with communication disorders. *Journal of Anxiety Disorders, 1,* 239–248.

Caspi, A., Henry, B., McGee, R. O., Moffit, T. E., & Silva, P. A. (1995). Temperamental origins of child and adolescent behavior problems: From age three to age fifteen. *Child Development, 66,* 55–68.

Cole, D., Peeke, L., Martin, J., Truglio, R., & Seroczynski, A. (1998). A longitudinal look at the relation between depression and anxiety in children and adolescents. *Journal of Consulting and Clinical Psychology, 66,* 451–460.

Compton, S. N., Nelson, A. H., & March, J. S. (2000). Social phobia and separation anxiety symptoms in community and clinical samples of children and adolescents. *Journal of the American Academy of Child and Adolescent Psychiatry, 39,* 1040–1046.

Conners, C. K., & Barkley, R. A. (1985). Rating scales and checklists for child psychopharmacology. *Psychopharmacology Bulletin, 21,* 809–815.

Costello, E. J., Edelbrock, C., & Costello, A. J. (1985). Validity of the NIMH Diagnostic Interview Schedule for Children: A comparison between psychiatric and pediatric referrals. *Journal of Abnormal Child Psychology, 13,* 579–595.

Dadds, M., & Barrett, P. (2001). Psychological treatments for anxiety disorders in children and adolescents. *Journal of Child Psychology, Psychiatry, and Allied Disciplines, 42,* 999–1011.

Dadds, M., Perrin, S., & Yule, W. (1999). Social desirability and self-reported anxiety in children: An analysis of the RCMAS Lie Scale. *Journal of Abnormal Child Psychology, 26,* 311–317.

Dadds, M., Spence, S., Holland, D., Barrett, P., & Laurens, K. (1997). Prevention and early intervention for anxiety disorders: A controlled trial. *Journal of Consulting and Clinical Psychology, 65,* 627–635.

Daleiden, E. L., Chorpita, B. F., Kollins, S. H., & Drabman, R. S. (1999). Factors affecting the reliability of clinical judgments about the function of children's school-refusal behavior. *Journal of Clinical Child Psychology, 28*(33), 396–406.

Damon, W., & Hart, D. (1982). The development of self-understanding from infancy through adolescence. *Child Development, 53,* 841–864.

Dawson, P. J. (1994). Philosophy, biology and mental disorder. *Journal of Advanced Nursing, 16,* 587–596.

Dobson, K. S. (1985). The relationship between anxiety and depression. *Clinical Psychology Review, 5,* 307–324.

Engel, N. A., Rodrigue, J. R., & Geffken, G. R. (1994). Parent-child agreement on ratings of anxiety in children. *Psychological Reports, 75,* 1251–1260.

Fallon, T., & Schwab-Stone, M. (1994). Determinants of reliability in psychiatric surveys of children aged 6–22. *Journal of Child Psychology and Psychiatry and Allied Disciplines, 35,* 1391–1408.

Fisher, P. W., Shaffer, D., Piacentini, J., Lapkin, J., Kafantaris, L. H., & Herzog, D. B. (1993). Sensitivity of the Diagnostic Interview Schedule for Children 2nd edition (DISC 2.1) for specific diagnoses of children and adolescents. *Journal of the American Academy of Child and Adolescent Psychiatry, 32,* 666–673.

Ginsburg, G. S., La Greca, A. M., & Silverman, W. K. (1998). Social anxiety in children with anxiety disorders: Relation with social and emotional functioning. *Journal of Abnormal Child Psychology, 26*(3), 175–185.

Gould, M. S., Shaffer, D., Rutter, M., & Sturge, C. (1988). UK/WHO study of *ICD-9.* In M. Rutter, A. H. Tuma, & I. S. Lann (Eds.), *Assessment and diagnosis in child psychopathology* (pp. 37–65). New York: Guilford Press.

Hagborg, W. J. (1991). The Revised Children's Manifest Anxiety Scale and social desirability. *Educational and Psychological Measurement, 51,* 423–427.

Harter, S. (1990). Issues in the assessment of the self-concept of children and adolescents. In A. M. La Greca (Ed.), *Through the eyes of the child: Obtaining self-reports from children and adolescents* (pp. 292–325). Boston: Allyn & Bacon.

Herjanic, B., & Reich, W. (1982). Development of a structured psychiatric interview for children: Agreement between child and parent on individual symptoms. *Journal of Abnormal Child Psychiatry, 10,* 307–324.

Hickling, E. J., & Blanchard, E. B. (1997). The private practice psychologist and manual-based treatments: Post-traumatic stress disorder secondary to motor vehicle accidents. *Behaviour Research and Therapy, 35*(3), 191–203.

Hodges, K., McKnew, D., Burbach, D. J., & Roebuck, L. (1987). Diagnostic concordance between the Child Assessment Schedule (CAS) and the Schedule for Affective Disorders and Schizophrenia for School-Age Children (K-SADS) in an outpatient sample using lay interviews. *Journal of the American Academy of Child and Adolescent Psychiatry, 26,* 654–661.

Hoehn-Saric, E., Maisami, M., & Wiegand, D. (1987). Measurement of anxiety in children and adolescents using semistructured interviews. *Journal of the American Academy of Child and Adolescent Psychiatry, 26,* 541–545.

Jensen, P., Martin, D., & Cantwell, D. P. (1997). Comorbidity in ADHD: Implications for research, practice, and *DSM-V. Journal of the American Academy of Child and Adolescent Psychiatry, 36*(8), 1065–1079.

Jensen, P., Roper, M., Fisher, P., Piacentini, J., Canino, G., Richters, J., Rubio-Stipee, et al. (1995). Test-retest reliability of the Diagnostic Interview Schedule for Children (DISC 2.1): Parent, child, and combined algorithms. *Archives of General Psychiatry, 52,* 61–71.

Kaufman, J., Birmaher, B., Brent, D., Rao, U., & Ryan, N. (1997). Schedule for Affective Disorders and Schizophrenia for School-Age Children–Present and Lifetime version (K-SADS-PL): Initial reliability and validity data. *Journal of the American Academy of Child and Adolescent Psychiatry, 36,* 980–988.

Kearney, C. A., & Silverman, W. K. (1993). Measuring the function of school refusal behavior: The School Refusal Assessment scale. *Journal of Clinical Child Psychology, 22,* 85–96.

Kearney, C. A., & Silverman, W. K. (1996). The evolution and reconciliation of taxonomic strategies for school refusal behavior. *Clinical Psychology: Science and Practice, 3*(4), 339–354.

Kendall, P., & Warman, M. (1996). Anxiety disorders in youth: Diagnostic consistency across *DSM-III-R* and *DSM-IV. Journal of Anxiety Disorders, 10,* 452–463.

King, N. J., & Gullone, E. (1990). Fear of AIDS: Self-reports of Australian children and adolescents. *Psychological Reports, 66,* 245–246.

King, N. J., Ollendick, T. H., & Gullone, E. (1991). Negative affectivity in children and adolescents: Relations between anxiety and depression. *Clinical Psychology Review, 11,* 441–459.

Kovacs, M., & Devlin, B. (1998). Internalizing disorders in childhood. *Journal of Child Psychology and Psychiatry and Allied Disciplines, 39,* 47–63.

Last, C., Hersen, M., Kazdin, A., Finkelstein, R., & Strauss, C. C. (1987). Comparison of *DSM-III* separation anxiety and overanxious disorders: Demographic characteristics and patterns of comorbidity. *Journal of the American Academy of Child and Adolescent Psychiatry, 26,* 527–531.

Last, C., Hersen, M., Kazdin, A., & Orvaschel, H. (1991). Anxiety disorders in children and their families. *Archives of General Psychiatry, 48,* 928–934.

Last, C., & Perrin, S. (1992). Anxiety disorders in African-American and White children. *Journal of Abnormal Child Psychology, 21,* 153–164.

Last, C., Perrin, S., Hersen, M., & Kazdin, A. E. (1992). *DSM-III-R* anxiety disorders in children: Sociodemographic and clinical characteristics. *Journal of the American Academy of Child and Adolescent Psychiatry, 31,* 1070–1076.

Last, C., Perrin, S., Hersen, M., & Kazdin, A. E. (1996). A prospective study of childhood anxiety disorders. *Journal of the American Academy of Child and Adolescent Psychiatry, 35,* 1502–1510.

Last, C., & Strauss, C. C. (1989). Panic disorder in children and adolescents. *Journal of Anxiety Disorders, 3,* 87–95.

Last, C., Strauss, C. C., & Francis, G. (1987). Comorbidity among childhood anxiety disorders. *Journal of Nervous and Mental Disease, 175,* 726–730.

Lewinsohn, P. M., Zinbarg, R., Seeley, J. R., Lewinsohn, M., & Sack, W. H. (1997). Lifetime comorbidity among anxiety disorders and between anxiety disorders and other mental disorders in adolescents. *Journal of Anxiety Disorders, 11,* 377–394.

March, J., Parker, J. D., Sullivan, K., Stallings, P., & Conners, C. K. (1997). The Multidimensional Anxiety Scale for Children (MASC): Factor structure, reliability, and validity. *Journal of the American Academy of Child and Adolescent Psychiatry, 36,* 554–565.

March, J., & Sullivan, K. (1999). Test-retest reliability of the Multidimensional Anxiety Scale for Children. *Journal of Anxiety Disorders, 13,* 349–358.

McCathie, H., & Spence, S. H. (1991). What is the Revised Fear Survey Schedule for Children measuring? *Behaviour Research and Therapy, 29,* 495–502.

McGee, R., Feehan, M., & Williams, S. (1990). Comorbidity of anxiety disorders in childhood and adolescence. In G. D. Burrows, M. Roth, & R. J. Noyes (Eds.), *Handbook of anxiety* (Vol. 5). Amsterdam, The Netherlands: Elsevier.

Perrin, S., & Last, C. (1992). Do childhood anxiety measures measure anxiety? *Journal of Abnormal Child Psychology, 20,* 567–578.

Piacentini, J., Schaffer, D., Fisher, P. W., Schwab-Stone, M., Davies, M., & Gioia, P. (1993). The Diagnostic Interview Schedule for Children–Revised Version (DISC-R): III. Concurrent criterion validity. *Journal of the American Academy of Child and Adolescent Psychiatry, 32,* 658–665.

Poland, J., Von Eckardt, B., & Spaulding, W. (1994). Problems with the *DSM* approach to classifying psychopathology. In G. Graham & L. Stephens (Eds.), *Philosophical psychopathology* (pp. 235–260). Cambridge: MIT Press.

Pollack, M. H., Otto, M. W., Sabatino, S., & Majcher, D. (1996). Relationship of childhood anxiety to adult panic disorder: Correlates and influence on course. *American Journal of Psychiatry,* 153, 376–381.

Pruis, A., Lahey, B. B., Thyer, B. A., & Christ, M. A. (1990). Separation anxiety disorder and overanxious disorder: How do they differ? *Phobia Practice and Research Journal, 3,* 51–59.

Quay, H. C., & La Greca, A. M. (1986). Disorders of anxiety, withdrawal, and dysphoria. In H. C. Quay, & J. S. Werry (Eds.), *Psychopathological disorders of childhood* (3rd ed., pp. 71–110). New York: Wiley.

Rapee, R. M., Barrett, P. M., Dadds, M. R., & Evans, L. (1994). Reliability of the *DSM-III-R* childhood anxiety disorders using structured interview: Interrater and parent-child agreement. *Journal of the American Academy of Child and Adolescent Psychiatry, 33,* 984–992.

Reynolds, C. R., & Richmond, O. B. (1978). What I think and feel: A revised measure of children's manifest anxiety. *Journal of Personality Assessment, 43,* 281–283.

Schniering, C. A., Hudson, J. L., & Rapee, R. M. (2000). Issues in the diagnosis and assessment of anxiety disorders in children and adolescents. *Clinical Psychology Review, 20*(4), 453–478.

Shaffer, D., Schwab-Stone, M., Fisher, P. W., Cohen, P., Piacentini, J., Davies, M., Conners, C. K., et al. (1993). The Diagnostic Interview Schedule for Children–Revised version (DISC-R): Preparation, field testing, interrater reliability, and acceptability. *Journal of the American Academy of Child and Adolescent Psychiatry, 32,* 643–650.

Silove, D., & Manicavasagar, V. (2001). Early separation anxiety and its relationship to adult anxiety disorders. In M. W. Vasey & M. R. Dadds (2001), *The developmental psychopathology of anxiety.* (pp. 459–479). Oxford, UK: Oxford University Press.

Silverman, W. K., & Albano, A. M. (1996). *Manual for the Anxiety Disorders Interview Schedule for DSM-IV: Child version.* Albany, NY: Graywind.

Silverman, W. K., & Eisen, A. R. (1992). Age differences in the reliability of parent and child reports of child anxious symptomatology using a structured interview. *Journal of the American Academy of Child and Adolescent Psychiatry, 31,* 117–124.

Silverman, W. K., & Rabian, B. (1995). Test-retest reliability of the *DSM-III-R* childhood anxiety disorders symptoms using the Anxiety Disorders Interview Schedule for Children. *Journal of Anxiety Disorders, 9,* 139–150.

Silverman, W. K., & Saavedra, L. M. (1998, October). Diagnosis and classification of anxiety disorders in youth. Paper presented at the symposium, *Treating anxiety disorders in youth: Current problems and future solutions.* Alexandria, VA.

Sonuga-Barke, E. J. S. (1998). Categorical models of childhood disorder: A conceptual and empirical analysis. *Journal of Child Psychology and Psychiatry, 39*(1), 115–133.

Spence, S. H. (1998). A measure of anxiety symptoms among children. *Behaviour Research and Therapy, 36,* 545–566.

Stone, W. L., & Lemanek, K. L. (1990). Developmental issues in children's self-reports. In A. M. La Greca (Ed.), *Through the eyes of the child: Obtaining self-reports from children and adolescents* (pp. 18–56). Boston: Allyn & Bacon.

Strauss, C. C., & Last, C. G. (1993). Social and simple phobias in children. *Journal of Anxiety Disorders, 7,* 141–152.

Strauss, C. C., Last, C. G., Hersen, M., & Kazdin, A. E. (1988). Association between anxiety and depression in children and adolescents with anxiety disorders. *Journal of Abnormal Child Psychology, 16,* 57–68.

Swedo, S. E., Rapoport, J. L., Leonard, H., Lenane, M., & Cheslow, D. (1989). Obsessive-compulsive disorder in children and adolescents: Clinical phenomenology of 70 consecutive cases. *Archives of General Psychiatry, 46,* 335–341.

Sylvester, C. E., Hyde, T. S., & Reichler, R. J. (1987). The Diagnostic Interview for Children and Personality Inventory for Children in studies of children at risk for anxiety disorders or depression. *Journal of the American Academy of Child and Adolescent Psychiatry, 26,* 668–675.

Taylor, J. A. (1953). A personality scale of manifest anxiety. *Journal of Abnormal Psychology, 48,* 285–290.

Tracey, S. A., Chorpita, B. F., Douban, J., & Barlow, D. H. (1997). Empirical evaluation of *DSM-IV* Generalized Anxiety Disorder criteria in children and adolescents. *Journal of Clinical Child Psychology, 26,* 404–414.

Turner, S., Beidel, D., & Costello, A. (1987). Psychopathology in the offspring of anxiety disorders patients. *Journal of Consulting and Clinical Psychology,* 55, 229–235.

Valleni-Basile, L. A., Garrison, C. Z., Jackson, K. L., Waller, J. L., McKeown, R. E., Addy, C. L., & Cuffe, S. P. (1994). Frequency of obsessive-compulsive disorder in a community sample of young adolescents. *Journal of the American Academy of Child and Adolescent Psychiatry, 33,* 782–791.

Vasey, M. W. (1993). Development and cognition in childhood anxiety: The example of worry. In T. H. Ollendick & R. J. Prinz (Eds.), *Advances in clinical child psychology,* (Vol. 15, pp. 1–39). New York: Plenum Press.

Vasey, M. W., & Dadds, M. (2001). *The developmental psychopathology of anxiety.* Oxford, UK: Oxford University Press.

Weissman, M., Wolk, S., Wickramaratne, P., Goldstein, R., Adams, P., Greenwald, S., Ryan, N., et al. (1999). Children with prepubertal-onset major depressive disorder and anxiety grown up. *Archives of General Psychiatry, 56,* 794–801.

Welner, Z., Reich, W., Herjanic, B., Jung, K. G., & Amado, H. (1987). Reliability, validity, and parent-child agreement studies of the Diagnostic Interview for Children and Adolescents (DICA). *Journal of the American Academy of Child and Adolescent Psychiatry, 26,* 649–653.

Werry, J. S. (1994). Diagnostic and classification issues. In T. H. Ollendick, N. J. King, & W. Yule (Eds.), *International handbook of phobic and anxiety disorders in children and adolescents* (pp. 21–42). New York: Plenum Press.

Werry, J. S., Reeves, J. C., & Elkind, G. S. (1987). Attention deficit, conduct, oppositional, and anxiety disorders in children: A review of research on differentiating characteristics. *Journal of the American Academy of Child and Adolescent Psychiatry,* 26, 133–143.

World Health Organization. (1975). *ICD-9: International statistical classification of diseases and related health problems* (9th rev.). Geneva, Switzerland: Author.

World Health Organization. (1992–1994). *ICD-10: International statistical classification of diseases and related health problems* (10th rev.). Geneva, Switzerland: Author.

2

ETIOLOGY OF FEAR
AND ANXIETY

MICHAEL SWEENEY & DANNY PINE

The term *emotion* refers to a brain state associated with signs of reward or punishment, a stimulus for which an animal will extend effort to approach or avoid. The term *fear* refers to a specific emotion elicited by potentially dangerous stimuli. Fear provides organisms with an internal early warning system that issues a call to action. Fear warns the organism of perceived impending danger and readies the organism for potential flight. *Anxiety* typically refers to emotional states that are analogous to fear. It differs from fear, however, in that anxiety refers to fearlike states that are out of proportion in terms of duration, degree of avoidance, or subjective distress, relative to the current level of danger provoked by potential fear stimuli.

Complications in developing a unified, comprehensive theory of fear or anxiety derive from the multiple factors that influence fear states. Genes, development, cognition, behavior, learning, physiology, and neuroanatomy interact to create the experience of fear (Taylor & Arnow, 1988). The situation is further confounded by the multifaceted manifestations of fear, given its cognitive, affective, behavioral, and physiological dimensions. Speculation about the purpose and mechanisms of fear has been at the center of the major theories of human development: evolutionary, biological, psychoanalytic, and behaviorist.

The current chapter is divided into two parts. The initial section presents a historical overview of four key theories as they apply to pathological anxiety: psychoanalysis, behaviorism, cognitive theories, and neuroscience. In the second section, findings from current areas of research are reviewed, because they inform refinements in etiologic theories.

THEORIES ON THE ETIOLOGY OF ANXIETY

Psychodynamic Theories

Freud coined the term *anxiety neurosis* in 1895. He viewed anxiety as the "fundamental phenomenon and the central problem of neurosis" (Freud, 1964). Freud's theory of anxiety evolved over time. The important aspects of early psychodynamic theory include the structural model of personality, the concept of psychosexual stages, and the notion that anxiety is a signal of underlying conflict. In 1903, Freud proposed psychosexual stages of development, for example, oral, anal, oedipal, latent, and phallic. Unsuccessful navigation through these stages would result in a fixation that would manifest itself in a symptom of anxiety. Each stage, because of the different developmental tasks, was posited to relate to a different type of anxiety.

In 1926, Freud devised the structural model and revisited his conceptualization of anxiety. The structural model posits a personality comprised of an id, ego, and superego, with anxiety resulting from conflict between these forces and the need to inhibit unacceptable thoughts and feelings from emerging into conscious awareness. If this "signal anxiety" does not adequately activate the ego's defensive resources, then intense, more persistent anxiety or other neurotic symptoms are thought to result (Gabbard, 1992).

Consequently, anxiety is a signal of unconscious fantasies of imagined dangerous situations. These fantasies are provoked by instinctual wishes or by perceptions of external situations (Michels, Frances, & Shear, 1985). Anxiety becomes problematic when defense mechanisms are no longer able to inhibit its manifestation adequately and symptoms therefore surface.

Learning Theory

Initial learning-based theories of anxiety developed from data on classical conditioning, also known as respondent conditioning, generated by Pavlov (1927). In a classical conditioning experiment, an unconditioned stimulus (UCS), such as an electric shock, refers to a stimulus that can elicit an unconditioned response (UCR), such as fear. If a second, neutral stimulus, such as a tone or a light, is repeatedly paired with the UCS, the previously neutral stimulus (referred to as a conditioned stimulus [CS]), can come to elicit a response similar to the one produced by the UCR. The effect the CS produces after conditioning is a conditioned response (CR).

Watson and Morgan (1917) argued that clinical anxiety is a conditioned response. Watson and Rayner (1920) tested this hypothesis in a now-famous experiment with an 11-month-old child who has come to be known as Little Albert. In the experiment, Albert initially demonstrated no fear of rabbits. Through repeated pairings of a rabbit with a startling noise, however, Albert began to fear the rabbit.

The Little Albert experiment and others suggest that humans can learn to be anxious, though a number of both scientific and ethical questions arise concerning these early experiments. Nevertheless, theories based on classical conditioning motivated development of a number of treatment approaches, including flooding, implosion, modeling, and systematic desensitization. Moreover, recent data in the neurosciences have raised new questions on the role played by classical conditioning in clinical anxiety.

Systematic desensitization is the process of pairing relaxation with progressive approximations of the feared situation (Wolpe, 1958). While studying the development of anxiety in cats, Wolpe observed that a cat that had received a shock in an experimental cage would appear nervous and refuse to eat while in the cage. Wolpe wondered if feeding might inhibit the anxiety, a process he termed reciprocal inhibition. Wolpe had the cats eat in rooms that were progressively more like the cage in which they were shocked. Once an animal appeared calm eating in one setting, it was moved to the next room in the hierarchy, until eventually the animal was comfortable in the cage where the fear was initiated. Such work relates to other research on instrumental conditioning, whereby an animal is trained to exert an active response to provoke one or another form of feedback, such as elicitation of a reward.

Classical conditioning was an important advancement in the understanding of the etiology and treatment development of anxiety disorders. However, classical conditioning alone could not account for the ways in which all fears are acquired. Mineka (1986) has outlined three shortcomings of classical conditioning. First, not every child exposed to the same classical conditioning paradigm will develop a fear reaction to the new stimuli. Second, many people demonstrate fears that have not been associated with any aversive event, such as a fear of dogs, though they have not had any negative contact with dogs. Third, anxiety problems do not develop in many people who have been repeatedly exposed to fearful situations. Many of these concerns were addressed in the development of social learning theory.

Social learning theory posits that behavior in a given situation is the result of the interplay of interpersonal, environmental, and behavioral factors. Social learning theory builds on the principles of classical and instrumental conditioning by adding the concepts of modeling, regulatory control, and self-efficacy (Bandura, 1986). Modeling is learning by observing others. An individual can surmise what is adaptive by learning from his or her observed experiences of others. Consequently, a parent who demonstrates relief after engaging in anxious avoidance teaches the child that some situations are dangerous and that avoidance is an adaptive strategy. Modeling is one mechanism that may contribute to the familial transmission of anxiety disorders. Self-efficacy is an individual's estimate of his or her ability to produce an outcome. Individuals with low self-efficacy hold that control over situations lies outside themselves. High self-efficacy individuals believe that they can impact or manage a situation. Individuals have low self-efficacy for the situations in which they feel anxious. For example, people who fear public speaking often believe that no amount of preparation will allow them to avoid the inevitable failure that is beyond their control. A greater belief in his or her abilities and a higher expectation of positive outcome would decrease the magnitude of the person's anxiety. Many aspects of social learning theory are incorporated into the cognitive model of anxiety.

Cognitive Theories

Behavioral theories of anxiety show strong overlap with cognitive theories, which place an emphasis on regulatory control; interactions of stimuli, thoughts, or cognition; and available reinforcement. Stimuli provide information about a situation, facilitating predictions about the future. For example, a traffic light provides information about when an individual can safely cross the street. Cognition refers to the thoughts about a situation. Reinforcement control is the notion that individuals act in accordance with the likely consequences. Cognitive-behavioral theories suggest that anxiety disorders are perpetuated by an interaction among these factors.

In the cognitive model of anxiety, the expectation and interpretation of events, and not simply events in themselves, govern one's experience. Cognition does not act alone. It functions synergistically with other primal systems, for example, affective, behavioral, and physiological. Primacy is attributed to the role of cognition because the cognitive system is responsible for integrating input, selecting an appropriate plan, and activating the other subsystems (Beck et al., 1985). In the cognitive model, anxiety disorders result from a chronic tendency to overestimate the likelihood of threat (Beck, 1976). For example, the person who fears elevators greatly overestimates the likelihood of being trapped in one. These misestimates of threat result in heightened levels of anxiety, triggering a set of responses designed to protect the individual from harm (Beck, 1976). These responses include changes in autonomic arousal (fight or flight), inhibition of ongoing behavior, and selectively scanning the environment for possible sources of danger. The autonomic arousal further increases heart rate and lends evidence to the initial fear. In addition to inappropriate reactions to new situations, the anxious individual remains geared for defensive action long after the situation has passed.

Cognitive theory differentiates between two levels of cognition: self-schemas and negative automatic thoughts. Self-schemas are general core assumptions or beliefs that people hold about themselves and the world. Dysfunctional assumptions make people prone to interpret situations in a maladaptive manner. For example, the adolescent who holds the belief that "everyone must like me" has tied his or her self-worth to social approval. As a result of this schema, the individual has heightened anxiety about all social contacts. There is likely a decrease in comfort and competency in social situations as well. Negative automatic thoughts function in the same manner but refer to certain thoughts and images that arise in a specific situation. For example, a child concerned about social evaluation may, during a lull in conversation, have a negative automatic thought such as "This group thinks I'm boring."

Neuroscience

In general, the past 20 years have been marked by a resurgence of interest in the biological aspects of emotion, and much of this interest has followed from insights on neuroscientific aspects of fear. Advances in neuroscience follow from the strong cross-species parallels, from rodents through humans, in the phenomenological, physiological, and neuroanatomical correlates of acute fear states (LeDoux, 1996, 1998). Much of this work extends insights into the instantiation of fear states through the fear conditioning experiment as described in learning theory, as previously noted. Fear conditioning involves pairing of an aversive UCS with a neutral CS. Conditioning results from changes in a neural circuit centered on the amygdala, a structure that lies in the brain's medial temporal lobe. Following advances in research on fear conditioning, recent studies have begun to examine related fear states, such as the states elicited by innate fear-provoking stimuli (Davis & Shi, 1999). These states engage both the amygdala and a range of other brain structures described later in this chapter.

Considerable diversity emerges in research relating particular neural circuits to distinct fear states (Davis & Shi, 1999). Despite such diversity, research on the neuroscientific aspects of fear states does provide some uniformity in the approach to fear as a normal adaptive construct and anxiety as a clinical problem. Namely, neuroscientific theories consistently explore the manner in which particular brain regions are engaged in specific fear states. Such a theoretical approach emphasizes the view that anxiety states represent outward manifestations of changes in brain systems. Nevertheless, such theories consider many factors, both socioenvironmental and genetic, that ultimately influence the manner in which changes in brain states relate to overt symptomatic manifestations of an anxiety disorder (Francis et al., 1999). As a result, a focus on brain states in such theories can lead to an emphasis in therapeutic research on environmental or social treatments as well as pharmacological treatments.

CURRENT RESEARCH

The previous section of this chapter provides a theoretical and historical framework for research on the etiology of anxiety. The current section reviews data in six areas that are likely to inform ongoing efforts to refine the available theories. These six areas are genetics, temperament, longitudinal course, neurochemistry, psychophysiology, and cognitive neuroscience.

Genetics

Anxiety disorders aggregate within families (Marks, 1986), and research has suggested that the development of childhood anxiety disorders may be genetically mediated (Biederman, Rosenbaum, Bolduc, Faraone, & Hirshfeld, 1991; Last, Hersen, Kazdin, Orvaschel, & Perrin, 1991). Many studies document such familial associations. For example, Weissman et al. (1984) found children of panic disordered probands to be at increased risk for anxiety disorders. Last et al. (1991) found a higher prevalence of anxiety disorders in the first degree relatives of affected children as compared to controls. Family aggregation, however, does not necessarily imply heritability, as common genes are confounded with common environment (Legrand, McGue, & Iacono, 1999). Twin or adoption studies must be employed to disentangle these effects.

Twin studies have been the most common method used to investigate the heritability of anxiety. Twin studies compare scores between monozygotic (MZ) twins and dizygotic (DZ) twins to estimate heritability. MZ twins are genetically identical, whereas DZ twins share, on average, half of their genes. Consequently, if a trait were due solely to genetics and measured without error, correlations between MZ twins, in theory, should be 1.0, whereas correlations between DZ twins should be 0.5. However, MZ and DZ twins also share aspects of their environment. Therefore, if shared aspects of the environment, such as social class, exert a substantial influence on a trait such as anxiety, the within-pair correlations for MZ and DZ twins on an anxiety measure should be similar. Hence, an examination of the degree to which within-pair correlations for MZ and DZ twins differ provides a measure of heritability.

Twin studies in juveniles are only beginning to emerge. Warren, Schmitz, and Emde (1999) investigated the heritability of anxiety in a sample of 7-year-old twins. The sample was comprised of 174 MZ and 152 DZ twin pairs. Participants completed the Revised Children's Manifest Anxiety Scale (RCMAS). The RCMAS has a total score and subscales for physiological anxiety, worry, and social concerns. The investigators found that within-pair correlations were significantly higher for MZ than DZ twins on both the physiological and social subscales. This suggested a genetic component for the attributes tapped by these subscales. However, the within-pair correlations for both the worry scale and the total anxiety score were more similar in MZ and DZ twins than the correlations for the physiological or social subscales. This suggests the presence of shared environmental influences. Specifically, these data suggest that genetic factors influence approximately one third of the variance for the physiological and social anxiety scores.

Legrand et al. (1999) investigated heritability in a large sample of twins: 311 twin pairs aged 11 (188 MZ pairs, 123 DZ pairs) and 236 twin pairs aged 17 (155 MZ, 81 DZ). Participants completed the State-Trait Anxiety Inventory (STAI) and the State-Trait Anxiety Inventory for Children (STAIC). Based on the pattern of correlations for MZ as contrasted with DZ twins, the investigators concluded that trait, but not state, anxiety symptoms are moderately heritable, with additive genes accounting for 45% of the variance.

Thapar and McGuffin (1995) found that parents' and children's reports disagreed on the magnitude of anxiety that can be attributed to heritable factors. The investigators obtained parental reports and adolescents' self-reports of anxiety on the RCMAS. Anxiety symptoms appeared highly heritable by parental report, with additive genes accounting for 59% of the variance. The adolescents' self-reports, however, provided very different results in that the shared environmental effects rather than genetic factors appeared to be of primary importance. This difference could be attributed to a variety of factors, and the findings raise major questions concerning the most appropriate interpretation of twin data. Anxiety is generally viewed as a unitary construct, reflective of some feature of the child. As a result, data documenting different heritability for parent- versus child-reported anxiety raise questions about which informant provides the most valid data from a family-genetic standpoint. Similarly, such divergence raises questions on the precise construct that is being modeled in twin studies of rating scales.

Attributes that are thought to be the precursors of anxiety disorders have also been the subject of investigation, though such studies typically have been conducted in adults. Anxiety sensitivity is the fear of anxiety-related sensations. Individuals with high anxiety sensitivity are more likely to experience anxiety symptoms as threatening, and high anxiety sensitivity has been found to be a risk factor for panic disorder. Stein, Jang, and Livesley (1999) investigated the heritability of anxiety sensitivity in adults. The study group was comprised of 179 MZ twin pairs and 158 DZ twin pairs. The investigators found that anxiety sensitivity has a strong heritable component, accounting for nearly half the variance in total anxiety-sensitivity scores. Similar conclusions have been generated in twin studies of other potential anxiety precursors, such as measures of respiratory dysfunction, as reviewed later in this chapter.

Finally, in contrast to most reports, some studies have found an overwhelming environmental influence. Topolski et al. (1999) investigated heritability in a sample of 1,412 twin pairs aged 8 to 16 years. As in the study by Warren et al. (1999), participants completed the RCMAS. The investigators concluded that environmental influences accounted for 80 to 90% of the variance.

Although findings from such genetic epidemiology studies generate consistent interest in genetic contributions of various complex behaviors, the sequencing of the human genome has accelerated interest in genetics research. Associations between several genes and various anxiety disorders have been reported. However, as in twin studies, inconsistencies or non-replications of findings have been common, and none of the associations between specific behaviors and one or another genetic factor have been clearly established (Smoller, Finn, & White, 2000).

Temperament

The term *temperament* refers to a relatively stable pattern of behavioral tendencies that emerges early in life. Chess, Thomas, Birch, and Hertzig (1960), in their seminal work on temperament, argued for the existence of an innate predisposition that renders some children more prone to problems with fear and anxiety. Work by Kagan (1989, 1994) and colleagues (Kagan, Reznick, & Gibbons, 1989; Kagan & Snidman, 1991, 1999; Kagan, Snidman, Zentner, & Peterson, 1999) over the past 20 years extended this view, demonstrating a consistent association between early-life temperament and later-life behavior, including anxiety symptoms. Kagan and colleagues conducted a series of prospective studies on the influence of temperament, following a sample of 462 healthy children from infancy through middle childhood. At 4 months of age, the children were presented with a variety of visual, auditory, and olfactory stimuli. Children were categorized as high- or low-reactive on the basis of their responses. About 20% of the sample was categorized as high reactive. When presented with the stimuli, they demonstrated a combination of frequent vigorous motor activity, fretting, and crying. About 40% of the sample demonstrated the opposite profile. These children, who had low activity and minimal distress to the same stimuli, were categorized as low reactive. Follow-up evaluations were conducted when the children were aged 14 and 21 months. The children were systematically exposed to a variety of unfamiliar social and nonsocial events. Unfamiliar stimuli included interaction with an examiner, placement of heart electrodes and a blood pressure cuff, an unfamiliar liquid placed on the child's tongue, and the appearance in different episodes of a stranger, a clown, and an odd-looking robot. Children who were categorized as high reactive at age 4 months demonstrated significantly more fears at both the 14- and 21-month assessments, as compared with children who were initially categorized as low reactive. Children in the high reactive group were also found to smile less frequently.

Signs of shyness and inhibition were evaluated again when the children were 4.5 years of age. The children interacted one-on-one with an examiner with whom they were unfamiliar in a playroom with two other children, while the parents of all three children were present. Videotapes of these interactions were coded for the occurrence of spontaneous comments and smiles. The children who were high reactive as infants were more likely to be classified as shy and demonstrated fewer spontaneous comments and smiles, compared with the group that had been low reactive as infants. The high- and low-reactive children were again evaluated when they were 7.5 years old. The presence of anxiety symptoms was assessed through parent and teacher reports. Anxiety symptoms included nightmares and fear of the dark, thunder, and lightning. Anxiety symptoms were present in 45% of the children who were high reactive as infants but in only 15% of the children who were low reactive as infants. Additionally, children in the high-reactive group demonstrated fewer spontaneous comments and smiles.

Kagan et al. (1999) concluded that temperament does not determine future behavior but limits the range of possible outcomes, that is, not every high-reactive child was consistently rated as inhibited at every evaluation. Not a single high-reactive child, however, was consistently rated as uninhibited at the follow-up assessments. Only 18% of high-reactive children were rated as inhibited at every evaluation. Although some high-reactive infants will have anxiety problems in childhood, it is important to note that most will not.

High reactivity in infancy does appear to increase the likelihood of inhibition in childhood. In turn, inhibited children may be more likely to develop anxiety disorders including simple phobia, social phobia, separation anxiety, and PTSD. In the samples followed by C. E. Schwartz, Snidman, and Kagan (1999), a specific association between inhibition and social anxiety disorder during adolescence was demonstrated. In terms of other anxiety disorders, a number of reports have demonstrated the influence of a preexisting inhibited style on risk for psychopathology. Pynoos et al. (1987) assessed all of the children in a Los Angles school one month after a sniper had killed one child and injured 13 other students. Anxiety problems were found in only 38% of the children. A preexisting inhibited style differentiated children who did and did not have a problem with anxiety in response to the tragedy (Terr, 1979).

Longitudinal Course

A series of studies have examined the longitudinal outcome of children with various forms of anxiety disorders. In general, these studies document a moderate level of stability among anxiety disorders present during childhood, adolescence, and adulthood (Pine, 1999). Pine, Cohen, Gurley, Brook, and Ma (1998) prospectively studied the continuity of adolescent to adult anxiety disorders in 776 young people evaluated on three occasions across a span of 9 years. For many but not most subjects, adolescent anxiety disorders persisted into adulthood. Most adult disorders, however, were preceded by adolescent disorders. The presence of an anxiety or depressive disorder in adolescence predicted a two- to threefold increased risk for adult anxiety or depressive disorder. Particular questions have arisen in these studies on the differential longitudinal course of specific anxiety disorders. There is some evidence to suggest specific outcomes for fears, panic attacks, social anxiety, and generalized anxiety disorder.

With respect to specific childhood fears, Muris, Merckelbach, Mayer, and Prins (2000) investigated a sample of 290 children (ages 8 to 13) who acknowledged current fears. The results indicated that childhood fears reflected an impairing anxiety disorder in a substantial minority (22.8%) of these children. For most children, fears cause transient upset and no enduring impairment. For many children, however, fear and anxiety problems beginning in childhood continue into adulthood (Pine, Cohen, & Brook, 2001) and may predict adolescent and adult episodes of major depression (Weissman et al., 1997).

Childhood fears are modified by developmental, environmental, and familial factors. As children grow, they enter new situations and acquire the ability to imagine future circumstances and new opportunities for fearful reactions. For example, fear of sleepovers becomes apparent when sleepovers become common in a child's peer group, and fear of death occurs when children are old enough to consider the notion of death.

With respect to other forms of anxiety, episodes of spontaneous panic in adolescents have been found to predict the onset of panic disorder in adulthood (Keyl & Eaton, 1990; Pine et al., 1998). Similarly, separation anxiety in childhood may also represent a precursor of panic disorder in adulthood. Adults with panic disorder, as compared with those who have other psychiatric disorders, report higher rates of separation anxiety as children (Berg, Butler, & Pritchard, 1974; D. F. Klein, Gittelman, Quitken, & Rifkin, 1980; R. Klein, Koplewicz, & Kanner, 1992). The offspring of adults with comorbid panic disorder and depression have been found to have higher rates of separation anxiety disorder than the offspring of adults with major depression without panic disorder (Capps, Sigman, Sena, & Henker, 1996; Weissman et al., 1984). Additional evidence comes from treatment trials showing that adults with panic disorder and children with separation anxiety have a positive response to the same medication (Gittelman-Klein & Klein, 1971).

Finally, Pine, Cohen, and Brook (2001) and Peterson et al. (2001) examined specificity in course for other anxiety disorders. Children and adolescents with social anxiety disorder faced an increased risk for social anxiety disorder but no other anxiety disorders as adults. Other anxiety disorders exhibited different longitudinal courses. For example, childhood or adolescent obsessive-compulsive disorder exhibited a particularly strong tie with later generalized anxiety disorder. Similarly, broad associations among overanxious, generalized anxiety, panic, and major depressive disorders were found. Adolescents with overanxious disorder were about as likely as adolescents with major depressive disorder to have an episode of major depression in adulthood. Adolescents with major depressive disorder were highly likely to have generalized anxiety as adults.

In conclusion, anxiety disorders with onset during childhood or adolescence persist into adulthood in many but not most cases. Most adult disorders, however, were preceded by adolescent disorders.

Neurochemistry

Rapid advances continue in our understanding of neurochemistry as it may apply to the causes and treatment of anxiety disorders. Research in this area may carry significant clinical insights by facilitating the development of effective pharmacological treatments. As a result, studies of neurochemistry are relevant to conceptualizations of both therapeutics and etiology.

Nerve cells communicate via chemical messengers known as neurotransmitters. At least three different groups of neurotransmitters have been implicated in anxiety. Recent studies have generated interest in a class of neurotransmitters known as neuropeptides. These substances include compounds such as substance-P and corticotropin-releasing hormone that have parallel effects in both nerve cell communication and hormonal regulation.

Although research on neuropeptides remains at the forefront of ongoing basic science studies, this subject is not reviewed in the current chapter, because this research has yet to generate clinical insights relevant to childhood anxiety disorders. Perhaps some of the most consistent interest in neurochemical aspects of anxiety pertains to studies of gamma-hydroxybutyric acid (GABA). Studies on this widely distributed neurotransmitter consistently note relationships to anxiety. Benzodiazepines, which exert their effects through the GABA receptor complex, reduce acute anxiety both in animal models and in various forms of clinical anxiety among adults. Because available randomized controlled trials in children generally do not document such beneficial effects for anxiety, this area is also not reviewed here. Finally, two specific monoamine neurotransmitters have been implicated in anxiety, both in animals and humans. Monoamines exert their effects by modulating activity in distributed neural circuits. Research on monoamines and their effects on neural circuits implicated in anxiety may carry significant implications for childhood anxiety disorders. As a result, research in this area is briefly reviewed.

The neurotransmitter serotonin appears particularly important to anxiety. Serotonin, as a monoamine, is involved in the mediation of a range of behaviors by affecting neural systems. These behaviors include emotional behaviors that relate to anxiety and related fear conditioning. Serotonergic neurons emerge from the raphe nuclei, with the median raphe providing innervation to the septohippocampal system as well as the cortex, which may play an important role in emotional cognition (Melik, Babar-Melik, Oezguenen, & Binokay, 2000).

Studies of genetically altered mice have been used successfully to investigate the influence of different neurotransmitter receptors on fear and anxiety. These are often referred to as knockout studies because a certain receptor site has been deleted or knocked out. Mice with a genetic deletion of various serotonin-related proteins, including both receptors and the reuptake transporter, have been shown to exhibit abnormal fear or anxiety responses in a number of behavioral conflict tests, confirming the important role of this receptor in modulating anxiety (Gross, Santarelli, Brunner, Zhuang, & Hen, 2000). Serotonin knockout mice, as compared with control mice, demonstrate increased anxiety to a variety of tasks, including tasks related to eating, locomotion, and heart rate. In response to a discrete aversive stimulus (e.g., foot shock), the knockout mice show increased freezing and increased tachycardia. Activation of the hypothalamic-pituitary-adrenal axis in response to stress appears to be slightly blunted in the knockout mice, however. Together, these data support the idea that serotonin modulates an important fear circuit in the brain. Serotonin is thought to serve a dual function as a presynaptic autoreceptor with the function of negatively regulating serotonin activity and as a postsynaptic heteroreceptor with the function of inhibiting the activity of nonserotonergic neurons in forebrain structures (Gross et al., 2000).

As noted above, the median raphe nucleus (MRN) provides key inputs to neural circuits in the brain that mediate fear and anxiety responses. Melik et al. (2000) investigated the role of the MRN in the development and maintenance of fear as measured by freezing behavior. A fear response was conditioned by pairing a foot shock with contextual cues. The contextual cues elicited the same fear response in MRN-lesioned rats and control rats directly following the conditioning. MRN-lesioned rats, however, showed a marked deficit in freezing behavior 48 hours after the conditioning. Findings indicate that the MRN-serotonergic septohippocampal pathway is involved in the regulation of anxiety related to fear conditioning triggered by contextual cues, suggesting that short-term contextual fear is independent of the MRN, whereas long-term contextual fear depends on the MRN.

Garpenstrand, Annas, Ekblom, Oreland, and Fredrikson (2001) investigated the role of serotonin and dopamine in the development and maintenance of fear in humans. A faster acquisition of fears was found among participants with a short serotonin transporter promoter allele or low monoamine oxidase activity in platelets as compared with participants with only long alleles or high monoamine oxidase activity. Concerning the maintenance of fears, participants with a long dopamine D4 receptor allele showed delayed extinction compared with those with only short alleles. The findings are consistent with animal studies and support the role of serotonin and dopamine in the development and maintenance of fears in humans.

Finally, perhaps the strongest evidence implicating serotonin in human forms of anxiety derives from research on psychopharmacology. Medications that alter functioning of the serotonergic nervous system exert considerable beneficial effects on various forms of anxiety. Perhaps the strongest evidence of such effects derives from studies of serotonin reuptake inhibitors. These medications show benefits in both children and adults for virtually all forms of anxiety.

The neurotransmitter noradrenaline also appears important in anxiety. Noradrenergic neurons arise from a region of the brain known as the locus coeruleus (LC), which is thought to serve as a relay center for warning or alarm. The LC releases stores of noradrenaline directly into the brain. Noradrenergic neurons, like serotonergic neurons, innervate diverse regions of the brain, such that this brain system exerts a widespread modulatory influence. This serves to increase the signal-to-noise ratio in ongoing processes. In animals, electrical and pharmacological activation of the LC increases norepinephrine turnover and fear-associated behaviors, whereas lesions and pharmacologic inhibition of the LC decreases fear-associated behavior and norepinephrine (NE) turnover (Boulenger & Uhde, 1982). Furthermore, exposure of rats to uncontrollable stress produces behavioral symptoms characteristic of depression and anxiety and results in decreased levels of norepinephrine in the LC (Simson & Weiss, 1994). Finally, the LC interacts closely with another set of neurons that use corticotrepin-releasing factor (CRF) as a neurotransmitter to regulate fear-related behaviors. Much like the data for the serotonergic nervous system, the strongest data implicating the LC and noradrenaline in human anxiety derives from pharmacological studies. Among adults, agents that alter noradrenergic functioning are powerful anxiolytics. Similarly, agents (such as yohimbine) that increase firing of the LC are potent anxiogenic compounds. Among children, available data less clearly document therapeutic effects of noradrenergic agents, though Sallee et al. (2000) did replicate, in children with separation anxiety disorder, the findings of enhanced anxiogenic response to yohimbine previously reported in adult panic disorder.

Psychophysiology

Considerable research examines the association between anxiety and various forms of autonomic regulation. For example, both adults and children with various forms of anxiety exhibit alterations in cardiovascular control. Despite the consistency of these findings, many questions remain. First, cardiovascular measures are regulated by a diverse array of neural structures and provide relatively indirect information concerning the state of brain systems presumably implicated in anxiety disorders. Second, abnormalities in cardiovascular control are not specific to anxiety disorders but also occur in a range of other conditions, including behavior disorders. Third, abnormalities in cardiovascular control can be heavily influenced by context and may be most apparent in anxiety-provoking situations. This raises a question as to the degree to which findings in this area represent epiphenomena. In contrast with data on cardiovascular control, data for respiratory indices address some of these limitations.

The relationship between anxiety and respiration has been supported by a wealth of research (McNally, 1994). The primary function of respiration is the exchange of oxygen (O_2) and carbon dioxide (CO_2) between the environment and the blood. This exchange requires effective movement of air into and out of the lungs. Minute ventilation is the amount of air breathed every minute and is determined by the size of each breath, known as tidal volume, multiplied by the number of breaths per minute, known as respiratory rate. Minute ventilation, tidal volume, and respiratory rate are regulated to ensure that adequate gas exchange occurs. For example, in response to high levels of CO_2, minute ventilation typically increases because of an increase in tidal volume, with respiratory rate remaining relatively unchanged. This response occurs reflexively and rapidly, as central chemoreceptors are extremely sensitive to chemical alterations produced by CO_2 in the brain's extracellular fluid. From a physiological standpoint, suffocation is associated with high levels of arterial CO_2, known as hypercapnia, and low levels of arterial O_2, known as hypoxia (McNally, 1994).

A leading theory holds that panic attacks are a suffocation alarm triggered by cues of impending suffocation (D. F. Klein, 1993). Studies utilizing CO_2 have contributed greatly to the understanding of anxiety and panic. The designs of respiratory challenge studies vary, but in the most common design, individuals with panic disorder or an anxiety disorder other than panic disorder (and normal controls) breathe air that has an increased concentration of CO_2 (McNally, 1994). Numerous studies have found that individuals with panic disorder experience high degrees of anxiety, panic attacks, and pronounced changes in respiratory parameters in response to CO_2 exposure, whereas nonanxious controls and individuals with major depression or generalized anxiety do not (Papp et al., 1993; Papp, Martinez, Klein, Coplan, & Gorman, 1995; Papp et al., 1997; see Table 2.1). Pine et al. (1998) extended this research to anxiety-disordered children (ages 7 to 17) and obtained results that parallel those obtained in adults. Hypersensitivity to CO_2 has not always been observed, however (Rapee, Brown, Antony, & Barlow, 1992; Woods & Charney, 1988).

Family studies have also supported the role of respiratory dysregulation and CO_2 sensitivity in the transmission of panic disorder. A stronger family loading for panic disorder is found in patients with evidence of regulatory dysregulation (Perna, Bertani, Arancio, Ronchi, & Bellodi, 1995). A hypersensitivity to CO_2 is found among the asymptomatic adult relatives of panic-disordered patients. Finally, respiratory indices linked to panic are heritable, raising the possibility of a shared genetic vulnerability for panic attacks and respiratory dysregulation (Coryell, 1997; Perna et al., 1995).

Cognitive models posit that CO_2 sensitivity results not from a biological switch but from panic-disordered individuals' hypersensitivity and catastrophic interpretation of internal sensations such as difficulty breathing (e.g., Barlow, 1988; Clark, 1986). In an examination of cognitive factors, McNally and Eke (1996) found that fears of bodily sensations are better predictors of response to CO_2 challenge than either behavioral sensitivity to carbon dioxide or general trait anxiety.

Because the interplay between physiological and psychological processes during a panic attack is practically instantaneous, it is difficult to determine whether physiological factors are a cause or a consequence of psychological factors involved in panic. Nevertheless, this paradigm has proven informative, in that it has demonstrated that physiological factors are a key component in panic disorder in a way that they are not in other anxiety disorders.

Neuroscience

Earlier neuroscientific approaches emphasized the role of the limbic system—which includes the hypothalamus, septum, hippocampus, amygdala, and cingulum—in anxiety. This view has lost favor in recent years, however, due to considerable imprecision in definitions of anatomical as well as functional aspects of the limbic system. Traditionally, the limbic system was thought to influence attentional processes, memory functions, affect, drive states, and olfaction (Lezak, 2000). Current research on fear conditioning and related fear states does emphasize a role for structures encompassed by older models of the limbic system (LeDoux, 1996). The amygdala in particular plays a central role in fear and anxiety. Evidence implicating the amygdala in anxiety disorders also exists. Much of this knowledge is derived from extensions of animal-based research as opposed to studies con-

Table 2.1.   Rate of Panic Attacks During CO_2 Exposure

Study	N	% CO_2	Panic-Disordered Subjects	Controls
				Not-Ill Controls:
Beck et al., 1999	28	5	29%	14%
Gorman et al., 1984	16	5	58%	0%
Gorman et al., 1988	56	5	39%	8%
Gorman et al., 1994	38	5	29%	0%
Gorman, 2001	115	5	52%	9%
Papp et al., 1997	98	5	54%	8%
Sasaki et al., 1996	28	5	38%	0%
Sinha et al., 1999	24	5	63%	0%
Papp, Martinez, Klein, Coplan, & Gorman, 1995	42	6	38%	5%
Bocola et al., 1998	19	7	89%	0%
Gorman et al., 1994	36	7	68%	12%
Gorman, 2001	115	7	67%	16%
Papp et al., 1997	98	7	58%	18%
Caldirola et al., 1997	68	35	69%	6%
Coryell, 1997	39	35	46%	0%
Coryell et al., 1999	46	35	42%	3%
Gorman et al., 1990	52	35	50%	21%
Perna, Bertani, Arancio, Ronchi, & Bellodi, 1995	59	35	55%	1%
Perna et al., 1995	86	35	46%	2%
Perna et al., 1999	15	35	80%	25%
Van De Hout et al., 1987	21	35	93%	12.5%
				Ill Controls:
Gorman et al., 1988	56	5	39%	0% (OAD)
Gorman, 2001	115	5	52%	50% (PMDD), 14% (MDD)
Gorman, 2001	115	7	67%	56% (PMDD), 35% (MDD)
Caldirola et al., 1997	68	35	69%	54% (PD + SOP), 43% (SOP)
Coryell, 1997	39	35	46%	0% (MDD)
Gorman et al., 1990	52	35	50%	36% (SOP)
Perna et al., 1995	59	35	55%	1% (MDD)
Perna et al., 1996	238	35	77%	90% (GAD + PD), 8% (GAD)
Verberg et al., 1998	35	35	65%	100% (PD + MDD)

Note. OAD = overanxious disorder; PMDD = premenstrual dysphoric disorder; SOP = social phobia; MDD = major depressive disorder; GAD = generalized anxiety disorder; PD = panic disorder.

ducted directly on humans (LeDoux, 1998). When the amygdala of a patient having brain surgery is stimulated, the patient often experiences realistic hallucinations, thoughts, or perceptions coupled with fear (Dozier, 1998). Damage to the amygdala can also effect fear states across a range of species, including humans, though such effects can appear relatively subtle or inconsistent (Lezak, 1995).

EEG STUDIES   Although considerable research has examined amygdala involvement in anxiety, other studies have examined activity in other brain
regions. For example, neural activity in the cortex can be monitored through
quantitative electroencephalography (qEEG). Children who are avoidant
of or fearful of unfamiliar events show greater desynchronization of alpha
frequencies over the right frontal area than the left frontal area under resting conditions (Davidson, 1992; Fox & Davidson, 1988). A subsequent
study of frontal area activation was conducted with high- and low-reactive
infants, characterized by vigorous motor activity, fretting, and crying versus
low activity and distress. This study demonstrated greater activation of the
right frontal area in high reactives when they were 9 and 24 months old,
whereas low reactives showed greater activation over the left frontal area
(Fox, Calkins, & Bell, 1994). Because neural activity in the amygdala can
effect frontal lobe activity via cholinergic fibers projecting from the basal
nucleus of Meynert, desynchronization of alpha frequencies in the right
frontal area may reflect greater activity in the right amygdala (Kapp, Supple,
& Whalen, 1994; Lloyd & Kling, 1991). Kagan and Snidman (1999) evaluated children from a longitudinal sample at 10 years of age and found that,
of 28 high reactives and 24 low reactives, the high reactives demonstrated
greater EEG activation over the right frontal area under resting conditions
(30% vs. 8%). The low reactives showed greater activation over the left frontal
area (55% vs. 25%). Nevertheless, in two studies of both qEEG and behavioral laterality profiles, no evidence emerged of abnormal asymmetries in
adolescents with anxiety disorders (Kentgen et al., 2000; Pine et al., 2000).

IMAGING STUDIES   Recent developments with functional magnetic resonance (fMRI) have made it possible to examine the relationship between
sensitivity for various danger cues in amygdala-based circuits and developmental changes in behaviors potentially related to anxiety disorders. This
includes behaviors possibly related to both social phobia and panic disorder (Pine, 1999). For example, in healthy adults, a selective response by
the amygdala to facial displays of aversive emotions, even when presented
below levels of conscious perception, has been demonstrated (Breiter et al.,
1996; Whalen et al., 1998). Other studies have shown social-phobic adults
facial stimuli at a conscious level to demonstrate amygdala hypersensitivity
in an fMRI paradigm (Birbaumer et al., 1998).
    Beyond the amygdala and cortex, the hippocampal formation has been
implicated in some aspects of anxiety as well as depression. Animal-based
studies on anxiety-related processes have implicated the hippocampus through
its connections with the amygdala in mediating an organism's response to
contextual stimuli in which fear cues are presented (Philips & LeDoux, 1992).
Furthermore, the effects of anxiolytics show parallels with the effects of
septohippocampal lesions in animal studies; both manipulations decrease bias
toward aversive stimuli (Gray & McNaughton, 1996). Hence, neural circuits
involved in aspects of anxiety may involve the hippocampal formation through
interactions with fear-relevant systems in the amygdala.

The thalamus participates in most exchanges between higher and lower brain structures, between sensory and motor or regulatory components at the same structural level, and between centers at the highest level of processing. In particular, the thalamus may play a key role in focusing attention on the source of threat (Dozier, 1998). The thalamus is one termination site for the ascending reticular activating system (RAS). Stimulation of the medial thalamus or dorsolateral thalamic nucleus may evoke feelings typical of anxiety (Delgado, 1972).

ANXIETY AND ATTENTION   Biases in information processing may play a role in the development and persistence of anxiety disorders (A. T. Beck & Emery, 1976; Daleiden & Vasey, 1997; Dalgleish & Watts, 1990; McNally, Riemann, Louro, Lukach, & Kim, 1992; Mineka & Sutton, 1992). Every day, we are bombarded by stimuli. We would be overwhelmed by extraneous stimuli if it were not for selective attention. Selective attention is the automatic and ubiquitous process of allocating greater attentional resources to some stimuli and less to others (Pick, Frankel, & Hess, 1975). The nature of the selected stimuli will affect experience. Anxious individuals may have a bias to selectively attend to stimuli perceived as threatening, which facilitates the development and maintenance of anxiety (A. T. Beck & Emery, 1976; Dalgleish and Watts, 1990; Mineka & Sutton, 1992).

Investigators have attempted to identify biases in the allocation of attention in anxious individuals (Dalgleish & Watts, 1990; McNally et al., 1992; Mineka & Sutton, 1992; Mogg, Gardiner, Stavrou, & Golombok, 1992). Self-report has been a common method of investigation. The limits of self-perception for an automatic process and the problems of response bias, however, circumscribe the utility of self-report. Consequently, there has been a move to study information processing in emotional disorders using paradigms taken from cognitive neuroscience (see Dalgleish & Watts, 1990, for a review). Paradigms from cognitive neuroscience offer a number of advantages over self-reports. These paradigms vary but some features are common. Anxious individuals and controls are exposed to a variety of stimuli, including anxiogenic and neutral stimuli; the presentation of stimuli may be masked in some manner so that perception is thought to be more reliant on automatic attentional processes. Often the outcome is an indirect measure of the attention to threat, such as speed to complete one or another task.

To investigate if anxious individuals allocate greater attention to threatening written words, investigators have employed an emotional Stroop task. In a Stroop task (Stroop, 1935), a participant is presented with a list of words and asked to name the color of the word while ignoring the meaning of the word. The color of a word can be named more quickly in congruent pairs (such as when green ink is used to print the word *green*) than in incongruent pairs (when green ink is used for the word *blue*). Attending to the meaning of a word is thought to be an automatic process, and the delay in processing incongruent word pairs is thought to result from the unintended deployment of attention to the meaning of the word. More recently, the Stroop test has been used to examine cognitive processing of emotional words. Williams, Mathews, and MacLeod, (1996) presented results from a meta-analysis examining the relationship between attention bias on emotional Stroop paradigms and clinical anxiety. This review convincingly documents an association between attention bias and clinical anxiety. For example, in one such study, Mogg and Marden (1990) investigated allocation of attention differences in a sample of high- and low-anxious subjects. Subjects were presented with one of three sets of words: general threat words (*mutilated*, *lonely*), achievement threat words (*stupid*, *ignorant*), or neutral words (*cooking*, *staircase*). The words were matched for length and frequency of use in common language. The words were colored red, yellow, green or blue. Subjects were instructed to name the color of the word as quickly as possible while ignoring the meaning of the word. Greater allocation of attention to threat words would result in slower completion of the threat-word lists. Mogg and Marden found that high-anxious subjects were slower in color-naming threat words than neutral words. As noted previously, the finding of longer response latencies for threat words than for neutral words among individuals with anxiety has been replicated in numerous studies with varied populations, including subjects with spider phobia (Watts, McKenna, F. P., Sharrock, R., & Trezise, 1986), generalized anxiety disorder (Martin, Williams, & Clark, 1991; Mathews & MacLeod, 1985; Mogg, Mathews, & Weinman, 1989), posttraumatic stress disorder (Foa et al., 2000; McNally et al., 1992), panic disorder (McNally, Riemann, & Kim, 1990), and social phobia (Hope, Rapee, Heimberg, & Dombeck, 1990; Lundh & Ost, 1996; Mattia, Heimberg, & Hope, 1993).

More direct investigations of the allocation of attention have been conducted with a dot-probe task, which measures the allocation of attention by measuring participants' reaction time to the appearance of a dot. In this task, two stimuli (such as words) are simultaneously flashed on a screen for milliseconds. A dot sometimes appears where a word had been. Faster reaction times to dots that follow threat words indicate a greater allocation of attention towards toward threat. This task eliminates the possibility of response-bias interpretations by requiring a neutral response (pressing a key) to a neutral stimulus (a dot).

In one of the first uses of the dot-probe task, MacLeod, Mathews, and Tata (1986) investigated differences in the allocation of attention in a sample of anxiety-disordered and not-ill adults. Subjects were presented with 288 word pairs; 48 of these pairs contained one threat word each. Examples of threat words included *criticized*, *humiliated*, *injury*, and *fatal*. The word pairs were presented briefly (500 milliseconds) and simultaneously on a computer screen, one on the top and the second on the bottom half of the screen. Following some word pair presentations, a dot would appear where the word had been. Subjects were instructed to strike a key immediately upon seeing the dot. Greater attention allocation to threat words would result in both faster response times to dots that followed threat words and slower response times to dots that followed the neutral stimuli. MacLeod et al. found that anxiety-disordered individuals shifted their attention in exactly this manner. These results have been replicated in numerous studies with varied populations, including high- and low-anxious medical students (Mogg et al., 1990) and anxiety-disordered individuals (Mogg et al., 1992; Mogg, Millar, & Bradley, 2000; Mogg, Bradley, & Williams, 1995; Taghavi et al., 2000; Vasey, El-Hag, & Daleiden, 1996).

Together, the above research indicates a relationship between clinical anxiety and attention allocation. This allocation of attention may occur at a preconscious level with the allocation of attention occurring automatically, without the awareness of the individual (Mineka & Sutton, 1992). Attention to threat is adaptive in truly threatening situations. If, however, the mechanism for the identification of threat were set too low, the result would be excessive and unnecessary anxiety. This could result in a sustained high level of arousal and maladaptive avoidance (Vasey, Daleiden, Williams, & Brown, 1995).

Selective attention toward material perceived as threatening clearly plays a role in the etiology and maintenance of anxiety; however, the nature of this role is unclear. It may be that biases in attention precede and provoke heightened arousal. Conversely, heightened arousal may result in greater vigilance for threatening material. A more complete view may be a synergistic process with attentional bias increasing arousal, and arousal increasing or maintaining a biased allocation of attention (A. T. Beck & Emery, 1976; Daleiden & Vasey, 1997; Dalgleish & Watts, 1990; McNally et al., 1992; Mineka & Sutton, 1992).

CONCLUSIONS

Fear and anxiety facilitate the survival of a species. Thus, these emotions have played a central role in evolution and natural selection. Fear provides a phylogenetic connection with our evolutionary ancestors and has been necessary for the propagation of a species. It is an emotion that shows relatively strong cross-species parallels, from humans through lower mammals. These parallels have facilitated animal research providing a basis for biological models.

Despite its necessary and adaptive function, the pathological manifestations of fear have garnered the greatest attention. Psychoanalysis provided the earliest (and as such, a highly influential) theory regarding the development and maintenance of anxiety. But psychodynamic notions of anxiety have lost favor to the more parsimonious and empirically grounded behavioral theories. Behavioral theories have provided the basis for effective treatments but have been criticized as reductionistic. The criticisms of strict behavioral theories include inadequate attention to the cognitive, social, and physiological aspects of human anxiety and the inability to explain all cases of anxiety. Social learning and cognitive theories evolved, in part, out of these concerns. Social learning theory stressed the continual interaction between behavior and its controlling influences, including vicarious and symbolic learning. Cognitive theories introduced the notion that expectation and interpretation of events, and not simply events in themselves, govern experience. These latter theories were also more inclusive of the growing information on the biological basis of behavior.

Temperament research has documented the presence of constitutional factors that may provide a persistent and influential bias toward a certain style of life, including the propensity for anxiety problems. Perception researchers have contributed the notion of biases in memory and attention that may influence an organism's assessment of the environment. Recent advances in neuroanatomy, psychophysiology, and respiration have helped to identify the physical structures, chemical messengers, and correlates of anxiety.

REFERENCES

Amir, N., McNally, R. J., Riemann, B.C., & Clements, C. (1996). Implicit memory bias for threat in panic disorder: application of the "white noise" paradigm. *Behaviour Research and Therapy, 34*(2), 157–162.

Bandura, A. (1986). *Social foundations of thought and action: A social cognitive theory.* Englewood Cliffs, NJ: Prentice-Hall.

Barlow, D. H. (1988). *Anxiety and its disorders: The nature and treatment of anxiety and panic.* New York: Guilford Press.

Beck, A. (1976). *Cognitive therapy and the emotional disorders.* New York: International Universities Press.

Beck, A., & Clark, D. (1997). An information processing model of anxiety: automatic and strategic processes. *Behaviour Research and Therapy, 35*(1), 49–58.

Beck, A. T., & Emory, G. (1985). *Anxiety disorders and phobias.* New York: Basic Books.

Beck, A. T., et al. (1985). In Musa, C. Z., & Lepine, J. P. (2000). Cognitive aspects of social phobia: a review of theories and experimental research. *European Psychiatry, 15,* 59–66.

Beck, J. G., Stanley, M. A., Averill, P. M., Baldwin, L. E., & Deagle, E. A., III. (1992). Attention and memory for threat in panic disorder. *Behaviour Research and Therapy, 30*(6), 619–629.

Becker, E., Rinck, M., & Margraf, J. (1994). Memory bias in panic disorder. *Journal of Abnormal Psychology, 103*(2), 396–399.

Becker, E. S., Roth, W. T., Andrich, M., & Margraf, J. (1999). Explicit memory in anxiety disorders. *Journal of Abnormal Psychology, 108*(1), 153–163.

Berg, I., Butler, A., & Pritchard, J. (1974). Psychiatric illness in the mothers of school phobic adolescents. *British Journal of Psychiatry, 125,* 466–467.

Biederman, J., Rosenbaum, J. F., Bolduc, E. A., Faraone, S. V., & Hirshfeld, D. R. (1991). A high risk study of young children of parents with panic disorder and agoraphobia with and without comorbid major depression. *Psychiatry Research, 37,* 333–348.

Birbaumer, N., Grodd, W., Diedrich, O., Klose, M., Erb, M., Lotze, M. Schneider, F., et al. (1998). fMRI reveals amgydala activation to human faces in social phobics. *NeuroReport, 9,* 1223–1226.

Boulenger, J., & Uhde, Thomas (1982). Biological peripheral correlates of anxiety. *Encephale, 8*(Suppl. 2), 119–130.

Bower, G. H. (1981). Mood and memory. *American Psychologist, 36*(2), 129–148.

Bradley, B. P., Mogg, K., & Williams, R. (1995). Implicit and explicit memory for emotion-congruent information in clinical depression and anxiety. *Behaviour Research and Therapy, 33*(7), 755–770.

Breiter, H. C., Etcoff, J. L., Whalen, P. J., Kennedy, W. A., Rauch, S. L., Buckner, R. L., Strauss, M. M., et al. (1996). Response and habituation of the human amygdala during visual processing of facial expression. *Neuron, 17,* 875–887.

Capps, L., Sigman, M., Sena, R., & Henker, B. (1996). Fear, anxiety, and perceived control in children of agoraphobia. *Journal of Child Psychology and Psychiatry, 37,* 445–452.

Chess, S., Thomas, A., Birch, H., & Hertzig, M. (1960). Implications of a longitudinal study of child development for child psychiatry. *American Journal of Psychiatry, 117,* 434–441.

Clark, D. M. (1986). A cognitive approach to panic. *Behaviour Research and Therapy, 24,* 461–470.

Cloitre, M., Cancienne, J., Heimberg, R. G., Holt, C. S., & Liebowitz, M. (1995). Memory bias does not generalize across anxiety disorders. *Behaviour Research and Therapy, 33*(3), 305–307.

Cloitre, M., & Liebowitz, M. R. (1991). Memory bias in panic disorder: An investigation of the cognitive avoidance hypothesis. *Cognitive Therapy and Research, 15*(5), 371–386.

Cloitre, M., Shear, M. K., Cancienne, J., & Zeitlin, S. B. (1994). Implicit and explicit memory for catastrophic associations to bodily sensation words in panic disorder. *Cognitive Therapy and Research, 18*(3), 225–240.

Coryell, W. (1997). Hypersensitivity to carbon dioxide as a disease-specific trait marker. *Biological Psychiatry, 41*(3), 259–263.

Daleiden, E. L., & Vasey, M. W. (1997). An information-processing perspective on childhood anxiety. *Clinical Psychology Review, 17*(4), 407–429.

Dalgleish, T., & Watts, F. N. (1990). Biases of attention and memory in disorders of anxiety and depression. *Clinical Psychology Review, 10*(5), 589–604.

Davidson, R. J. (1992). Anterior cerebral asymmetry and the nature of emotion. *Brain Cognition, 20,* 125–151.

Davis, M., & Shi, C. (1999). The extended amygdala: Are the central nucleus of the amygdala and the bed nucleus of the stria terminalis differentially involved in fear versus anxiety? In J. F. McGinty et al. (Eds.), *Annals of the New York Academy of Sciences: Vol. 877. Advancing from the ventral striatum to the extended amygdala: Implications for neuropsychiatry and drug use* (pp. 281–291).

Delgado, J. M. R. (1972). Physical control of the mind. In E. M. Karlins & L. M. Andrews (Eds.), *Man controlled: Readings in the psychology of behavior control.* New York: Free Press.

Eysenck, M. W. (1985). Anxiety and the worry process. *Bulletin of Psychonomic Society, 22,* 545–548.

Eysenck, M. W. (1992). *Anxiety: The cognitive perspective.* Hillsdale, NJ: Erlbaum.

Foa, E. B., Gilboa-Schechtman, E., Amir, N., & Freshman, Melinda. (2000). Memory bias in generalized social phobia: Remembering negative emotional expressions. *Journal of Anxiety Disorders, 14*(5), 501–519.

Foa, E. B., & Kozak, M. J. (1986). Emotional processing of fear: Exposure to corrective information. *Psychological Bulletin, 99*(1), 20–35.

Foa, E. B., & McNally, R. J. (1986). Sensitivity to feared stimuli in obsessive-compulsives: A dichotic listening analysis. *Cognitive Therapy and Research, 10,* 477–485.

Foa, E. B., McNally, R., & Murdock, T. B. (1989). Anxious mood and memory. *Behaviour Research and Therapy, 27,* 141–147.

Fox, N. A., Calkins, S. D., & Bell, M. A. (1994). Neural plasticity and development in the first two years of life. *Development and Psychopathology, 6,* 677–696.

Fox, N. A., & Davidson, R. J. (1988). Pattern of brain electrical activity during facial signs of emotion in ten month old infants. *Developmental Psychology, 24,* 230–236.

Francis, D., Caldji, C., Champagne, F., Plotsky, P., & Meaney, M. (1999). The role of corticotropin-releasing factor–norepinephrine systems in mediating the effects of early experience on the development of behavioral and endocrine responses to stress. *Biological Psychiatry, 46*(9), 1153–1166.

Freud, S. (1964). In J. Strachey (Ed. and Trans.), *Standard edition of the complete psychological works of Sigmund Freud,* 24 vols. London: Hogarth Press. (Original works published 1886–1939)

Gabbard, G. O. (1992). Psychodynamics of panic disorder and social phobia. *Bulletin of the Menninger Clinic, 56*(2, Suppl. A), A3–A13.

Garpenstrand, H., Annas, P., Ekblom, J., Oreland, L., & Fredrikson, M. (2001). Human fear conditioning is related to dopaminergic and serotonergic biological markers. *Behavioral Neuroscience, 115*(2), 358–364.

Gittelman-Klein, R., & Klein, D. F. (1971). Controlled imipramine treatment of school phobia. *Archives of General Psychiatry, 25,* 204–207.

Graf, P., & Schacter, D. L. (1985). Implicit and explicit memory for new associations in normal and amnesic subjects. *Journal of Experimental Psychology: Learning, Memory, &Cognition, 11*(3), 501–518.

Gray, J. A., and McNaughton, N. (1996). The neuropsychology of anxiety: Reprise. In D. A. Hope (Ed.), *Nebraska Symposium on Motivation: Vol. 43. Perspectives on anxiety, panic, and fear* (pp. 61–134). Omaha: University of Nebraska Press.

Gross, C., Santarelli, L., Brunner, D., Zhuang, X., & Hen, R. (2000). Altered fear circuits in 5–HT-sub(1A) receptor KO mice. *Biological Psychiatry, 48*(12), 1157–1163.

Hope, D. A., Rapee, R. M., Heimberg, R. G., & Dombeck, M. J. (1990). Representations of the self in social phobia: Vulnerability to social threat. *Cognitive Therapy and Research, 14*(2), 177–189.

Kagan, J. (1989). Temperamental contributions to social behavior. *American Psychologist, 44,* 668–674.

Kagan, J. (1994). *Galen's prophecy.* New York: Basic Books.

Kagan, J., Reznick, J. S., & Gibbons, J. (1989). Inhibited and uninhibited types of children. *Child Development, 60,* 838–845.

Kagan, J., & Snidman, N. (1991). Infant predictors of inhibited and uninhibited profiles. *Psychological Science, 2*(1), 40–44.

Kagan, J., & Snidman, N. (1999). Early childhood predictors of adult anxiety disorders. *Biological Psychiatry, 46,* 1536–1541.

Kagan, J., Snidman, N., Zentner, M., & Peterson, E. (1999). Infant temperament and anxious symptoms in school age children. *Development and Psychopathology, 11*, 209–224.

Kapp, B. S., Supple, W. F., & Whalen, P. J. (1994). Effects of electrical stimulation of the amygdaloid central nucleus on neurocortical arousal in the rabbit. *Behavioral Neuroscience, 108*, 81–93.

Kentgen, L., Tenke, C. E., Pine, D., Fong, R., Klein, R., & Bruder, G. (2000). Electroencephalographic asymmetries in adolescents with major depression: Influence of comorbidity with anxiety disorders. *Journal of Abnormal Psychology, 109*(4), 797–802.

Keyl, P. M., & Eaton, M. W. (1990). Risk factors for the onset of panic disorder and other panic attacks in a prospective, population-based study. *American Journal of Epidemiology, 131*, 301–311.

Klein, D. F. (1993). False suffocation alarms, spontaneous panics, and related conditions: an integrative hypothesis. *Archives of General Psychiatry, 50*, 306–317.

Klein, D. F., Gittelman, R., Quitken, F., & Rifkin, A. (1980). *Diagnosis and drug treatment of psychiatry disorders: Adults and children* (2nd ed.). Baltimore: Williams and Wilkins.

Klein, R., Koplewicz, H., & Kanner, A. (1992). Imipramine treatment of children with separation anxiety disorder. *Journal of the American Academy of Child & Adolescent Psychiatry, 31*(1), 21–28.

Lang, P. J. (1978). A bio-informational theory of emotional imagery. *Psychophysiology, 16*(6), 495–512.

Last, C., Hersen, M., Kazdin, A., Orvaschel, H., & Perrin, S. (1991). Anxiety disorders in children and their families. *Archives of General Psychiatry, 48*, 928–934.

LeDoux, J. E. (1996). *The emotional brain*. New York: Simon and Schuster.

LeDoux, J. E. (1998). Fear and the brain: Where have we been; where are we going? *Biological Psychiatry, 44*, 1229–1238.

Legrand, L. N., McGue, M., & Iacono, W. G. (1999). A twin study of state and trait anxiety in childhood and adolescence. *Journal of Child Psychology and Psychiatry, 40*(6), 953–958.

Lezak, M. (1995). *Neuropsychological assessment* (3rd ed.). New York: Oxford University Press.

Lezak, M. (2000). Nature, applications, and limitations of neuropsychological assessment following traumatic brain injury. In A.-L. Christensen, B. P. Uzzell, et al. (Eds.), *International handbook of neuropsychological rehabilitation: Critical issues in neuropsychology* (pp. 67–79). New York: Kluwer Academic/ Plenum Publishers.

Lloyd, R. L., & Kling, A. S. (1991). Delta activity from amygdala in squirrel monkeys (*Saimiri sciureus*): Influence of social and environmental contexts. *Behavioral Neuroscience, 105*, 223–229.

Lundh, L., & Ost, L. (1996). Stroop interference, self-focus, and perfectionism in social phobics. *Personality and Individual Differences, 20*, 725–731.

Lundh, L., & Ost, L. (1997). Explicit and implicit memory bias in social phobia: The role of subdiagnostic type. *Behaviour Research and Therapy, 35*(4), 305–317.

MacLeod, C., Mathews, A., & Tata, P. (1986). Attentional bias in emotional disorders. *Journal of Abnormal Psychology, 95*(1), 15–20.

MacLeod, C., & McLaughlin, K. (1995). Implicit and explicit memory bias in anxiety: A conceptual replication. *Behaviour Research and Therapy, 33*(1), 1–14.

Marks, I. M. (1986). Genetics of fear and anxiety disorders. *British Journal of Psychiatry, 149,* 406–418.

Martin, M., Williams, R. M., & Clark, D. M. (1991). Does anxiety lead to selective processing of threat-related information? *Behaviour Research and Therapy, 29,* 147–160.

Mathews, A. (1990). Why worry? The cognitive function of anxiety. *Behaviour Research and Therapy, 28,* 455–468.

Mathews, A., & MacLeod, C. (1985). Selective processing of threat cues in anxiety states. *Behaviour Research and Therapy, 23,* 563–569.

Mathews, A., & MacLeod, C. (1986). Discrimination of threat cues without awareness in anxiety states. *Journal of Abnormal Psychology, 95,* 131–138.

Mathews, A., & MacLeod, C. (1994). Cognitive approaches to emotion and emotional disorders. *Annual Review of Psychology, 45,* 25–50.

Mathews, A., Mogg, K., May, J., & Eysenck, M. (1989). Implicit and explicit memory bias in anxiety. *Journal of Abnormal Psychology, 98*(3), 236–240.

Mattia, J. I., Heimberg, R. G., & Hope, D. A. (1993). The revised Stroop color-naming task in social phobics. *Behaviour Research and Therapy, 31*(3), 305–313.

McCabe, R. E. (1999). Implicit and explicit memory for threat words in high- and low-anxiety-sensitive participants. *Cognitive Therapy and Research, 23*(1), 21–38.

McNally, R. J. (1994). Cognitive bias in panic disorder. *Current Directions in Psychological Science, 3*(4), 129–132.

McNally, R. J. (1995). Automaticity and the anxiety disorders. *Behaviour Research and Therapy, 33*(7), 747–754.

McNally, R. J., & Eke, M. (1996). Anxiety sensitivity, suffocation fear, and breath-holding duration as predictors of response to carbon dioxide challenge. *Journal of Abnormal Psychology, 105,* 146–149.

McNally, R. J., Foa, E. B., & Donnell, C. D. (1989). Memory bias for anxiety information in patients with panic disorder. *Cognition and Emotion, 3*(1), 27–44.

McNally, R. J., Riemann, B. C., & Kim, E. (1990). Selective processing of threat cues in panic disorder. *Behaviour Research and Therapy, 28,* 407–412.

McNally, R. J., Riemann, B. C., Louro, C. E., Lukach, B. M., & Kim, E. (1992). Cognitive processing of emotional information in panic disorder. *Behaviour Research and Therapy, 30,* 143–149.

Melik, E., Babar-Melik, E., Oezguenen, T., & Binokay, S. (2000). Median raphe nucleus mediates forming long-term but not short-term contextual fear conditioning in rats. *Behavioural Brain Research, 112*(1–2), 145–150.

Michels, R., Frances, A., & Shear, M. K. (1985). Psychodynamic models of anxiety. In A. H. Tuma & J. D. Maser (Eds.), *Anxiety and the anxiety disorders.* Hillsdale, NJ: Erlbaum.

Mineka, S. (1986). The frightful complexity of the origins of fears. In J. B. Overmier & F. R. Brush (Eds.), *Affect, conditioning, and cognition: Essays on the determinants of behavior.* Hillsdale, NJ: Erlbaum.

Mineka, S., & Sutton, S. K. (1992). Cognitive biases and the emotional disorders. *Psychological Science, 3*(1), 65–69.

Mogg, K., Gardiner, J. M., Stavrou, A., & Golombok, S. (1992). Recollective experience and recognition memory for threat in clinical anxiety states. *Bulletin of the Psychonomic Society, 30*(2), 109–112.

Mogg, K., & Marden, B. (1990). Processing of emotional information in anxious subjects. *British Journal of Clinical Psychology, 29*(2), 227–229.

Mogg, K., Mathews, A., & Weinman, J. (1987). Memory bias in clinical anxiety. *Journal of Abnormal Psychology, 96*(2), 94–98.

Mogg, K., Mathews, A., & Weinman, J. (1989). Selective processing of threat cues in anxiety states: A replication. *Behaviour Research and Therapy, 27,* 317–323.

Mogg, K., Millar, N., & Bradley, B. P. (2000). Biases in eye movements to threatening facial expressions in generalized anxiety disorder and depressive disorder. *Journal of Abnormal Psychology, 109*(4), 695–704.

Mogg, K., Bradley, B., & Williams, R. (1995). Attentional bias in anxiety and depression: The role of awareness. *British Journal of Clinical Psychology, 34,* 17–36.

Muris, P., Merckelbach, H., Mayer, B., & Prins, E. (2000). How serious are common childhood fears? *Behaviour Research and Therapy, 38*(3), 217–228.

Neidhardt, E., & Florin, I. (1998). Do patients with a panic disorder show a memory bias? *Psychotherapy & Psychosomatics, 67,* 71–74.

Nunn, J. D., Stevenson, R. J., & Whalan, G. (1984). Selective memory effects in agoraphobic patients. *British Journal of Clinical Psychology, 23,* 195–20.

Oatley, K., & Johnson-Laird, P. (1987). Towards a cognitive theory of emotions. *Cognitive Emotion, 1,* 29–50.

Papp, L. A., Klein, D. F., Martinez, J., Schneier, F., Cole, R., Liebowitz, M. R., Hollander, E., et al. (1993). The diagnostic and substance specificity of carbon-dioxide-induced panic. *American Journal of Psychiatry, 150,* 250–257.

Papp, L. A., Martinez, J. M., Klein, D. F., Coplan, J., & Gorman, J. M. (1995). Rebreathing tests in panic disorder. *Biological Psychiatry, 38,* 240–245.

Papp, L. A., Martinez, J. M., Klein, D. F., Coplan, J. D., Norman, R. G., Cole, R., DeJesus, M. J., et al. (1997). Respiratory psychophysiology of panic disorder: Three respiratory challenges in 98 subjects. *American Journal of Psychiatry, 154,* 1557–1565.

Parrott, W. G., & Sabini, J. (1990). Mood and memory under natural conditions: Evidence for mood incongruent recall. *Journal of Personality and Social Psychology, 59,* 321–326.

Pavlov, I. P. (1927). *Conditioned reflexes.* London, UK: Oxford University Press.

Perna, G., Bertani, A., Arancio, C., Ronchi, P., & Bellodi, L. (1995). Laboratory response of patients with panic and obsessive-compulsive disorder to 35% CO_2 challenges. *American Journal of Psychiatry, 152,* 85–89.

Perrig, W. J., & Perrig, P. (1988). Mood and memory: Mood-congruity effects in the absence of mood. *Memory & Cognition, 16,* 102–109.

Philips, R. G., & LeDoux, J. E. (1992). Differential contribution of amygdala and hippocampus to cued and contextual fear conditioning. *Behavioral Neuroscience, 106,* 274–285.

Pick, A. D., Frankel, D. G., & Hess, V. 1. (1975). Children's attention: The development of selectivity. In E. M. Hetherington (Ed.), *Review of child developmental research* (Vol. 5). Chicago: University of Chicago Press.

Pine, D. (1999). Pathophysiology of childhood anxiety disorder. *Biological Psychiatry, 46,* 1555–1566.

Pine, D., Cohen, P., & Brook, J. (2001). Adolescent fears as predictors of depression. *Biological Psychiatry, 50*(9), 721–724.

Pine, D., Cohen, P., Gurley, D., Brook, J., & Ma, Y. (1998). The risk for early-adulthood anxiety and depressive disorders in adolescents with anxiety and depressive disorders. *Archives of General Psychiatry, 55,* 56–64.

Pine, D. S., Kentgen, L. M., Bruder, G. E., Leite, P., Bearman, K., Ma, Y., & Klein, R. G. (2000). Cerebral laterality in adolescent major depression. *Psychiatry Research, 93*(2), 135–144.

Pynoos, R. S., Frederick, C., Neder, K., Arroyo, W., Steinberg, A., Eth, F., Nunez, F., et al. (1987). Life threat and posttraumatic stress disorder in school-age children. *Archives of General Psychiatry, 44,* 1057–1063.

Rapee, R. M., Brown, T. A., Antony, M. M., & Barlow, D. H. (1992). Response to hyperventilation and inhalation of 5.5% carbon dioxide-enriched air across the *DSM-III-R* anxiety disorders. *Journal of Abnormal Psychology, 101,* 538–552.

Rapee, R. M., McCallum, S. L., Melville, L. F., Ravenscroft, H., & Rodney, J. M. (1994). Memory bias in social phobia. *Behaviour Research and Therapy, 32*(1), 89–99.

Sallee, F. R., Sethuraman, G., Sine, L., & Liu, H. (2000). Yohimbine challenge in children with anxiety disorders. *American Journal of Psychiatry, 157*(8), 1236–1242.

Schwartz, C. E., Snidman, N., & Kagan, J. (1999). Adolescent social anxiety as an outcome of inhibited temperament in childhood. *Journal of the American Academy of Child and Adolescent Psychiatry, 38,* 1008–1015.

Schwartz, N., & Clore, G. L. (1983). Mood, misattribution, and judgments of well-being: Informative and directive functions of affective states. *Journal of Personality and Social Psychology, 45,* 513–523.

Simson, P., & Weiss, J. (1994). *Catecholamine function in posttraumatic stress disorder: emerging concepts.* Washington, DC: American Psychiatric Press.

Smoller, J. W., Finn., C., & White, C. (2000). The genetics of anxiety disorders: An overview. *Psychiatric Annals, 30*(12), 745–753.

Stein, M. B., Jang, K. L., & Livesley, W. J. (1999). Heritability of anxiety sensitivity: A twin study. *American Journal of Psychiatry, 156*(2), 246–251.

Stroop, J. R. (1935). Studies of interference in serial verbal reactions. *Journal of Experimental Psychology, 18,* 643–662.

Taghavi, M. R, Moradi, A. R., Neshat-Doost, H. T., Yule, W., & Dalgleish, T. (2000). Interpretation of ambiguous emotional information in clinically anxious children and adolescents. *Cognition and Emotion, 14*(6), 809–822.

Taylor, C., & Arnow, B. (1988). *The nature and treatment of anxiety disorders.* New York: Free Press.

Terr, L. C. (1979). Children of Chowchilla. *Psychoanalytic Study of the Child, 34,* 547–627.

Thapar, A., & McGuffin, P. (1995). Are anxiety symptoms in childhood heritable? *Journal of Child Psychology and Psychiatry, 36*(3), 439–447.

Topolski, T., Hewitt, J., Eaves, L., Meyer, J., Silberg, J., Simonoff, E., & Rutter, M. (1999). Genetic and environmental influences on ratings of manifest anxiety by parents and children. *Journal of Anxiety Disorders, 13,* 371–397.

Vasey, M. W., Daleiden, E. L., Williams, L. L., & Brown, L. M. (1995). Biased attention in childhood anxiety disorders: A preliminary study. *Journal of Abnormal Child Psychology, 23*(2), 267–279.

Vasey, M. W., El-Hag, N., & Daleiden, E. L. (1996). Anxiety and the processing of emotionally threatening stimuli: Distinctive patterns of selective attention among high- and low-test-anxious children. *Child Development, 67,* 1173–1185.

Warren, S. L., Schmitz, S., & Emde, R. N. (1999). Behavioral genetic analyses of self-reported anxiety at seven years of age. *Journal of the American Academy of Child and Adolescent Psychiatry, 38*(11), 1403–1408.

Watson, J. B., & Morgan, J. B. (1917). Emotional reactions and psychological experimentation. *American Journal of Psychology, 28,* 163–174.

Watson, J. B., & Rayner, R. (1920). Conditioned emotional reactions. *Journal of Experimental Psychology, 3,* 1–14.

Watts, F. N., McKenna, F. P., Sharrock, R., & Trezise, L. (1986). Colour naming of phobia related words. *British Journal of Psychology, 77,* 97–108.

Weissman, M. M., Gershon, E. S., Kidd, K. K., Prusoff, B. A., Leckman, J. F., Dibble, E., Hamovit, J., et al. (1984). Psychiatric disorders in the relatives of probands with affective disorders: With Yale-NIMH collaborative family study. *Archives of General Psychiatry, 41,* 13–21.

Wells, A., & Matthews, G. (1994). *Attention and emotion: A clinical perspective.* Hillsdale, NJ: Erlbaum.

Whalen, P. J., Rauch, S. L., Etcoff, J. L., McInerney, S. C., Lee, M. B., & Jenike, M. A. (1998). Masked presentation of emotional facial expressions modulate amygdala activity without explicit knowledge. *Journal of Neuroscience, 18,* 411–418.

Williams, J. M. G., Mathews, A., & MacLeod, C. (1996). The emotional Stroop task and psychopathology. *Psychological Bulletin, 120,* 3–24.

Williams, J. M. G., Watts, F. N., MacLeod, C., & Mathews, A. (1988). *Cognitive psychology and emotional disorders.* Chichester, UK: Wiley.

Wolpe, J. (1958). *Psychotherapy by reciprocal inhibition.* Stanford, CA: Stanford University Press.

Woods, S. W., & Charney, D. S. (1988). Applications of the pharmacologic challenge strategy in panic disorders research. *Journal of Anxiety Disorders, 2,* 31–49.

3

DEVELOPMENTAL EPIDEMIOLOGY OF ANXIETY DISORDERS

E. Jane Costello, Helen L. Egger, & Adrian Angold

The task of epidemiology is to establish "patterns of disease distribution in time and space" (Kleinbaum, Kupper, & Morgenstern, 1982). Understanding these patterns is fundamental both for scientific understanding of the causes of disease and for public health interventions to prevent and control them. Epidemiologic research involves both clinical and community samples. Although clinical samples are a vital source of observations for generating hypotheses and for treatment efficacy studies, we know that the majority of cases of child psychiatric disorder receive no treatment (Burns et al., 1995; Lavigne et al., 1998; Leaf et al., 1996). For example, in the Great Smoky Mountains Study (GSMS), a longitudinal community study of 1,420 children and adolescents, only 14.3% of those with an anxiety disorder were seen by a mental health professional (E. J. Costello, 2001). Furthermore, we know that the subgroup of children with disorders who receive treatment is not a random sample of the population with the illness. Factors that affect the probability of receiving treatment, such as insurance status (Burns et al., 1995) or comorbidity (Berkson, 1946), can confound the relationships between causes and illness that our research is trying to unravel. Epidemiologic research uses representative population-based samples to ensure that findings are not biased by such confounding factors. This review concentrates on such population-based research.

It is nearly 2 decades since the first major review of the epidemiology of childhood anxiety disorders (Orvaschel & Weissman, 1986), and almost a decade since the second (E. J. Costello & Angold, 1995b). No population-based studies of children were available to inform the first review. The most important change between the first and second reviews was the release of findings from several population-based studies from around the world that contained diagnostic information on the prevalence of anxiety disorders in children and adolescents using the criteria of the *International Classification of Diseases,* or *ICD* (U.S. Department of Health and Human Services, 1980) or the diagnostic and statistical manuals of the American Psychiatric Association (*DSMs*). A summary of these studies in the second review revealed a considerable degree of unanimity about the extent of the problem of anxiety disorders in general, despite differences in the samples' age, gender, and race/ethnicity distributions, sources of information, taxonomies, and data collection methods.

Since 1995 there have been several developments. First, *DSM-IV* (American Psychiatric Association [APA], 1994) made some significant changes to the *DSM* taxonomy of childhood anxiety disorders. Overanxious disorder (OAD) had been introduced in *DSM-III* (APA, 1980) to capture the core childhood symptoms of what might become generalized anxiety disorder (GAD) in adulthood: excessive worry about the past or future, concern with competence, need for reassurance, self-consciousness, somatic complaints, tension. GAD in *DSM-III* and *DSM-III-R* (APA, 1987) used the same criteria for children as for adults. It had four symptom clusters: "apprehensive expectation" or unrealistic worry, motor tension, autonomic hyperactivity, and vigilance or scanning. *DSM-III* required 3 out of 4 symptoms, and *DSM-III-R* required worry plus 6 out of 18 symptoms from the other three categories. One effect of these criteria was that, although OAD was quite commonly diagnosed in community studies of children or adolescents using *DSM-III* or *DSM-III-R* criteria, GAD was very rarely diagnosed in this age group. For example, analysis of the public access National Comorbidity Survey (NCS) data, from a probability sample of the noninstitutionalized population of the United States, showed that there were only two cases of *DSM-III-R* GAD among the 479 adolescents aged 15 to 17 years old in the sample (OAD was not included in the interviews). Similarly, in GSMS, GAD diagnosed using *DSM-III-R* criteria occurred in only 0.7% of children (E. J. Costello et al., 1996).

With the advent of *DSM-IV*, avoidant disorder and OAD of childhood disappeared, and the core symptoms of OAD (excessive worry about the past or future, concern with competence, need for reassurance, self-consciousness) were subsumed under Criterion A of GAD: "excessive anxiety and worry (apprehensive expectation) . . . about a number of events (such as work or school performance)" (APA, 1994, p. 435). Criterion C for GAD was revised to include several symptoms (restlessness, fatigue, difficulty concentrating, irritability, sleep disturbance) that are very difficult to separate from symptoms of depression. Although three such symptoms from Criterion C are required for adults, only one is required for children. In the next section, we examine the impact of these changes on rates of diagnosis.

The second major change since the last review is that child psychiatric epidemiology has begun to take on board the accumulation of knowledge about normal development and developmental psychopathology now available to inform our understanding of patterns of disease distribution. *Developmental epidemiology* is a term increasingly used to describe how, in trying to map and understand patterns of disease distribution, research is incorporating many decades of careful work on the developmental tasks confronting children at each stage, the environmental supports that they need to achieve mastery, the range of normal development, and the consequences of failure. Just as the prevention of cardiovascular disease needs as a background an understanding of the development, structure, and functioning of a normal cardiovascular system, so the prevention of psychiatric disorders, anxiety disorders among them, needs as a basis an understanding of physiological, psychological, and social development.

In the past few years, several longitudinal studies of child psychopathology have begun to yield an incredible wealth of information about the developmental course of psychiatric disorders. Children first studied at birth in the 1970s—for example, in the Dunedin and Christchurch studies in New Zealand (Anderson, Williams, McGee, & Silva, 1987; Fergusson, Horwood, & Lynskey, 1993), the Isle of Wight study in Britain (Rutter, Tizard, & Whitmore, 1970), and the New York State study in the United States (Velez, Johnson, J., & Cohen, 1989)—are now adults, and many are parents of a new generation of potential subjects. This has enormous implications for epidemiologic research. We no longer need to infer causality from cross-sectional surveys but can set up rigorous tests of cause and effect. We no longer need to rely on retrospective reports of risk exposure, such as adult recollections of exposure to childhood sexual abuse, in trying to follow the pathways from risk to outcome. We can map age at onset and continuity and desistance of disorders, as well as of specific symptoms, and begin to identify different groups of children with acute, chronic, and recurrent types of the same disorder. We can study homotypic and heterotypic disorders over time: for example, whether childhood separation anxiety predicts adolescent generalized anxiety. We can create case-control studies from our longitudinal, community samples to study the prodromal symptoms of adolescent-onset disorders. In this chapter, we present examples of this wealth of new knowledge.

The third major change is that studies of the genetics of child and adolescent psychopathology are quantifying the heritability of psychiatric disorders and, more important, how and when gene expression is under environmental influence. In a few cases, promising candidate genes have even been identified. The expansion of a *genetic epidemiology* of psychiatric disorders not only adds to our substantive understanding, but also redirects the design of future epidemiologic research.

Fourth, links between epidemiology and mental health services research have been forged and are beginning to shed light on the gap between need for and availability of treatment (Burns et al., 1995; Lavigne et al., 1998; Leaf et al., 1996), and even on the effectiveness of treatment at the population level (Angold, Costello, Burns, Erkanli, & Farmer, 2000). An important component of this research is dealing with the *pharmacoepidemiology* of childhood disorders, monitoring the ways in which drugs are used to treat child psychopathology, including over- and underprescribing and geographic differences in prescribing patterns. This work has yet to be extended to the anxiety disorders.

Fifth, neuroscientific research is just beginning to yield ideas about how the neural circuitry involved in emotional regulation may function, or, in the anxiety disorders, malfunction. This is of particular importance for epidemiology and taxonomy. It has been suggested (Pine & Grun, 1999) that there may be "three interrelated limbic brain circuits—amygdala-based, the septohypocampally-based [*sic*], and brainstem-hypothalamic-based circuits—in three adult anxiety disorders, comprising phobias, generalized anxiety, and panic disorders" (p. 4). Pine and Grun present evidence that the same three brain circuits may be active in three related areas of child psychopathology: phobias, generalized anxiety, and separation anxiety.

So far, the epidemiologic literature has had little to say about any theory-driven groupings of this kind. With the growth of large, longitudinal data sets, we can now look in more detail at both individual diagnoses and at the three conceptual groupings described by Pine and Grun (1999) and shown in Table 3.1: worry disorders (GAD, OAD), unconditioned fear disorders (panic disorder, separation anxiety disorder [SAD], obsessive-compulsive disorder [OCD]), and conditioned fear disorders (specific phobias, agoraphobia, social phobia, posttraumatic stress disorder [PTSD]).

Several of the topics to which epidemiology can contribute are dealt with in detail elsewhere in this volume. In this chapter, we review current evidence about prevalence and comorbidity, examine what recent studies can tell us about the homotypic and heterotypic continuity of anxiety disorders and syndromes, and discuss the evidence from recent epidemiologic studies that relates to the idea that there may be three clusters of anxiety disorders.

Table 3.1. Hypothesized Groupings of Anxiety Disorders Based on Brain Structure and Function (Pine & Grun, 1999)

Group	Hypothesized Common Biological Pathway	DSM-III-R or DSM-IV Diagnoses
Worry disorders	Septohippocampus	Overanxious disorder Generalized anxiety disorder
Unconditioned fear disorders	Brainstem-hypothalamus	Panic disorder, separation anxiety disorder, obsessive compulsive disorder
Conditioned fear disorders	Amygdala	Specific phobias, agoraphobia, social phobia, posttraumatic stress disorder

PREVALENCE AND COMORBIDITY

It has taken a long time for the change from *DSM-III-R* to *DSM-IV* to be translated into revised assessment instruments and scoring algorithms and to trickle down into the literature in the form of epidemiologic studies reporting prevalence, comorbidity, and risk. Many epidemiologic studies have reported on anxiety in general, without distinguishing among the specific categories set out in, for example, *DSM-III-R* or *DSM-IV*, and it is often unclear how many different diagnoses have been included in the research protocol. In this chapter, we review the epidemiologic literature published since the last edition (E. J. Costello & Angold, 1995b). We include published data on anxiety disorder in general and, where specified, on SAD, GAD, OAD, specific phobias, panic disorder, agoraphobia, social phobia, PTSD, and OCD. We have also included some unpublished data from our own studies—GSMS and Caring for Children in the Community (CCC)—and from the public access data made available from the NCS (Kessler, 1994).

Table 3.2 summarizes information on prevalence from recent epidemiologic studies. It includes all published studies using *DSM-III-R* (the earliest published in 1992) or *DSM-IV* (1996 onward). Thus, it includes some studies covered in the last review (E. J. Costello & Angold, 1995b), in which *DSM-III-R* was used, and those for which new data have become available. Studies are listed in order of their period of reference (current, 3 months, 6 months, 12 months, lifetime).

Any Anxiety Disorder

Studies with a short assessment interval and a single data wave had the lowest prevalence; for example, the current prevalence of one or more anxiety disorders was 2.8% in the Oregon Adolescent Depression Study (OADS) (Lewinsohn et al., 1993). Three-month estimates ranged from 2.2% to 8.6%, with a median of 5.0%. Six-month estimates ranged from 5.5% to 17.7%, 12-month estimates from 8.6% to 20.9%, and lifetime estimates from 8.3% to 27.0%. Not surprisingly, use of a lifetime criterion on the oldest samples generated the highest estimates. Compared with the last review, this one generates a similarly wide range of estimates, but it is more nuanced in showing how prevalence is affected by time frame and age. Most studies show modestly higher rates of "any anxiety" in girls than in boys.

When trying to get an estimate of the burden of disease associated with anxiety disorders, it is worth noting that across the studies reviewed in Table 3.2, the 6-month, 12-month, and lifetime estimates are about two to three times as high as the 3-month estimates. For example, in a single study—the NCS—the lifetime prevalence of any anxiety disorder was 24.7%, whereas the 12-month prevalence was 20.9%; in the Munich study (Wittchen, Nelson, & Lachner, 1998), the equivalent estimates were 14.4% and 9.3%. This suggests a very long duration of disease, or rapid cycling, or forget-

Table 3.2. Summary of *DSM-IIIR, DSM-IV,* and *ICD-10* Studies of Prevalence of Anxiety Disorders: Prevalence Percentages

	Separation Anxiety Disorder	Panic Disorder	Obsessive-Compulsive Disorder	Specific Phobias	Agoraphobia With or Without Panic Disorder	Social Phobia	Posttraumatic Stress Disorder	Avoidant Disorder	Overanxious Disorder	Generalized Anxiety Disorder	Any Anxiety Disorder
1. Lewinsohn et al., 1997; Lewinsohn, Lewinsohn, Gotlib, Seeley, & Allen, 1998: Oregon Adolescent Depression Study (OADS) DSM-III-R K-SADS, age 14–18, N = 1,709											
Current	0.2										2.8
Lifetime		0.3	0.1	1.3	0.1	0.9			0.5		8.3
Lifetime by age 19											27%
2. Simonoff et al., 1997: Virginia Twin Study of Adolescent Behavioral Development (VTSABD) DSM-III-R CAPA, 3-month, age 8–17, N = 2,824	1.2			4.4	1.1	2.5			4.4		8.6
3. Angold et al., : Caring for Children in the Community (CCC) DSM-III-R and DSM-IV CAPA, 3-month, age 9–12, N = 388	3.6	0.2	0.1	0.3	0.4	0.8	2.6	0.0	1.5	1.4	5.0

4. E. J. Costello et al., 1996: Great Smoky Mountains Study (GSMS) DSM-III-R and DSM-IV CAPA, 3-month, age 9–12, N = 2,709	2.1	0.1	0.1	0.1	0.2	0.3	0.5	0.0	0.6	1.4	2.9
5. Angold et al., 2000: Caring for Children in the Community (CCC) DSM-III-R and DSM-IV CAPA, 3-month, age 13–17, N = 532	2.6	1.8	0.3	0.5	0.6	1.7	4.0	0.1	3.6	3.9	5.9
6. E. J. Costello et al., 1996: Great Smoky Mountains Study (GSMS) DSM-III-R and DSM-IV CAPA, 3-month, age 13–16, N = 3,895	0.4	0.3	0.2	0.3	0.3	0.7	1.0	0.1	1.5	2.3	2.2
7. Breton, Bergeron, Valla, Berthiaume, & Gaudet, 1999: Quebec Child Mental Health Survey DSM-III-R DISC 2.25, 6-month, age 6–14, N = 2,400											
Child	2.6			4.9					3.1		9.1
Parent	1.6			11.5					3.8		14.7
8. Shaffer, Fisher, Dulcan, & Davies, 1996: Methods for the Epidemiology of Child and Adolescent Mental Disorders (MECA) DSM-III-R DISC 2.3, 6-month (Dx + CGAS < 71), age 9–17, N = 1,285	3.9			2.6	3.3	5.4			5.7		13.0

(continued)

67

Table 3.2. (continued)

	Separation Anxiety Disorder	Panic Disorder	Obsessive-Compulsive Disorder	Specific Phobias	Agoraphobia With or Without Panic Disorder	Social Phobia	Posttraumatic Stress Disorder	Avoidant Disorder	Overanxious Disorder	Generalized Anxiety Disorder	Any Anxiety Disorder
9. E. J. Costello, Angold, & Keeler, 1999: Health Maintenance Organization study (HMO) DSM-III-R DISC 2.3, 6-month, age 12–18, N = 278	3.2	1.1		3.6	2.2	5.1		1.8	7.1	4.6	17.7
10. Verhulst, van der Ende, Ferdinand, & Kasius, 1997: Random sample, Holland. DSM-III-R DISC 2.3, 6-month, age 13–18, N = 274	1.8	0.4	1.0	12.7	2.6	9.2		4.0	3.1	1.3 wCGAS < 71	
11. Beals et al., 1997: Northern Plains Study DISC 2.1C DSM-III-R, 6-month, child only, age 14–16, N = 109	1.9			2.9		2.0			1.9		5.5
12. Fergusson, Horwood, & Lynskey, 1993: Christchurch Longitudinal Study DSM-III-R DISC 23. 6-month, age 15, N = 1,000											12.8%

Study	(1)	(2)	(3)	(4)	(5)	(6)	(7)	(8)
13. Wittchen, Nelson, & Lachmer, 1998: Early Developmental Stages of Psychopathology (EDSP) DSM-IV CIDI, age 14–24, N = 3,021								
12-month	1.2	0.6	1.8	1.6 w/o panic	2.6	0.7	0.5	9.3
Lifetime	1.6	0.7	2.3	2.6 w/o panic	3.5	1.3	0.8	14.4
14. Brady, Killeen, Brewerton, & Lucerini, 2000; Kessler, 1994: National Comorbidity Survey (NCS) DSM-III-R CIDI, age 15–17, N = 479								
12-month	3.0		11.8	4.0	12.4		0.3	20.9
Lifetime	3.1		12.2	9.1	13.1		0.6	24.7
15. Douglass, Moffitt, Dar, McGee, & Silva, 1995; Feehan, McGee, & Williams, 1993: Dunedin Longitudinal Study DSM-III-R DIS DISC and DIS, 12-month, age 18, N = 993		4.0			11.1			12.4
16. Newman, Moffitt, Caspi, & Silva, 1998: Dunedin Longitudinal Study DSM-III-R DISC, 12-month, DIS 12-month, age 21, N = 960	0.6	7.1	8.4	3.8	9.7		1.9	20.3

(continued)

69

Table 3.2. (continued)

	Separation Anxiety Disorder	Panic Disorder	Obsessive-Compulsive Disorder	Specific Phobias	Agoraphobia With or Without Panic Disorder	Social Phobia	Posttraumatic Stress Disorder	Avoidant Disorder	Overanxious Disorder	Generalized Anxiety Disorder	Any Anxiety Disorder
17. Rueter, Scaramella, Wallace, & Conger, 1999: Iowa Family Study DSM-III-R UM-CIDI, any onsets between ages 15 and 19, N = 303		1.3 (attack)		2.6	1.7	5.0					8.6
18. Essau, Conradt, & Petermann, 1998, 1999a, 1999b, 1999c; Essau, Karpinski, Petermann, & Conradt, 1998: Bremen study DSM-IV CIDI, lifetime, age 12–17, N = 1,035		0.5		3.5		1.6	1.6				
19. Warren, Huston, Egeland, & Sroufe, 1997: Minnesota Parent-Child Project K-SADS-RMPE DSM-III-R, lifetime, age 17.5, N = 172	4.6	1.7	1.7			5.8		1.7	4.6		15.1
20. Kasen, Cohen, Skodol, Johnson, & Brook, 1999: New York State Longitudinal Study DSM-III-R DISC, by age 18, N = 551											15.1
21. Giaconia et al., 1995: Boston Longitudinal Study DSM-III-R, lifetime, age 21, N = 384							6.0				

ting, or some combination of these. Without knowing the length of episodes and the number of episodes in the same individual, it is not possible to calculate the extent to which the differences in rates for different time periods result from true persistence versus faulty memory. However, it is worth noting that, in the NCS, 85% of "lifetime" anxiety disorders reported by 15- to 17-year-olds were reported as occurring in the past 12 months, compared with 70% of the lifetime anxiety disorders reported by 18- to 54-year-olds. Yet the lifetime prevalence rates of older and younger participants were not very different. This suggests either a sudden epidemic of anxiety disorders, striking young and old alike in the 12 months before the survey, or highly chronic disorders, or (more likely) a tendency for people to forget earlier episodes and report a more recent one as the first. This points to the importance of longitudinal *prospective* studies, if the full burden of disease is to be measured accurately.

Specific Anxiety Disorders

Recent studies have provided much new information about the prevalence of *specific* anxiety disorders. *DSM-III-R* OAD, and GAD using *DSM-IV* criteria, were the most common anxiety diagnoses, and panic disorder and agoraphobia (separately or together) the least common. In the earlier studies reviewed in 1995, the reported prevalence of specific phobias ("simple phobias" in *DSM-III*) was extremely high, but most diagnostic instruments for children have now resolved this problem by taking disability into account in making the diagnosis (see discussion later in this chapter). Two studies using adult instruments still reported high rates of specific phobias, and also of social phobias and agoraphobia. This suggests that attention needs to be paid to the use of adult measures when assessing phobias in children. On the other hand, the Bremen study of 12- to 17-year-olds, which also used an adult instrument, reported rates of specific and social phobia well within the range found in other studies of children and adolescents.

Anxiety and Disability

One of the most hotly debated areas in child psychopathology in the past few years has been the relationship between psychiatric diagnosis and level of functioning. When the first versions of the Diagnostic Interview Schedule for Children (DISC) were introduced in the 1980s, they were found to generate extremely high prevalence rates for some disorders, among them some anxiety disorders (A. J. Costello, Edelbrock, Dulcan, Kalas, & Klaric, 1984; Shaffer, Fisher, Dulcan, Davies, Piacentini, et al., 1996). For example, according to data from the four-site Methods for the Epidemiology of Child and Adolescent Mental Disorders (MECA) study, 39.5% of the children had at least one anxiety diagnosis in the past 12 months (Shaffer, Fisher, Dulcan, Davies, Piacentini, et al., 1996). At the same time, health maintenance organizations (HMOs), insurance companies, and government agen-

cies were concerned about whether all these children really needed treatment (E. J. Costello, Burns, Angold, & Leaf, 1993).

One solution to both problems was to require that, to receive a diagnosis, a child should show a significant degree of functional impairment or
disability (to use the World Health Organization's preferred term). Some
writers of structured diagnostic interviews began to incorporate disability
into their measures and scoring algorithms. In 1993, the *Federal Register*
defined a new class of psychiatric disorders called *serious emotional disturbance* (SED) that required significantly impaired functioning or disability
in addition to a diagnosis. SED was to be used as the criterion for assessing
the prevalence of child psychiatric disorder in each state, for the purpose of
allocating federal block grants. Work began to add disability criteria to
psychiatric diagnoses.

Disability can be measured at several different levels. Each symptom
can require impaired functioning, or disability can be evaluated at the level
of the syndrome or diagnosis or in the presence of any diagnosis, irrespective of which one causes impaired functioning. Or the interviewer can rate
the child's level of functioning without making a diagnosis, using a separate measure (e.g., Hodges, Doucette-Gates, & Liao, 1999; Shaffer, 1992).
Or, of course, more than one method can be used.

The effects on the prevalence of anxiety disorders of assessing disability in different ways can been seen in Table 3.3, which presents data from
the four-site MECA study using the DISC 2.3. The study used two kinds
of disability assessment: (a) one attached to each symptom cluster, such that
the interviewer asked about disability if the child or parent endorsed "half
plus one" symptoms (i.e., one more than half of the symptoms needed for
the diagnosis), and (b) one that required the interviewer to rate the child
on a scale of 0 to 100 on level of functioning, using the Children's Global
Assessment Scale (C-GAS; Shaffer, 1992) after the interview was ended.
Adding either diagnosis-specific impairment or *mild impairment* (70 or less)

Table 3.3. Effect of Different Rules for Defining Impairment on the
Percentage of Prevalence of Any Anxiety Disorder (Parent or Child Interview)
Using the DISC 2.3 (Shaffer, Fisher, Dulcan, & Davies, 1996)

	Diagnosis Without Diagnosis-Specific Impairment Criteria			
	Criteria only	*C-GAS ≥ 70 (Mild)*	*C-GAS ≥ 60 (Moderate)*	*C-GAS ≥ 50 (Severe)*
Any anxiety diagnosis	39.5	18.5	9.6	4.3
	Diagnosis With Diagnosis-Specific Impairment Criteria			
	Criteria only	*C-GAS ≥ 70 (Mild)*	*C-GAS ≥ 60 (Moderate)*	*C-GAS ≥ 50 (Severe)*
Any anxiety diagnosis	20.5	13.0	7.2	3.2

Note. C-GAS = score on the Children's Global Assessment Scale.

on the C-GAS halved the prevalence rate; adding both reduced it by two thirds; requiring both diagnosis-specific impairment and *severe* (50 or below) impairment on the C-GAS reduced it by almost 90% (Shaffer, Fisher, Dulcan, & Davies, 1996). Anxiety was, of all diagnoses, the area most severely affected by requiring impairment, and among the anxiety disorders, simple phobia was the most affected; the prevalence estimate fell from 21.6% (no impairment requirements) to 0.7% (diagnosis-specific plus C-GAS. 50).

Sex and Age Differences

A review of the most recent studies does not change earlier conclusions about the sex and age distribution of anxiety disorders in general. Girls were still somewhat more likely than boys to report an anxiety disorder of some sort. However, at the level of individual diagnoses, very few of the sex differences were large. If we assume that the difference is likely to be clinically and statistically meaningful if twice as many girls as boys reported a diagnosis, then only eight studies reported any meaningful sex differences. Three studies reported more specific phobias in girls; two reported more panic disorders; two, more agoraphobia; and one each reported more SAD and OAD. Lewinsohn, Lewinsohn, Gotlib, Seeley, and Allen (1998), in one of the few studies to examine the effects of potentially confounding factors associated with both sex and anxiety, found that controlling for 15 such factors did not eliminate the excess of anxiety disorders in girls.

It is difficult to draw conclusions about age trends from this review, because in many cases, age of subjects was confounded with the time frame of the interview. (Clearly, lifetime data are not helpful here.) Thus, the 3-month studies had both the lowest prevalence rates and the youngest subjects, whereas the 12-month studies tended to have the highest prevalence as well as the oldest subjects. Readers who want to know more about age effects are better advised to go back to the individual studies that can provide cross-sectional (NCS, CCC, VTSABD) or longitudinal (GSMS, HMO) data by age. It is worth noting that Lewinsohn et al. (1998), using retrospective data, identified the female preponderance in anxiety disorders as emerging by age 6.

Conclusions

Anxiety disorders have been among the most difficult to assess reliably and validly in epidemiologic studies (Angold & Costello, 1995b; Shaffer, Fisher, Dulcan, Davies, Piacentini, et al., 1996). Requiring disability as a criterion for making the diagnosis brings the rates down to levels that certainly make provider institutions more comfortable. However, there is growing evidence that disability can be associated with anxiety symptoms that do not reach the threshold for a diagnosis (Angold, Costello, Farmer, Burns, & Erkanli, 1999). There is also evidence that, even controlling for comorbidity with other psychiatric disorders, anxiety disorders are associated with a high degree of disability (Ezpeleta, Erkanli, Costello, Keeler, & Angold, in press). The true burden to children, families, and society associated with these conditions is still unclear and needs further longitudinal research.

COMORBIDITY AMONG ANXIETY DISORDERS

Comorbidity among anxiety disorders has historically been a problem, not only for nosology and epidemiology, but also for diagnosis and treatment. This is an area in which the high level of comorbidity found in clinical samples is mirrored in community samples. A review of published studies yields inconclusive results because (a) not all diagnoses were included in every study, and the number of anxiety disorders included in the analyses of comorbidity varies from study to study; (b) there is a lack of consensus about whether to control for comorbidity with other anxiety disorders, or with other diagnoses, when examining the strength of a particular association; and (c) concurrent and sequential comorbidity are not always distinguished clearly. The two published papers to explore the issue of comorbidity among anxiety disorders (Lewinsohn, Zinbarg, Seeley, Lewinsohn, & Sack, 1997; Simonoff et al., 1997) used bivariate analyses (corrected for sex and age in the latter case), so it is hard to interpret their finding that the majority of comparisons yielded significant odds ratios.

We attempted to conduct a meta-analysis of the available data sets, along the lines of work on psychiatric comorbidity that we have previously published (Angold, Costello, & Erkanli, 1999). However, for many of the diagnostic comparisons, there were too few data sets for such analyses to be feasible. Therefore, we can only draw some very tentative conclusions, based mainly on studies for which we had direct access to the data (GSMS, CCC, HMO, NCS).

We first grouped all anxiety diagnoses into the three broad groups described in Table 3.1 as possibly having some basis in brain structure and functioning: the worry disorders (GAD, OAD), the unconditioned fear disorders, and the conditioned fear disorders. We looked across studies at the extent of difference or association among the three broad groupings of anxiety disorders. There was a great deal of comorbidity but little support for specificity or differentiation at this level. The odds ratios between worry disorders as a group and unconditioned fear disorders as a group were positive and significant, as were most of those linking conditioned with unconditioned fear disorders, and conditioned fear disorders with worry disorders. Next, we looked at the evidence for comorbidity within each of the three groupings.

GAD and OAD   A question of nosologic interest is the extent to which the old OAD category overlaps with the *DSM-IV* generalized anxiety diagnosis. The intention was that children who would formerly have received a diagnosis of OAD of childhood would be subsumed into the new GAD category. The criteria for GAD were loosened for children, who could receive the diagnosis if they had only one of the six symptoms of Criterion C—restlessness, fatigue, difficulty concentrating, irritability, muscle tension, sleep disturbance. However, with one exception, these symptom classes are very different from those defined for OAD (worries about the past or future, concerns about one's competence, need for reassurance, somatic symptoms, self-consciousness, muscle tension). Although mentioned briefly in the description of Criterion A (excessive anxiety or worry), the latter are not set out in the new formal diagnostic criteria. On the other hand, five of the six new Criterion C symptoms are very similar to symptoms of major depressive episode; it is very difficult to write diagnostic questions that reliably capture the subtle differences between, for example, the fatigue associated with depression and that associated with GAD. Thus, any examination of the overlap between OAD and GAD should take into account the possibility of their overlap with depression.

Only three data sets (GSMS, CCC, HMO) permitted a comparison of GAD, OAD, and depression in the same children (only two adolescents from the NCS sample had GAD, probably because the highly restrictive *DSM-III-R* criteria were used). Here we use GSMS data to examine *concurrent* comorbidity among OAD using *DSM-III-R* criteria, GAD using *DSM-IV* criteria, and *DSM-IV* depression. Figure 3.1 shows the results for GSMS. Over the course of the study, 182 children (11.6% of the sample) had one or more of the three diagnoses by the age of 16. Of those who were

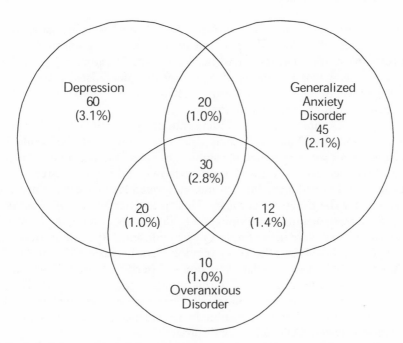

Figure 3.1. Comorbidity among OAD, GAD, and depression by age 16 from the Great Smoky Mountains Study

comorbid (5.4% of the sample, or 47% of those with any of the three diagnoses), more than half (52%) had all three disorders. Because GAD was supposed to subsume OAD, one might expect this combination to be quite common. In fact, only 12 children (16% of those with either GAD or OAD) had both of the worry disorders, without depression, over the course of the study. Of the children with OAD without GAD, 36 of 88 (weighted 42%) also had depressive disorders, not far from the 135 of 296 (weighted 34%) of children with GAD but not OAD. As noted earlier, there is a great deal of similarity between many of the symptoms of MDD and GAD in *DSM-IV*. So one might have expected more comorbidity between depression and GAD than between depression and OAD, but this did not occur. In summary, although there is evidence for considerable comorbidity among the worry disorders (and depression), tracing the extent to which this degree of comorbidity is real rather than methodological will require detailed longitudinal investigation.

Comorbidity Among the Conditioned Fear Disorders   All or almost all the studies confirmed significant comorbidities among the phobias: specific phobia, social phobia, and agoraphobia. However, the one study that permitted a testing of the link with PTSD—another diagnosis hypothesized to be one of the group of conditioned fear disorders (Pine & Grun, 1999)—showed no association between PTSD and any of the phobias after controlling for other anxiety comorbidities.

Comorbidity Among the Unconditioned Fear Disorders   The association between panic disorder and separation anxiety was nonsignificant in three of the four studies that measured it. The clinical literature suggests that separation anxiety is a predictor of later panic disorder (Black, 1994; Klein, 1995; Silove, Manicavasagar, Curtis, & Blaszczynski, 1996), but to date we lack community studies to test this.

Figure 3.2 summarizes the findings about significant associations (depicted as solid lines) among anxiety disorders, from the studies available. Having found some evidence for significant comorbidities among members of the theoretical groups of disorders in two of the three clusters (worries and conditioned fears, but not unconditioned fears), we examined the evidence for the necessary corollary: lack of association among disorders across the three diagnostic groupings. The dotted lines on Figure 3.2 show associations that were never found to be significant. Little connection was found between SAD and the group of phobias, or between SAD and OAD. GAD and OAD were unrelated to simple/specific phobias. There was, however, a consistent pattern of significant association between OAD and social phobia. In light of the clinical data suggesting a *developmental* link, it is of interest that there was absolutely no evidence of a *cross-sectional* association between SAD and panic disorder.

All of the other possible links between disorders in Figure 3.2 are areas of conflicting evidence. For example, the connection between panic disor-

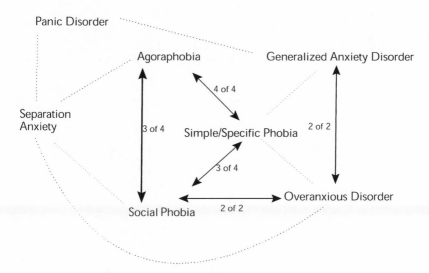

Figure 3.2. Comorbidity among anxiety disorders: Summary of six studies

der and any of the phobias was highly inconsistent. However, it must be emphasized that the evidence is often patchy; some pathways were only represented in two or three studies.

Conclusions

Although too few studies are available for formal meta-analysis, a few general conclusions may be ventured. First, almost all studies found significant comorbidity among the conditioned fear disorders, although the association with PTSD needs more research. Second, although the association between OAD and GAD was intentional, the two did not overlap entirely. Third, GAD and OAD were linked to the fear disorders largely through social phobia, whereas their links to the panic disorders were inconclusive. Fourth, the hypothesized association between separation anxiety and panic disorder was not evident in the data. Fifth, most studies were cross sectional and could not test for possible sequential or developmental relationships.

COMORBIDITY WITH OTHER DISORDERS

Table 3.4 summarizes the available information on comorbidity between any anxiety disorder and (a) attention-deficit/hyperactivity disorder (ADHD), (b) conduct disorder/oppositional defiant disorder (CD/ODD), (c) depression, and (d) substance abuse disorders (SUD). Most of the table comes from our reviews of psychiatric comorbidity (Angold & Costello, & Erkanli, 1999) and of comorbidity with substance use and abuse (Armstrong & Costello, 2002). We have also included data not available when those studies were written.

Table 3.4. Rates of Diagnosis and Comorbidity in General Population Studies

Study	DSM Edition	N	Age	Time Frame	Pop. Rate of a (%)	Pop. Rate of b (%)	Rate of a in b (%0)	Rate of a in not b (%)	Rate of b in a (%)	Rate of b in not a (%)	Odds Ratio	Confidence Internal	p
a = ADHD, b = Anxiety													
1	DSM-IV	920	9–17	3 mo	1.1	5.6	2.7	1.0	13.2	5.5	2.0	0.4–9.1	NS
3	DSM-III-R	278	12–18	6 mo	12.2	14.4	21.1	10.7	25.0	13.0	2.24	1.0–5.1	NS
8	DSM-III-R	1,015	9–13	3 mo	1.9	5.5	4.3	1.7	12.8	5.3	2.63	1.0–6.7	**
9	DSM-IV	970	10–14	3 mo	1.02	3.7	4.7	0.9	17.2	3.6	5.6	1.9–16.2	**
10	DSM-IV	928	11–15	3 mo	.9	2.8	5.3	.7	17.2	2.7	7.4	1.7–33.3	**
11	DSM-IV	820	12–16	3 mo	.6	1.0	0	.6	0	1.0	—	—	—
12	DSM-III-R	323	9–13	3 mo	1.3	5.3	0	1.3	0	5.4	—	—	—
13	DSM-IV	317	10–14	3 mo	1.3	3.8	0	1.3	0	3.9	—	—	—
14	DSM-IV	304	11–15	3 mo	1.0	2.0	16.7	.7	33.3	1.7	29.2	2.3–377	**
15	DSM-IV	289	12–16	3 mo	.4	3.9	0	.4	0	3.9	—	—	NS
16	DSM-III-R	986	15	6 mo	4.8	12.8	—	—	—	—	1.0	0.4–2.5	NS
17	DSM-III-R	2,762	8–16	3 mo	1.4	4.4	—	—	—	—	2.6	0.5–8.6	NS
a = CD/ODD, b = Anxiety													
1	DSM-IV	920	9–17	3 mo	7.0	5.6	13.3	5.0	16.6	6.4	1.9	0.9–4.3	NS
2	DSM-III-R	930	18	1 yr	5.5	19.7	7.1	5.1	25.5	19.3	1.4	0.7–2.7	NS
3	DSM-III-R	278	12–18	6 mo	13.9	14.4	2.08	12.8	21.6	13.3	1.8	0.8–3.9	NS
8	DSM-III-R	1,015	9–13	3 mo	5.2	5.5	18.3	4.4	19.2	4.7	4.81	2.1–10.9	***
9	DSM-IV	970	10–14	3 mo	4.9	3.8	13.0	4.6	9.9	3.4	3.1	1.4–6.9	**
10	DSM-IV	928	11–15	3 mo	3.4	2.8	7.9	3.2	6.6	2.7	2.6	0.8–7.7	NS
11	DSM-IV	820	12–16	3 mo	2.9	0.98	16.2	2.8	5.5	0.9	6.8	1.6–29.6	**
12	DSM-III-R	323	9–13	3 mo	6.5	5.3	5.9	6.5	4.8	5.3	.89	.11–7.1	NS
13	DSM-IV	317	10–14	3 mo	8.2	3.8	33.3	7.2	15.4	2.8	6.4	1.8–23.0	**
14	DSM-IV	304	11–15	3 mo	5.3	2.0	33.3	4.7	12.5	1.4	10.1	1.7–60.2	*
15	DSM-IV	289	12–16	3 mo	4.2	3.8	27.3	3.2	25.0	2.9	11.2	2.5–49.4	**

16	DSM-III-R	986	15	6 mo	10.8	12.8	—	—	—	—	3.2	1.8-5.5	*
17	DSM-III-R	2,762	8-16	3 mo	4.3	4.4	—	—	—	—	3.7	1.9-6.8	*
19	DSM-III-R	479	15-17	Life	14.4	24.7	26.8	10.3	46.1	21.2	3.2	1.6-6.2	***

a = Depression, b = Anxiety

1	DSM-IV	920	9-17	3 mo	2.9	5.6	26.0	5.0	13.4	2.3	5.1	201-12.5	***
2	DSM-III-R	930	18	1 yr	18.0	19.7	45.9	11.1	50.3	13.0	6.8	4.7-9.8	***
3	DSM-III-R	278	12-18	6 mo	4.2	14.4	12.3	2.8	42.4	13.2	4.9	1.5-15.6	**
4	DSM-IV	776	9-18	1 yr	3.4	19.6	7.2	2.5	42.3	18.8	3.2	–1.4-7.6	**
5	DSM-III-R	776	11-20	1 yr	2.8	10.4	11.1	2.1	40.9	9.5	6.6	2.7-16.2	***
6	DSM-IV	1,710	14-18	1 yr	2.9	3.2	16.7	18.0	18.0	2.7	7.9	3.6-17.2	***
7	DSM-III-R	1,170	15-18	Current	20.4	8.8	48.7	17.6	21.0	5.7	4.4	3.1-6.3	***
8	DSM-III-R	1,015	9-13	Life	1.5	5.5	8.01	1.1	28.6	5.09	7.5	2.6-21.7	***
9	DSM-IV	970	10-14	3 mo	3.1	3.8	17.0	2.5	20.9	3.2	7.9	2.2-28.5	**
10	DSM-IV	928	11-15	3 mo	3.2	2.8	23.7	2.6	2.07	2.2	11.5	3.2-40.6	***
11	DSM-IV	820	12-16	3 mo	2.7	1.0	58.5	2.1	21.5	.42	65.2	12.5-341	***
12	DSM-IV	323	9-13	3 mo	.31	5.3	0	.33	0	5.3	—	—	—
13	DSM-IV	317	10-14	3 mo	1.6	3.8	16.7	1.0	40.0	3.2	20.1	3.0-134	**
14	DSM-IV	304	11-15	3 mo	4.3	2.0	33.3	3.7	15.4	1.4	13.0	2.2-79.0	**
15	DSM-IV	289	12-16	3 mo	1.7	3.8	18.2	1.1	40.0	3.2	20.4	3.0-137	**
16	DSM-III-R	986	15	6 mo	6.6	12.8	—	—	—	—	4.6	2.6-8.0	*
17	DSM-III-R	2,762	8-16	3 mo	1.2	4.4	—	—	—	—	4.6	2.6-8.0	*
19	DSM-III-R	479	15-17	Life	15.1	42.7	54.3	19.5	33.2	9.2	4.9	2.5-9.5	***

a = Substance abuse disorder b = Anxiety

1	DSM-IV	920	9-17	3 mo	4.7	5.6	11.4	5.4	9.6	4.5	1.7	0.7-4.6	NS
2	DSM-III-R	930	18	1 yr	10.6	19.7	21.8	8.2	40.4	17.7	3.1	—	—
3	DSM-III-R	278	12-18	6 mo	1.8	14.4	1.5	1.9	11.7	14.5	0.8	0.05-11.9	NS
5	DSM-III-R	698	11-20	1 yr		10.4					1.15	1.0-1.28	*

(continued)

Table 3.4. Rates of Diagnosis and Comorbidity in General Population Studies

Study	DSM Edition	Age	N	Time Frame	Pop. Rate of a (%)	Pop. Rate of b (%)	Rate of a in b (%0)	Rate of a in not b (%)	Rate of b in a (%)	Rate of b in not a (%)	Odds Ratio	Confidence Internal	p
6	DSM-III-R	14–18	1,507	Life	9.8	8.2	19.3	—	16.2	—	2.7	—	—
8	DSM-III-R	9–13	1,015	3 mo	0.1	5.5	0	0.1	0	5.5	—	—	—
9	DSM-IV	10–14	970	3 mo	0.4	3.8	1.5	0.4	8.9	2.3	4.2	0.2–112.4	NS
10	DSM-IV	11–15	928	3 mo	0.9	2.8	3.3	0.9	8.0	2.2	3.9	0.4–39.9	NS
11	DSM-IV	12–16	820	3 mo	2.5	1.0	0	2.5	0	1.0	—	—	—
12	DSM-III-R	9–13	323	3 mo	1.2	5.3	25.0	4.1	7.1	1.0	7.8	1.1–56.8	*
13	DSM-IV	10–14	317	3 mo	1.6	3.8	0	2.9	0	1.6	—	—	—
14	DSM-IV	11–15	304	3 mo	3.5	2.0	0	1.3	0	3.6	—	—	—
15	DSM-IV	12–16	289	3 mo	3.1	3.8	11.1	0.7	33.3	2.8	17.4	2.7–110.6	**
18	DSM-III-R	14–17	401	6 mo	6.2	—	—	—	20.0	15.7	1.5	0.5–4.4	NS
19	DSM-III-R	15–17	479	Life	11.1	24.7	15.3	9.7	34.1	23.5	1.7	0.8–3.7	NS

Study 1. Angold et al. Includes unpublished analyses.
Study 2. Feehan, McGee, Raja, & Williams, 1994.
Study 3. E. J. Costello, Angold, & Kealer, 1999. Includes unpublished analyses.
Study 4. Brook, Cohen, & Brook, 1998; Velez, Johnson, & Cohen, 1989.
Study 5. Velez, Johnson, & Cohen, 1989; a follow-up of Study 7.
Study 6. Rohde, Lewinsohn, & Seeley, 1991; Lewinsohn, Rohde, & Seeley, 1995.
Study 7. Lewinsohn, Hops, Roberts, Seeley, & Andrews, 1993.
Studies 8–15. E. J. Costello, Farmer, Angold, Burns, & Erkanli, 1997; includes unpublished analyses.
Study 16. Fergusson, Horwood, & Lynskey, 1993.
Study 17. Simonoff et al., 1997.
Study 18. Kandel et al., 1999.
Study 19. Kessler et al., 1994; includes unpublished analyses.
*p < .05 **p < .01 ***p < .001

The two review papers also included meta-analyses of the available community studies, summarizing the available data on comorbidity. Controlling for other comorbid conditions, the highest level of anxious comorbidity was with depression, with a median odds ratio of 8.2 ($p < .05$, confidence interval [CI] = 5.8 to 12.0). This means that, across all available studies, depression was 8.2 times as likely in children with anxiety disorders as in children without anxiety disorders, and that 95 times out of 100 the increase in likelihood of depression in the presence of anxiety would lie between 5.8 times and 12 times. The odds ratio for comorbidity with CD/ODD was 3.1 ($p < .05$, CI = 2.2 to 4.6), and that with ADHD was 3.0 ($p < .05$, CI = 2.1 to 4.3). These confidence intervals all exclude 1, indicating a statistically and substantively significant degree of comorbidity. In the case of substance use or abuse, although the bivariate odds ratios were significant in some studies, the association disappeared once comorbidity between anxiety and other psychiatric disorders was controlled (Armstrong & Costello, 2002). However, Weissman et al.'s (1999) high-risk sample of prepubertal children of anxious parents did show an association between early anxiety disorders and *later* SUD, suggesting that although there is little sign of concurrent comorbidity, early anxiety may predict later substance abuse.

There are very few published papers that permit a review of comorbidity between *specific* anxiety disorders and other psychiatric diagnoses. Comorbidity analyses of the OADS data set (Lewinsohn et al., 1997), looking at lifetime diagnoses, showed that depression was significantly associated with each of the anxiety disorders except OCD, controlling for other disorders. Other lifetime associations found were ADHD with simple phobia, ODD with OCD, bipolar disorder with SAD (in males), and alcohol abuse/dependence with OAD. The importance of a more detailed approach is shown by Kaplow, Curran, Angold, and Costello's (2001) reanalysis of the data from GSMS described above. This showed that different anxiety disorders had different relationships to risk of beginning substance use. Children with SAD symptoms were *less* likely than other children to begin drinking alcohol, and did so later than others, whereas those with GAD symptoms were *more* likely than other children to begin drinking and did so earlier.

Analyses of the GSMS and CCC data sets also found that the only consistent pattern of comorbidity with specific anxiety disorders was between depression and GAD, OAD, panic disorder, and PTSD. Depression and the other conditioned fear disorders (apart from PTSD) showed little association, once other diagnoses were controlled, and the behavioral disorders showed no consistent patterns of association with any of the anxiety disorders.

Conclusions

The most recent data sets confirm the strong association between the anxiety disorders and depression. Evidence for any specificity of association is not strong. *DSM-IV* creates a strong methodological link between depression and the worry disorders; to show whether there is a real association beyond the methodological requires further research. The relationship of specific anxiety disorders to SUD warrants further investigation. There is little evidence for any association between anxiety disorders and the disruptive behavior disorders, once comorbidity among other psychiatric disorders is controlled. However, there are hardly any studies that deal thoughtfully with issues of concurrent versus sequential comorbidity (but see Orvaschel, Lewinsohn, & Seeley, 1995), or with sex differences in the role of anxiety disorders as precursors of later psychopathology.

COURSE AND DEVELOPMENT

The natural history of anxiety disorders is another topic that requires population-based, preferably longitudinal, research. Findings about onset and course of disease based on clinical studies using referred or treated samples are liable to be affected by characteristics that brought these children with anxiety disorders, rather than the rest of the population with anxiety disorders, into the clinic, and by the point at which a child's anxiety symptoms create problems for parents or teachers, rather than for the child.

In both clinic-based and population-based studies, there are problems about the accuracy with which parents and children report age at onset of specific symptoms and disorders, and the relative timing of putative risk factors and the onset of disorder. For example, we have shown that the test-retest reliability of the dating of specific psychiatric symptoms was unreliable if the onset occurred more than 3 months before the interview (Angold, Erkanli, Costello, & Rutter, 1996). On the other hand, the *relative* timing of onsets (i.e., whether one occurred before another) was more reliable. This suggests that even if we cannot trust the actual date given by a parent or a child for the onset of a specific symptom, we can be (cautiously) confident in the rank ordering of these dates.

Lewinsohn et al. (1997) analyzed the order of onsets for major depressive disorder (MDD) and several anxiety disorders in the OADS data set. They found that simple phobia, SAD, social phobia, and OAD nearly always preceded the onset of MDD, whereas panic disorder and MDD showed no systematic temporal ordering. In the Dunedin, New Zealand, longitudinal study, two thirds of those who had an anxiety disorder by age 21 had a previous anxiety diagnosis, but the likelihood of a previous nonanxiety diagnosis was no higher in those with early adult anxiety than in those without (Newman, Silva, & Stanton, 1996). Table 3.5 shows the age of onset of anxiety disorders in GSMS, in youth who developed a disorder by age 16. The average age at onset of the anxiety disorder varied widely. Figure 3.3 shows the mean age at onset, standard deviation, and interquartile range (i.e., the ages between which the middle 50% of cases had their onset.) Specific phobias, GAD, and social phobia all began to appear at about the time that children started grade school. Another group of disorders (SAD, agoraphobia, OAD and OCD) all appeared first at about age 9 to 11. Then there was a gap until the onset of panic disorder in the mid-teens (mean

Table 3.5. Mean Age at Onset of Anxiety Disorders and Depression, Standard Deviation, and Interquartile Range (Great Smoky Mountains Study)

	Mean Age (SD) and Interquartile Range Female	Mean Age (SD) and Interquartile Range Male	Mean Age (SD) and Interquartile Range Total
Any anxiety disorder	8.0 (4.7) 2–11	5.7 (3.5) 2–10*	7.0 (4.2) 2–10
Generalized anxiety disorder	6.8 (5.9) 0–13	4.6 (5.3) 1–11	5.8 (5.7) 0–12
Specific phobias	3.6 (4.3) 0.5–11	9.4 (5.0) 0–12	6.3 (5.2) 0–11
Social phobia	7.4 (5.6) 5–11	6.9 (3.7) 0–9	7.3 (4.8) 1–10
Separation anxiety disorder	9.4 (1.9) 7–11	8.0 (2.2) 7–11*	8.8 (2.1) 7–11
Agoraphobia	10.5 (1.9) 8–11	8.1 (4.4) 0–10	9.5 (3.6) 2–11
Obsessive-compulsive disorder	9.4 (2.7) 8–13	10.8 (3.1) 9–12.5	10.4 (2.8) 8–13
Overanxious disorder	10.2 (4.3) 9–14	12.3 (4.3) 5.5–15	11.0 (4.4) 7–15
Panic disorder	13.8 (1.3) 12–15	11.9 (1.2) 11–14	13.4 (1.3) 11.5–14.5
Unipolar depressive disorder	14.0 (1.8) 11–15	14.5 (1.5) 11–15	14.2 (1.7) 11–15

*Mean onset for males earlier than mean onset for females, $p < .05$.

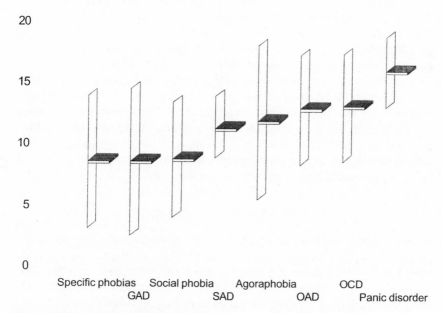

Figure 3.3. Mean age of onset by age 16, and interquartile range, anxiety disorders (Great Smoky Mountains Study)

age 13.4). The mean age of onset of unipolar depression was 14.2, so the 3-month data are consistent with Lewinsohn et al.'s lifetime data in showing that all anxiety disorders except panic disorder preceded depression, and that there was no consistent temporal ordering of panic and depression.

Also of note in Figure 3.3 is the relative length of the interquartile ranges around the mean ages at onset. This variability itself varied widely, from 4 years for SAD to 12 years for GAD. This was not just an effect of sample size, for there were more children with GAD than with SAD. It appears that SAD may have a relatively short window, running for most children through the grade-school years. On the other hand, the narrow onset range for panic disorders in this sample may be due to the subjects' youth; they had not yet passed through the full period of risk for onset of the disorder.

Another aspect of the timing of anxiety disorders is the effect of comorbidity on age at onset. This is an important question for clinicians, because early intervention strategies depend on our knowing the age or developmental stage at which disorders are likely to emerge. There are two questions here: Does psychiatric comorbidity affect age at onset of anxiety disorders, and do anxiety disorders affect the age at onset of other psychiatric disorders?

In answer to the first question, again the data are sparse. In GSMS, the only anxiety disorder whose onset was affected by comorbidity was panic disorder, and the only comorbid condition that affected it was depression. In youth with panic disorder who had a depressive episode at some time before age 16, the age at onset of panic disorder was almost 3 years earlier than it was in youth with panic disorder but no history of depression, controlling for sex and other comorbidities (13.3 years [$SD = 1.6$] vs. 16.2 years [$SD = 1.9$], $z = 2.7$, $p = .003$).

With regard to the second question: Despite the growing evidence that anxiety is often a precursor to depression, data are lacking about the effect of anxiety on the *timing* of other psychiatric disorders. The GSMS data showed very little effect of anxiety on the timing of depression or the disruptive behavior disorders (E. J. Costello, 2001). However, the exception to this discussed earlier—the contradictory effects of SAD and GAD symptoms on the onset of alcohol use (Kaplow et al., 2001)—warns us to be careful in jumping to hasty conclusions. More work, with larger comorbid samples, is needed to examine this important issue.

SUMMARY AND CONCLUSIONS

In this chapter, we have brought together current knowledge about the prevalence, comorbidity, and developmental course of the major anxiety disorders. Space limitations preclude dealing with other issues often treated in chapters on the epidemiology of disorders, such as risk factors and prevention strategies. These are addressed elsewhere in this volume.

The evidence on prevalence is stronger than it was in 1995, although estimates still vary. Current or 3-month estimates for the prevalence of any anxiety disorder are in the 2% to 4% range, whereas the median 6-month and 12-month estimates are mainly between 10% and 20%. The lifetime estimates are only modestly higher than this, suggesting either that anxiety is extremely chronic or that children and adolescents tend to forget earlier episodes after a gap of several months. We still lack information at the diagnostic level about prevalence and onset in children below the age of 8 or 9.

At the level of the specific anxiety disorders, the variability of estimates is still unacceptably high, but the rank ordering shows a certain stability. The worry diagnoses OAD and GAD (*DSM-IV* variety) are among the most common diagnoses, followed by SAD and specific phobias. Panic disorders, OCD, and agoraphobia rarely reach more than 1% prevalence in population samples, although panic disorders are more common in adolescents.

High levels of comorbidity with depression are consistently found (although the methodological problems of the overlap between the *DSM-IV* criteria for GAD and depression need sorting out). The two studies that have examined developmental progression of anxiety disorders agree that, in cases with child or adolescent onset, all except panic disorder precede the onset of depression. The association with behavioral disorders is much less consistent across studies. Comorbidity was significant with CD/ODD in 4 out of 13 studies, with ADHD in 3 out of 6 studies, and with SUD in 3 out of 8 studies. Meta-analysis shows that, controlling for other comorbidities, the association with ADHD is modest but significant (odds ratio [OR] = 3.1), as is that with ADHD (OR = 3.0), but that with SUD is not significant. Comorbidity among anxiety disorders needs much more work, with attention to unraveling the sequential as well as the cross-sectional links and the methodological problems (for example, it is clear that children meeting *DSM-III-R* criteria for OAD are far from being subsumed under *DSM-IV* GAD, as was intended). There is some evidence for two of the three hypothetical groupings discussed earlier; worry disorders are highly comorbid (for real or methodological reasons), and several of the conditioned fear disorders—agoraphobia, specific phobias, and social phobia—frequently co-occur. However, few studies have found the hypothesized link between the unconditioned fear disorders, SAD, and panic disorder. Few studies have looked at comorbidity with OCD and PTSD.

Recent research confirms the 2 to 1 (girls to boys) sex ratio for anxiety disorders, although this varies from diagnosis to diagnosis. It does not, however, appear to show the sex-specific age change seen in depression (i.e., a postpubertal increase for girls but not for boys.) Nor are patterns of comorbidity, either concurrent or sequential, markedly different in boys and girls.

Apart from the usual pleas for more research, the main conclusion that we draw from this review is that it is time for epidemiologic studies to stop reporting on anxiety as if it were a single phenomenon and to pay more attention to its different manifestations at different ages, in relation to different risk factors and correlates, and in conjunction with other disorders.

In particular, as the neurosciences trace possible genetic and neurological pathways that are (on one hand) shared across the emotional disorders, and (on the other) are specific to certain groups among them, careful phenomenological work at the population level will be critical to the task of testing hypotheses about correlates, risk factors, and—dare we say it—the causes of anxiety.

NOTE

This research was supported in part by (5K02–MH-01167–07, 1K23–MH-02016–01, 5P30–MH-57761–02, 5R01–DA-11301–04, 5P01–HL-36587–13). Some sections of the chapter are based on "The Development of Anxiety Disorders: Analyses From the Great Smoky Mountains Study," an article by E. J. Costello, Egger, and Angold that has been submitted for publication.

REFERENCES

Alloy, L. B., Kelly, K. A., Mineka, S., & Clements, C. M. (1990). Comorbidity in anxiety and depressive disorders: A helplessness-hopelessness perspective. In J. D. Maser & C. R. Cloninger (Eds.), *Comorbidity of mood and anxiety disorders* (pp. 499–544). Washington, DC: American Psychiatric Press.

American Psychiatric Association. (1968). *Diagnostic and statistical manual of mental disorders* (2nd ed.). Washington, DC: Author.

American Psychiatric Association. (1980). *Diagnostic and statistical manual of mental disorders* (3rd ed.). Washington, DC: Author.

American Psychiatric Association. (1987). *Diagnostic and statistical manual of mental disorders: DSM-III-R* (3rd ed., rev.). Washington, DC: Author.

American Psychiatric Association. (1994). *Diagnostic and statistical manual of mental disorders: DSM-IV* (4th ed.). Washington, DC: Author.

Anderson, J. C., Williams, S., McGee, R., & Silva, P. A. (1987). *DSM-III* disorders in preadolescent children: Prevalence in a large sample from the general population. *Archives of General Psychiatry, 44,* 69–77.

Angold, A., & Costello, E. J. (1995a). Developmental epidemiology. *Epidemiologic Reviews, 17,* 74–82.

Angold, A., & Costello, E. J. (1995b). A test-retest reliability study of child-reported psychiatric symptoms and diagnoses using the Child and Adolescent Psychiatric Assessment (CAPA-C). *Psychological Medicine, 25,* 755–762.

Angold, A., Costello, E. J., Burns, B. J., Erkanli, A., & Farmer, E. M. Z. (2000). The effectiveness of non-residential specialty mental health services for children and adolescents in the "real world." *Journal of the American Academy of Child and Adolescent Psychiatry, 39,* 154–160.

Angold, A., Costello, E. J., & Erkanli, A. (1999). Comorbidity. *Journal of Child Psychology and Psychiatry, 40,* 57–87.

Angold, A., Costello, E. J., Farmer, E. M. Z., Burns, B. J., & Erkanli, A. (1999). Impaired but undiagnosed. *Journal of the American Academy of Child and Adolescent Psychiatry, 38,* 129–137.

Angold, A., Erkanli, A., Costello, E. J., & Rutter, M. (1996). Precision, reliability and accuracy in the dating of symptom onsets in child and adolescent psychopathology. *Journal of Child Psychology and Psychiatry, 37,* 657–664.

Angold, A., Erkanli, A., Egger, H. L., & Costello, E. J. (2000). Stimulant treatment for children: A community perspective. *Journal of the American Academy of Child and Adolescent Psychiatry, 39*, 975–984.

Angold, A., Erkanli, A., Farmer, E. M. Z., Fairbank, J. A., Burns, B. J., Keeler, G., & Costello, E. J. (2002). Psychiatric disorder, impairment and service use in rural African American and white youth. *Archives of General Psychiatry, 59*, 893–901.

Armstrong, T. D., & Costello, E. J. (2002). Community studies on adolescent substance use, abuse, or dependence and psychiatric comorbidity. *Journal of Consulting and Clinical Psychology, 71*, 1224–1239.

Beals, J., Piasecki, J., Nelson, S., Jones, M., Keane, E., Dauphinais, P., Shirt, R. R., Sack, W. H., & Manson, S. M. (1997). Psychiatric disorder among American Indian adolescents: Prevalence in Northern Plains youth. *Journal of the American Academy of Child and Adolescent Psychiatry, 36*, 1252–1259.

Berkson, J. (1946). Limitations of the application of fourfold table analysis to hospital data. *Biometrics Bulletin, 2*, 47–52.

Black, B. (1994). Separation anxiety disorder and panic disorder. In J. March (Ed.), *Anxiety disorders in children and adolescents*. New York: Guilford Press.

Brady, K. T., Killeen, T. K., Brewerton, T., & Lucerini, S. (2000). Comorbidity of psychiatric disorders and posttraumatic stress disorder. *Journal of Clinical Psychiatry, 61*(Suppl. 7), 22–32.

Breslau, N., Schultz, L., & Peterson, E. (1995). Sex differences in depression: A role for preexisting anxiety. *Journal of Psychiatric Research, 58*, 1–12.

Breton, J.-J., Bergeron, L., Valla, J.-P., Berthiaume, C., & Gaudet, N. (1999). Quebec child mental health survey: Prevalence of *DSM-III-R* mental health disorders. *Journal of Child Psychology and Psychiatry, 40*, 375–384.

Brook, J. S., Cohen, P., & Brook, D. W. (1998). Longitudinal study of co-occurring psychiatric disorders and substance use. *Journal of the American Academy of Child and Adolescent Psychiatry, 37*, 322–330.

Burns, B. J., Costello, E. J., Angold, A., Tweed, D., Stangl, D., Farmer, E. M. Z., & Erkanli, A. (1995). Children's mental health service use across service sectors. *Health Affairs, 14*, 147–159.

Costello, A. J., Edelbrock, C. S., Dulcan, M. K., Kalas, R., & Klaric, S. H. (1984). *Development and Testing of the NIMH Diagnostic Interview Schedule for Children in a clinic population: Final report (Contract no. RFP-DB-81–0027)*. Rockville, MD: NIMH Center for Epidemiologic Studies.

Costello, E. J. (2001). [Longitudinal community study: Incidence of professional mental health treatment of children and adolescents with anxiety disorders]. Unpublished raw data.

Costello, E. J., & Angold, A. (1995a). Developmental epidemiology. In D. Cicchetti & D. Cohen (Eds.), *Developmental psychopathology* (Vol. 1, pp. 23–56). New York: Wiley.

Costello, E. J., & Angold, A. (1995b). Epidemiology. In J. March (Ed.), *Anxiety disorders in children and adolescents* (pp. 109–124). New York: Guilford Press.

Costello, E. J., Angold, A., Burns, B. J., Stangl, D. K., Tweed, D. L., Erkanli, A., & Worthman, C. M. (1996). The Great Smoky Mountains Study of Youth: Goals, designs, methods, and the prevalence of *DSM-III-R* disorders. *Archives of General Psychiatry, 53*, 1129–1136.

Costello, E. J., Angold, A., & Keeler, G. P. (1999). Adolescent outcomes of childhood disorders: The consequences of severity and impairment. *Journal of the American Academy of Child and Adolescent Psychiatry, 38,* 121–128.

Costello, E. J., Burns, B. J., Angold, A., & Leaf, P. J. (1993). How can epidemiology improve mental health services for children and adolescents? *Journal of the American Academy of Child and Adolescent Psychiatry, 32,* 1106–1113.

Costello, E. J., Costello, A. J., Edelbrock, C., Burns, B. J., Dulcan, M. K., Brent, D., & Janiszewski, S. (1988). Psychiatric disorders in pediatric primary care: Prevalence and risk factors. *Archives of General Psychiatry, 45,* 1107–1116.

Costello, E. J., Farmer, E. M., Angold, A., Burns, B. J., & Erkanli, A. (1997). Psychiatric disorders among American Indian and White youth in Appalachia: The Great Smoky Mountains Study. *American Journal of Public Health, 87,* 827–832.

Douglass, H. M., Moffitt, T. E., Dar, R., McGee, R., & Silva, P. (1995). Obsessive-compulsive disorder in a birth cohort of 18-year-olds: Prevalence and predictors. *Journal of the American Academy of Child and Adolescent Psychiatry, 34,* 1424–1431.

Essau, C. A., Conradt, J., & Petermann, F. (1998). Frequency and comorbidity of social anxiety and social phobia in adolescents: Results of a Bremen adolescent study. *Fortschritte der Neurologie-Psychiatrie, 66,* 524–530.

Essau, C. A., Conradt, J., & Petermann, F. (1999a). Frequency and comorbidity of social phobia and social fears in adolescents. *Behaviour Research and Therapy, 37,* 8321–843.

Essau, C. A., Conradt, J., & Petermann, F. (1999b). Frequency of panic attacks and panic disorder in adolescents. *Depression and Anxiety, 9,* 19–26.

Essau, C. A., Conradt, J., & Petermann, F. (1999c). Incidence of post-traumatic stress disorder in adolescents: Results of the Bremen Adolescent Study. *Zeitschrift fur Kinder- und Jugendpsychiatrie und Psychotherapie, 27,* 37–45.

Essau, C. A., Karpinski, N. A., Petermann, F., & Conradt, J. (1998). Frequency and comorbidity of psychological disorders in adolescents: Results of the Bremen Adolescent Study. *Zeitschrift fur Klinische Psychologie, Psychopathologie, und Psychotherapie, 46,* 105–124.

Ezpeleta, L., Erkanli, A., Costello, E. J., Keeler, G., & Angold, A. (2001). Epidemiology of psychiatric disability in childhood and adolescence. *Journal of Child Psychology and Psychiatry, 42,* 901–904.

Feehan, M., McGee, R., Raja, S. N., & Williams, S. M. (1994). *DSM-III-R* disorders in New Zealand 18-year-olds. *Australian and New Zealand Journal of Psychiatry, 28,* 87–99.

Feehan, M., McGee, R., & Williams, S. M. (1993). Mental health disorders from age 15 to age 18 years. *Journal of the American Academy of Child and Adolescent Psychiatry, 32,* 1118–1126.

Fergusson, D. M., Horwood, L. J., & Lynskey, M. T. (1993). Prevalence and comorbidity of *DSM-III-R* diagnoses in a birth cohort of 15 year olds. *Journal of the American Academy of Child and Adolescent Psychiatry, 32,* 1127–1134.

Giaconia, R. M., Reinherz, H. Z., Silverman, A. B., Pakiz, B., Frost, A. K., & Cohen, E. (1995). Traumas and posttraumatic stress disorder in a community population of older adolescents. *Journal of the American Academy of Child and Adolescent Psychiatry, 34,* 1369–1380.

Hodges, K., Doucette-Gates, A., & Liao, Q. (1999). The relationship between the Child and Adolescent Functional Assessment Scale (CAFAS) and indicators of functioning. *Journal of Child and Family Studies, 8,* 109–122.

Kandel, D. B., Johnson, J. G., Bird, H. R., Weissman, M. M., Goodman, S. H.,

Lahey, B. B., Regier, D. A., et al. (1999). Psychiatric comorbidity among adolescents with substance use disorders: Findings from the MECA study. *Journal of the American Academy of Child and Adolescent Psychiatry, 38,* 693–699.

Kaplow, J. B., Curran, P. J., Angold, A., & Costello E. J. (2001). The prospective relation between dimensions of anxiety and the initiation of adolescent alcohol use. *Journal of Clinical Child Psychology, 30,* 316–326.

Kasen, S., Cohen, P., Skodol, A. E., Johnson, J. G., & Brook, J. S. (1999). Influence of child and adolescent psychiatric disorders on young adult personality disorder. *American Journal of Psychiatry, 156,* 1529–1535.

Kellam, S. G., & Werthamer-Larsson, L. (1986). Developmental epidemiology: A basis for prevention. In M. Kessler & S. E. Goldston (Eds.), *A decade of progress in primary prevention* (pp. 154–180). Hanover, NH: University Press of New England.

Kendler, K. S., Heath, A. C., Martin, N. G., & Eaves, L. J. (1987). Symptoms of anxiety and symptoms of depression: Same genes, different environments? *Archives of General Psychiatry, 122,* 451–457.

Kendler, K. S., Neale, M. C., Kessler, R. C., Heath, A. C., & Eaves, L. J. (1992). Major depression and generalized anxiety disorder: Same genes, (partly) different environments? *Archives of General Psychiatry, 49,* 716–722.

Kessler, R. C. (1994). The National Comorbidity Survey of the United States. *International Review of Psychiatry, 6,* 365–376.

Kessler, R. C., McGonagle, K. A., Zhao, S., Nelson, C. B., Hughes, M., Eshleman, S., Wittchen, H. U., et al. (1994). Lifetime and 12–month prevalence of *DSM-III-R* psychiatric disorders in the United States: Results from the National Comorbidity Study. *Archives of General Psychiatry, 51,* 8–19.

Klein, R. G. (1995). Is panic disorder associated with childhood separation anxiety disorder? *Clinical Neuropharmacology, 18,* S7–S14.

Kleinbaum, D. G., Kupper, L. L., & Morgenstern, H. (1982). *Epidemiologic research: Principles and quantitative methods.* New York: Van Nostrand Reinhold.

Lavigne, J. V., Arend, R., Rosenbaum, D., Binns, H. J., Christoffel, K. K., Burns, A., & Smith, A. (1998). Mental health service use among young children receiving pediatric primary care. *Journal of the American Academy of Child and Adolescent Psychiatry, 37,* 1175–1183.

Leaf, P. J., Alegria, M., Cohen, P., Goodman, S. H., Horwitz, S., Hoven, C. W., Narrow, W. E., et al. (1996). Mental health service use in the community and schools: Results from the four-community MECA study. *Journal of the American Academy of Child and Adolescent Psychiatry, 35,* 889–897.

Lewinsohn, P. M., Hops, H., Roberts, R. E., Seeley, J. R., & Andrews, J. A. (1993). Adolescent psychopathology: I. Prevalence and incidence of depression and other *DSM-III-R* disorders in high school students. *Journal of Abnormal Psychology, 102,* 133–144.

Lewinsohn, P. M., Lewinsohn, M., Gotlib, I. H., Seeley, J. R., & Allen, N. B. (1998). Gender differences in anxiety disorders and anxiety symptoms in adolescents. *Journal of Abnormal Psychology, 107,* 109–117.

Lewinsohn, P. M., Rohde, P., & Seeley, J. R. (1995). Adolescent psychopathology: III. The clinical consequences of comorbidity. *Journal of the American Academy of Child and Adolescent Psychiatry, 34,* 510–519.

Lewinsohn, P. M., Zinbarg, R., Seeley, J. R., Lewinsohn, M., & Sack, W. H. (1997). Lifetime comorbidity among anxiety disorders and between anxiety disorders and other mental disorders in adolescents. *Journal of Anxiety Disorders, 11,* 377–394.

Newman, D. L., Moffitt, T. E., Caspi, A., & Silva, P. A. (1998). Comorbid mental disorders: Implications for treatment and sample selection. *Journal of Abnormal Psychology, 107,* 305–311.

Newman, D. L., Silva, P. A., & Stanton, W. R. (1996). Psychiatric disorder in a birth cohort of young adults: Prevalence, comorbidity, clinical significance, and new case incidence from ages 11 to 21. *Journal of Consulting and Clinical Psychology, 64,* 552–562.

Orvaschel, H., Lewinsohn, P. M., & Seeley, J. R. (1995). Continuity of psychopathology in a community sample of adolescents. *Journal of the American Academy of Child and Adolescent Psychiatry, 34,* 1525–1535.

Orvaschel, H., & Weissman, M. M. (1986). Epidemiology of anxiety disorders in children: A review. In R. Gittelman (Ed.), *Anxiety disorders of childhood* (pp. 58–72). New York: Guilford Press.

Pine, D. S., & Grun, J. S. (1999). Childhood anxiety: Integrating developmental psychopathology and affective neuroscience. *Journal of Child and Adolescent Psychopharmacology, 9,* 1–12.

Rohde, P., Lewinsohn, P. M., & Seeley, J. R. (1991). Comorbidity of unipolar depression: II. Comorbidity with other mental disorders in adolescents and adults. *Journal of Abnormal Psychology, 100,* 214–222.

Rueter, M. A., Scaramella, L., Wallace, L. E., & Conger, R. D. (1999). First onset of depressive or anxiety disorders predicted by the longitudinal course of internalizing symptoms and parent-adolescent disagreements. *Archives of General Psychiatry, 56,* 726–732.

Rutter, M., Tizard, J., & Whitmore, K. (1970). *Education, health, and behaviour.* London: Longmans.

Safer, D. J., Zito, J. M., & Fine, E. M. (1996). Increased methylphenidate usage for attention deficit disorder in the 1990s. *Pediatrics, 98,* 1084–1088.

Shaffer, D. (1992). A Children's Global Assessment Scale (C-GAS).

Shaffer, D., Fisher, P., Dulcan, M. K., & Davies, M. (1996). The NIMH Diagnostic Interview Schedule for Children Version 2.3 (DISC 2.3): Description, acceptability, prevalence rates, and performance in the MECA study. *Journal of the American Academy of Child and Adolescent Psychiatry, 35,* 865–877.

Shaffer, D., Fisher, P. W., Dulcan, M., Davies, M., Piacentini, J., Schwab-Stone, M., Lahey, B. B., Bourdon, K., Jensen, P., Bird, H., Canino, G., & Regier, D. (1996). The NIMH diagnostic interview schedule for children (DISC 2.3): Description, acceptability, prevalences, and performance in the MECA study. *Journal of the American Academy of Child and Adolescent Psychiatry, 35,* 865–877.

Silberg, J., Neale, M., Rutter, M., & Eaves, L. (2001). Genetic moderation of environmental risk for depression and anxiety in adolescent girls. *British Journal of Psychiatry, 179,* 116–121.

Silberg, J., Rutter, M., & Eaves, L. (2001). Genetic and environmental influences on the temporal association between earlier anxiety and later depression in girls. *Biological Psychiatry, 49,* 1040–1049.

Silove, D., Manicavasagar, V., Curtis, J., & Blaszczynski, A. (1996). Is early separation anxiety a risk factor for adult panic disorder? A critical review. *Comprehensive Psychiatry, 37,* 167–179.

Simonoff, E., Pickles, A., Meyer, J. M., Silberg, J. L., Maes, H. H., Loeber, R., Rutter, M., et al. (1997). The Virginia Twin Study of adolescent behavioral development: Influences of age, sex and impairment on rates of disorder. *Archives of General Psychiatry, 54,* 801–808.

U.S. Department of Health and Human Services. (1980). *The international classification of diseases, 9th revision, clinical modification: ICD-9-CM. Vol. 1.* (2nd ed.) Washington, DC: U.S. Government Printing Office.

U.S. Department of Health and Human Services. (1993). *Federal Register, 58,* 29425.

Velez, C. N., Johnson, J., & Cohen, P. (1989). A longitudinal analysis of selected risk factors of childhood psychopathology. *Journal of the American Academy of Child and Adolescent Psychiatry, 28,* 861–864.

Verhulst, F. C., van der Ende, J., Ferdinand, R. F., & Kasius, M. C. (1997). The prevalence of *DSM-III-R* diagnoses in a national sample of Dutch adolescents. *Archives of General Psychiatry, 54,* 329–336.

Warren, S. L., Huston, L., Egeland, B., & Sroufe, L. A. (1997). Child and adolescent anxiety disorders and early attachment. *Journal of the American Academy of Child and Adolescent Psychiatry, 36,* 637–644.

Weissman, M. M., Wolk, S., Wickramaratne, P., Goldstein, R. B., Adams, P., Greenwald, S., Ryan, N. D., et al. (1999). Children with prepubertal-onset major depressive disorder and anxiety grown up. *Archives of General Psychiatry, 56,* 794–801.

Wittchen, H.-U., Nelson, C. B., & Lachner, G. (1998). Prevalence of mental disorders and psychosocial impairments in adolescents and young adults. *Psychological Medicine, 28,* 109–126.

Zito, J. M., Daniel, J. S., dos Reis, S., Gardner, J. F., Boles, M., & Lynch, F. (2000). Trends in the prescribing of psychotropic medications to preschoolers. *Journal of the American Medical Association, 283,* 1025–1030.

Zito, J. M., Riddle, M. A., Safer, D., Johnson, R., Fox, M., Speedie, S., & Scerbo, M. (1995). Pharmacoepidemiology of youth with treatments for mental disorders. *Psychopharmacology Bulletin, NCDEU ABSTRACTS,* 540.

Zito, J. M., Safer, D. J., dos Reis, S., & Riddle, M. A. (1998). Racial disparity in psychotropic medications prescribed for youths with Medicaid insurance in Maryland. *Journal of the American Academy of Child and Adolescent Psychiatry, 37,* 179–184.

4

DEVELOPMENTAL
ISSUES

SUSAN L. WARREN & L. ALAN SROUFE

WHAT IS THE VALUE OF A
DEVELOPMENTAL PERSPECTIVE?

A developmental perspective not only involves an understanding of the evolution of maladaptive behaviors and their course, but also includes an understanding of the ties between maladaptive behavior and adaptive developmental processes. It is often difficult to determine where typical development ends and illness begins, but the perspective of examining the linkages between the two allows us to identify the factors that cause some individuals to develop problems whereas others do not. A developmental perspective also takes into account developmental issues at different ages. In addition, such an approach provides attention to nonpathological childhood patterns as they may forecast later disorder and patterns that generally are predictive of disorder but that, for reasons yet to be discovered, do not do so with a particular subgroup of individuals (Sroufe & Rutter, 1984).

Rutter (1980) has provided additional insight into the importance of a developmental perspective:

> It is not just that some disorders involve a distortion of personality development, or that some have their roots in physical or experiential traumata in childhood or that some involve a genetically determined interference with the normal developmental process, or that some last for so many years that considerations of developmental causes and consequences are unavoidable. Rather it is that the process of development constitutes the crucial link between genetic determi-

nants and environmental variables, between sociology and individual psychology, and between physiogenic and psychogenic causes. Development thus encompasses not only the roots of behavior in prior maturation, in physical influences (both internal and external) and in the residues of earlier experiences, but also the modulation of that behavior by the circumstances of the present. (p. 1)

A developmental approach may thus help us to combine or integrate various perspectives, including biological and environmental ones as well as individual and societal or relational ones.

Three features of a developmental perspective are noteworthy. The first entails viewing psychopathology as developmental deviation, that is, psychopathology is viewed against the backdrop of typical development, as adaptive developmental processes gone awry. In looking at fear and anxiety, for example, in a developmental approach, one would consider both the usual functions of these emotions and the typical course of development of children's fears and anxieties. One then examines how such typical processes become distorted.

Second, from a developmental perspective, cause is viewed as probabilistic, not deterministic. A particular set of risk factors, in interaction with supportive or protective factors, is viewed as initiating a pathway, the outcome of which is probabilistically related to a family of outcomes, only some of which are pathological. Moreover, understanding cause must also include considering factors that maintain or deflect the individual from any one pathway.

Finally, development is viewed as cumulative, that is, hierarchical in nature. Current challenges and opportunities are always processed in terms of previously established patterns of adaptation, a stress for one person being benign for another. In this view, behavior is not simply determined by genes or environment, or even genes and current environment together, but at every point by genes, environment, and past developmental history. Because of this cumulative, hierarchical feature, early adaptation is afforded special attention in examining the development of psychopathology.

A developmental perspective provides powerful implications for clinicians. By thoroughly understanding the factors that pull individuals toward or away from increased risk at various age periods, we can gain valuable information for primary prevention. Knowledge about development, moreover, can provide insights about treatment interventions. This chapter aims to explicate a developmental approach to anxiety disorders and provide potential insights that may benefit clinicians.

WHAT ARE THE SEQUENCE AND TIMING FOR THE ONSET OF FEARS AND ANXIETY DURING TYPICAL DEVELOPMENT?

Several researchers have studied, in predominantly cross-sectional study designs, which fears children tend to experience at which ages. Young infants fear heights; loss of support; and sudden, loud, and unpredictable stimuli (Ball & Tronick, 1971; Bronson, 1972; Campbell, 1986; Jersild & Holmes, 1935). Toward the end of the first year, infants may fear strange people and novel objects (Bronson, 1972; Scarr & Salapatek, 1970). They also begin to evidence distress at separation from their mother or primary caretakers (Bowlby, 1969). These separation fears tend to peak between the ages of 9 to 18 months and decrease after about 2½ years of age for most children (Marks, 1987; Thyer, 1993).

In the early preschool years, children fear animals, the dark, doctors, storms, and imaginary creatures (Bauer, 1976; Jersild & Holmes, 1935; Lapouse & Monk, 1959; Lentz, 1985; Maurer, 1965). Most of these fears tend to disappear during the school years (Angelino, Dollins, & Mech, 1956; Bauer, 1976; Jersild & Holmes, 1935; Lapouse & Monk, 1959; Maurer, 1965). In support of this, Strayer (1986) found that 4- to 5-year-olds were more likely to say that fear was caused by fantasy events (e.g., "if a monster came in") than 8-year-olds.

From an evolutionary, developmental perspective, all of these early manifestations of anxiety are part of normal human adaptation (Bowlby, 1973). The young human in the environment in which we evolved was extremely vulnerable to predation. This was especially so in conditions of unfamiliarity, when sensory information was curtailed (as in darkness), and, especially when separated from the protective adult caregiver and alone. Thus, fear or anxiety is functional in such circumstances, prompting closeness with the attachment figure. It is only problematic when such experiences of anxiety are pervasive, persist beyond the typical age, and are independent of genuine threat.

Fears of bodily injury, physical danger, loss, natural hazards, and anxiety about school performance and social relations increase with age in the middle school years and into adolescence (Angelino et al., 1956; Bauer, 1976; Croake, 1969; Maurer, 1965). Older adolescents and adults show anxiety in relation to achievement (test anxiety, fear of failure), social acceptance (social anxiety), physical danger, dread of being alone, and death (Bernstein & Allen, 1969; Lewis & Volkmar, 1990).

Abe and Masui (1981) obtained information on 2,500 individuals between the ages of 11 and 23. They found that fear of going outdoors alone and fear of impending death tended to become much less common in the older age groups. However, fears of blushing, being looked at, tremulousness of hands, disease, fainting spells or faintness, and constriction or a lump in the throat seemed to peak between the ages of 13 and 20.

Miller, Barrett, Hampe, and Noble (1972) obtained parents' ratings of specific fears in 179 children aged 6 to 16 years old. A factor analysis revealed that the children's fears fell into three main categories: physical injury (including fear of loss or abandonment), natural and supernatural events (including storms, dark, animals, ghosts) and psychic stress (including separation, school, and social relations). Miller et al. noted that comparison with factor studies of adult fears suggested that fear of physical injury and psychic stress continued through much of the life span, whereas fear of natural events decreased with age. Unfortunately, Miller and colleagues did not report analyses of specific types of fears with smaller age groupings (e.g., early school age versus later school age and adolescence).

Ollendick (1979) has suggested that if the categories of animal fears and inanimate objects were combined into Miller's natural and supernatural factor, perhaps younger children could be described as showing two of the same fears as older children, with physical injury emerging somewhat later.

In another study, Ollendick, King, and Frary (1989) found that children aged 7 to 10 endorsed significantly more specific fears than 11- to 13-year-olds or 14- to 16-year-olds. The eight most common fears endorsed by all ages were being hit by a car or truck, not being able to breathe, a bombing attack or being invaded, getting burned by fire, falling from a high place, a burglar breaking into the house, earthquake, and death. Younger children (aged 7 to 10) endorsed getting lost in a strange place and being sent to the principal more frequently than older children (11 to 16 years old). The oldest children (14 to 16 years old) were more afraid of failing a test. These common fears were similar to those reported by Scherer and Nakamura (1968), using the Fear Survey Schedule for Children, and were consistent throughout the different cultural groups studied (Ollendick et al., 1989). This suggests that, despite some differences in fears at different ages, there may be some core fears that are present at many ages but vary in degree.

It is interesting to speculate on why children experience different fears at different ages. One theory is that cognitive and environmental changes are the cause. Infants and young children tend to be fearful of events that occur in their immediate presence. Their level of sensorimotor and cognitive maturation restricts the range of fears they can experience (Ferrari, 1986). In the early preschool years, as they can move around more and become aware of a larger world, children begin to worry about things that are not in their immediate environment or that they have not directly experienced (Campbell, 1986; Jersild & Holmes, 1935). In the early school years, fears of monsters and imaginary creatures may decline and fears of true physical dangers may increase because of increased cognitive development (Bauer, 1976). This may be the result of increased differentiation (from a global state to more differentiated representations of objective reality) or of an increased understanding of genuine physical cause-and-effect reasoning (Bauer, 1976). Moreover, as children in the early school years begin to anticipate the future and become more aware of themselves as individuals, their fears may become more internalized and directed towards future situations such as school or physical well-being (Kennedy, 1965; Simon & Ward, 1974). As children develop greater experience and increased control over their environment, their fears become more realistic (Bauer, 1976; Campbell, 1986; Maurer, 1965). In adolescence, as they struggle with philosophical and sexual issues, they tend to have more moral, religious, and sexual fears (Miller, 1983).

Breger (1974) has provided an integrative perspective on the development of normal anxiety. He argues that all anxiety represents a threat to the integrity of the self, beginning in infancy with threats to the caregiving relationship, which could result in literal demise of the corporal self. With development, the source of anxiety becomes more distal, internalized, and abstract. Thus, the toddler may experience anxiety in the face of scolding (which raises the specter of separation), and the preschooler by a transgression even when there is no caregiver present (again because this could alienate the caregiver and perhaps result in a breach in the relationship). Later sources of anxiety (e.g., concerning achievement or a moral transgression), although transformed and not obvious, relate back to the original core in separation. Now, however, it is loss of the sense of integrity of the psyche that is at center stage. Although failing to achieve may displease a parent, a truly moral transgression assaults one's self-concept.

HOW DO THE SEQUENCE AND TIMING FOR THE ONSET OF ANXIETY DISORDERS IN CHILDREN AND ADOLESCENTS RELATE TO THE SEQUENCE AND TIMING OF FEARS AND ANXIETY DURING NORMAL DEVELOPMENT?

It is quite interesting to see that there is a clear correspondence between the typical age for the development of a normal fear or anxiety and the typical age for the development of a related anxiety disorder, in keeping with the notion of disorder as development gone awry. For example, phobias seem to vary in onset, depending on the type of fear. Marks and Gelder (1966), in a retrospective study, reported that specific animal phobias start before 5 years of age, whereas social phobias have an onset with puberty. This seems to fit with a developmental perspective, because younger children show more fears of animals, and older children show more anxieties in relation to social situations. Agoraphobia and other specific situational phobias, such as fear of heights, darkness, and storms, were reported by Marks and Gelder as having a variable age of onset.

The age of onset of the other anxiety disorders is also interesting. Last, Perrin, Hersen, and Kazdin (1992) found, in a clinical sample, the following ages of onset: 7.5 years (separation anxiety disorder, or SAD), 8.2 years (avoidant disorder), 8.4 years (simple phobia), 8.8 years (overanxious disorder, or OAD), 11.3 years (social phobia), and 14.1 years (panic disorder, or PD). Similarly, in a community sample, Keller et al. (1992) found a median age of onset of 8 years for SAD and 10 years for OAD. Werry (1991), when reviewing the literature on OAD, reported that, overall, the studies suggest that OAD could begin at any age in childhood. In any case, SAD seems to begin more commonly at a younger age and social phobia tends to occur later. This probably relates to normal developmental changes.

Kashani and Orvaschel (1990) studied children aged 8, 12, and 17 years, from a community sample. As would be expected from a developmental perspective, they found higher rates of SAD in the 8-year-olds and similar rates of phobic disorders in all three groups. Social fears were also more prevalent among the older ages, and physiological symptoms were significantly less common in the 12- and 17-year-olds. OAD was most common in the 17-year-olds.

Developmental differences have also been reported for the expression of SAD in children. Francis, Last, and Strauss (1987) studied children diagnosed with SAD and found that children 5 to 8 years old were most likely to report worry concerning harm befalling an attachment figure, worry that a calamitous event would separate the child from the attachment figure, and reluctance and/or refusal to go to school. Children 9 to 12 years old more commonly reported excessive distress with separation and withdrawal, apathy, sadness, and/or poor concentration when separated. Adolescents aged 13 to 16 most frequently reported physical complaints during school days and reluctance and/or refusal to go to school. Nightmares focusing on separation were found to be significantly more likely in children aged 5 to 8 than in children aged 9 to 12. Moreover, children aged 5 to 12 were significantly more likely to report excessive distress with separation than were adolescents. In addition, children aged 5 to 8 years old were significantly more likely to present with 4 or more total SAD symptoms than were children aged 9 to 12. Thirty-one percent of the children aged 9 to 12 years old received the diagnosis based on the minimum number of criteria (three symptoms; Francis et al., 1987). These results seem to parallel findings in the literature (concerning nonclinical children) in which younger children seem to have more concerns about separation from attachment figures than adolescents, and older children show more school-related concerns.

Similarly, children with OAD report different levels of anxiety at different ages. Strauss, Lease, Last, and Francis (1988) found that 66% of children aged 12 to 19 reported more than five symptoms, compared with 35% of children aged 5 to 11 years ($p < .05$). Twenty-eight percent of the older children met all seven criteria for OAD, compared with only 4% of the younger children ($p < .06$). Furthermore, the criterion of worry about past behavior was more common in the older group (Strauss et al., 1988).

Differences have also been found between the types of fears reported by children with SAD versus those reported by children with OAD. This may relate to the differences in age of onset of the two disorders. Last, Francis, and Strauss (1989) administered the Fear Survey Schedule for Children–Revised (FSSC-R; Ollendick, 1983) to children with SAD and OAD. Although both groups reported the same number of fears, children with SAD most commonly reported a fear of getting lost. They also reported fears of germs/illness and bee stings. Overanxious children most often reported fears of being criticized, being teased, and making mistakes. The authors noted that none of these fears were as common in nonpsychiatrically referred youngsters (Last et al., 1989).

Using a psychosocial developmental theory, Westenberg, Berend, and Treffers (2001) have described why the age of onset for SAD could differ from that of OAD on the basis of ego developmental transitions. Summarizing the ego models of Loevinger (1976), moralization of judgment model of Kohlberg (1969), and social cognition model of Selman (1980), among others, Westenberg and colleagues have described several developmental levels of importance for anxiety disorders. The lowest relevant level is the impulsive level in which individuals are vulnerable, dependent, and live in the moment of their immediate wishes and emotions. Others are expected to set and enforce the rules and take care of the impulsive-level individuals. Individuals at the conformist level, in contrast, are more interested in meeting social expectations or standards for achievement. The focus is less on potential loss of others who provide basic supports and more on judging oneself through the eyes of others. Westenberg and colleagues have found that SAD is related to the impulsive level and OAD is related to the conformist levels, regardless of age. Thus, differing onsets of these disorders may depend on ego developmental processes, more so than on age per se.

The onset of PD in childhood is a somewhat controversial issue (see chapter 11, this volume). Several researchers have stated that PD cannot occur in preadolescents because younger children tend to attribute external causes to physical symptoms and are not capable of cognitive symptoms of panic such as fear of dying and fear of going crazy (Nelles & Barlow, 1988). However, Moreau and Weissman (1992) have described several studies that report the onset of panic attacks in pubertal and prepubertal children. Though some children seem to experience the onset of their attacks at an early age, the review indicates that in general, the mean age of onset of PD in childhood is about 13 to 14 years. Ollendick, Mattis, and King (1994) similarly have reported that panic attacks are common in adolescents and that both panic attacks and PD appear to be present, but less frequent, in children. Moreover, Mattis and Ollendick (1997) have found children to be capable of reporting cognitive symptoms, albeit less catastrophic ones. Ollendick and colleagues (1994) have suggested that modification of the criteria for younger children may be useful. In addition, two studies have shown that agoraphobia tends to have an earlier age of onset than PD (Biederman et al., 1997; Wittchen, Reed, & Kessler, 1998).

Table 4.1 provides a simplified summary of some of the salient developmental issues hypothesized to relate to specified anxiety disorders. It is interesting to see how the anxiety disorders generally seem to develop in conjunction with corresponding normative developmental challenges. It is therefore possible that:

1. Anxiety disorders develop as a result of difficulties mastering challenges associated with a particular developmental phase.
2. Anxiety disorders compromise development in subsequent phases.
3. Anxiety disorders may be manifestations of an underlying diathesis in which the disorders are transformed from one to another as development progresses. The disorders appear to be

Table 4.1. Simplified Summary of Salient Developmental Issues Hypothesized to Relate to Anxiety Disorders

Age	Developmental Issues[1]	Hypothesized Common Fears and Concerns	Associations With Anxiety Disorders
0–6 months	• Biological regulation	• Startlelike response to loud noises or loss of support	• High reactivity • Low regulation
6–18 months	• Object permanence • Formation of attachment relationship	• Fear of strange people and situations • Separation anxiety	• Behavioral inhibition • Fearful shyness • Anxious/resistant attachment
2–3 years	• Exploration of material object world • Individuation and autonomy	• Fear of animals	• Animal phobia
3–6 years	• Self-reliance • Initiative • Development of symbolic thought and representation	• Fears of dark, imaginary creatures, storms, and loss of caregivers	• Separation anxiety disorder • Self-conscious shyness
6–10 years	• Sense of industry or competence • School adjustment	• Concerns about bodily injury, physical danger, and school	• Overanxious disorder • Generalized anxiety disorder
10–12 years	• Social understanding • Same-sex friends	• Concerns about friendships	• Social phobia
13+ years	• Flexible perspective taking • Beginning heterosexual relationships • Emancipation • Identity	• Concerns about heterosexual relationships, independence, and life plans	• Agoraphobia • Panic disorder

[1]See Sroufe and Rutter (1984).

associated with certain developmental levels because the specific developmental levels provide opportunities for manifesting specific behaviors that can be diagnosed as particular anxiety disorders.

CAN WE DEFINE ANY DEVELOPMENTAL PATHWAYS FOR ANXIETY DISORDERS?

At this time, there are no well-defined pathways for anxiety disorders, tracing continuity and change over time. However, several areas of research are beginning to provide information that may inform creation of a developmental account. Some risk factors in the early years that are pertinent to later anxiety have been defined, and these represent a starting point for exploration.

Temperament

Several issues are important to consider before embarking on a discussion of temperament. One issue, which has been controversial in the literature, is the definition of temperament (Goldsmith et al., 1987). Garrison and Earls (1987) have noted the lack of agreement about the specific nature of this construct. Some researchers, such as Buss and Plomin (1975), have described temperament as a consistent inherited characteristic of the individual, whereas others, such as Thomas and Chess (1977), have focused on an interactional style.

From a developmental perspective, temperament can be viewed as a descriptive construct referring to the *how* of behaviors, that is, differences in behavioral style. Such features, like all behaviors, are assumed to develop through a transactional process in which child and environment are inseparable and mutually influencing one another. Even in infancy, and certainly in childhood, it is overly simplistic to describe such characteristics as merely inherent in the child. Temperamental characteristics are subject to change and may be influenced by experience (Belsky, Fish, & Isabella, 1991).

Nonetheless, it is of interest to see how such descriptions of children are associated with anxiety problems. Behavioral inhibition (BI) is the temperamental construct that has been most extensively studied in relation to anxiety disorders. BI is a temperament feature that has been defined by Kagan (1994) as an enduring tendency to exhibit quiet withdrawal in novel situations. When a child so designated is presented with an unfamiliar person, object or situation, the child is quiet, retreats to mother or withdraws from unfamiliar stimuli. Kagan (1994) has measured BI by examining the latency of the child to talk to and interact with an unfamiliar examiner, physical retreat from an unfamiliar person, the tendency to retreat from novel objects, cessation of vocalization in new situations, and long periods of proximity to mother, especially when not playing. What follows is a description of the research relating BI to anxiety disorders.

In initial studies, after screening several hundred children, Kagan and colleagues (Kagan & Reznick, 1986; Kagan, Reznick, & Snidman, 1987, 1988) identified several cohorts of children who were consistently inhibited or uninhibited in their behavior when exposed to novel situations. Approximately 10 to 15% of the children screened were determined to be behaviorally inhibited. When placed in novel situations, inhibited children had higher heart rates and less heart-rate variability than noninhibited children. Heart-rate patterns were stable in at least two cohorts for up to 5 years (Kagan et al., 1987, 1988). Kagan and colleagues (1987) also found inhibited children's salivary cortisol levels measured at home and in the lab to be higher than those of noninhibited children. Moreover, the inhibited children with elevated salivary cortisol levels frequently had fears and somatic and behavioral symptoms often associated with anxiety states such as gastrointestinal distress, chronic constipation, nightmares, and sleeplessness, though comprehensive clinical interviews were not conducted (Kagan et al., 1987). Unusual fears at ages 5.5 and 7.5 (violence on television and in movies, being kidnapped, and going into the bedroom alone) were also most frequent in the inhibited children with high heart rates and least frequent in the uninhibited children with low heart rates (Kagan et al., 1988). Although this research did not establish specific linkages been BI and anxiety disorders, it did pique interest in this area.

A number of studies have demonstrated associations between parental anxiety and depressive disorders and increased BI in their young children (Kochanska, 1991; Rosenbaum et al., 1988; Rosenbaum et al., 2000; Rubin, Both, Zahn-Waxler, Cummings, & Wilkinson, 1991). Although this relation may be due a variety of factors (both genetic and neurological), it nonetheless attests to the presumed validity of the BI construct. It remains to be shown whether these predictions are specific to internalizing disorders or whether they pertain to various forms of adult psychopathology.

In terms of specific associations between BI and childhood and adolescent anxiety disorders, Biederman and colleagues (1990) examined children with BI for anxiety disorders and found that inhibited children of parents with psychiatric disorders (the same parents from the Rosenbaum et al. [1988] study, who had panic disorder with agoraphobia [PDAG]) had higher rates of multiple anxiety disorders and OAD than normal controls. Biederman and colleagues (1990) also examined children in one of Kagan and colleagues' longitudinal cohorts, who were identified as behaviorally inhibited. (This cohort had not been identified by parental psychopathology.) They found that these children had higher rates of phobic disorders than uninhibited children.

Rosenbaum and colleagues (1991) examined the parents of that same longitudinal cohort (of Kagan and colleagues) and found that the parents of children identified as inhibited at 21 months had an increased incidence of social phobia, childhood avoidant disorder and OAD, and continuing anxiety disorders (as indicated by both childhood and adulthood anxiety disorder diagnoses), compared with parents of uninhibited children or control parents. It is interesting that social phobia was the only adult anxiety disorder identified in the parents of the inhibited children.

In a later analysis, Rosenbaum et al. (1992) examined the parents (from both cohorts) of children with inhibition and anxiety disorders, inhibition alone, and neither inhibition nor anxiety disorders. They found a significant difference between the first two groups in parental anxiety disorders and continuing anxiety disorders. This study suggests that children with inhibition who have parents with anxiety disorders (particularly continuing anxiety disorders) may be at greater risk for developing anxiety disorders than children with either factor alone.

Hirshfeld et al. (1992) conducted an additional analysis concerning the children in Kagan and colleagues' longitudinal sample who were consistently inhibited at 21 months, 4 years, 5½ years, and 7½ years. Seventy percent ($n = 41$) of the original sample remained in the study at that time. Of these, 12 were *stable inhibited* (BI at all four ages), 10 were *unstable inhibited* (originally classified as inhibited but later classified as uninhibited during at least one later assessment), 9 were *stable uninhibited* (uninhibited at all of the assessments), and 10 were *unstable uninhibited* (initially classified as uninhibited but later classified as inhibited during at least one later assessment). The stable inhibited children who still had BI at age 7 were found to have significantly greater single and multiple anxiety disorders and phobic disorders than the other three groups of children (Hirshfeld et al., 1992). Although this may suggest that stable inhibition confers a greater risk for anxiety disorders, it is also possible that BI at age 7 accounts for this relation and that BI at this age is simply a manifestation of anxiety itself.

The most compelling work examining associations between BI and anxiety disorders has been based on longitudinal studies. In a 3-year follow-up study of the same cohorts of children with and without BI, Biederman and colleagues (1993) found that BI in the children (Kagan's cohort and cohort of children of parents with PDAG combined) was associated with significantly higher rates of multiple anxiety disorders, avoidant disorder, SAD, and agoraphobia. In addition, the increase in anxiety disorder rates from baseline was significantly greater for BI than for non-BI children. Moreover, children who were inhibited over multiple assessment points (stable inhibition) demonstrated higher rates of anxiety disorders.

Although concerns may be raised with the preceding studies, Schwartz, Snidman, and Kagan (1999) reported the results of a 12-year follow-up of samples studied by Kagan (1994). Seventy-nine 13-year-olds who had been classified as inhibited or uninhibited at 2 years of age were assessed with direct observation in a laboratory procedure and a diagnostic interview. Although there were no significant differences between the adolescents who had been inhibited or uninhibited in terms of performance anxiety, separation anxiety, and specific fears, there was a significant difference in terms of generalized social anxiety. Adolescents who had been behaviorally inhibited at 2 years of age were significantly more likely at 13 years of age to have generalized social anxiety, compared with adolescents who had been uninhibited at 2 years of age. Behavioral data obtained during a laboratory procedure also supported these results, with significantly decreased spontaneous comments in the adolescents with generalized social anxiety who had been behaviorally inhibited at 2 years of age. This research is particularly instructive and extremely compelling, because it follows a nonclinical sample longitudinally over many years.

Prior, Smart, Sanson, and Oberklaid (2000) also examined the relations between shy-inhibited temperament in childhood and anxiety problems in adolescents, using a longitudinal data set from a community sample in Australia. Children were identified as shy if they were at least one standard deviation above the mean for parental ratings of low approach behavior. Children who were at least one standard deviation above the mean on combined parental and child questionnaire ratings of anxiety were classified as having anxiety problems. Although the relation between shyness in infancy and later anxiety was modest (odds ratio [OR] = 1.42; confidence interval [CI] = 1.05 to 1.92), the relation became stronger across development (OR = 3.44; CI = 2.40 to 4.93 at 12 to 13 years of age). Persistent shyness predicted anxiety most strongly (χ^2 = 69.55, p < .00001). Almost half of the children classified as anxious, however, had never been rated shy. Unfortunately, the researchers did not report specific findings for social anxiety. This research is interesting because it focuses on a different community sample than that identified by Kagan (1994) and supports associations over time between low approach behaviors and anxiety disorders. However, parental report was used for both the temperament measure and as part of the anxiety measure, which represents an important limitation of this research.

In another longitudinal study, Hayward, Killen, Kraemer, and Taylor (1998) prospectively evaluated the risk of childhood BI for later onset of social phobia in a large nonclinical sample of adolescents over 4 years. Social avoidance and fearfulness, as measured with the Retrospective Self-Report of Inhibition questionnaire, served as a marker for the onset of social phobia in the adolescents, as measured with diagnostic interviews. This research again supported associations between BI and social phobia.

In summary, there appears to be an association between temperament and internalizing disorders including anxiety and depression. Children of parents with PD, major depressive disorder, or both are at risk for BI, and children with BI are more frequently diagnosed later with anxiety disorders. These associations are very modest in the first 2 years and become stronger for older children. One question that demands attention at this time is whether early BI is really most specifically associated with later generalized social phobia. Retrospective data (Mick & Telch, 1998), along with many of the studies described above, support this conclusion. Children who show persistent BI may be presenting early indications that will be diagnosed later as generalized social phobia.

From a developmental perspective, these findings regarding temperament are interpreted in probabilistic terms of initiating conditions or markers of a pathway. Whatever the origins of temperamental variations in BI, children who are showing extreme inhibition may be thought of as manifesting signs that an anxiety pathway has been enjoined. Remaining on the pathway for a number of years, as indicated by continuity of BI to later childhood, is more strongly associated with anxiety disorders, as would be predicted by a pathways model.

The Attachment Relationship

Grounding his ideas in evolutionary theory, including the vital functions of emotions, Bowlby (1969) proposed that management of typically occurring fear and anxiety was the key to evaluating attachment relationships. In well-functioning relationships, infants use caregivers as havens, retreating to them in the face of threat and using them as a base of security for venturing forth. Attachment behaviors become organized around a specific caregiver during the second half of the first year of life. After that time, an infant will become threatened if there is danger in the immediate environment or if the attachment figure is not readily available. In a threatening situation, the infant will seek help from the attachment figure. Behaviors include crying, clinging, signaling, and (with locomotion) proximity seeking. The goal in infancy is to balance exploration with proximity to the caregiver.

The development of adaptive and maladaptive anxiety is a central construct in attachment theory. Bowlby (1973) noted that, once infants become attached to the caregiver, there is a period during which they are made anxious by brief separations. This typical, adaptive response protects the infant from harm by ensuring that the infant stays close to a protective adult.

In contrast, maladaptive anxiety may develop in the context of repeated experiences of anxiety that do not appear to be resolvable from the perspective of the child. As discussed earlier, separation anxiety is one of the earliest forms of anxiety experienced by children. If the caregiver routinely comes to the child's aid when the child is in need, the child develops confidence that the caregiver will help and protect the child. Such a child is less likely to feel chronically anxious and is said to have a *secure* attachment relationship. In contrast, a child who has not experienced sensitive and responsive care, and thus does not believe that the caretaker will come to his or her aid, is said to have an *insecure* attachment relationship. An insecurely attached child may be anxious frequently, even in benign circumstances. Chronic vigilance and anxiety may set the stage for the development of an anxiety disorder.

Ainsworth, Blehar, Waters, and Wall (1978) described two types of insecure attachment relationships and the corresponding mother-infant interactions that preceded them. Infants with mothers who responded consistently to their needs were found to have *secure* attachment relationships (B classification; 66%). Such infants were easily comforted and explored confidently in their mother's presence in an unfamiliar situation. Infants whose mothers frequently rejected them when the infant sought contact were found to have *anxious/avoidant* attachment relationships (A classification; 22%). These infants tended to avoid their caregiver on reunion after a brief separation, perhaps as a way of avoiding the feelings they experienced in relation to their mother's unavailability (Sroufe, 1996). Infants who had experienced inconsistent or intrusive caregiving were found to have an *anxious/resistant* attachment (C classification; 12%). These infants showed angry, resistant, and ambivalent behavior on reunion and appeared to experience and display both anxiety and anger at the mother. Both A and C infants were said to be anxiously attached, though one type showed explicit anxiety (Type C) and the other did not (Type A).

Note that these attachment classifications are characterizations of a relationship, not of a child (Sroufe, 1985). The child may have different relationships with different parents—for example, being secure with one and anxious with the other. Moreover, these classifications are not defined by temperament, and they have been shown to change with alterations in parental life stress and social support (Vaughn & Sroufe, 1979).

Main and Solomon (1986) have described a third type of insecure relationship that is called *disorganized* attachment (D classification). Infants in these types of relationships are not able to maintain an organized strategy for obtaining parental comfort, and they can sometimes show mixed strategies (both A and C). Infants in disorganized attachment relationships can also show fear of the mother, freezing, and other unusual behaviors (hitting mother or self) that suggest that the child does not feel that he or she can rely upon the mother for help.

Over time, the child constructs models of relationships, which are called *internal working models* (Main, Kaplan, & Cassidy, 1985). These are mental representations of the child's view of self, intimate others, and world experiences. Representations that have consolidated can guide appraisals of experience and interpersonal behavior and may be slow to change if they are unconscious. Internal working models have been examined in children by using narratives (Cassidy, 1988) and drawings (Fury, Carlson, & Sroufe, 1997), and in adults by using the Adult Attachment Interview (Main & Goldwyn, 1991).

Several studies have examined associations between representations of the attachment relationship and anxiety disorders. With adults, Cassidy (1995) found that adolescents and adults with generalized anxiety disorder reported more caregiver unresponsiveness, role-reversal/enmeshment, and feelings of anger/vulnerability toward their mothers than did controls; although, as with all retrospective data, caution must be used in interpreting these results. In a prospective study with children, Warren, Emde, and Sroufe (2000) found that 5-year-olds who ended stories negatively and did not anticipate help from their caregivers in their play narratives showed higher levels of anxiety at 6 years of age.

In two very interesting studies, Manassis, Bradley, Goldberg, Hood, and Swinson (1994, 1995) examined 18 mothers with anxiety disorders (14 with PD, 3 with generalized anxiety disorder, and 1 with obsessive-compulsive disorder) and their 20 children (18 to 59 months of age). No mothers were found to be secure with respect to their own attachment (as measured with the Adult Attachment Interview; Main & Goldwyn, 1991). In terms of the children, five were found to be anxious/avoidant (25%), nine were secure (45%), and six were anxious/resistant (30%). This represents significantly more anxious/resistant attachment relationships than in typical samples. Thirteen of the children (65%) were also classified as disorganized. In addition, 13 (65%) of the children showed BI. No relation between BI and security of attachment was found, however, with roughly equal proportions of inhibited and noninhibited children classified as insecure. Table 4.2 describes the characteristics of the three children who were found to have clinical diagnoses. All three children demonstrated insecure

Table 4.2. Data From Manassis, Bradley, Goldberg, Hood, and Swinson (1994, 1995) Examination of Children of Mothers With Anxiety Disorders

Diagnoses of Children	Attachment Relationship	Temperament Classification
Separation anxiety disorder (2 children)	Avoidant and resistant/disorganized attachment	Not behaviorally inhibited
Avoidant disorder (1 child)	Avoidant/disorganized attachment	Behaviorally inhibited

attachment relationships. One child who was diagnosed with avoidant disorder was found to be behaviorally inhibited as well. This is an extremely small sample, so it is difficult to draw firm conclusions. Nonetheless, the findings suggest that insecure attachment is a precursor of childhood anxiety disorders and that BI may operate independently and may be a more specific risk factor for avoidant disorder or social phobia.

Using data from a longitudinal study conducted by L. Alan Sroufe and Byron Egeland, Warren and colleagues (Warren, Huston, Egeland, & Sroufe, 1997) examined the relation between the attachment relationship measured in infancy and anxiety disorders measured 16 years later in the same children. Mothers were from a high-risk sample (mostly consisting of women who had unplanned pregnancies, were unmarried, and were of low socioeconomic status) and were recruited during pregnancy. The Strange Situation procedure (Ainsworth et al., 1978), a laboratory-based procedure involving two brief parent-child separations, was administered when the infants were 12 months of age. Diagnostic interviews using the Schedule for Affective Disorders and Schizophrenia for School-Age Children (K-SADS) were conducted with the adolescents at 17 years of age. Twenty-six adolescents were diagnosed with past or current anxiety disorders. More adolescents with anxiety disorders were, as infants, classified as having an anxious/resistant attachment relationship. Thirteen percent of the children who were not classified as having an anxious/resistant attachment relationship developed anxiety disorders, whereas 28% of the children who were classified as having an anxious/resistant attachment relationship developed anxiety disorders. This represented a twofold increase in risk. In addition, the infant-parent attachment relationship significantly predicted adolescent anxiety disorders, even after controlling for maternal anxiety and infant temperament.

The relation between infant anxious/resistant attachment and later anxiety disorders can be explained developmentally. Children who feel insecure and tend to express their feelings of insecurity may evolve a pattern of adaptation in infancy that initially serves them and is adaptive. Extreme vigilance and expressions of distress may initially help these children to obtain attention and comfort from their caretakers. Over time, however, these behaviors may become maladaptive and put the children at risk. Children may later demonstrate anxiety disorders because they have continued to be vigilant, have continued to experience and express their distress, and do not feel that they can obtain comfort from others or themselves.

This research indicates that an anxious attachment relationship may initiate a pathway to the development of anxiety disorders. Manassis (2001) has proposed several potential developmental pathways toward the development of anxiety disorders. She states that infants who show anxious/avoidant attachment may not only avoid their parents but may also come to avoid other social situations. Over time, temperamentally vulnerable infants who show anxious/avoidant attachment could develop social phobia as they repeatedly avoid social encounters. In contrast, temperamentally vulnerable infants with an anxious/resistant attachment relationship could develop SAD because they are ambivalent about remaining close to their caregivers. Manassis (2001) hypothesizes that all types of insecure attachment relationships may predispose toward the development of anxiety disorders of various forms.

HOW CAN THESE RESEARCH FINDINGS BE INTEGRATED IN A DEVELOPMENTAL MODEL?

The integrative nature of a developmental perspective is its greatest potential strength. Thus, the temperament and attachment literatures may be brought together into a more encompassing and coherent model. They are united in the concept of initiating pathways to psychopathology. When this is done, more powerful predictive results are obtained than when they are considered separately (Warren et al., 1997).

Sameroff (1993) has described four different models of development based on the work of Riegel (1978). These models focus on combinations of passive and active contributions of the individual and the environment to developmental outcomes.

1. *Passive person–passive environment.* In this category, both the individual and environment are passive. Sameroff (1993) describes this model as being the basis for learning theories in which factors such as the contiguity, frequency, or recency of stimuli determine how they will be coded in the receiving mind.
2. *Passive person–active environment.* This category includes Skinnerian approaches and behavior modification therapy in which the environment is actively changed to influence the person's behavior and the person is assumed to make no independent contributions to the outcome.
3. *Active person–passive environment.* This category includes the work of Piaget and Chomsky. The environment plays a

necessary role in development but does not have an active role in structuring the outcome; rather, the individual is active in organizing experience in response to the environment.

4. *Active person–active environment.* In the final category, both the individual and the environment actively contribute to the developmental outcome. For example, in the transactional model described by Sameroff (1993), the development of the child is seen as a product of a continuous dynamic interaction between the child and the experience provided by family interactions and the social context.

The active person–active environment category appears most conducive to the integration of the research concerning the development of anxiety disorders, and is most compatible with a developmental psychopathology perspective. In this model, a dynamic interplay between the child and environmental/relationship contributions is hypothesized. For example, an infant may develop a high sensitivity to novel stimuli for a variety of reasons. Then, as described by Kagan (1994), the child may show "high reactivity" or high cry and high motor activity in response to novel stimuli. Because of the high motor activity and other factors, parents may be reluctant to hold the child to calm the child and may instead try to distract the child. Regardless of whether these parental behaviors contributed to child characteristics in the first place, they nonetheless contribute now in an ongoing transactional loop. As a result, the child may continue to have difficulty in self-calming. The child may learn to withdraw and avoid novel stimuli and new situations, thus showing inhibited behavior. Such a child has not learned how to depend on the caregiver for comfort, and thus will not have a secure attachment relationship. Over time, as these processes continue, childhood anxiety disorders may develop, because the child has learned to avoid new situations and has developed internal working models of others as not supportive and the self as incompetent to handle new situations.

IS ANY OF THIS USEFUL CLINICALLY?

This section summarizes some take-home messages that may be useful clinically.

- *It's important to take the developmental level into account when evaluating children for anxiety disorders.*

The criteria in the *Diagnostic and Statistical Manual of Mental Disorders: DSM-IV* (American Psychiatric Association, 1994) indicate that developmental level is important when diagnosing anxiety disorders, because certain fears and anxieties are developmentally expected at certain ages. Thus, understanding the typical course of fear/anxiety development can be helpful in making these distinctions. When anxieties and fears develop, they may be transient reactions to internal and external changes. Diagnosing these as an anxiety disorder depends on the context of the behaviors, level of distress, and degree of impairment.

A developmental understanding can also be useful in identifying further areas for exploration that may be needed to treat individual patients. For example, a 12-year-old who exhibits fears of monsters is unusual. Because fear of monsters is usually associated with the impulsive level as described by Westenberg and colleagues (2001), such an adolescent could also be experiencing SAD, which is thought to be associated with the impulsive level. Thus, understanding the developmental progression may help with easier identification of possible additional difficulties. In addition, noticing that certain children or adolescents are unusual in their developmental trajectories can prompt even further exploration, which may be important. For example, the 12-year-old who exhibits fears of monsters could have cognitive delays or could have experienced trauma that has delayed development.

- *Children who are extremely shy on multiple occasions or who are shy and have a parent with an anxiety disorder or depression may have an anxiety disorder.*

Biederman, Rosenbaum, Chaloff, and Kagan (1995) state that clinicians should consider an inhibited young child of a parent with an anxiety disorder as likely to develop an anxiety disorder over time. Again, even in advance of the detailed developmental research needed to understand the transactional processes that underlie the emergence of anxiety problems, we know that this combination of features is probabilistically linked to disorder. Studies also indicate that inhibited children of parents with depression may also be at risk (Rosenbaum et al., 2000). In addition, children with BI that is stable over multiple assessments may be more likely to develop anxiety disorders (Biederman et al., 1995). Thus, clinicians who observe that a child is persistently extremely shy, or who observe a shy child with a parent who has an anxiety disorder or depression, should evaluate the child for an anxiety disorder, even if the presenting problem seems unrelated.

Clinicians who are treating adults with major depression and PD should similarly think about evaluating the children of those adults for anxiety disorders, especially if the children seem to be inhibited. It is important for clinicians to be aware that although shyness may be normative in some contexts and often fades, in some situations shyness may signal the fact that the child is struggling with painful feelings that could benefit from intervention.

- *Children who have anxiety disorders may have difficulties with close personal relationships.*

Research indicates that an insecure attachment relationship is a risk factor for the development of anxiety disorders. Because children and adolescents develop certain kinds of internal working models over time, children with anxiety disorders may struggle to feel comfortable in close personal relationships. Research focused on children with anxiety disorders supports the view that such children can have difficulties in relationships with others (Beidel & Turner, 1999). Thus, it could be quite useful for clinicians who are treating children and adolescents with anxiety disorders to explore the quality of parent-child and peer relationships. Children and adolescents with anxiety disorders may benefit from discussing their relationships and using the therapist as a secure base. Clinicians should also be aware that children and adolescents with anxiety disorders may also have great difficulty feeling comfortable in a therapeutic setting.

- *The best treatment approaches may vary with development.*

Ollendick and Vasey (1999) discuss how the developmental perspective may help to inform the treatment process in terms of the selection of specific interventions. For example, although standard desensitization has been found to be effective with adults and adolescents, studies with children have shown a need for revision in those procedures. Ollendick (1979) has noted that young children may be unable to achieve deep relaxation (perhaps due to a lack of attentiveness or cooperation) and may also have difficulty achieving vivid images in order to adequately imagine the feared stimuli in sufficient detail to allow for deconditioning to occur. As a result, Ollendick suggests that other counterconditioning agents such as play, music, food, emotive imagery, and interpersonal relationships be substituted for muscular relaxation and that the anxiety-arousing scenes be presented in games or in vivo rather than in imagination. Similar developmental adaptations may be necessary when using self-instruction procedures with younger children (Ollendick & Vasey, 1999). For example, Ollendick and Vasey describe how younger children (in Piaget's preoperational stage) may benefit from simple task-oriented self-instructions in terms of improved task performance but are unlikely to generalize across tasks. In contrast, older children (in Piaget's concrete operational stage) may benefit more from generalized self-instruction, both in task performance and generalization across tasks.

In addition, several research studies indicate that younger children may benefit more from behavioral parent training than adolescents (Ollendick & Vasey, 1999). In the treatment of anxiety disorders, Barrett, Dadds, and Rapee (1996) found that combined family-based intervention was more effective for 7- to 10-year-old children than 11- to 14-year-old preadolescents. In contrast, individual treatment was found to be as effective with 11- to 14-year-old preadolescents as the combined treatment. It is therefore quite likely that enhancing parenting skills may be more important for younger children, but for older children and preadolescents, individual child cognitive work and exposure to fear stimuli may be sufficient.

Additional research is needed to explore the effectiveness of differing treatment interventions at different ages. Incorporating a developmental perspective into this research could greatly aid our understanding of the prevention and treatment of child and adolescent anxiety disorders.

NOTE

This research was supported by funds from NIMH Scientist Development Award for Clinicians 1K08MH01532 to Dr. Warren and NIMH MH40864 to Byron Egeland, Ph.D.

REFERENCES

Abe, K., & Masui, T. (1981). Age-sex trends of phobic and anxiety symptoms. *British Journal of Psychiatry, 138,* 297–302.

Ainsworth, M. B. S., Blehar, M., Waters, E., & Wall, S. (1978). *Patterns of attachment.* Hillsdale, NJ: Erlbaum.

American Psychiatric Association. (1994). *Diagnostic and statistical manual of mental disorders: DSM-IV* (4th ed.). Washington, DC: Author.

Angelino, H., Dollins, J. & Mech, E. V. (1956). Trends in the fears and worries of school children as related to socioeconomic status and age. *Journal of Genetic Psychology, 89,* 263–276.

Ball, W., & Tronick, E. (1971). Infant responses to impending collision: Optical and real. *Science, 171,* 818–820.

Barrett, P. M., Dadds, M. R., & Rapee, R. M. (1996). Family treatment of childhood anxiety: A controlled trial. *Journal of Consulting and Clinical Psychology, 64,* 333–342.

Bauer, D. H. (1976). An exploratory study of developmental changes in children's fears. *Journal of Child Psychology and Psychiatry, 17,* 69–74.

Beidel, B. C., & Turner, T. M. (1999). The natural course of shyness and related syndromes. In L.A. Schmidt & J. Schulkin (Eds.). *Extreme fear, shyness, and social phobia* (pp. 203–223). New York: Oxford University Press.

Belsky, J., Fish, M., & Isabella, R. (1991). Continuity and discontinuity in infant negative and positive emotionality: Family antecedents and attachment consequences. *Developmental Psychology, 27,* 421–431.

Bernstein, D. A., & Allen, G. J. (1969). Fear Survey Schedule: II. Normative data and factor analyses based upon a large college sample. *Behaviour Research and Therapy, 7,* 403–407.

Biederman, J., Faraone, S. V., Marrs, A., Moore, P., Garcia, J., Ablon, S., Mick, E., et al. (1997). Panic disorder and agoraphobia in consecutively referred children and adolescents. *Journal of the American Academy of Child and Adolescent Psychiatry, 36*(2), 214–223.

Biederman, J., Rosenbaum, J. F., Bolduc, E. A., Faraone, S. V., Chaloff, B. A., Hirshfeld, D. R. & Kagan, J. (1993). A 3-year follow-up of children with and without behavioral inhibition. *Journal of the American Academy of Child and Adolescent Psychiatry, 32,* 814–822.

Biederman, J., Rosenbaum, J. F., Chaloff, J., & Kagan, J. (1995). Behavior inhibition as a risk factor for anxiety disorders. In J. S. March (Ed.) *Anxiety disorders in children and adolescents* (pp. 61–81). New York: Guilford Press.

Biederman, J., Rosenbaum, J. F., Hirshfeld, D. R., Faraone, S. V., Bolduc, E. A., Gersten, M., Meminger, S. R., et al. (1990). Psychiatric correlates of behavioral inhibition in young children of parents with and without psychiatric disorders. *Archives of General Psychiatry, 47,* 21–26.

Bowlby, J. (1969). *Attachment and loss: Vol. I. Attachment*. New York: Basic Books.

Bowlby, J. (1973). *Attachment and loss: Vol. II. Separation: Anxiety and anger*. New York: Basic Books.

Breger, L. (1974). *From instinct to identity*. Englewood Cliffs, NJ: Prentice-Hall.

Bronson, G. W. (1972). Infants' reactions to unfamiliar persons and novel objects. *Monographs of the Society for Research Child Development, 37*(3, Serial No. 148).

Buss, A. H., & Plomin, R. (1975). *A temperament theory of personality development*. New York: Wiley.

Campbell, S. B. (1986). Developmental issues in childhood anxiety. In R. Gittelman (Ed.), *Anxiety disorders of childhood*. New York: Guilford Press.

Cassidy, J. (1988). Child-mother attachment and the self in six-year-olds. *Child Development, 59*, 121–134.

Cassidy, J. (1995). Attachment and generalized anxiety disorder. In D. Cicchetti & S. L. Toth (Eds.), *Emotion, cognition and representation: Rochester symposium on developmental psychopathology VI* (Vol. 6). Rochester, NY: University of Rochester Press.

Croake, J. W. (1969). Fears of children. *Human Development, 12*, 239–247.

Ferrari, M. (1986). Fears and phobias in childhood: Some clinical and developmental considerations. *Child Psychiatry Human Development, 17*, 75–87.

Francis, G., Last, C. G., & Strauss, C. C. (1987). Expression of separation anxiety disorder: The roles of age and gender. *Child Psychiatry and Human Development, 18*, 82–89.

Fury, G., Carlson, E., & Sroufe, L.A. (1997). Children's representations of attachment relationships in family drawings. *Child Development, 68*, 1154–1164.

Garrison, W. T., & Earls, F. J. (1987). *Temperament and child psychopathology*. Newbury Park, CA: Sage.

Goldsmith, H. H., Buss, A. H., Plomin, R., Rothbart, M. K., Thomas, A., Chess, S., Hinde, R. A., et al. (1987). Roundtable: What is temperament? Four approaches. *Child Development, 58*, 505–529.

Hayward, C., Killen, J. D., Kraemer, H. C., & Taylor, C. B. (1998). Linking self-reported childhood behavioral inhibition to adolescent social phobia. *Journal of the American Academy of Child and Adolescent Psychiatry, 37*, 1308–1316.

Hirshfeld, D. R., Rosenbaum, J. F., Biederman, J., Bolduc, E. A., Faraone, S. V., Snidman, N., Reznick, J. S., et al. (1992). Stable behavioral inhibition and its association with anxiety disorder. *Journal of the American Academy of Child and Adolescent Psychiatry, 31*, 103–111.

Jersild, A. T., & Holmes, F. B. (1935). *Children's fears* (Child Development Monographs, 20). New York: Teachers College, Columbia University.

Kagan, J. (1994). *Galen's prophecy*. New York: HarperCollins.

Kagan, J., & Reznick, J. S. (1986). Shyness and temperament. In W. H. Jones, J. M. Cheak, & S. R. Briggs (Eds.), *Shyness* (pp. 47–70). New York: Plenum.

Kagan, J., Reznick, J. S., & Snidman, N. (1987). The physiology and psychology of behavioral inhibition in children. *Child Development, 58*, 1459–1473.

Kagan, J., Reznick, J. S., & Snidman, N. (1988). Biological bases of childhood shyness. *Science, 240*, 167–171.

Kashani, J. H., & Orvaschel, H. (1990). A community study of anxiety in children and adolescents. *American Journal of Psychiatry, 147*, 313–318.

Keller, M. B., Lavori, P. W., Wunder, J., Beardslee, W. R., Schwartz, C. E., &

Roth, J. (1992). Chronic course of anxiety disorders in children and adolescents. *Journal of the American Academy of Child and Adolescent Psychiatry, 31,* 595–599.

Kennedy, W. A. (1965). School phobia: Rapid treatment of fifty cases. *Journal of Abnormal Psychology, 70,* 285–290.

Kochanska, G. (1991). Patterns of inhibition to the unfamiliar in children of normal and affectively ill mothers. *Child Development, 62,* 250–263.

Kohlberg, L. (1969). Stage and sequence: The cognitive-developmental approach to socialization. In D. A. Goslin (Ed.), *Handbook of socialization theory and research* (pp. 347–480). Chicago: Rand McNally.

Lapouse, R., & Monk, M. A. (1959). Fears and worries of a representative sample of children. *American Journal of Orthopsychiatry, 29,* 803–818.

Last, C. G., Francis, G., & Strauss, C. C. (1989). Assessing fears in anxiety-disordered children with the Revised Fear Survey Schedule for Children (FSSC-R). *Journal of Clinical Child Psychology, 18,* 137–141.

Last, C. G., Perrin, S., Hersen, M., & Kazdin, A. E. (1992). *DSM-III-R* anxiety disorders in children: Sociodemographic and clinical characteristics. *Journal of the American Academy of Child and Adolescent Psychiatry, 31,* 1070–1076.

Lentz, K. A. (1985). The expressed fears of young children. *Child Psychiatry and Human Development, 16,* 3–13.

Lewis, M., & Volkmar, F. R. (1990). *Clinical aspects of child and adolescent development.* Philadelphia: Lea & Febiger.

Loevinger, J. (1976). *Ego development: Conceptions and theories.* San Francisco: Jossey-Bass.

Main, M., & Goldwyn, R. (1991). Adult attachment classification system. In M. Main (Ed.), *Behavior and the development of representational models of attachment: Five methods of assessment.* Cambridge, UK: Cambridge University Press.

Main, M., Kaplan, N., & Cassidy, J. (1985). Security in infancy, childhood, and adulthood: A move to the level of representation. *Monographs of the Society for Research in Child Development, 50*(1–2, Serial No. 209), 66–104.

Main, M., & Solomon, J. (1986). Discovery of an insecure-disorganized/disoriented attachment pattern. In T. B. Brazelton & M. Yogman (Eds.), *Affective development in infancy.* Norwood, NJ: Ablex.

Manassis, K. (2001) Child-parent relations: Attachment and anxiety disorders. In W. K. Silverman & P. D. A Treffers (Eds.), *Anxiety disorders in children and adolescents* (pp. 255–273). New York: Cambridge University Press.

Manassis, K., Bradley, S., Goldberg, S., Hood, J., & Swinson, R. P. (1994). Attachment in mothers with anxiety disorders and their children. *Journal of the American Academy of Child and Adolescent Psychiatry, 33,* 1106–1113.

Manassis, K., Bradley, S., Goldberg, S., Hood, J., & Swinson, R. P. (1995). Behavioural inhibition, attachment and anxiety in children of mothers with anxiety disorders. *Canadian Journal of Psychiatry, 40,* 87–92.

Marks, I. (1987). The development of normal fear: A review. *Journal of Child Psychology and Psychiatry and Allied Disciplines, 28,* 667–697.

Marks, I. M., & Gelder, M. G. (1966). Different ages of onset in varieties of phobia. *American Journal of Psychiatry, 123,* 218–221.

Mattis, S. G., & Ollendick, T. H. (1997). Children's cognitive responses to the somatic symptoms of panic. *Journal of Abnormal Child Psychology, 25,* 47–57.

Maurer, A. (1965). What children fear. *Journal of Genetic Psychology, 106,* 265–277.

Mick, M.A., & Telch, M. J. (1998). Social anxiety and history of behavioral inhibition in young adults. *Journal of Anxiety Disorders, 12,* 1–20.

Miller, L. C. (1983). Fears and anxieties in children. In C. E. Walker & M. C.
Roberts (Eds.), *Handbook of clinical child psychology.* New York: Wiley.

Miller, L. C., Barrett C. L., Hampe, E., & Noble, H. (1972). Factor structure of
childhood fears. *Journal of Consulting and Clinical Psychology, 39,* 264–268.

Moreau, D., & Weissman, M. M. (1992). Panic disorder in children and adolescents: A review. *American Journal of Psychiatry, 149,* 1306–1314.

Nelles, W. B., & Barlow, D. H. (1988). Do children panic? *Clinical Psychology
Review, 8,* 359–372.

Ollendick, T. H. (1979). Fear reduction techniques with children. In M. Hersen,
R. M. Eisler, & P. M. Miller (Eds.), *Progress in behavior modification* (Vol.
8, pp. 127–168). New York: Academic Press.

Ollendick, T. H. (1983). Reliability and validity of the Revised Fear Survey Schedule for Children (FSSC-R). *Behaviour Research and Therapy, 21,* 395–399.

Ollendick, T. H., King, N. J., & Frary, R. B. (1989). Fears in children and adolescents: Reliability and generalizability across gender, age and nationality.
Behaviour Research and Therapy, 27, 19–26.

Ollendick, T. H., Mattis, S., & King, N. J. (1994) Panic in children and adolescents: A review. *Journal of Child Psychology and Psychiatry, 35,* 113–134.

Ollendick, T. H., & Vasey, M. (1999). Developmental theory and the practice of
child clinical psychology. *Journal of Clinical Child Psychology, 28,* 457–466

Prior, M., Smart, D., Sanson, A., & Oberklaid, F. (2000). Does shy-inhibited
temperament in childhood lead to problems in adolescence? *Journal of the
American Academy of Child and Adolescent Psychiatry, 39,* 461–468.

Riegel, K. F. (1978). *Psychology, mon amour: A countertext.* Boston: Houghton
Mifflin.

Rosenbaum, J. F., Biederman, J., Bolduc, E. A., Hirshfeld, D. R., Faraone, S. V.,
& Kagan, I. (1992). Comorbidity of parental anxiety disorders as risk for
childhood-onset anxiety in inhibited children. *American Journal of Psychiatry, 149,* 475–481.

Rosenbaum, J. F., Biederman, J., Gersten, M., Hirshfeld, D. R., Meminger, S. R.,
Herman, J. B., Kagan, J., et al. (1988). Behavioral inhibition in children of
parents with panic disorder and agoraphobia. *Archives of General Psychiatry,
45,* 463–470.

Rosenbaum, J. F., Biederman, J., Hirshfeld, D. R., Bolduc, E. A., Faraone, S. V.,
Kagan, J., Snidman, N., et al. (1991). Further evidence of an association
between behavioral inhibition and anxiety disorders: Results from a family
study of children from a non-clinical sample. *Journal of Psychiatric Research,
25,* 49–65.

Rosenbaum, J. F., Biederman, J., Hirshfeld-Becker, D. R., Kagan, I., Snidman,
N., Friedman, D., Nineberg, A., et al. (2000). A controlled study of behav-
ioral inhibition in children of parents with panic disorder and depression.
American Journal of Psychiatry, 157, 2002–2020.

Rubin, K. H., Both, L., Zahn-Waxler, C., Cummings, E. M., & Wilkinson, M.
(1991). Dyadic play behaviors of children of well and depressed mothers.
Development and Psychopathology, 3, 243–251.

Rutter, M. (1980). Introduction. In M. Rutter (Ed.), *Scientific foundations of
developmental psychiatry.* London: Heinemann.

Sameroff, A. J. (1993). Models of development and developmental risk. In C. H.

Zeanah, Jr. (Ed.), *Handbook of infant mental health* (pp. 3–13). New York: Guilford Press.

Scarr, S., & Salapatek, P. (1970). Patterns of fear development during infancy. *Merrill-Palmer Quarterly, 16,* 53–90.

Scherer, M. W., & Nakamura, C. Y. (1968). A Fear Survey Schedule for Children (FSS-FC): A factor analytic comparison with manifest anxiety (CMAS). *Behaviour Research and Therapy, 6,* 173–182.

Schwartz, C. E., Snidman, N., & Kagan, J. (1999) Adolescent social anxiety as an outcome of inhibited temperament in childhood. *Journal of the American Academy and Child and Adolescent Psychiatry, 38,* 1008–1015.

Selman, R. L. (1980). *The growth of interpersonal understanding: Developmental and clinical analyses.* New York: Academic Press.

Simon, A., & Ward, L. (1974). Variables influencing the sources, frequency, and intensity of worry in secondary school pupils. *British Journal of Social and Clinical Psychology, 13,* 391–396.

Sroufe, L. A. (1985). Attachment classification from the perspective of infant-caregiver relationships and infant temperament. *Child Development, 56,* 1–14.

Sroufe, L. A. (1996). *Emotional development.* New York: Cambridge University Press.

Sroufe, L. A., & Rutter, M. (1984). The domain of developmental psychopathology. *Child Development, 55,* 17–29.

Strauss, C. C., Lease, C. A., Last, C. G., & Francis, G. (1988). Overanxious disorder: An examination of developmental differences. *Journal of Abnormal Child Psychology, 16,* 433–443.

Strayer, J. (1986). Children's attributions regarding the situational determinants of emotion in self and others. *Developmental Psychology, 22,* 649–654.

Thomas, A., & Chess, S. (1977). *Temperament and development.* New York: Brunner/Mazel.

Thyer, B. A. (1993). Childhood separation anxiety disorder and adult-onset agoraphobia: Review of evidence. In C. G. Last (Ed.), *Anxiety across the lifespan: A developmental perspective* (pp. 128–147). New York: Springer.

Vaughn, B., & Sroufe, L.A. (1979). The temporal relationship between infant HR acceleration and crying in an aversive situation. *Child Development, 50,* 565–567.

Warren, S. L., Emde, R. N. & Sroufe, L. A. (2000). Internal representations: Predicting anxiety from children's play narratives. *Journal of the American Academy of Child and Adolescent Development, 39,* 100–107.

Warren, S. L., Huston, L., Egeland, B., & Sroufe, L. A. (1997). Child and adolescent anxiety disorders and early attachment. *Journal of the American Academy of Child and Adolescent Psychiatry, 36,* 637–644.

Werry, J. S. (1991). Overanxious disorder: A review of its taxonomic properties. *Journal of the American Academy of Child and Adolescent Psychiatry, 30,* 533–544.

Westenberg, P. M., Berend, S. M., & Treffers, P. D. A. (2001). Psychosocial developmental theory in relation to anxiety and its disorders. In W. K. Silverman & P. D. A Treffers (Eds.), *Anxiety disorders in children and adolescents* (pp. 72–89). New York: Cambridge University Press.

Wittchen, H.-U., Reed, V., & Kessler, R. C. (1998). Social fears and social phobia in a community sample of adolescents and young adults. *Archives of General Psychiatry, 55,* 1017–1024.

5

COMORBIDITY OF CHILDHOOD AND ADOLESCENT ANXIETY DISORDERS

Prevalence and Implications

JOHN F. CURRY, JOHN S. MARCH,
& AARON S. HERVEY

With one exception, the categorization and description of anxiety disorders in the most recent diagnostic system, the *DSM-IV* (American Psychiatric Association [APA], 1994) is identical for adults and for younger people. The single anxiety disorder specific to children or adolescents is separation anxiety disorder (SAD). In contrast to the previous diagnostic system (*DSM-III-R*, APA, 1987), the current system omits childhood-specific overanxious disorder (OAD) and avoidant disorder (AD). The former has been subsumed under the category of generalized anxiety disorder (GAD), and the latter proved indistinguishable from social phobia (Francis, Last, & Strauss, 1992).

In this chapter, we begin by describing briefly each of the *DSM-IV* anxiety disorders. Because the base rate of individual disorders influences the probability of comorbidity, we then review studies pertaining to the prevalence of each disorder and of associated comorbid conditions. This review includes, first, comorbidity among the anxiety disorders, and second, comorbidity of anxiety disorders with other types of disorders. Because much of this research was conducted using *DSM-III-R* categories, we include studies on the prevalence of OAD, as well as more recent studies using GAD as a childhood disorder. In the final section of the chapter, we outline and discuss salient issues that are raised by the empirical findings on comorbidity.

DSM-IV ANXIETY DISORDERS

In this section, we describe each of the anxiety disorders in *DSM-IV*. More extensive discussions of these disorders are included in other chapters of this book. SAD is characterized by excessive and developmentally inappropriate anxiety about separating from the home or from attachment figures. SAD has its onset in the developmental period, before age 18, but may continue into adulthood. By contrast with SAD, GAD is characterized by excessive anxiety and poorly controlled worry, accompanied by physiological symptoms, poor concentration, or irritability. In adults, three of six possible associated symptoms are required, but in children, only one is required. The delineation of specific age features makes it clear that this category subsumes the former OAD. Such age-related features may include excessive reassurance seeking and worry about school performance or athletic competence, each of which had previously been construed as a possible symptom of OAD.

The remaining anxiety disorders include agoraphobia, panic disorder, specific phobia, social phobia, obsessive-compulsive disorder, posttraumatic stress disorder, and acute stress disorder. Each has a central or defining feature accompanied by indices of avoidance or by associated symptoms. Agoraphobia (AGOR) is diagnosed when the central anxiety concerns being in a setting from which escape might be difficult or in which help may be unavailable if panic erupts. Indices of associated avoidance may be actual avoidance or painful endurance of such situations or the need for a companion in such situations. The central feature of panic disorder (PD) is the experience of recurrent panic attacks followed by worry about additional attacks. These attacks represent discrete episodes of intense fear accompanied by cognitive symptoms, physiological symptoms, or both. PD may or may not be accompanied by AGOR. AGOR is associated either with a history of and fear of PD, or with a history of and fear of panic symptoms that are below the diagnostic threshold for PD.

A specific phobia (SP) is the excessive and unreasonable fear of a certain object or situation. Associated avoidance or painful endurance leads to interference in functioning.

Social phobia (SOP) has as its core feature a significant and persistent fear of social or performance situations in which the person may feel embarrassed or humiliated. Exposure to the situation provokes anxiety, and the situation is consequently avoided or painfully endured. Either functional interference or marked distress is an associated feature. A child would not be given this diagnosis unless it is clear that he or she has the ability to relate socially to familiar people and that the social anxiety occurs with peers as well as adults.

Obsessive-compulsive disorder (OCD) has as core features obsessions, compulsions, or both. Obsessions are recurrent and persistent thoughts, images, or impulses that are intrusive. Compulsions are repetitive behavioral or mental actions in response to an obsession or to rigid rules. Obsessions or compulsions must be time-consuming or must interfere with functioning in order to rise to the level of a diagnosable disorder.

Posttraumatic stress disorder (PTSD) requires that the person has been exposed to an event involving the threat to self or to another of death, injury, or loss of physical integrity, as well as the accompanying experience of intense anxiety or helplessness. Associated symptoms may include disturbing dreams, memories, experiencing the recurrence of the trauma, or psychological or physiological responses to cues associated with the event. Avoidance and increased arousal are assessed through symptomatic manifestations. Acute stress disorder (ASD) is similar to PTSD, but by definition it resolves within 1 month from the time of onset and has fewer symptoms. ASD is not reviewed in this chapter, because little is known about it in children or adolescents.

PREVALENCE OF AND COMORBIDITY AMONG THE ANXIETY DISORDERS

Epidemiological studies with community samples have repeatedly demonstrated that the anxiety disorders have the highest or second-highest prevalence of any psychiatric disorders in children and adolescents. In addition to high prevalence, childhood anxiety disorders are also associated with significant impairment, causing distress that interferes with school performance, family, and social functioning (Ialongo, Edelsohn, Werthamer-Larsson, Crockett, & Kellam, 1994, 1995).

In 1988, Kashani and Orvaschel studied a community sample of 14- to 16-year-olds and found that anxiety disorders were the most commonly diagnosed conditions, occurring in 17% of the sample. Subsequently, the same authors (1990) interviewed 210 young people, ages 8, 12, and 17 years, and once again found that anxiety was the most frequently reported form of psychopathology.

Cohen et al. (1993) assessed *DSM-III-R* disorders in a sample of nearly 800 children and adolescents in New York. Anxiety disorders were the most common diagnoses among preadolescent girls, and OAD showed stable rates among females until age 20. Among boys, OAD declined with age, as did SAD in both sexes. At each age, anxiety disorders were more common than depression in both sexes but less prevalent than disruptive behavior disorders in adolescents and in prepubertal boys.

The Great Smoky Mountains Study of Youth (Costello et al., 1996) included screening of 4,500 9-, 11-, and 13-year-olds, followed by diagnostic interviewing of over 1,000 children who scored high on screening instruments. Three-month prevalence of *DSM-III-R* disorders was highest for behavior disorders (6.56%), followed by anxiety disorders (5.69%).

Anxiety disorders were the most prevalent psychiatric conditions among 15-year-olds in the Dunedin, New Zealand, study (McGee et al., 1990). In the Oregon Adolescent Depression Project (Lewinsohn, Hops, Roberts, Seeley, & Andrews, 1993), based on diagnostic interviews with over 1,500 U.S. high school students, anxiety disorders had higher point prevalence than depression, substance use, or disruptive behavior disorders but lower lifetime prevalence than depression.

Extending their research from adolescence into adulthood, Kessler and his colleagues (1994) reported lifetime and 12-month prevalence of *DSM-III-R* disorders from the National Comorbidity Survey of over 8,000 15- to 54-year-olds. Lifetime diagnoses of any anxiety disorder characterized 25% of the sample, slightly below the rate for substance use disorders (27%) but above the rate for affective disorders (19%). By contrast, the 12-month prevalence of anxiety disorders (17%) surpassed that of substance use or affective disorders (both 11%).

DEVELOPMENTAL TRENDS IN PREVALENCE

In our review of the specific anxiety disorders of childhood and adolescence, we rely primarily on cross-sectional studies focused on particular disorders. However, when data are available, we also comment on developmental trends in disorder prevalence and comorbidity. For example, Compton, Nelson, and March (2000), using self-report data on the prevalence of SOP or SAD symptoms in a community sample, found that preadolescents were more likely than adolescents to report elevated levels of both types of symptoms. Preadolescents were also more likely to report elevated SAD symptoms in the absence of elevated SOP symptoms. Conversely, adolescents more often reported symptoms of SOP than did preadolescents. Such findings are consistent with the developmental trend of a decrease in SAD reported by Cohen and colleagues (1993), but only partially consistent with the expected adolescent age of onset of SOP reported by Last, Perrin, Hersen, and Kazdin (1992). It appears that, in preadolescent cases where symptoms of SAD are already present, comorbid SOP symptoms should also be assessed.

OVERANXIOUS DISORDER OR
GENERALIZED ANXIETY DISORDER

Community Samples   Keller and his colleagues (1992) recruited 275 children for a study of prevalence and course of anxiety disorders. Of this sample, 14% had an anxiety disorder. OAD was the most common diagnosis, characterizing 11% of the sample. OAD occurred in 26 (12%) of the 210 preadolescents and early adolescents interviewed in the Missouri study (Kashani & Orvaschel, 1990). Similar but somewhat higher rates were obtained by Cohen and colleagues (1993) with females from age 10 to 20 (14–15%) in New York. Among boys, the prevalence of OAD was 13% at ages 10 to 13, declining to 5% later in adolescence. In the Great Smoky Mountains Study (Costello et al., 1996), both OAD and GAD were diagnosed in the pre-adolescent and early adolescent sample. This yielded a combined prevalence of about 3%. OAD was the most prevalent disorder in mid-adolescence in the Dunedin Study, occurring in 6% of the sample. Girls were twice as likely as boys to have OAD (McGee et al., 1990). In the Oregon Adolescent study, which involved high school students in mid-adolescence, point prevalence of OAD was only approximately .5% (Lewinsohn et al., 1993). These studies varied in the time period considered for prevalence, in diagnostic interview methods, and in the age range sampled, any of which may have contributed to varying estimates. Although prevalence rates across studies range from less than 1% to approximately 13%, some trends are suggested. Girls are more likely than boys to have OAD, especially among adolescents. In most studies, the rates of OAD were lower in adolescents than in children. However, among adults, GAD was the third most frequent anxiety disorder, had a 12-month prevalence of 3.1%, and was twice as likely to occur in females as in males (Kessler et al., 1994).

Comorbidity in Community Samples   Few community studies report rates of comorbidity among specific anxiety disorders, focusing instead on co-morbidity among classes of disorders (affective, anxiety, disruptive behavior). However, Kashani and Orvaschel (1990) found that the most common comorbid anxiety disorders among young people with OAD were SAD, which was diagnosed in almost half of OAD subjects, and simple phobia, diagnosed in about 20%. Benjamin, Costello, and Warren (1990) investigated 1-year prevalence and comorbidity of anxiety disorders in a pediatric sample. Of these 7- to 11-year-olds, 15% had an anxiety disorder, with approximately 5% demonstrating OAD. Again the most common comorbid anxiety disorders were SAD and SP, each occurring in half of the children with OAD.

Comorbidity in Clinical Samples   As Caron and Rutter (1991) pointed out, clinical samples always contain a larger proportion of subjects demonstrating comorbid conditions as well as an index disorder, because not all subjects in the population who have the index disorder will be referred to clinical care (Berkson's bias). This caution must be kept in mind when reviewing comorbidity rates in clinic samples. Last, Strauss, and Francis (1987) studied 73 outpatients, ages 5 to 18, in an anxiety treatment clinic. OAD occurred in 11 subjects (15% of the sample). More than half had a comorbid diagnosis, the most common of which was SOP or AD. Subsequently, Last and her colleagues (Last et al., 1992) found that a primary diagnosis of OAD characterized 13% of a larger clinical sample. Again the most common comorbid diagnosis was SOP, which characterized over half of OAD subjects.

Kendall and Brady (1995) interviewed 106 children and early adolescents (ages 9–13) at the Temple Anxiety Disorders Clinic. OAD was by far the most common diagnosis, occurring in 90% of this sample. Almost 75%

of OAD children had second anxiety diagnoses. The most common of these were SOP and AD, which occurred in nearly half of OAD children, followed by SAD, which occurred in over one third of OAD children. Masi, Mucci, Favilla, Romano, and Poli (1999) investigated comorbidity of *DSM-IV* GAD in a sample of 19 children and 39 adolescents with this diagnosis. GAD was rarely the only diagnosis, because 87% of GAD patients had another diagnosis. SP (29%) and SAD (21%) were the most common comorbid anxiety disorders, but the age trends for these two conditions moved in opposite directions. SAD was much more common in children than in adolescents, but SP was much more common in adolescents than in children. Among GAD symptoms, brooding was more common in adolescents and reassurance seeking more common in children.

In summary, OAD is very frequently accompanied by one or more additional anxiety disorders. Estimates of comorbidity in clinical samples range from 50% to over 80%. Even in community samples, rates of a comorbid anxiety diagnosis stand at about 50%. OAD appears to have a typical age of onset in middle childhood. Last and colleagues (1992) reported mean age of onset as 8.8 years, whereas Keller and colleagues (1992) found typical age of onset to be 10 years.

SEPARATION ANXIETY DISORDER

Community Samples   Among the anxiety disorders affecting children, SAD is generally found to be the second most frequently diagnosed disorder after OAD/GAD (Bell-Dolan & Brazeal, 1993). The Missouri study (Kashani & Orvaschel, 1990) reported a prevalence rate of 12.9%, with the diagnosis 4 times more likely among girls than among boys. In New York, Cohen and colleagues (1993) reported a similar prevalence rate among 10- to 13-year-olds of both sexes (11% for boys and 13% for girls), but with rates declining markedly after age 13. In the 14- to 16-year-old age range, girls were 4 times as likely as boys to have this disorder, but after age 16 both sexes had low prevalence (2% to 3%). Benjamin and colleagues (1990) reported that SAD occurred in 4% of their pediatric sample, with a 1.7 to 1 female-to-male ratio. SAD was the most common anxiety disorder in the Great Smoky Mountains Study, occurring in 3.5% of the sample, with a 1.6 to 1 female-to-male ratio (Costello et al., 1996). In mid-adolescence, McGee and colleagues (1990) reported a prevalence of 2%, with a 2 to 1 female-to-male ratio, but Lewinsohn's group (1993) found point prevalence below .20%, with the disorder virtually absent among boys. Again, despite varying estimates, there is clear evidence that SAD declines with age and that it is more prevalent in girls than in boys.

Comorbidity in Community Samples   The comorbidity of SAD with other anxiety disorders is common. About half (52%) of those with SAD in the Kashani and Orvaschel (1990) study met criteria for a second anxiety disorder, the most frequent of which were OAD (40%) and SP (18%). Of those with SAD, 7% had both OAD and SP. Benjamin and colleagues (1990) found SP to be the most prevalent additional anxiety disorder in children with SAD (46%), followed by OAD and AGOR (26% each).

Comorbidity in Clinical Samples   Using a sample of 5- to 18-year-olds referred to an anxiety disorders clinic, Last et al. (1987) found that 41% of children with SAD had one or more additional anxiety disorders. The most common concurrent diagnosis was OAD (33%), followed by SP and AD (12.5% each) and SOP (8%). In a second study from the same clinic (Last et al., 1992), SP was the most common comorbid lifetime diagnosis (37%), followed by OAD (23%) and SOP (19%). Kendall and Brady (1995) found that 82% of children with SAD also had SP, 60% had OAD, and 30% had SOP. Taken together, these three studies indicate that SP, OAD, and SOP occur with very high frequency in children with SAD. SAD has an early age of onset (7.5 years on average; Last et al., 1992) and declines very significantly during adolescence.

PANIC DISORDER AND AGORAPHOBIA

By the mid-1990s, it had been established that panic attacks and PD occurred not only in adolescents, but also less frequently in prepubertal children (Moreau & Weissman, 1992; Ollendick, Mattis, & King, 1994). Evidence in support of the existence of prepubertal PD came from retrospective reports of adults with PD, from clinical case studies, and from surveys of U.S. and Australian high school students. PD, AGOR, or both have been assessed in selected epidemiological and clinical studies.

Community Samples   In the Great Smoky Mountains Study (Costello et al., 1996), PD was found in .03% of the sample and AGOR in .07%. It is interesting that all cases occurred in males. A large high school survey study in New Jersey found a lifetime prevalence rate for PD of .6% (Whitaker et al., 1990). Point prevalence among adolescents in the Oregon study was .35% for PD and .41% for AGOR, with females about twice as likely as males to have PD and about 5 times more likely to have AGOR (Lewinsohn et al., 1993). By adulthood, 12-month prevalence rates were 2.3% for PD and 2.8% for AGOR (Kessler et al., 1994). Females were about twice as likely as males to have either disorder.

Comorbidity in Community Samples   King, Gullone, Tonge, and Ollendick (1993) found that adolescents reporting panic attacks had higher levels of physiological tension and worry than those without panic, suggesting the possibility that generalized anxiety may predispose to panic attacks. AGOR, but not PD, was assessed and reported in the pediatric sample study conducted by Benjamin and his colleagues (1990). Four of the five children with AGOR also had SAD, three had SP, one had OAD, and one had SOP.

Comorbidity in Clinical Samples   Among 188 children and adolescents referred to an anxiety disorders clinic, 10% had PD. Of these youngsters, 62% had another anxiety disorder, most commonly OAD (Last et al., 1992). Strikingly similar results were found in an Italian study (Masi, Favilla, Mucci, & Millepiedi, 2000b). Among 220 children and adolescents referred to an outpatient clinic, 10.4% had PD. GAD was diagnosed in 74% of these PD youngsters. SP and AGOR were each present in over half of those with PD (56%). Although current SAD was diagnosed in only 22% of PD young-sters, a past diagnosis of SAD was reported in another 44%. Other studies of inpatient, outpatient, or high-risk samples of adolescents or children have shown that the most common anxiety disorder comorbid with PD was SAD (reviewed in Ollendick et al., 1994). Thus, there appear to be at least two anxiety disorders of childhood that are associated with and may raise the risk for development of PD: OAD and SAD. Mean age of onset of PD in young people was 14 years in the study by Last and her colleagues (1992). Among adults with PD, the Epidemiological Catchment Area Study (Rob-ins, Croughan, Williams, & Spitzer, 1981) found the peak age of onset to fall between 15 and 19 years of age. Prepubertal onset does occur, how-ever, as documented in a number of clinical samples (Ollendick et al., 1994).

SOCIAL PHOBIA

Community Samples   Kashani and Orvaschel (1990) found few cases of SOP in their sample of 8-, 12-, and 17-year-olds in Missouri. There were no cases among 8-year-olds, and only two among older children. Benjamin and colleagues (1990), in their study of 7- to 11-year-old pediatric cases, found a 1-year prevalence of 1% for SOP. Costello and colleagues (1996) in the Great Smoky Mountains Study found the 3-month prevalence of SOP among 9- to 13-year-olds to be .58%, substantially lower than for SAD or GAD/OAD. In the mid-adolescent (age 15) Dunedin study (McGee et al., 1990), prevalence of SOP was 1.1%, lower than OAD, SAD, or simple phobia. Similarly, the point prevalence of SOP in the Oregon Adolescent Depression Project (Lewinsohn et al., 1993) was .94%. In striking contrast, the adult sample in the National Comorbidity Study (Kessler et al., 1994) had a 12-month prevalence of SOP of 7.9%, second only to SP among adult anxiety disorders. These studies suggest that SOP becomes more preva-lent with age: Previous reviewers have found that it is rarely diagnosed in children younger than age 10 (Albano, Chorpita, & Barlow, 1996). Data on gender differences is conflicting, but the majority of the community studies (Benjamin et al., 1990; Costello et al., 1996; Kessler et al., 1994; Lewinsohn et al., 1993) show a higher prevalence in females.

Comorbidity in Community Samples   Prior to *DSM-IV* (APA, 1994), sev-eral clinical studies assessed SOP and AD independently. Keller et al. (1992) found that 2 of their sample of 275 children had AD, but both of them also had OAD. Kashani and Orvaschel (1990) found that one of their two children with SOP also had OAD. Benjamin et al. (1990) reported that two of the three children in their pediatric sample who had SOP also had OAD, and two of the three had SP.

Comorbidity in Clinical Samples Last and colleagues (1987) reported that 15% of 5- to 18-year-olds in an anxiety disorders clinic had primary SOP, and 1.4% had AD. Of those with SOP, 64% had some additional diagnosis. Last et al. (1992) subsequently reported on a larger sample from the same clinic. Primary SOP was diagnosed in 15%, and 2.7% had primary AD. SOP had a relatively late mean age of onset (11 years of age), but AD had an extraordinarily early age of onset (2.2 years of age). Of those with AD, 65% had lifetime diagnoses of SOP, and 60% had OAD. Of those with SOP, nearly half (48%) had OAD. Francis and colleagues (1992), reporting from the same clinic, assessed differences between children and adolescents with SOP and those with AD. They found the previously noted difference in age but no differences in gender, socioeconomic background, rates of comorbid anxiety or mood disorders, or additional fears. They concluded that there was little evidence to support the validity of AD as a diagnosis separate from SOP.

Kendall and Brady (1995) combined SOP and AD in their anxiety disorders clinic. Of this 9- to 13-year-old sample, 48% had such a diagnosis. There was no comorbid anxiety diagnosis in 10%, but 90% had OAD, and 23% had SAD.

SPECIFIC PHOBIAS

Community Samples Prior to *DSM-IV*, SPs were termed *simple phobias,* so the latter diagnosis was assessed in epidemiological studies conducted prior to 1994. Kashani and Orvaschel (1990) diagnosed simple phobia in 3.3% of their sample, but the disorder was much more prevalent among girls than among boys (5.7% versus 1.0%, respectively). In the Great Smoky Mountains Study (Costello et al., 1996) SP had an overall prevalence of .27%, occurring about 3 times as often in girls as in boys (.42% versus .13%). Among anxiety disorders SP was less frequent than SAD, OAD/GAD, or SOP. Similarly, McGee and colleagues (1990) reported that the disorder was 3 times as prevalent in mid-adolescent girls as in boys. The prevalence overall was 3.6%, exceeded only by OAD among the anxiety disorders. The Oregon project found a point prevalence of 1.4%, making it the most common current anxiety disorder in this high school sample (Lewinsohn et al., 1993). Again a gender ratio of approximately three females to each male was noted. SP is the most common anxiety disorder among adults (Kessler et al., 1994), with a 12-month prevalence of 4.4% in males and 13.2% in females.

Comorbidity in Community Samples Kashani and Orvaschel (1990) reported that 86% of SP children and adolescents had another anxiety disorder, either SAD or OAD (43% each). Benjamin et al. (1990) found that

33% of SP children had SAD, 19% had OAD, 14% had AGOR, and 10% had SOP.

Comorbidity in Clinical Samples Last et al. (1992) found that children and adolescents with SP had frequent lifetime diagnoses of SAD (39%), SOP (31%), or OAD (27%). Diagnoses occurring in less than 20% of SP young people included OCD (16%), PD (10%), and AD (5%). As noted previously, Kendall and Brady (1995) found SP to be very common in children with diagnoses of OAD, SOP, or SAD, but they did not report converse rates of these three disorders among all children with SP.

SP has an average age of onset in middle childhood (8.4 years; Last et al., 1992). It is not the most commonly diagnosed anxiety disorder among children, but review of cross-sectional studies and the National Comorbidity Study suggest that it becomes the most common such disorder by adulthood.

POSTTRAUMATIC STRESS DISORDER

Community Samples Among the anxiety disorders in children and adolescents, PTSD has received perhaps the most belated attention. Only one general childhood epidemiological study has assessed its frequency. In the Great Smoky Mountains Study, Costello and her colleagues (1996) found a 3-month prevalence of only .02% among 9- to 13-year-olds. Thus, the epidemiology of PTSD in children and adolescents has not been widely studied. The National Comorbidity Study of adults, however, estimated a lifetime prevalence rate of PTSD in the general population of 7.8% (Kessler, Sonnega, Bromet, Hughes, & Nelson, 1995).

In a longitudinal study examining the prevalence of both traumatic experiences and PTSD in a community sample of 384 participants, Giaconia and her associates (1995) found that 6.3% of their sample of 18-year-old participants had received a lifetime diagnosis of PTSD. Although the likelihood of experiencing a trauma did not differ by gender, overall rate of PTSD did differ, with the rate of PTSD in females 6 times that in males.

Comorbidity in Community Samples Giaconia et al. (1995) found several notable relationships between a diagnosis of PTSD and other comorbid disorders. Adolescents diagnosed with PTSD were 4 times as likely as those who experienced trauma without a PTSD diagnosis, and 7 times as likely as those who did not experience a trauma, to meet *DSM-III-R* criteria for at least one of five other disorders. Indeed, approximately 80% of those with a lifetime diagnosis of PTSD qualified for at least one other disorder. Comorbidity rates were 29.2% and 33.3% for simple phobia and SOP, respectively.

Comorbidity in Clinical Samples Studies using clinical or high-risk samples of children and adolescents with PTSD are more extant in the literature, and data regarding comorbidity more available. However, some of these

studies are retrospective in nature and therefore do not always utilize structured measures, but instead depend on unstructured clinical interview notes
to determine diagnosis. Koltek, Wilkes, and Atkinson (1998) looked at the
comorbidity of PTSD and other anxiety disorders in a retrospective study
of 187 adolescent inpatients with a mean age of 15 years. The overall rate
of PTSD in the sample was 42%. Patients with PTSD were significantly more
likely than those without this diagnosis to have an additional anxiety disorder or a depressive disorder. Brent et al. (1995) evaluated a sample of adolescents with PTSD who were peers of suicide victims. Although their PTSD
sample was small ($n = 8$) relative to the comparison group of peers who did
not develop PTSD ($n = 138$), they found that the PTSD group was significantly more likely to have a history of AGOR (12.5%) than was the comparison group (0.7%).

OBSESSIVE-COMPULSIVE DISORDER

Community Samples   Three-month prevalence of obsessive-compulsive
disorder (OCD) was .17% among the 9- to 13-year-olds in the Great Smoky
Mountains Study (Costello et al., 1996). Point prevalence was .06% in the
Oregon Adolescent Depression Project (Lewinsohn et al., 1993). Other
epidemiological studies identify lifetime prevalence rates between 2% and
4% (Douglass, Moffitt, Dar, McGee, & Silva, 1995; Flament et al., 1988;
Valleni-Basile et al., 1994). In addition, whereas OCD in adults is fairly
equally expressed in both genders, males are diagnosed more frequently
among those under 18 years of age (Geller et al., 1998).

Comorbidity in Community Samples   Valleni-Basile and her colleagues
(1994) utilized a community sample of 488 mother-child dyads. They found
that 34% of children with OCD also met the criteria for SAD, and 29% met
criteria for some type of phobia. Similarly, a study investigating self-reported
OCD at age 18 in an unselected birth cohort of 930 individuals found that,
in those with OCD, 38% received a comorbid diagnosis of SOP, 19% had
SP, 16% had AGOR, and 5% had GAD (Douglass et al., 1995).

Comorbidity in Clinical Samples   Last and her colleagues (1992) found
that OCD was the primary diagnosis in 7% of admissions to an anxiety disorders clinic. Mean age of onset was almost 11 years of age. The most common comorbid condition was SP, present in nearly half of the children or
adolescents with OCD. Leonard, Lenane, and Swedo (1993) also found
SP to be the most common comorbid anxiety disorder in pediatric OCD
patients evaluated at the National Institute of Mental Health, affecting 17%
of those with OCD. OAD was another common comorbidity (16%), with
SAD occurring in 7%.

Geller, Biederman, Griffin, Jones, and Lefkowitz (1996) utilized a relatively small clinical sample ($N = 30$) from an OCD specialty clinic to conduct a comprehensive retrospective study investigating the rates of OCD

and comorbid disorders. Overall, 70% of those with OCD received at least one other anxiety disorder diagnosis, and 43% at least two others. The most common comorbid anxiety disorders were OAD (38%), SAD (33%), PD (28%), AGOR (23%), SP (17%), and SOP (10%). Often, the emergence of other anxiety disorders predated that of OCD.

COMORBIDITY OF ANXIETY AND DEPRESSION

The depressive disorders include major depression (MDD) and dysthymia (DD). Both are characterized by sad, unhappy, irritable, or depressed mood of a duration and severity that exceeds normal reactions to life events. MDD includes an array of significant biological and cognitive symptoms lasting at least 2 weeks. Symptoms in DD are milder, but duration is at least 1 year. A significant proportion of children with anxiety disorders also have depressive disorders. Angold and Costello (1993) found, however, that the rates of comorbid anxiety and depression varied widely across studies. In part, this variation is a function of sample characteristics. As expected, comorbidity rates are higher in clinical than community samples. Rates are also higher among older children than younger ones (Kendall, Kortlander, Chansky, & Brady, 1992).

Community Samples   Anderson, Williams, McGee, and Silva (1987) diagnosed depression in 17% of preadolescent children with anxiety disorders. Similarly, the Great Smoky Mountains Study of 9- to 13-year-olds reported that 14% of anxious children were depressed (Costello et al., 1996). McGee and colleagues (1990) found a similar rate among New Zealand adolescents (13%), but Lewinsohn's (1993) study of U.S. youths found a much higher rate of depression in anxious adolescents (49%). By contrast to analyses of depression among anxious children, several studies show markedly higher rates of anxiety disorder among depressed participants (71%, Anderson et al., 1987, and 44%, Costello et al., 1996), but this pattern was not found in the Oregon study.

Clinical Samples   Clinical studies suggest that depression occurs in between 30% and 50% of anxious youths. Kovacs and Devlin (1998) reviewed clinical studies and found that the average rate of depression among those with anxiety disorders was 41%.

Rates may vary according to the specific anxiety disorder under consideration. However, considerably more research is needed to determine whether this is the case. Last and colleagues (1987) reported that one third of clinical children with OAD had depressive disorder. Masi, Favilla, Mucci, and Millepiedi (2000a) reported that 50% of those with GAD had depressive disorder. Last et al. (1992) found that 30% of patients diagnosed with SAD also received a diagnosis of depression.

Kovacs, Gatsonis, Paulauskas, and Richards (1989) followed depressed children and found that comorbid SAD or OAD was more frequent than comorbid SP, OCD, or PD. However, studies of children with primary OCD show higher rates of comorbid depression. Swedo, Rapoport, Leonard, Lenane, and Cheslow (1989) found that depression occurred in 39% of 70 children and adolescents with OCD. Even higher rates are reported in more recent studies (45%, Valleni-Basile et al., 1994; 62%, Douglass et al., 1995; and 73%, Geller et al., 1996).

Among children and adolescents with PTSD, the rate of depression may again be in the range calculated by Kovacs and Devlin, approximately 42% (Giaconia et al., 1995). Goenjian et al. (1995) studied a group of 218 Armenian school-aged children 1½ years after a severe earthquake struck their communities. Looking at three communities, the authors found that as the distance from the epicenter of the quake decreased, rates of comorbid PTSD and depressive disorders increased, with overall comorbidity rates of 50%, 57.7%, and 78.9% respectively at three decreasing distances.

Anxious children with comorbid depression are older than those without depression and have more functional impairment (Kendall et al., 1992; Masi et al., 2000a). Kovacs and Devlin (1998) reported that mean age of onset of an anxiety disorder was 7.2 years, that of dysthymic disorder was 10.8 years, and that of major depression was 13.8 years. Not surprisingly, then, in most clinical cases, the anxiety disorder precedes the depression, although childhood onset dysthymia more often precedes an anxiety disorder (Kovacs et al., 1989). Angold, Costello, and Erkanli (1999) calculated mean odds ratios for several common comorbid conditions, based on community samples. They found that the odds ratio for comorbid anxiety and depression was significantly higher than those for comorbid anxiety and conduct disorder or for comorbid anxiety and attention deficit hyperactivity disorder. Given the high prevalence of comorbid anxiety and depression and the associated functional impairment, this comorbidity is deserving of particular theoretical and clinical attention.

ANXIETY, DISRUPTIVE BEHAVIOR DISORDERS, AND SUBSTANCE USE DISORDERS

The disruptive behavior disorders include attention-deficit/hyperactivity disorder (ADHD), conduct disorder (CD), and oppositional defiant disorder (ODD). The first is characterized by inattention, hyperactivity, and impulsivity; the second by violations of major societal rules; and the third by refusal to comply with requests, annoying and irritating behavior, and frequent anger or irritability. Substance use disorders include abuse and dependence, with the latter more severe and equivalent to addiction.

Community Samples   Angold et al. (1999) found that the odds ratios for comorbid anxiety and conduct disorder and for comorbid anxiety and attention deficit hyperactivity disorder were essentially equal (3.1 and 3.0, respectively), but lower than those for comorbid anxiety and depression (8.2) in community samples. Anderson and colleagues (1987) reported that

23% of anxious children had ADHD, and 32% had CD or ODD. Similarly, in the Great Smoky Mountains Study (Costello et al., 1996), 29% of anxious children had a disruptive behavior disorder. The Cohen et al. (1993) community sample found 36% of those diagnosed with either OAD, SAD, or both also qualified for a comorbid disruptive disorder. Studies of adolescents report somewhat lower rates of comorbidity. McGee et al. (1990) reported that 4% of anxious 15-year-olds had ADHD, and 6% had CD or ODD. In the Oregon project (Lewinsohn et al., 1993), 13% of anxious adolescents had lifetime disruptive behavior disorder diagnoses. In these same studies, the rates of anxiety disorder among those with disruptive behavior disorders ranged from about 15% to about 30%. Because substance use disorders rarely have onset before adolescence, child studies have not assessed their frequency or comorbidity. Lewinsohn et al. (1993) found that, among anxiety disordered adolescents, 15% had lifetime substance use disorders.

Clinical Samples   Last, Perrin, Hersen, and Kazdin (1996) followed 84 children who had been seen in an anxiety disorders clinic. During the 3- to 4-year follow-up period, over 80% of the children recovered from their initial disorders. However, 7% developed a behavior disorder, a figure that was lower than the rate for development of a new anxiety disorder (15%) or a new depressive disorder (13%). Regarding specific anxiety disorders, children with SAD, OCD, or PD appeared to be more likely to develop a behavior disorder than those with other index anxiety disorders. Douglass and her colleagues (1995) identified 16% of the OCD patients in their study as also having conduct disorder. Geller's research group (1996) found that 53% of their OCD sample met criteria for at least one disruptive behavior disorder, most commonly ODD (43%) or ADHD (33%). The symptoms of these two disorders frequently preceded OCD. Koltek et al. (1998) found high rates of comorbidity between PTSD and both ADHD (33%) and conduct disorders (36%). Glod and Teicher (1996) found that abused children who received a diagnosis of PTSD were much more likely than those without this diagnosis to have comorbid ADHD, with about one third of the PTSD children demonstrating ADHD.

In the recently completed NIMH Multimodal Treatment Study of Children with ADHD (MTA; March et al., 2000), 35% of ADHD children also had an anxiety disorder. The MTA compared medication management, behavioral treatment, and their combination to a community treatment condition. For the sample as a whole, medication and combined treatment were superior to behavioral treatment alone or community treatment. However, for children with ADHD and comorbid anxiety disorder, behavioral treatment was as efficacious as medication or combined treatment, with all three conditions superior to community treatment. In contrast to findings from some early, smaller studies, the MTA results did not indicate that the presence of anxiety had an adverse effect on the response of core ADHD symptoms to stimulant medication (March et al., 2000).

The hypothesis that anxious or distressed individuals are at risk for development of substance use disorders has received support in adult studies, and adolescents frequently cite tension reduction as a reason to use substances (Bukstein, Brent, & Kaminer, 1989). Douglass and colleagues (1995) evaluated alcohol and marijuana dependence among young people with OCD and controls, finding higher rates of dependence for both substances in the OCD group (reporting 24% for alcohol and 19% for marijuana).

There is emerging evidence suggesting that certain anxiety disorders may be more likely than others to be associated with substance use disorders. D. B. Clark and Neighbors (1996) reviewed clinical studies of adolescents in treatment for substance use disorders and concluded that SOP and PD are most likely to be the associated anxiety disorders. Deykin and Buka (1997) evaluated 297 adolescents aged 15 to 19 years who met the *DSM-III-R* criteria for dependence on alcohol or other drugs. Overall, the lifetime prevalence of PTSD was 30%, and the point prevalence was 19%. Rates differed by gender. Lifetime and point prevalence rates were 24% and 12% for males, but 45% and 40% for females.

Certain anxiety disorders may even offer protection against initiation of substance use. Kaplow, Curran, Angold, and Costello (2001) analyzed longitudinal data from the Great Smoky Mountains Study, finding that early GAD was associated with increased risk for onset of drinking, but early SAD was associated with decreased risk.

ISSUES RAISED BY COMORBIDITY FINDINGS

Theoretical Issues

IS THE CURRENT NOSOLOGY OF ANXIETY DISORDERS ADEQUATE?   As Caron and Rutter (1991) pointed out, the clinical ideal in medicine is for a single diagnosis to be made. Child and adolescent psychiatric comorbidity rates imply that this ideal is relatively rarely attained in clinical settings. The frequency of comorbidity among the anxiety disorders, and between anxiety and other disorders, therefore raises questions about the adequacy of contemporary (*DSM*) diagnostic systems. As early as 1987, Last and her colleagues raised the question of whether the many subdivisions among the anxiety disorders are warranted. The first theoretical issue, then, is whether comorbidity is simply an epiphenomenon of an inadequate diagnostic nomenclature.

First, it is clear that, although comorbidity rates are higher in clinical samples, comorbidity is also found in studies of community samples. This indicates that the phenomenon is not purely a function of referral processes. Second, as Caron and Rutter (1991) demonstrated, comorbidity cannot be explained simply as a function of intersecting base rates: The rate of Disorder B in the presence of Disorder A exceeds what would be predicted simply by the base rate of B in the population. These two points suggest that comorbidity reflects a real rather than an artificial process.

However, it still remains difficult to understand how a single patient could demonstrate symptoms of two or three disorders simultaneously. One approach to the problem of multiple categorical diagnoses is to conceptualize psychopathology along dimensional lines rather than in categorical terms. If psychopathology is conceptualized as an extreme manifestation of normal personality traits, then comorbidity exists when a person has two or more extreme traits.

Would such an approach obviate the problem of comorbidity? It is true that such an approach would remove the conceptual difficulty of assuming that multiple independent disorders or illnesses are simultaneously causing current symptomatology in a patient. However, this solution to the problem may be largely illusory. Obviously, if one conceptualizes psychopathology along dimensions rather than in categories, there will be no instances of multiple categorical disorders. However, the problem of explaining comorbidity is simply transferred from a categorical to a dimensional model. So long as certain combinations of extreme traits are more likely to occur than are other combinations, the phenomenon of comorbidity still remains to be explained. To take just one example, the revised Minnesota Multiphasic Personality Inventory (MMPI-2) was normed on a large nationally representative sample of U.S. adults (Butcher, 1996). In the normative sample, certain pairs of the 10 clinical scales on the MMPI-2 are more likely to be simultaneously elevated than are other pairs, an example of dimensional comorbidity.

A second approach to the problem of comorbidity is to conceptualize psychopathology in broader categories. For example, the categories included in the nosologies of *ICD* (*International Statistical Classification of Diseases and Related Health Problems;* World Health organization, 1992–1994) include both broad and combined categories, such as depression-plus-conduct disorder. However, as Caron and Rutter (1991) noted, this approach may blur actual comorbidity, because two separate processes are combined, and therefore, each is relatively neglected. Moreover, broader categories, in themselves, do not explain why certain combinations of those categories occur with more frequency than other combinations.

A third approach is to consider the high rates of apparent comorbidity as an opportunity rather than a problem (Angold et al., 1999). More specifically, Angold and his colleagues view comorbidity as an opportunity to enhance our understanding of developmental psychopathology. One need not assume that every current diagnostic category is a valid description of an independent pathological process in order to use the nosology as a provisional heuristic device to understand the development and course of psychopathology during childhood and adolescence. Nor need one assume that each current diagnostic category is representative of the same level of abstraction or type of psychopathological process. Certain categories may reflect processes that are more fundamental, general, or pervasive than others.

WHAT DOES COMORBIDITY SUGGEST ABOUT PSYCHOPATHOLOGY AND ITS DEVELOPMENT?   Initial clues about comorbidity and its developmental processes may be found in the chronological onset of various disorders of child-hood. Kovacs and Devlin (1998) reviewed seven studies reporting mean age of onset. The more common anxiety disorders (SAD, OAD, SP) had the earliest age of onset, typically between ages 6 and 9. Next in sequence were the disruptive behavior disorders, with average age of onset about 8. Other anxiety disorders (SOP, OCD) tended to begin between ages 10 and 13. Depressive disorders had typical onset at ages 10 to 15, with DD arising earlier than MDD, on average.

These findings suggest that comorbidity rates are in part a function of relative base rates in different age groups. For example, since SOP rarely has onset before age 10, it is less likely to be a comorbid condition in young children. Rates of comorbid SOP in community or clinical studies will also be lower if the sample includes few adolescents.

In addition, the chronology of disorders' mean age of onset raises the question of whether the first disorder's occurrence raises the risk for development of a second disorder. In the anxiety disorders, for example, both OAD and SAD (early childhood onset disorders) are frequent comorbid diagnoses with PD (most typically an adolescent-onset disorder). Although neither is essential to pave the way for onset of PD, it may be the case that risk of PD is elevated in youngsters with a history of OAD or SAD.

Certain anxiety disorders have shown a specific course from adolescence into early adulthood. Pine, Cohen, Gurley, Brook, and Ma (1998) found that adolescent SP predicted adult SP, and that adolescent SOP predicted either adult SOP or SP. However, there was a broader associative link among the more generalized anxiety disorders (OAD, GAD) and depression. Adolescent OAD predicted not only adult GAD, but also adult SOP and major depression.

When considering depression and comorbid anxiety disorders and depression, it is most commonly the case that the anxiety disorder precedes the depression. Does this suggest that anxiety raises the risk for subsequent depression? Such a hypothesis is supported by data from the Dunedin study (Feehan, McGee, & Williams, 1993). Following adolescents from age 15 to age 18, these authors found that a depressive disorder at 18 was twice as likely in adolescents who had had an anxiety disorder at age 15 (22%) as in those with no diagnosis at 15 (11%).

A second clue to understanding comorbidity and its psychopathological processes comes from the relative rates of comorbidity across classes of disorders. As Kovacs and Devlin (1998) noted, the disorder most likely to be comorbid with an index anxiety disorder is another anxiety disorder. The next most likely would be a depressive disorder, and then a disruptive behavior disorder. This raises the question of why the various anxiety disorders are so likely to co-occur, and why anxiety and depression are so often comorbid conditions.

Based on data from adults with anxiety disorders, Barlow (2000) has proposed a hierarchical theory of the anxiety and mood disorders. In Barlow's model, there are three levels of vulnerabilities for development of anxiety,

anxiety disorders, and mood disorders. At the most basic level, there is a biological vulnerability. In personality psychology, this vulnerability is variously termed neuroticism, negative affect, or behavioral inhibition, and it has a genetic component (L. A. Clark, Watson, & Mineka, 1994). Based on a review of studies of personality and psychopathology, Barlow proposes that this vulnerability forms a common basis for most of the anxiety disorders, as well as depression.

The second vulnerability is development of a diminished sense of personal control. In animal studies, early experience of lack of control has been demonstrated to lead to behavioral inhibition, agitation, restlessness or tension, and (in more recent studies) permanent neurobiological changes. The third vulnerability is the key to specificity of the anxiety disorder: learning where to focus anxious apprehension. General anxiety may constitute the most basic type of anxiety disorder (OAD, GAD; Brown & Barlow, 1992). This would be consistent with the high rates of comorbid OAD among children with another index anxiety disorder. However, Barlow proposes that early experiences lead some to focus anxiety on specific objects (SP), and others to focus on somatic (interoceptive) sensations (PD), social evaluation (SOP), or internal thoughts (OCD).

An additional factor has been proposed to account for the distinction between anxiety and depression in this and related models (L. A. Clark & Watson, 1991). Specifically, although both anxious and depressed individuals share high levels of negative affect, depression is also characterized by low levels of positive affect. This trait approach to the question, buttressed by considerable data from adult studies, is limited by its inability to account for chronology of onset. The relatively later onset of depressive disorders and of certain anxiety disorders may, however, be accounted for by developmental factors, including biological and neuroendocrine development, and the increased cognitive capacity for self-reflection (including rumination) and abstract thinking (Kovacs & Devlin, 1998).

Clinical Issues

What are the implications of comorbidity for assessment and treatment? In this section, it is assumed that clinical assessment will include systematic review of symptoms through a semistructured interview. In addition, because anxiety is an internalizing disorder, the review of symptoms should include the child or adolescent as the major informant. The high rates of comorbidity among the anxiety disorders indicate that, in the assessment of children or adolescents presenting with anxiety symptoms, a range of possible disorders should be assessed routinely. Knowledge of base rates and comorbidity rates can guide such assessment. With young children, for example, assessment of OAD, SAD, and SP is essential. If one of these disorders is present, SOP should also be assessed. Among adolescents, on the other hand, the clinician should routinely inquire about the later onset anxiety disorders (SOP, PD), as well as the earlier onset disorders. Lower base rate disorders, such as OCD, may best be addressed in the initial assessment by screening questions.

Relations between anxiety disorders and depression and between anxiety disorders and disruptive behavior disorders suggest additional assessment guidelines. Regarding depression and anxiety, comorbidity rates are so high that routine assessment of MDD and DD is essential in the assessment of anxious young people. Comorbidity with disruptive behavior disorders (ADHD, ODD, CD) is less frequent, suggesting that screening questions or use of parent rating scales may be the most efficient method to determine whether additional inquiry is indicated. Among adolescents, the high rate of comorbidity between anxiety and substance use disorders leads to the conclusion that substance use patterns (especially for nicotine, marijuana, and alcohol) should be inquired about routinely with teenagers.

Assuming that the clinician has conducted a thorough assessment, there remains the problem of deciding what disorder should be the primary focus of treatment. Brown and Barlow (1992) delineated three meanings of the notion that one diagnosis among two or more is the primary diagnosis: the disorder that occurred first in the patient's lifetime, the disorder that contributed to or caused the other(s), or the disorder that is currently causing the most functional impairment.

Consider two cases in which a child with OCD later develops a depressive disorder. The clinician may judge that the OCD was primary in the first sense (i.e., chronology of onset). In addition, the OCD may also be primary in the second sense, if OCD is a major source of the child's distress and self-critical, depressive thinking. Should the OCD then be the primary treatment target? The answer to this question depends on the issue of functional impairment. If the depression is a relatively mild one (DD), OCD may be the best initial treatment target. However, if the child has developed MDD, which may include suicidal ideation, for example, it would be imperative to treat the depression first before addressing OCD. In general, the third conceptualization of primary diagnosis, based on functional impairment, appears to be the most compelling in clinical practice and in treatment research.

Comorbidity of disorders presents a particular challenge to the treating clinician. In psychosocial treatment, comorbidity can cloud the focus of treatment and lead to therapist drift in treatment goals. Sessions may focus on one disorder, then the next, in response to patient material, but without allowing sufficient time or attention to resolve either disorder. Treatment for comorbid anxious children and adolescents, then, requires that the clinician decide on one of three possible systematic approaches. The treatment can target the primary disorder first and the comorbid condition second (sequential treatment). The treatment can target common processes underlying both disorders (common process treatment). The treatment can be an integrated approach to both disorders addressing processes that are relatively specific to each disorder (modular treatment).

Sequential treatment with psychosocial intervention is illustrated by a case in which a 7-year-old boy presents with OCD and ADHD. At the time of assessment, it is clear that the OCD is causing the most functional impairment and family distress, and that the ADHD is mild. In such a case, an empirically supported treatment for OCD, such as exposure and response prevention, would reasonably be implemented first. After improvement in the primary disorder is achieved, treatment for ADHD could be started.

Common process treatment can be illustrated with reference to anxiety and depression (Kendall et al., 1992). Kendall and colleagues delineated a cognitive-behavioral treatment approach based on the affective, behavioral, and cognitive processes common to both disorders. In the affective domain, children with anxiety and children with depression share the need to become comfortable with labeling and expressing a range of emotions and to learn the connections between their emotions, thoughts, and behaviors. In the behavioral domain, both can benefit from relaxation training, with comorbid children needing to enhance both the capacity to control physiological arousal and the capacity to generate positive imagery. In the cognitive domain, anxious and depressed children both benefit from learning to generate solutions to problems and to reinforce themselves for progress toward goals. For comorbid children, clinicians need to attend to the full sequence of cognitions that precede and follow a distressing event, because anxiety is associated with negative anticipatory cognitions and depression with self-critical subsequent cognitions.

Common process treatment may also be illustrated by the use of a single medication to treat both anxiety and depression. For example, OCD and major depression may both respond to the use of a selective serotonin reuptake inhibitor.

Modular treatment is illustrated in a cognitive-behavioral approach to primary depression with secondary anxiety (Curry et al., 2000). Modular treatment assumes that certain processes must be addressed in treating the primary disorder, and that others may be addressed as a function of comorbidity. For instance, in treating primary depression, such processes as mood monitoring, goal setting, increasing involvement in pleasant activities, problem solving, and cognitive restructuring are common to almost all cognitive-behavioral treatments and may be considered essential. Some of these processes are also included in CBT for anxiety, so their inclusion here is similar to their inclusion in common process treatment. However, other processes, such as relaxation training and affect regulation, are not essential components in treating depression. In the case of a comorbid anxious and depressed adolescent, these latter processes would be included in the treatment plan based on the judgment of the treating clinician.

SUMMARY

The anxiety disorders in children and adolescents are very frequently accompanied by additional disorders. In decreasing order of frequency, these additional disorders are likely to be a second anxiety disorder, a depressive disorder, or a disruptive behavior disorder. Although the very high frequency of comorbidity calls into question the adequacy of the current U.S. diagnostic system, the phenomenon of comorbidity also presents an opportunity to study the course and processes of developmental psychopathology in a more finely honed manner than was possible using more broadly defined diagnostic categories. For the practicing clinician and the clinical researcher, comorbidity presents challenges in assessment and especially in treatment. Much recent work in the development of treatments for child and adolescent disorders has focused on ameliorating specific disorders. The frequency of comorbidity, however, indicates that clinicians who apply empirically supported treatments for specific disorders to the care of young people will need to meet the needs of their patients by such methods as sequential, common process, or modular treatments.

REFERENCES

Albano, A. M., Chorpita, B. F., & Barlow, D. H. (1996). Childhood anxiety disorders. In E. J. Mash & R. A. Barkley (Eds.), *Child psychopathology* (pp. 196–242). New York: Guilford Press.

American Psychiatric Association. (1987). *Diagnostic and statistical manual of mental disorders: DSM-III-R* (3rd ed., rev.). Washington, DC: Author.

American Psychiatric Association. (1994). *Diagnostic and statistical manual of mental disorders: DSM-IV* (4th ed.). Washington, DC: Author.

Anderson, J. C., Williams, S. M., McGee, R., & Silva, P. A. (1987). *DSM-III* disorders in preadolescent children. *Archives of General Psychiatry, 44,* 69–76.

Angold, A., & Costello, E. J. (1993). Depressive comorbidity in children and adolescents: Empirical, theoretical, and methodological issues. *American Journal of Psychiatry, 150*(12), 1779–1791.

Angold, A., Costello, E. J., & Erkanli, A. (1999). Comorbidity. *Journal of Child Psychology and Psychiatry, 40*(1), 57–87.

Barlow, D. H. (2000). Unraveling the mysteries of anxiety and its disorders from the perspective of emotion theory. *American Psychologist, 55*(11), 1247–1263.

Bell-Dolan, D., & Brazeal, T. J. (1993). Separation anxiety disorder, overanxious disorder, and school refusal. In H. L. Leonard (Ed.), *Anxiety disorders: Child and Adolescent Psychiatric Clinics of North America* (pp. 563–580). Philadelphia: W. B. Saunders.

Benjamin, R. S., Costello, E. J., & Warren, M. (1990). Anxiety disorders in a pediatric sample. *Journal of Anxiety Disorders, 4,* 293–316.

Brent, D. A., Perper, J. A., Moritz, G., Liotus, L., Richardson, D., Canobbio, R., Schweers, J., et al. (1995). Posttraumatic stress disorder in peers of adolescent suicide victims: Predisposing factors and phenomenology. *Journal of the American Academy of Child and Adolescent Psychiatry, 34*(2), 209–215.

Brown, T. A., & Barlow, D. H. (1992). Comorbidity among anxiety disorders: Implications for treatment and *DSM-IV. Journal of Consulting and Clinical Psychology, 60*(6), 835–844.

Bukstein, O., Brent, D., & Kaminer, Y. (1989). Comorbidity of substance abuse and other psychiatric disorders in adolescents. *American Journal of Psychiatry, 146,* 1131–1141.

Butcher, J. N. (1996). Interpretation of the MMPI-2. In L. Beutler and M. Berren (Eds.). *Integrative assessment of adult personality* (pp. 206–239). New York: Guilford Press.

Caron, C., & Rutter, M. (1991). Comorbidity in child psychopathology: Concepts, issues, and research strategies. *Journal of Child Psychology and Psychiatry, 32*(7), 1063–1080.

Clark, D. B., & Neighbors, B. (1996). Adolescent substance abuse and internalizing disorders. *Child and Adolescent Psychiatric Clinics of North America, 5*(1), 45–55.

Clark, L. A., & Watson, D. (1991). Tripartite model of anxiety and depression: Psychometric evidence and taxonomic implications. *Journal of Abnormal Psychology, 107,* 74–85.

Clark, L. A., Watson, D., & Mineka, S. (1994). Temperament and personality in mood and anxiety disorders. *Journal of Abnormal Psychology, 103,* 103–116.

Cohen, P., Cohen, J., Kasen, S., Velez, C. N., Hartmark, C., Johnson, J., Rojas, M., Brook, J., et al. (1993). An epidemiological study of disorders in late childhood and adolescence: I. Age- and gender-specific prevalence. *Journal of Child Psychology and Psychiatry, 34*(6), 851–867.

Compton, S. N., Nelson, A. H., & March, J. S. (2000). Social phobia and separation anxiety symptoms in community and clinical samples of children and adolescents. *Journal of the American Academy of Child and Adolescent Psychiatry, 39,* 1040–1046.

Costello, E. J., Angold, A., Burns, B., Stangl, D. K., Tweed, D. L., Erkanli, A., & Worthman, C. M. (1996). The Great Smoky Mountains Study of Youth: Goals, design, methods, and the prevalence of *DSM-III-R* disorders. *Archives of General Psychiatry, 53,* 1129–1136.

Curry, J. F., Wells, K. C., Brent, D. A., Clarke, G. N., Rohde, P., Albano, A. M., Reinecke, M.A., et al. (2000). *Treatment for adolescents with depression study (TADS): Cognitive behavior therapy manual.* Unpublished manuscript, Duke University Medical Center, Durham, NC.

Deykin, E. Y., & Buka, S. L. (1997). Prevalence and risk factors for posttraumatic stress disorder among chemically dependent adolescents. *American Journal of Psychiatry, 154,* 752–757.

Douglass, H. M., Moffitt, T. E., Dar, R., McGee, R., & Silva, P. A. (1995). Obsessive-compulsive disorder in a birth cohort of 18–year-olds: Prevalence and predictors. *Journal of the American Academy of Child and Adolescent Psychiatry, 34*(11), 1424–1431.

Feehan, M., McGee, R., & Williams, S. M. (1993). Mental health disorders from age 15 to 18 years. *Journal of the American Academy of Child and Adolescent Psychiatry, 32*(6), 1118–1126.

Flament, M. F., Whitaker, A., Rapoport, J. L., Berg, C. Z., Kalikow, K., Sceery, W., & Shaffer, D. (1988). Obsessive compulsive disorder in adolescence: An epidemiological study. *Journal of the American Academy of Child and Adolescent Psychiatry, 27*(6), 764–771.

Francis, G., Last, C. G., & Strauss, C. C. (1992). Avoidant disorder and social phobia in children and adolescents. *Journal of the American Academy of Child and Adolescent Psychiatry, 31,* 1086–1089.

Geller, D. A., Biederman, J., Griffin, S., Jones, J., & Lefkowitz, T. R. (1996). Comorbidity of juvenile obsessive-compulsive disorder with disruptive behavior disorders. *Journal of the American Academy of Child and Adolescent Psychiatry, 35*(12), 1637–1646.

Geller, D. A., Biederman, J., Jones, J., Shapiro, S., Schwartz, S., & Park, K. S. (1998). Obsessive-compulsive disorder in children and adolescents: A review. *Harvard Review of Psychiatry, 5,* 260–273.

Giaconia, R. M., Reinherz, H. Z., Silverman, A. B., Pakiz, B., Frost, A. K., & Cohen, E. (1995). Traumas and posttraumatic stress disorder in a community population of older adolescents. *Journal of the American Academy of Child and Adolescent Psychiatry, 34*(10), 1369–1380.

Glod, C. A., & Teicher, M. H. (1996). Relationship between early abuse, posttraumatic stress disorder, and activity levels in prepubertal children. *Journal of the American Academy of Child and Adolescent Psychiatry, 34*(10), 1384–1393.

Goenjian, A. K., Pynoos, R. S., Steinberg, A. M., Najarian, L. M., Asarnow, J. R., Karayan, I., Ghurabi, M., et al. (1995). Psychiatric comorbidity in children after the 1988 earthquake in Armenia. *Journal of the American Academy of Child and Adolescent Psychiatry, 34*(9), 1174–1184.

Ialongo, N., Edelsohn, G., Werthamer-Larsson, L., Crockett, L., & Kellam, S. (1994). The significance of self-reported anxious symptoms in first-grade children. *Journal of Abnormal Child Psychology, 22,* 441–455.

Ialongo, N., Edelsohn, G., Werthamer-Larsson, L., Crockett, L., & Kellam, S. (1995). The significance of self-reported anxious symptoms in first-grade children: Prediction to anxious symptoms and adaptive functioning in fifth grade. *Journal of Child Psychology & Psychiatry & Allied Disciplines, 36,* 427–437.

Kaplow, J. B., Curran, P. J., Angold, A., & Costello, E. J. (2001). The prospective relation between dimensions of anxiety and the initiation of adolescent alcohol use. *Journal of Clinical Child Psychology, 30,* 316–326.

Kashani, J. H., & Orvaschel, H. (1988). Anxiety disorders in mid-adolescence: A community sample. *American Journal of Psychiatry, 145,* 960–964.

Kashani, J. H., & Orvaschel, H. (1990). A community study of anxiety in children and adolescents. *American Journal of Psychiatry, 147*(3), 313–318.

Keller, M. B., Lavori, P. W., Wunder, J., Beardslee, W. R., Schwartz, & Roth, J. (1992). Chronic course of anxiety disorders in children and adolescents. *Journal of the American Academy of Child and Adolescent Psychiatry, 31,* 595–599.

Kendall, P. C., & Brady, E. U. (1995). Comorbidity in the anxiety disorders of childhood. Implications for validity and clinical significance. In K. Craig (Ed.), *Anxiety and depression in adults and children* (pp. 3–36). Thousand Oaks, CA: Sage.

Kendall, P. C., Kortlander, E., Chansky, T. E., & Brady, E. U. (1992). Comorbidity of anxiety and depression in youth: Treatment implications. *Journal of Consulting and Clinical Psychology, 60,* 869–880.

Kessler, R. C., McGonagle, K. A., Zhao, S., Nelson, C. B., Hughes, M., Eshleman, S., Wittchen, H.-U., et al. (1994). Lifetime and 12–month prevalence of *DSM-III-R* psychiatric disorders in the United States. *Archives of General Psychiatry, 51,* 8–19.

Kessler, R. C., Sonnega, A., Bromet, E., Hughes, M., & Nelson, C. B. (1995). Posttraumatic stress disorder in the National Comorbidity Survey. *Archives of General Psychiatry, 52,* 1048–1060.

King, N. J., Gullone, E., Tonge, B. J., & Ollendick, T. H. (1993). Self-reports of panic attacks and manifest anxiety in adolescents. *Behavior Therapy and Research, 31,* 111–116.

Koltek, M., Wilkes, T. C. R., & Atkinson, M. (1998). The prevalence of post-traumatic stress disorder in an adolescent inpatient unit. *Canadian Journal of Psychiatry, 43,* 64–68.

Kovacs, M., & Devlin, B. (1998). Internalizing disorders in childhood. *Journal of Child Psychology and Psychiatry, 39*(1), 47–63.

Kovacs, M., Gatsonis, C., Paulauskas, S., & Richards, C. (1989). Depressive disorders in childhood: Vol. IV. A longitudinal study of comorbidity with and risk for anxiety disorders. *Archives of General Psychiatry, 46,* 776–782.

Last, C. G., Perrin, S., Hersen, M., & Kazdin, A. E. (1992). *DSM-III-R* anxiety disorders in children: Sociodemographic and clinical characteristics. *Journal of the American Academy of Child and Adolescent Psychiatry, 31*(6), 1070–1076.

Last, C. G., Perrin, S., Hersen, M., & Kazdin, A. E. (1996). A prospective study of childhood anxiety disorders. *Journal of the American Academy of Child and Adolescent Psychiatry, 35*(11), 1502–1510.

Last, C. G., Strauss, C. C., & Francis, G. (1987). Comorbidity among childhood anxiety disorders. *Journal of Nervous and Mental Disease, 175,* 726–730.

Leonard, H. L., Lenane, M. C., & Swedo, S. (1993). Obsessive-compulsive disorder. In H. L. Leonard (Ed.), *Anxiety Disorders: Child and Adolescent Psychiatric Clinics of North America* (vol. 2, pp. 655–666). Philadelphia: W. B. Saunders.

Lewinsohn, P. M., Hops, H., Roberts, R. E., Seeley, J. R., & Andrews, J. A. (1993). Adolescent psychopathology: I. Prevalence and incidence of depression and other *DSM-III-R* disorders in high school students. *Journal of Abnormal Psychology, 102*(1), 133–144.

March, J. S., Swanson, J. M., Arnold, L. E., Hoza, B., Conners, C. K., Hinshaw, S. P., Hechtman, L., et al. (2000). Anxiety as a predictor and outcome variable in the multimodal treatment study of children with ADHD (MTA). *Journal of Abnormal Child Psychology, 28*(6), 527–541.

Masi, G., Favilla, L., Mucci, M., & Millepiedi, S. (2000a). Depressive comorbidity in children and adolescents with generalized anxiety disorder. *Child Psychiatry and Human Development, 30*(3), 205–215.

Masi, G., Favilla, L., Mucci, M., & Millepiedi, S. (2000b). Panic disorder in clinically referred children and adolescents. *Child Psychiatry and Human Development, 31*(2), 139–151.

Masi, G., Mucci, M., Favilla, L., Romano, R., & Poli, P. (1999). Symptomatology and comorbidity of generalized anxiety disorder in children and adolescents. *Comprehensive Psychiatry, 40*(3), 210–215.

McGee, R., Feehan, M., Williams, S. M., Partridge, F., Silva, P. A., & Kelly, J. (1990). *DSM-III* disorders in a large sample of adolescents. *Journal of the American Academy of Child and Adolescent Psychiatry, 29*(4), 611–619.

Moreau, D., & Weissman, M. M. (1992). Panic disorder in children and adolescents: A review. *American Journal of Psychiatry, 149*(10), 1306–1314.

Ollendick, T. H., Mattis, S. G., & King, N. J. (1994). Panic in children and adolescents: A review. *Journal of Child Psychology and Psychiatry, 35*(1), 113–134.

Pine, D. S., Cohen, P., Gurley, D., Brook, J., & Ma, Y. (1998). The risk for early-adulthood anxiety and depressive disorders in adolescents with anxiety and depressive disorders. *Archives of General Psychiatry, 55,* 56–64.

Robins, L. N., Croughan, J., Williams, J. B. W., & Spitzer, R. L. (1981). *The NIMH Diagnostic Interview Schedule: Version III* (Publication ADM-T-42-3). Washington, DC: U.S. Public Health Service.

Swedo, S. E., Rapoport, J. L., Leonard, H., Lenane, M., & Cheslow, D. (1989). Obsessive-compulsive disorder in children and adolescents: Clinical phenomenology of 70 consecutive cases. *Archives of General Psychiatry, 46,* 335–341.

Valleni-Basile, L. A., Garrison, C. Z., Jackson, K. L., Waller, J. L., McKeown, R. E., Addy, C. L., & Cuffe, S. P. (1994). Frequency of obsessive-compulsive disorder in a community sample of young adolescents. *Journal of the American Academy of Child and Adolescent Psychiatry, 33*(6), 782–791.

Whitaker, A., Johnson, J., Shaffer, D., Rapoport, J. L., Kalikow, K., Walsh, B. T., Davies, M., et al. (1990). Uncommon troubles in young people: Prevalence estimates of selected psychiatric disorders in a nonreferred adolescent population. *Archives of General Psychiatry, 47,* 487–496.

World Health Organization. (1992–1994). *ICD-10: International statistical classification of diseases and related health problems* (10th rev.). Geneva, Switzerland: Author.

6

INTEGRATED PSYCHOSOCIAL AND PHARMACOLOGICAL TREATMENT

JOHN S. MARCH & THOMAS H. OLLENDICK

The marriage of molecular neuroscience and cognitive psychology is driving a revolution in how we understand the diagnosis and treatment of anxiety disorders across the life span (Kandel & Squire, 2000). It is increasingly clear that psychotropic medications work by biasing specific central nervous system information processes; it is less commonly acknowledged but no less true that psychosocial treatments also have both a somatic substrate and psychosocial valence. Put simply, drugs and psychotherapy work at least in part because they act on the brain (Hyman, 2000). Hence, when selecting a treatment strategy that is appropriate to the needs of children with anxiety disorders, the treating clinician must consider both medication and psychosocial treatment strategies, either alone or in combination with one another.

In a perfectly evidence-based world, selecting an appropriate treatment from among the many possible options would be reasonably straightforward. However, in the complex world of clinical practice, choices are rarely so clear-cut. Even when a comprehensive assessment produces an unambiguous diagnosis and readily defined target symptoms, expected outcomes vary by disorder, by treatment modality, and certainly by factors specific to the child, the clinician, and the setting(s) in which they live and work. Depending on the theoretical underpinning and nature of the treatment, psychotherapeutic options are generally more narrowly defined than drug treatments, which often have a broader spectrum of action. Implementing two distinct treatments can be complicated when they differ in dose and the time it takes to reach a desired outcome. Clinicians, children, and their families sometimes differ (and rightly so) in their preferences regarding choices of appropriate treatments. These, and other factors outlined below, complicate the choice of treatment strategy for many if not most families.

Matching treatment(s) to clinical problems also has become more complicated (albeit also more effective) as the field has moved from global, nonspecific interventions toward specific, problem-focused treatments keyed to particular *DSM-IV* diagnoses (Kazdin, 1997). In particular, the past 40 years has seen the emergence of diverse, sophisticated, empirically-supported, cognitive-behavioral, and pharmacological interventions that cover the range of childhood-onset anxiety disorders. Many clinicians and researchers now believe that the combination of disorder-specific cognitive-behavioral therapy (CBT) and medication administered in an evidence-based, disease-management model is the initial treatment of choice for many if not most children and adolescents with diagnosable anxiety disorders (see, for example, March, Frances, Kahn, & Carpenter, 1997).

In this context, it is often said that 50% of what we know about treating mentally ill children will be out of date and the other 50% will be wrong within 5 to 10 years. Sometimes it is hard to tell the two scenarios apart, but the message is clear: Although keeping up with a rapidly expanding evidence base is extraordinarily difficult (Sackett, Richardson, Rosenberg, & Haynes, 2000), keep up we must, because new developments point toward the improved outcomes that we and our patients desire (Barlow, Levitt, & Bufka, 1999). Nowhere is this truer than when divergent treatment options—be they medication or psychosocial—are on the menu.

An empirical literature on the value and place of combined versus unimodal treatment is just beginning to emerge in the pediatric and adult literatures. For example, randomized controlled trials in adults with panic disorder (Barlow, Gorman, Shear, & Woods, 2000) suggest advantages for combined drug and CBT over the respective monotherapies. Illustrating the fact that we cannot simply take for granted the assumption that two treatments are better than one, however, combination treatment does not appear to offer a significant advantage over CBT alone, at least in adults with obsessive-compulsive disorder, or OCD (Edna Foa, personal communication). With the notable exception of the Multimodal Treatment Study of Children with ADHD (MTA; Arnold et al., 1997a) there are no studies in mentally ill youth that have compared single modality treatments to each other or their combination against a control condition in the same patient population, though such studies are currently underway in OCD and teenage major depression.

In a stages-of-treatment model that emphasizes the practice of evidence-based medicine (EBM), this chapter provides a conceptual framework for how best to approach combining drug and psychosocial treatments at the level of the individual patient. The reader interested in exploring EBM should begin with the text by Sackett and colleagues (1997) before moving on to the excellent "User's Guides" series in the *Journal of the American Medical Association* (Guyatt & Rennie, 1993). The reader interested in how best to combine specific treatments for particular disorders would be well advised to consult the American Academy of Child and Adolescent Psychiatry practice parameters series (Dunne, 1997), textbooks that address the relative benefits of psychosocial and medication management (Hersen & Bellack, 1999; Pollack, Otto, & Rosenbaum, 1996; Van Hasselt & Hersen, 1993), and the few available empirically derived practice guidelines that include children and adolescents (Conners, March, Frances, Wells, & Ross, 2001; March et al., 1997; Pliszka et al., 2000a, 2000b).

COMBINING TREATMENTS IN A MULTIDISCIPLINARY FRAMEWORK

Disease-Management Model

Although it will be some time before stakeholder issues yield to a unifying body of widely accepted, scientific evidence concerning the etiopathogensis and treatment of the pediatric anxiety disorders, it was clear by the late 1970s that a biopsychosocially-oriented disease-management model is as powerful a change strategy in psychiatry as it is in other areas of medicine (Ludwig & Othmer, 1977). More specifically, the three features of the disease-management model—the concept of disease and diagnosis, the concept of etiology and treatment, and the nature of the doctor-patient relationship—come into play in clinical psychiatry and psychology just as they do in medicine more generally. Consistent with a biopsychosocial approach, combined treatment is the rule rather than the exception across most of medicine (cf. the treatment of hypertension with antihypertensives and weight reduction or the treatment of juvenile rheumatoid arthritis with ibuprofen and physical therapy). In this regard, the treatment of the anxious child can be thought of as partially analogous to the treatment of juvenile-onset diabetes, with the caveat that the target organ—the brain, in the case of major mental illness—requires psychosocial interventions of much greater complexity. The treatment of diabetes and anxiety disorder both involve medications: insulin for diabetes, and for anxiety, typically, a serotonin reuptake inhibitor. Each also involves an evidence-based psychosocial intervention that works in part by biasing the somatic substrate of the disorder toward more normal function. In diabetes, the psychosocial treatment of choice is diet and exercise, and in anxiety, it is exposure-based CBT. Success depends on the presence of risk and protective factors; not every patient has the same outcome. Bright youngsters from well-adjusted two-parent families typically do better with either diabetes or anxiety than those beset with tremendous psychosocial adversity. Thus, adversity when present appropriately becomes a target for intervention, usually to increase compliance with treatment for the primary illness. Finally, not everybody recovers completely, even with the best of available treatments, so some interventions need to target coping with residual symptoms, such as diabetic foot care in diabetes and helping patients and their families cope skillfully with residual symptoms in anxiety disorders.

Why Combine Psychosocial and Drug Treatments?

Psychosocial treatments usually are combined with medication for one of three reasons. First, in the initial treatment of the severely ill child, two treatments provide a greater "dose" and thus may promise a better and perhaps speedier outcome. For this reason, many patients with OCD opt for combined treatment, even though CBT alone may offer equal benefit (March & Leonard, 1998). Second, comorbidity frequently but not always requires two treatments, because different targets may require different treatments. For example, treating an 8-year-old who has attention-deficit/hyperactivity disorder (ADHD) and mild separation anxiety disorder with a psychostimulant and CBT is a reasonable treatment strategy (March et al., 2000). Even in a single anxiety disorder, important functional outcomes may vary in response to treatment. For example, anticipatory anxiety in the acutely separation-anxious child may be especially responsive to a benzodiazepine and reintroduction to school via gradual exposure (Kratochvil, Kutcher, Reiter, & March, 1999). Third, in the face of partial response, an augmenting treatment can be added to the initial treatment to improve the outcome in the symptom domain targeted by the initial treatment. For example, CBT can be added to an selective serotonin reuptake inhibitor (SSRI) for OCD to improve OCD-specific outcomes. In an adjunctive treatment strategy, a second treatment can be added to a first one to positively impact one or more additional outcome domains. For example, an SSRI can be added to CBT for OCD to handle comorbid depression or panic disorder.

Cognitive-Behavioral Therapy in a Medical Context

Most mental health clinicians are familiar with treatments that assume that psychological distress represents the outcome of historical and current relationship problems that must be uncovered and addressed in therapy. In contrast to these more story-oriented approaches to psychotherapy, CBT asks the clinician to adopt a problem-solving model in which he or she acts as a coach to teach the patient a set of adaptive coping skills (while at the same time assisting the patient in unlearning unskillful coping behaviors) for specific symptoms that are associated with distress and impairment in the present tense (March 2000; Ollendick & Seligman, 2000). Thus, CBT (unlike most other psychotherapeutic approaches) fits beautifully into a disease-management framework in which the symptoms of the illness and associated functional impairments are specifically targeted for treatment. The cornerstone of CBT is a careful functional analysis of problem behaviors that is governed by several important assumptions.

1. Behavior (normal as well as problem) is primarily governed by environmental contingencies (and in cognitive theory, by thoughts and emotions), such that the relationship between

thoughts, feelings, and behaviors is the primary focus of assessment and treatment.

2. The antecedents and consequences of target behaviors, as well as target behaviors themselves, must be operationally defined and accurately measured.

3. Behavior may differ across settings so that multi-informant, multimodal, multi-domain assessment is critical.

4. Treatment planning depends on careful assessment, including periodic reassessment of how behaviors have changed, with revision of treatment interventions as necessary.

Whereas these assumptions and procedures are not necessarily incompatible with pharmacological management, the level of specificity for functional outcomes is generally greater for CBT than for medication management. On the other hand, the level of monitoring for change should be roughly equal for both pharmacological and psychosocial interventions, because it is symptomatic change and improvement in functional outcomes that govern patient and clinician assessment of degree of improvement. To put it experimentally, CBT lends itself to viewing the treatment of each patient through the lens of one of several possible single-case designs (Ollendick & Cerny, 1981), which makes combining pharmacological and cognitive-behavioral interventions relatively straightforward.

Using a Stages-of-Treatment Model

As a general rule, it is always best to use the simplest, least risky, and most cost-effective treatment intervention available and to do so in a stages-of-treatment model to identify key decision points in the everyday treatment of patients with anxiety disorders. In particular, to be useful to clinicians, a treatment review must addresses the following:

1. *Selection of initial treatment.* Given evidence-based psychotherapy and pharmacotherapy and very few studies of combined versus unimodal treatment, the clinician must make a judgment about the relative benefits and risks of single versus combined treatment over the short and long terms. Besides relative effectiveness, the feasibility, acceptability, and tolerability of the treatment must also be considered. Additionally, the evidence base is often stronger for older, perhaps less optimal treatments, whereas newer treatments often are favored by experts even though the evidence base is weaker. The transition from tricyclic antidepressants to the SSRIs in the treatment of panic disorder provides an excellent example of how the introduction of a newer treatment complicates the selection of initial therapy solely on the basis of existing literature (Ballenger, 1993).

2. *Management of partial response.* Most patients improve substantially with current treatment. However, it is likely that most will not normalize, especially when functional outcomes rather than symptoms are considered. Furthermore, when a primary disorder remits, secondary problems often come to the fore. Thus, combining treatments is often more common as treatment progresses and the limits of initial treatment become apparent.

3. *The treatment-refractory patient.* When a patient has had two trials of different medications, and, when appropriate, combinations of medications as well as optimal psychosocial treatment, and when these trials are adequate in dose and duration, and the patient still shows little or no improvement, it is justifiable to label the patient as treatment resistant. In this situation, newer treatments, treatments with a lower probability of success, heroic treatments, and riskier combinations of treatment are all warranted.

4. *Maintenance treatment.* Finally, when a patient is a responder, it is critical from a personal and public health perspective to know how long to continue treatment at what dose and visit schedule before trying, if appropriate, to discontinue treatment. If discontinuation is desirable, and it may not be in the face of persisting symptoms or previous relapses, then the optimal schedule for discontinuing medications versus psychosocial treatment, given that these two modalities may show differences in durability of benefit, must be considered.

Most of the time, the extant treatment literature and, typically, unsystematic reviews of the treatment literature, do not provide much guidance past the choice of initial unimodal treatment. This is especially true for treatment reviews that focus on either medication or psychotherapy alone and hence cannot address the issue of combining treatments—in part because the authors reflect different treatment traditions (see, for example, March, 1999, and Turner & Heiser, 1999). Because this leaves out the majority of patients for whom combined treatment is appropriate if not de rigueur—namely those who are partial responders to initial treatment, those who have failed to respond to several treatments, and/or those who require a combination of treatments because of comorbidity (all crucial clinical decision nodes that are seldom studied under controlled scientific conditions)—typical unsystematic treatment reviews are of less use in clinical practice. To better standardize best practice at crucial clinical decision points that are not presently covered by general scientific knowledge, this chapter presents rules for combining information from studies of unimodal treatment and the use of expert-based practice guidelines to provide guidance in these clinically common and important situations, whereas the treatment chapters that follow use an expert-based, consciously multidisciplinary stages-of-treatment approach.

Being Consciously Multidisciplinary

Although cognitive-behavioral and pharmacological treatment strategies for anxious children readily combine, psychology and psychiatry are often at odds over stakeholder issues. We believe strongly that it is not possible to practice competent and ethical psychopharmacology without the availability of empirically supported psychotherapy. Similarly, it is not possible to practice competent and ethical psychotherapy without the availability of empirically supported psychopharmacology. Physicians (who typically write prescriptions) and psychologists (who, for the most part, have developed CBT and are better versed in it) must join hands in the care of individual patients, if for no other reason than that the complexity of modern mental health care is beyond the capacity of any one individual to master (March, Mulle, Stallings, Erhardt, & Conners, 1995). In this regard, the current generation of comparative treatment trials (see, for example, Jensen, 1999) nicely models both the benefits and the difficulties of multidisciplinary practice in which practitioners of both disciplines become stakeholders for the experiment (the research question) or the benefit of the individual patient (the clinical question). Without this commitment to multidisciplinary practice, we shortchange our patients.

USING EVIDENCE-BASED MEDICINE AS A FRAMEWORK FOR CONSIDERING WHETHER AND HOW TO COMBINE TREATMENTS

What Is Evidence-Based Medicine?

One of the more common criticisms of an evidence-based approach to clinical practice is that clinical trials and clinical practice are only weakly related. In research language, the external validity of many efficacy studies—defined as the extent to which the results of the research are generalizable to clinical populations—is limited by filters imposed by the methods for sample selection, assessment, and treatment. External validity is often contrasted with internal validity, that is, the extent to which a study is methodologically sound. Without internal validity, it is hard to argue for the external validity of a study. Nonetheless, many internally valid studies are not fully relevant to clinical practice, because the treatments used or the nature of the patients enrolled in these studies are dissimilar to clinical practice, and thus the results do not transfer easily to clinical practice settings. This is one of the reasons why the National Institute of Mental Health (NIMH) recently moved away from funding efficacy trials conducted in "relatively pure" patients toward effectiveness trials, such as the MTA, conducted with "messy" clinical samples and in "messy" clinical settings (Norquist & Magruder, 1998).

From the point of view of an individual practitioner hoping to conform to best-practice standards in caring for anxious children, it is critical therefore to quickly decide whether and how the results of a particular study are clinically relevant to clinical practice. EBM provides a simple, straightforward framework for accomplishing this task. Not an invocation to slavish adherence to an ill-defined gold standard, EBM is simply a set of tools that allows the conscientious, explicit, and judicious use of current best evidence in making decisions about the care of the individual patient through integrating individual clinical expertise with the best available external clinical evidence from systematic research (Guyatt, Sackett, & Cook, 1993, 1994; Guyatt, Sinclair, Cook, & Glasziou, 1999).

Steps in Evaluating the Usefulness of a Treatment Study

Whether used in approaching diagnosis, prognosis, or treatment, EBM always begins with selecting a specific question from among the panoply of clinically relevant questions presented by the care of a specific patient. As summarized in Table 6.1, the first step in evaluating a treatment question is to frame the question as a PECO: What are the *population*, the *exposure* to active treatment, the *control or comparison* condition, and the desired *outcome*? A simple PECO might be as follows: In children with OCD, what is the evidence that a serotonin reuptake inhibitor is better than placebo in reducing symptoms of OCD? Having framed the question as a PECO, the clinician can then turn for an answer to the increasingly EBM-optimized resources available on the Internet, such as the clinical queries algorithm on PubMed (http://www.ncbi.nlm.nih.gov/entrez/query.fcgi). More specifically, EBM provides a clear hierarchy of search strategies that move from EBM reviews, which mean that the clinician's work is already done, because all the relevant literature is already summarized, to critically appraised topics (CATs), which summarize one or two relevant articles, to the clinician's searching and critiquing the literature on his or her own. Full-text articles for many journals can be retrieved from OVID (http://www.ovid.com/site/index.jsp), which is available either as a subscription service or free from most academic libraries. Assuming that the designs and

Table 6.1. What Is a PECO?

Term	Definition	Example
Population	The target population to whom the treatment is intended to generalize	In children with separation anxiety disorder . . .
Exposure	The active treatment or treatments	is a selective serotonin reuptake inhibitor (SSRI) . . .
Control/Comparison	The control (inactive) or comparison (active) condition	better than pill PBO (a control) or treatment as usual (an active comparator) . . .
Outcome	The desired outcome (benefit) or undesired outcome (harm)	in reducing symptoms of separation anxiety?

outcomes are similar, the most recent or most powerful study likely is sufficient to construct a CAT. Conversely, when the literature is rich in randomized evidence, an up-to-date EBM review might be the most important source of information (Guyatt et al., 1999; see also Sackett et al., 2000, for a more detailed discussion of search strategies, systematic reviews, and CATs).

Having identified an article that is directly relevant to the question of interest, the next step is to evaluate the article for its validity and applicability to your patient. Table 6.2 summarizes the EBM approach to reviewing an article about treatment, which requires only a reasonably close reading of (a) the abstract, to get an overall summary of the question, method, and results; (b) the methods section, to assess validity and to identify the population studied; and (c), the results section, to understand the direction and clinical importance of the outcome. In the opposite of the usual approach, the introduction and discussion often can be skipped as an inefficient use of time (although such information might be extremely useful for other purposes).

Four relatively easy and commonsensical steps then provide an answer to the question of clinical relevance to your patient:

Step 1: Is the Study Valid?   Did the investigators use a randomized, controlled, blind design in which all patients were followed up at the end? Apart from intrinsic differences in the treatments themselves, were all the patients treated the same way? Without affirming these relatively straightforward parameters, it is impossible to know whether differences in the outcome reflect true differences in the impact of the treatments or some other characteristic of the study.

Step 2: What Were the Results?   Ideally, the results should be presented both dimensionally, using standardized and normed rating scales so that the reader can judge improvement toward or into the normal range, and categorically, to allow easy calculation of magnitude of clinical improvement. If the results are presented as change scores (the mean at posttreatment minus the mean at pretreatment for each treatment group), the actual mean scores for each treatment group at baseline should also be included so that the clinician can judge whether the amount of change moved the average patient into the normal range. If comorbidity is a factor, initial levels of comorbid symptomatology and changes in comorbidity over time should also be presented. Finally, the same questions that are asked about treatment effectiveness can be asked about harm, to answer the critical question: Is the treatment safe? (Levine et al., 1994).

Step 3: Are the Results Clinically Meaningful?   This is an important variable for clinicians desiring to ascertain whether the results of a clinical trial can be applied at the patient level. Traditionally, in psychiatry and psychology (Weisz, 2000), the magnitude of the effect has been portrayed in terms of small (.3), medium (.5) *or* large (> .8) effect sizes in standard deviation

Table 6.2. Evidence-Based Medicine (EBM) Applied to Treatment

Steps in Evaluating a Treatment Article	Main Points	Hints
Is there a clear question?	Frame the question as a PECO?	For any patient, there will be many possible questions. Hence, as an astute clinician, you must weigh the possible questions and, having done so, choose one or two. Then, having framed the question as a PECO, search the literature for (a) a systematic review; (b) a meta-analysis, (c) a relevant article, or (d) a treatment guideline that includes the question being asked, using EBM principles to evaluate the chosen article.
Are the results of the study valid?	Randomized controlled design? Investigators blind to treatment assignment? All patients treated the same way? All patients followed up?	After reading the abstract to get the big picture, quickly review the methods section to see if the research design meets minimal standards for interpretability.
What are the results?	Dimensional and categorical outcomes? Movement into the normal range? Comorbidity? Subgroup analyses? A safe treatment?	To quickly calculate an *NNT* (number needed to treat), look first for categorical results for the main outcome measure in the study, then for dimensional outcomes, and finally for other outcomes besides the main ones. If the results are presented as change scores, look for the baseline mean score to see how far the patient moved toward the normal range. Use this information to establish the *NNT*.

| *How strong was the effect?* | Calculate the *NNT*. Adjust the *NNT* for factors that might improve or decrease the expected response. The equivalent statistic for harm is the *NNH* (number needed to harm). | The *NNT* can be calculated without a special software program to do so, but confidence intervals and many other EBM statistics, although conceptually simple, are more easily done by using such a program. A widely used program with an EBM add-in is Syncalc (www. syncalc.com). Depending on the nature of and methods for detecting adverse events, the ratio of the *NNH* and *NNT* can be though of as the risk/benefit ratio. |
| *Are the results applicable to your patient?* | Is your patient represented? Were the clinically important outcomes considered? How long did the treatment last? Are the treatments worth the potential benefits, harms and costs? Can you provide the treatment? Will the patient accept the treatment? | In the methods section, quickly scan the inclusion and exclusion criteria to see if your patient falls within the types of patient entered into the study. If necessary, adjust the *NNT* so that the expectations for benefit match the divergence of your patient from the average patient in the study population. Factor in your preferences and expectations and preferences of your patient and family. |

Note. PECO = population/exposure/condition/outcome

units (Cohen, 1977). EBM uses a much simpler rubric, the number needed to treat, or *NNT*. In practice, the *NNT* represents the number of patients that need to be treated with the active treatment to produce one additional good outcome beyond that obtainable with the control or comparison condition. For example, an *NNT* of 10 means that you would have to treat 10 patients with the active treatment to find one that wouldn't have done just as well if assigned to the control treatment.[1] A very small *NNT* (that is, an *NNT* that approaches 1) means that a favorable outcome occurs in nearly every patient who receives the treatment and in relatively few patients in the comparison group. An *NNT* of 2 or 3 indicates that a treatment is quite effective. In contrast, *NNTs* above 30 or 40 fall in the realm of public health effects, although they may still be considered clinically relevant. Tables 6.3 and 6.4 present *NNT* calculations for *responders* (defined as those with a 25% reduction in Children's Yale-Brown Obsessive-Compulsive Scale [CY-BOCS] scores) and *excellent responders* (defined as those with normal scores, or CY-BOCS scores of less than 10) in children and adolescents with OCD treated with sertraline (March et al., 1998). *NNTs* of 5 and 10, respectively, confirm the implications in the change in mean score in the sertraline group, namely, that an average 6-point CY-BOCS drop (a pre- to posttreatment drop from 24 to 18), which parenthetically is consistent across pediatric and adult OCD SSRI trials (Greist, Jefferson, Kobak, Katzelnick, & Serlin, 1995; Leonard, March, Rickler, & Allen, 1997), leaves most patients in the clinically ill range. Used in this fashion, the *NNT* can help in making decisions between treatment options, for example, what to put in (which treatment is best) and when to take it out (how big is the effect) of the black bag.

Step 4: Is the Result Applicable to My Patient?   Before applying the results of this study to the care of an individual patient, it is important to understand the similarities between the research study and the particular clinical situation faced in the office. This can be accomplished quickly by asking the following questions:

> Is my patient represented in the research sample or were patients like mine excluded from the trial?
>
> Were the clinically important outcomes both functional (e.g., return to school) and disorder-specific (e.g., less anxiety)?
>
> How were the outcomes measured? Are they clinically meaningful, and can I apply these measures in my practice?
>
> To the extent that my patient has a better or worse prognosis that the average patient in the study, would an adjusted[2] *NNT* bias my choice of treatments (for example, toward combined drug and psychosocial treatment in a very ill multiply comorbid patient)?
>
> Are the treatments worth the potential benefits, harms, and costs?

Table 6.3. Response to Selective Serotonin Reuptake Inhibitors (SSRIs) in Pediatric Obsessive-Compulsive Disorder (OCD)

Response to SSRIs in OCD		*Relative Risk Reduction (RRR)*	*Absolute Risk Reduction (ARR)*	*Number Needed to Treat (NNT)*
Usual Control Event Rate (CER)	*SSRI Experimental Event Rate (EER)*	$\frac{EER\text{-}CER}{EER}$	EER-CER	1/AAR
25%	45%	$\frac{45\%\text{-}25\%}{45\%} = 44\%$	45%–25% = 20%	$\frac{1}{0.2}$ = 5 patients

Note. Using data from March (1998), responders were defined as having a decrease greater than 25% in Children's Yale-Brown Obsessive-Compulsive Scale scores (CY-BOCS), from baseline to end of treatment. Assuming, for simplicity's sake, 100 patients in each group, the 95% confidence interval (*CI*) for an *NNT* = 1 divided by limits on the *CI* of its *ARR* = 3 to 14, calculated

as $\pm 1.96 \sqrt{\frac{\text{CER} \times (1 - \text{CER})}{\text{\# of control pts.}} + \frac{\text{EER} \times (1 - \text{EER})}{\text{\# of exper. pts.}}} =$

> Can I and a colleague work together to provide the treatment in our treatment setting(s)?
>
> Will the patient accept the treatment?

The answers to these questions bring the research study to the level of direct patient care.

Example 1: Combined Treatment for Internalizing Disorders and School Refusal

The treatment of teenagers with severe anxiety, depression, and associated school refusal provides an excellent example of how EBM can be used to

Table 6.4. Excellent Response to Selective Serotonin Reuptake Inhibitors (SSRIs) in Pediatric Obsessive-Compulsive Disorder (OCD)

Response to SSRIs in OCD		*Relative Risk Reduction (RRR)*	*Absolute Risk Reduction (ARR)*	*Number Needed to Treat (NNT)*
Usual Control Event Rate (CER)	*SSRI Experimental Event Rate (EER)*	$\frac{EER\text{-}CER}{EER}$	EER-CER	1/AAR
5%	15%	$\frac{15\%\text{-}5\%}{5\%} = 44\%$	15%–5% = 10%	$\frac{1}{0.1}$ = 10 patients

Note. Using data from March (1998), excellent responders can be defined as having an end-of-treatment score of less than or equal to 10 on the Children's Yale-Brown Obsessive-Compulsive Scale (CY-BOCS). Assuming, for simplicity's sake, 100 patients in each group, the 95% confidence interval (*CI*) on an *NNT* = 1 divided by limits on the *CI* of its *ARR* = 5 to 55, calculated as in Table 6.3.

guide the combination of medication and psychosocial treatments in clinical practice. One of the most challenging clinical problems in pediatric psychiatry and psychology, these patients present with multiple behavioral and family problems and are often, if inappropriately, thought of as treatment refractory, even before treatment has begun (Bernstein, Borchardt, & Perwien, 1996; Bernstein, Warren, Massie, & Thuras, 1999). In a recently published study, Bernstein and colleagues (2000) asked the following question, framed as a PECO: "In school-refusing teenagers with combined anxiety and depressive disorders (the population), is imipramine plus CBT (the exposure) more effective than CBT plus pill PBO (the control) in returning patients to school (the outcome) after 8 weeks of treatment?" They used a balanced randomized parallel group design, complete follow-up, an intent-to-treat analysis, blind assessment, and (given pill PBO to balance the CBT-alone condition) equal treatment characteristics in each group, apart from the intervention. Over 8 weeks, they found a statistically significant difference favoring combined treatment over CBT alone for depression outcomes and in returning patients to school. The magnitude and precision of the NNT (NNT = 3, confidence interval [CI] = 1 to 4) for this notoriously difficult-to-treat population were quite impressive, indicating that combined CBT and medication is better than CBT alone for anxious-depressed school refusers.

The study by Bernstein and colleagues was initiated before SSRIs came into wide use in children and adolescents. A large number of studies have shown that the tricyclic antidepressants (TCAs) are not effective, on average, for children and adolescents with major depression (the results of a different EBM search) and that, apart from effectiveness, the TCAs are riskier and more complicated to use than the SSRIs (Birmaher, 1998; Leonard et al., 1997). Thus, we might want to ask, can we substitute an SSRI for the TCA imipramine, in combination with CBT, in this patient population? A recently published study from the Research Unit on Pediatric Psychopharmacology (RUPP) Anxiety Study Group (2001) network that compared fluvoxamine to PBO in children and adolescents with generalized, social, and separation anxiety disorders provides an unambiguous affirmative answer. With an NNT of 2 (CI = 1 to 3) in this study, we could reasonably assume that the Bernstein findings would have been as good or even better had they used fluvoxamine, though of course there is as yet no randomized evidence pointing in that direction. Given this new evidence and substantial expert opinion favoring the SSRIs over the TCAs in this patient population (Bernstein & Shaw, 1997; March, 1999), the substitution of an SSRI for imipramine seems eminently reasonable.

Example 2: Treatment for Children Exhibiting ADHD Comorbid With Anxiety

A large body of literature suggests that treatment with a psychostimulant is effective for externalizing symptoms in children with ADHD (Swanson,

1993). However, it has long been speculated that comorbid anxiety may adversely influence the outcome of drug treatment for ADHD (Pliszka, 1998). Whether this is true or would confer an advantage for behavioral or combined treatment was, until recently, unknown (Jensen, Martin, & Cantwell, 1997). Thus, given a patient with ADHD and anxiety, we might wish to know (framing the question as a PECO) whether, in the treatment of young children with ADHD comorbid with an anxiety disorder (the population), combined treatment (the exposure) has an advantage over treatment with medication or parent training alone (the comparison condition). A search of PubMed using the clinical queries option and the search terms *ADHD, anxiety, child,* and *combined treatment* would identify the primary outcome papers from the NIMH Collaborative Multimodal Treatment Study of Children with ADHD (MTA; MTA Cooperative Group, 1999a, 1999b) and a subsequent secondary analysis from the MTA Cooperative Group specifically addressing the impact of anxiety on treatment outcome (March et al., 2000).

The MTA study was designed to addresses a priori questions about the individual and combined effects of pharmacological and psychosocial (behavioral) treatment for children aged 7 to 9 with ADHD (Arnold et al., 1997b). The rationale and design of the MTA, which serves as a heuristically valuable example of how CBT and medication can and should be combined, have been reported elsewhere (Arnold et al., 1997b). Briefly, 579 children aged 7 to 9 meeting dimensional criteria for hyperactivity and *DSM-IV* criteria for ADHD, combined subtype, were randomly assigned to an intensive behavior therapy program (Beh), a titration-adjusted optimized medication management strategy (MedMgt), an interactive combination of Beh and MedMgt (Comb) in which dose and timing of interventions were adjusted for one treatment depending on response to the other, and a comparison group that was assessed and then referred to local community care resources (CC). Children and parents received comprehensive assessments at baseline, 3, 9, and 14 months, the treatment end point (Hinshaw et al., 1997). The Beh treatment consisted of 14 months of parent training, using both group and individual parent sessions, 4 months of classroom behavioral management by a trained paraprofessional working with the teacher, and an intensive 8-week summer treatment program (Wells et al., 2000). Optimal medication dosage was attained by acutely titrating medication (starting with methylphenidate and moving on as needed to other drugs) and subsequently adjusting the dose and timing of drug administration based on teacher and parent symptom ratings over the course of the study (Greenhill et al., 1996).

As recently summarized by Jensen and colleagues (2001), Comb and MedMgt interventions proved substantially superior to Beh and CC interventions for ADHD symptoms (MTA Cooperative Group, 1999a). Despite the fact that CC children were frequently medicated, these effects were clinically meaningful, with an *NNT* for Comb or MedMgt relative to CC of 2, indicating clearly that well-delivered treatment that includes medication is superior to less intensive community standard care. For other functioning domains (social skills, academics, parent-child relations, oppositional behavior, anxiety/depression), results suggested modest incremental benefits of the Comb intervention over the single component (MedMgt, Beh) treatments and community care (MTA Cooperative Group, 1999b).

Initial moderator analyses of MTA findings suggested that child anxiety ascertained by parent report on the Diagnostic Interview Schedule for Children 2.3 (DISC) differentially moderated the outcome of treatment (MTA Cooperative Group, 1999b). Left unanswered were questions regarding the nature of DISC anxiety, the impact of comorbid conduct problems on the moderating effect of DISC anxiety, and the clinical significance of DISC anxiety as a moderator of treatment outcome. Exploratory analyses by March and colleagues (2000) suggested that DISC Anxiety reflected parental attributions regarding child negative affectivity and associated behavior problems, particularly in the area of social interactions, rather than fearfulness, another core component of anxiety that is more typically associated with phobic symptoms. Analyses using hierarchical linear modeling (HLM) indicated that the moderating effect of DISC Anxiety continued to favor the inclusion of psychosocial treatment for anxious ADHD children irrespective of the presence or absence of comorbid conduct problems. This effect, although clinically meaningful, was confined primarily to parent-reported outcomes involving disruptive behavior, internalizing symptoms, and inattention, and was generally stronger for combined than unimodal treatment. Contravening earlier studies, no adverse effect of anxiety on medication response for core ADHD or other outcomes in anxious or nonanxious ADHD children was demonstrated (March et al., 2000). In particular, the effect sizes for the comorbid group were often double that for the nonanxious group (large versus small) irrespective of treatment modality, with Comb intervention more often showing large and Beh and MedMgt showing medium effects.[3] Thus, granting defensible (Jensen, 1999) limitations in generalizibility (Boyle & Jadad, 1999), the MTA would suggest that the clinician, when confronted with a child with ADHD comorbid with anxiety, would be wise to recommend a combination of intensive MedMgt and, at a minimum, parent training, whereas for the uncomplicated youngster, MedMgt alone will likely suffice at least as the initial treatment of choice.

Example 3: Managing Partial Response to an SSRI in OCD

Many patients in clinical practice have already failed to respond or have had a partial response to one or more initial treatments, especially when treatment was unimodal. Though robust responses may still occur, on probabilistic grounds such patients may be expected to have a poorer response to another unimodal treatment in the same class. For example, an OCD patient on a third SSRI trial is likely to have as much as a threefold-lower chance of responding than a treatment-naive patient (Greist et al., 1995; March et al., 1998). If your patient falls into this group, the NNT will be higher than the average research subject. Taking $F = .3$, the *NNT* for an excellent response from monotherapy with an SSRI would be 30 (or 10 divided by 0.3), illustrating the fact that repeated SSRI trials are unlikely to result in full remission of symptoms. The corresponding *NNT* from open trials in which CBT was added to medication is approximately 2 (Franklin et al., 1998; March, Mulle, & Herbel, 1994). Hence, if full remission is the aim, the EBM-informed clinician would likely opt for adding CBT to an SSRI early in the course of partial response in preference to switching to another SSRI.

LESSONS FROM THE CLINIC

Although a full discussion of treatment planning procedures for each anxiety disorder is beyond the scope of this chapter (see Part II, chapters 7 to 15, this volume), several important principles merit elaboration insofar as they apply to combining drug and psychosocial interventions. The discussion here is primarily clinical in orientation. A seminal discussion of methodological issues that arise in comparative treatment trials can be found in a series of articles describing the MTA study (Arnold et al., 1997a; Greenhill, Pine, March, Birmaher, & Riddle, 1998; Hinshaw et al., 1997; Wells, 2001)

Importance of Differential Therapeutics

In the disease-management model, differential therapeutics—identifying treatment interventions that are appropriate to differing treatment targets—can be seen as something like a game of pickup sticks. To function effectively, the clinician has to correctly identify the targets of treatment at the symptom level (the sticks) before sequencing a set of target-specific interventions (picking up the sticks in the proper order) to help the patient get better. Put in terms of the disease-management model, current best-practice treatment requires clear specification of the behavioral/emotional syndrome (e.g., separation anxiety disorder); the problems within that syndrome (afraid to leave home for school); and within those problems, the symptoms (e.g., won't sleep alone) targeted for intervention. Both behavioral/symptomatic (clinician-assigned) and functional (usually parent- and child-assigned) outcomes must be factored into the selection of psychosocial and drug treatments. Depending on the nature of the problem, some outcomes will be more easily approached with medication, and others with psychosocial interventions. Some will require both to be successful (e.g., that the treatments interact rather than simply providing an additive or complimentary impact).

Rating Scales: The Sphygmomanometers of Psychiatry and Psychology

Most children present for mental health care because of problematic behaviors either in their relationships or in the school setting. Starting with the presenting complaint, the clinician's task is to understand these behaviors in the context of the constraints to normal development that underlie them and, in doing so, to construct a differential diagnostic hierarchy that informs a thoughtfully constructed treatment regimen. In this sense, the task of the psychiatric diagnostician is much like that of the cardiologist confronted with a patient with chest pain. Based on the presenting complaint and probabilities attending important demographic factors, he or she identifies the most likely diagnosis, possible comorbid conditions, and the important diagnoses to rule out in the process of reaching a decision regarding differential therapeutics. Of all the assessment technologies available to us, gender-, age-, and race-normed rating scales perhaps offer the most efficient way to collect information regarding both internalizing and externalizing behavioral disturbances at home and school. Excellent scales with good psychometric properties are now available for self-report of conduct problems (Conners, 1995), fear (Ollendick, 1983), anxiety (March, 1998), and depression (Kovacs, 1985). Besides assessing an overall construct (e.g., anxiety), a child self-report measure such as the Multidimensional Anxiety Scale for Children (March, 1998) also provides useful information at the factor (e.g., physical anxiety symptoms) and item (e.g., suffocation anxiety) level. Clinician-administered ratings scales, such as CY-BOCS (Scahill et al., 1997) also are de rigueur for some disorders, such as OCD. Using reliable and valid rating scales both speeds the interview and begins a dialogue between clinician and patient about the patient's most troubling symptoms, thereby facilitating treatment planning. Such a procedure is consistent with medical evaluation procedures across other medical specialties and meets goals for guidelines-based practice in managed care, irrespective of whether a disease is conceptualized categorically (e.g., schizophrenia) or dimensionally (e.g., generalized anxiety). For example, just as hypertension is the extreme of blood pressure abnormalities and presages multiple adverse medical outcomes, anxiety disorders can be conceptualized dimensionally, with the extreme of the distribution presaging functional impairments now and in the future, rendering rating scales something like the sphygmomanometer: an essential tool for best practice.

Not All Treatments Can or Should Be Tailored

Although some argue that tailored treatment is the optimum treatment for all children (see Hickling & Blanchard, 1997, and Ollendick & King, 2000, for discussion), not all treatment interventions can be matched to specific targets, no matter how obvious such a match ought to be. For example, because behavior therapy reduces impulsivity in ADHD (a change usually attributed to medication) and psychostimulants reduce negative parent-child interactions (a change readily attributable to behavioral treatment) these two conceptually divergent treatment and outcome dimensions may not be separable when it comes to matching treatments to individual patients (Wells, 2001). In some domains, even theoretically reasonable treatment interventions do not necessarily impact the match targeted outcomes. For example, cognitive therapy (with the exception of anger management) has not been found to be effective in controlled studies of children with ADHD, despite ample evidence for cognitive deficits in children with ADHD (Abikoff, 1991). Given that developmentally sensitive, face-valid interventions don't necessarily work and that treatment effects are not always highly specific, the public health benefit of empirically supported, standardized treatment packages will likely be greater than using theoretically-driven tailored treatments in most, if not all, circumstances. The exception is when a treatment component can be clearly shown to have a negative or no effect in the care of an individual child, in which case it should, of course, be omitted. However, there is no literature to suggest that unmatched treatment ingredients provided to mentally ill children in the context of a comprehensive treatment intervention produce negative effects (for example, the provision of family interventions to nonanxious or dysfunctional parents; the empirical literature simply provides little or no guidance on this topic).

Pay Careful Attention to Dose-Response and Time-Response Issues

When initiating pharmacological treatment, the ability to construct a dose-response curve and to analyze time-action effects is critical. The former refers to the relationship between dose of drug and the presence of benefits and adverse effects. Establishing these relationships depends on understanding time-action parameters, namely the relationship between the timing of administration and onset of response, maximum responsiveness, and loss or offset of drug effect. Departures from a linear dose-response pattern are common, with some children showing a threshold effect (no response below a threshold level) and others a quadratic response (linear at lower doses and degradation at higher doses). Thus, each child requires an individually constructed dose-response curve, taking into consideration the time-action effects of the drug at each dose before making dosage adjustments. With a single-drug treatment, many clinicians start with the lowest possible dose, working upward toward the end of the expected time-response window until benefits are maximized or the patient shows prohibitive side effects. Using this strategy, which assumes that enough drug is enough, eliminates the possibility of undertreatment while minimizing potential adverse events.

Psychosocial treatments also exhibit distinctive dose-response and time-response characteristics. For example, the average number of weekly CBT sessions is 12 to 16, irrespective of anxiety disorder targeted; or, stated differently, the dose- and time-response parameters for expected benefit are about 16 sessions over 16 weeks with a range of 6 to 24 weeks (March, 2000). Thus, when combining drug and psychosocial treatments, it is often possible to capitalize on between-treatment differences in dose-response and time-response parameters. With respect to dose response, there is some evidence that treatments can be additive (i.e., the impact of the dose of both treatments is the same as the impact of each treatment separately added together) or multiplicative (two treatments act synergistically, i.e., the benefit of the combination is greater than the additive combination). This may be the case for OCD, for which partial response to medication is the rule rather than the exception (March et al., 1997, 1998). Similarly, when combining treatments, a lower dose of one or both treatments may be necessary, with a resultant decrease in expense, inconvenience, or adverse events. For example, the MTA study implemented a very high dose behavioral condition—a 14-month combination of parent training, a summer treatment program, and a classroom intervention (Wells et al., 2000)—that resulted in a slightly lower methylphenidate dose in the combined group (28 mg per day in divided doses) as compared with the methylphenidate does in the medication-alone group (36 mg per day in divided doses). Even when dose does not differ, capitalizing on differences in time-response parameters can lead to reduced patient suffering. By blocking full panic episodes and quelling anticipatory anxiety, combining clonazepam with an SSRI in the acutely separation-anxious youngster allows more-rapid reintroduction to school than CBT or an SSRI alone might permit (Birmaher, Yelovich, & Renaud, 1998; March, 1999). Finally, even when not divergent, time-response parameters can be matched to the patient's benefit, such as when the patient experiences maximum benefit from an SSRI just at the time he or she reaches the top of the stimulus hierarchy in CBT (March, 1998).

Monitor Desired and Undesirable Outcomes

Once treatment has started, the clinician inevitably will need to conduct additional assessments to collect detailed data on the patient's specific symptomatology and its impact on his or her day-to-day functioning. Such data will serve as a basis for evaluating the progress and rate of treatment and, when possible, for differentiating response to behavioral as contrasted with pharmacological interventions. This is why most CBT manuals include detailed mapping of triggers, responses, and problem-maintaining factors (including family, peer, and school problems) as a routine part of treatment planning. Why evaluate outcome? First, tracking symptoms requires the clinician to periodically update the problem target list, minimizing the possibility that new or reemerging symptoms will be missed. Second, child and parent ratings allow the clinician to address discrepant views of the child's progress or differential treatment response across different settings where they exist. Third, rating scales provide a detailed view of how the child is progressing in treatment. In this regard, disorder-specific rating scales, whether standardized or tailored to the patient's problems, provide a far richer source of information than global measures, which simply involve therapist ratings of general outcome. Using OCD as an example, patient symptomatology can be tracked with the CY-BOCS symptoms checklist, OCD symptoms with the CY-BOCS itself, specific CBT targets with a stimulus hierarchy, and reductions in anxiety in response to successive exposure trials (e.g., habituation curves), using a fear thermometer.

Think Developmentally

As with academic skills, children normally acquire social-emotional (self and interpersonal) competencies across time. The failure to do so, relative to age-, gender-, and culture-matched peers, may reflect capacity limitations; individual differences in the rate of skill acquisition for specific competencies; environmental factors; the development of a major mental illness; or a combination of these (Ollendick, Grills, & King, 2001; Ollendick & Vasey, 1999). The task of the mental health practitioner considering how to combine drug and psychosocial treatment(s) is to understand the presenting symptoms in the context of constraints to normal development, and to devise a tailored target-specific treatment program that eliminates those constraints so that the youngster can resume a normal developmental trajectory insofar as is possible. Depending on the nature of the symptoms and the capacity of the child and family to make use of target-specific psychosocial interventions, the blend of treatments may vary in a developmental context. For example, irrespective of medication treatment, school avoidance in a separation-anxious 6-year-old will require dyadic CBT in which control is transferred from the therapist to the parent and then to the child, whereas a school-avoidant teen with panic disorder likely will do best with individual CBT, perhaps in association with behavioral family therapy (Silverman & Kurtines, 1996; Wells, 1995).

Emphasize Psychoeducation

Despite our best intentions, parents and children sometimes come away with only a limited appreciation of the complexity of their situation as we (clinicians) appreciate it at the end of the diagnostic process. In this context, one of the primary goals of the assessment stage is to use the diagnostic process as a vehicle for psychoeducation regarding the rationale for combining treatments. When initiating or elaborating treatment in the context of partial response, the intention must always be to implement interventions that present a logically consistent and compelling relationship between the disorder, the treatment, and the specified outcome. In particular, it is critical to keep the various treatment targets (the nails) distinct with respect to the various treatment interventions (the hammers) so that aspects of the symptom picture that are likely to require or respond to psychosocial intervention, as distinct from psychopharmacological intervention, are kept clear insofar as is possible. This emphasis encourages a detailed review of the indications, risks, and benefits of proposed and alternative treatments, after which parents and patient generally chose a treatment protocol consisting of a monotherapy (typically either CBT or medication) or CBT in combination with an appropriate medication intervention.

It is important to note that a number of complexities are present when treating pediatric patients that are not present with most adults, and that these may influence whether and how to combine treatments. For example, children rarely seek treatment themselves (Ollendick & Cerny, 1981). Alternatively, parents are sometimes cornered into treatment by pressure from school or social service agencies. Children commonly fear being labeled as mental patients by peers or extended family, and parents often have strong preferences regarding psychosocial or psychopharmacological treatment. Thus, exploring the meaning of the diagnosis and resultant medication or psychosocial interventions to the child and to his or her parents is important. Placing medication in the context of an overall treatment plan that includes psychosocial treatment may ease the route to using medications, as when the OCD patient is willing to try medication because concomitant CBT offers not only improved outcomes but also a lesser chance of relapse when medication is discontinued. Finally, despite the power of pharmacological treatments, it is clear that the outcome of major mental illness is heavily dependent on the ability of the supporting environment to facilitate access to and compliance with effective treatment. This is the opposite of biological determinism, and the savvy clinician who understands this perspective takes pains to point out that the greater the degree of CNS dysregulation, the more important becomes skillful coping by the child and by the child's environment.

PRACTICE GUIDELINES

When the empirical literature and expert opinion agree regarding best practice—what treatment or combination of treatments likely will work best for most if not all patients—it usually is not acceptable to substitute a less for a more empirically supported treatment, as doing so would not be in the patient's best interest. For example, initiating treatment for newly diagnosed OCD with other than CBT, an SSRI, or the combination of the two would be difficult to justify (King, Leonard, & March, 1998; March et al., 1997). Because clinician, family, and patient preferences all come in to play when choosing between these treatments, any one of the three options is acceptable as initial treatment, although the clinician ought to suggest that the probability of acute and long-term remission is greater if CBT is included in the treatment mix (King et al., 1998; March et al., 1997).

Furthermore, for many clinically important decisions, it is unlikely that there will ever be randomized evidence. For example, how many SSRI trials should precede a clomipramine trial in the partially responsive child with OCD? How long does one wait before adding an SSRI when treating a child with OCD who is not particularly responsive to weekly CBT? Under conditions of uncertainty (e.g., absent data-driven agreement regarding best practice), there is little reason to be dogmatic regarding treatment choice and more reason to weight the available treatment options in light of clinician and patient preference. How, then, do we define best practice when the available literature provides little guidance? Although their ultimate utility will depend on improving the evidence base (Chambless & Ollendick, 2001; Weisz & Hawley, 1998), treatment guidelines offer one increasingly attractive option (Dunne, 1997; Frances, Kahn, Carpenter, Frances, & Docherty, 1998). In the EBM framework, guidelines are defined as systematically developed statements to assist practitioners and patients in making decisions about appropriate health care for specific clinical circumstances (Sackett et al., 2000). In contrast to unsystematic clinical reviews, which typically focus on a content area rather than on a specific clinical question or set of questions linked to clinical decision nodes, a systematically assembled guideline begins with a clear question (e.g., what CBT components are effective as initial treatment for the depressed teenager?) or set of decision nodes (e.g., specification of best-practice treatment for OCD in a stages-of-treatment model), uses an explicit search strategy, specifies criteria for evaluating the evidence, provides a clear statement of real or potential biases in interpretation of the review, and concludes with a recommendation for use of the guideline in making decisions about the care of individual patients. As a result, an empirically based guideline provides expert consultation (without the expert) regarding best-practice options at the "bedside." Note that consultation in a subspecialty clinic may be the recommended option, for example, when a patient fails to respond to standard interventions in the primary care setting (Conners et al., 2001).

Guidelines of varying quality are available, and more are under development as the idea of *care maps* gains increasing credence in psychiatric practice, as it has in pediatrics (Bergman, 1999). The practice parameters of the American Academy of Child and Adolescent Psychiatry (AACAP), which tend to focus on content surveys for initial treatment, are perhaps the best known to child and adolescent psychiatrists (Dunne, 1997); similar efforts are underway in psychology (Ammerman, Hersen, & Last, 1999; Weisz, 2000; Weisz & Hawley, 1998). Empirically based guidelines that systematically poll the experts and employ a stages-of-treatment framework are available for ADHD (Conners et al., 2001; Pliszka et al., 2000a, 2000b) and OCD (March et al., 1997). The Expert Consensus Guidelines Series for OCD (March et al., 1997), which heavily influenced the AACAP Practice Parameters on OCD (King et al., 1998), provides an excellent example of a comprehensive guideline that includes both psychosocial and medication management in the context of a stages-of-treatment model (the full guideline is available for downloading at http://www.psychguides.com). As shown in Figure 6.1, which presents the guideline in flowchart format, the experts (an even mixture of psychiatrists and psychologists) recommend starting with CBT or CBT plus an SSRI, depending on severity and pattern of comorbidity; both recommend that patients started on SSRI monotherapy who are partial responders be augmented with CBT. Thus, experts generally consider CBT a first-line augmentation strategy and medication augmentation a second-line option. Options for treatment resistant OCD include high (intensive) dosing strategies for both CBT and medications, aggressive polypharmacy, and, in some cases, neurosurgery. Maintenance treatment recommendations depend on severity of symptoms, residual symptoms, and previous relapse history, all of which bias toward longer treatment even in the presence of CBT, which is generally believed to be of more durable benefit than medication once medication is withdrawn.

OVERALL STRATEGIES FOR ACUTE PHASE TREATMENT OF OCD

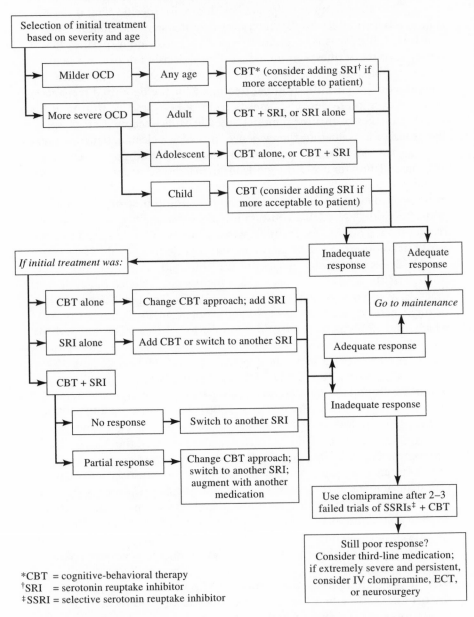

Figure 6.1. Expert consensus treatment guidelines for OCD

TACTICS FOR DURATION AND INTENSITY OF TREATMENT DURING ACUTE AND MAINTENANCE PHASES

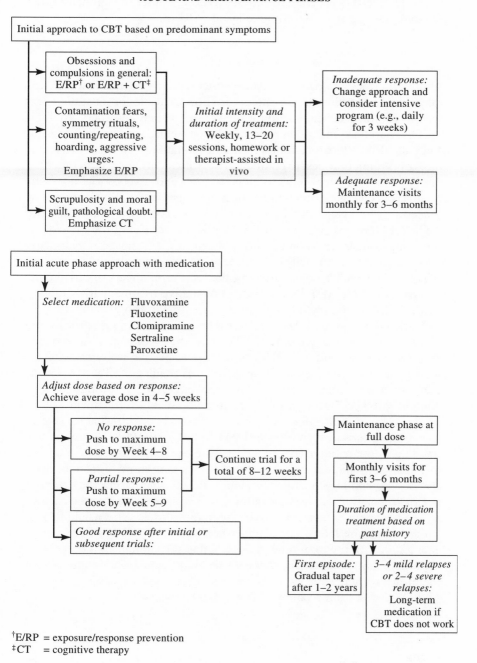

Initial approach to CBT based on predominant symptoms

Obsessions and compulsions in general: E/RP† or E/RP + CT‡

Contamination fears, symmetry rituals, counting/repeating, hoarding, aggressive urges: Emphasize E/RP

Scrupulosity and moral guilt, pathological doubt. Emphasize CT

Initial intensity and duration of treatment: Weekly, 13–20 sessions, homework or therapist-assisted in vivo

Inadequate response: Change approach and consider intensive program (e.g., daily for 3 weeks)

Adequate response: Maintenance visits monthly for 3–6 months

Initial acute phase approach with medication

Select medication: Fluvoxamine Fluoxetine Clomipramine Sertraline Paroxetine

Adjust dose based on response: Achieve average dose in 4–5 weeks

No response: Push to maximum dose by Week 4–8

Partial response: Push to maximum dose by Week 5–9

Good response after initial or subsequent trials:

Continue trial for a total of 8–12 weeks

Maintenance phase at full dose

Monthly visits for first 3–6 months

Duration of medication treatment based on past history

First episode: Gradual taper after 1–2 years

3–4 mild relapses or 2–4 severe relapses: Long-term medication if CBT does not work

†E/RP = exposure/response prevention
‡CT = cognitive therapy

165

Finally, illustrating the importance of systematically derived expert opinions, the experts (answering the questions posed earlier) recommend a trial of clomipramine after two to three failed SSRI trials.

CONCLUSION

Although cynics bemoan our relatively incomplete evidence base, empirically supported unimodal treatments are now available for most disorders seen in clinical practice, including the various anxiety disorders, ADHD, OCD, Tourette's, major depression, schizophrenia, and autism (see King and Ollendick, 2000, for a review). Despite limitations in the research literature concerning how best to combine acute treatments, long-term outcome of combined treatment, effectiveness of drugs and psychosocial interventions across divergent outcome domains and ages, and optimal assessment procedures for selecting whether and how to combine treatments, the empirical literature also is increasingly positive regarding the benefits of short- and longer-term combinations of drug and psychosocial treatments for some, if not all, mentally ill children and adolescents. In addition to the MTA study, which is now examining the long-term impact of early intensive treatment for ADHD, multisite comparative treatment trials funded by the NIMH that include a combined treatment arm are underway in pediatric OCD and in adolescent depression. (For more information on the Pediatric OCD Treatment Study [POTS] and the Treatment of Adolescents with Depression Study [TADS], visit their respective websites: http://www2.mc.duke.edu/pcaad and http://www.nimh.nih.gov.) Taken together, these studies and others about to be undertaken (in anxiety, eating, and conduct disorders) begin to approach the question of which treatment—drug, psychosocial or combination—is best for which child with what set of predictive characteristics (Jensen, 1999; March & Curry, 1998). As our understanding of the pathogenesis of mental illness in youth increases, dramatic treatment innovations inevitably will accrue, including knowledge about when and how to combine treatments. Hence, the clinician facing the daunting task of keeping up with the rapid advances in evidence regarding the diagnosis and treatment of mental illness in children and adolescents would be well advised to acquire at least a basic understanding of the tools of EBM (Sackett et al., 2000). In the meantime, it is likely that the combination of targeted medication and psychosocial therapies skillfully applied across time affords the most plausible basis for sustained benefit in children, adolescents, and adults suffering from a variety of major mental illnesses.

NOTES

This research was supported by NIMH Grants 1 K24 MHO1557 to Dr. March and by contributions from the Robert and Sarah Gorrell family. This material was adapted from a chapter by March and Wells on an evidence-based approach to combining pharmacotherapy and psychotherapy in March (2002).

1. Starting with a dimensional response metric, ES is a measure of the average response in standard deviation units calculated as MC minus ME divided by SD_{pooled}, where ME represents the mean of the experimental treatment, MC represents the mean of the control treatment, and SD_{pooled} represents pooling of the standard deviations from within both groups at the end of treatment. Starting with a categorical response metric, NNT is a measure of the average response presented as the probability of response in single patient units. Arithmetically, the NNT is the inverse of the absolute risk reduction $(1/ARR)$ defined as the percentage of response in the experimental group minus the percentage of response in the control condition. When benefit (a positive response) rather than risk (e.g., mortality) is the outcome, the ARR is often rephrased as the absolute benefit increase or ABI. For example, if 80% of patients respond to Treatment X and 30 percent to a PBO control condition, the ABI is 50% and the NNT is 2, a very robust response. As shown in Tables 6.3 and 6.4, confidence intervals can be calculated for the NNT to estimate the precision of the treatment effect. Confidence intervals are a useful measure of the certainty that, you, the clinician can provide when informing your patient about the expected outcome of treatment. The wider the CI, the less confident you can be about predicting correctly.

2. Modifications to the NNT can be introduced depending on the extent to which the individual patient resembles the patients assembled in the treatment study. Specifically, the NNT can be adjusted for a specific patient by estimating the patient's likelihood of change relative to the average control patient in the trial report, expressing the likelihood as a decimal fraction, F, and then dividing the reported NNT by F. For example, if your patient is judged to have half of the probability of a positive response as the average control patient, then F equals 0.5 and the NNT divided by F equals twice the unadjusted NNT.

3. It is straightforward but arithmetically complex to obtain an NNT from Cohen's absent data on categorical response (Furukawa, 1999; Guyatt, Juniper, Walter, Griffith, & Goldstein, 1998). However, by referring to standard statistical tables, it is relatively easy to obtain the proportions of the normal distribution above and below a specified ES (e.g., the proportion of the control group scores that are less than the average score in the experimental group: $ES = 0$ [50%], $ES = .4$ [66%], $ES = .8$ [79%], $ES = 1$ [84%], and $ES = 1.6$ [95%]). Assuming this to represent a minimum clinically significant difference—an almost certain overstatement—yields corresponding $NNTs$ that range from approximately 10 to 1, which in turn reflects the fact that most published treatments work at least in some patients.

REFERENCES

Abikoff, H. (1991). Cognitive training in ADHD children: Less to it than meets the eye. *Journal of Learning Disabilities, 24*(4), 205–209.

Ammerman, R., Hersen, M., & Last, C. (1999). *Handbook of prescriptive treatments for children and adolescents* (2nd ed.). New York: Allyn & Bacon.

Arnold, L. E., Abikoff, H. B., Cantwell, D. P., Conners, C. K., Elliott, G., Greenhill, L. L., Hechtman, L., et al. (1997a). National Institute of Mental Health Collaborative Multimodal Treatment Study of Children with ADHD (the MTA): Design challenges and choices. *Archives of General Psychiatry, 54*(9), 865–870.

Arnold, L. E., Abikoff, H. B., Cantwell, D. P., Conners, C. K., Elliott, G., Greenhill, L. L., Hechtman, L., et al. (1997b). NIMH Collaborative Multimodal Treatment Study of Children with ADHD (the MTA): Design, methodology and protocol evolution. *Journal of Attention Disorders, 2*(3), 141–158.

Ballenger, J. C. (1993). Panic disorder: Efficacy of current treatments. *Psychopharmacology Bulletin, 29*(4), 477–486.

Barlow, D. H., Gorman, J. M., Shear, M. K., & Woods, S. W. (2000). Cognitive-behavioral therapy, imipramine, or their combination for panic disorder: A randomized controlled trial [see comments]. *Journal of the American Medical Association, 283*(19), 2529–2536.

Barlow, D. H., Levitt, J. T., & Bufka, L. F. (1999). The dissemination of empirically supported treatments: A view to the future. *Behaviour Research and Therapy, 37*(Suppl. 1), S147–S162.

Bergman, D. A. (1999). Evidence-based guidelines and critical pathways for quality improvement. *Pediatrics, 103*(1 Suppl. E), 225–232.

Bernstein, G. A., Borchardt, C. M., & Perwien, A. R. (1996). Anxiety disorders in children and adolescents: A review of the past 10 years. *Journal of the American Academy of Child and Adolescent Psychiatry, 35*(9), 1110–1119.

Bernstein, G. A., Borchardt, C. M., Perwien, A. R., Crosby, R. D., Kushner, M. G., Thuras, P. D., & Last, C. G. (2000). Imipramine plus cognitive-behavioral therapy in the treatment of school refusal. *Journal of the American Academy of Child and Adolescent Psychiatry, 39*(3), 276–283.

Bernstein, G. A., & Shaw, K. (1997). Practice parameters for the assessment and treatment of children and adolescents with anxiety disorders: American Academy of Child and Adolescent Psychiatry. *Journal of the American Academy of Child and Adolescent Psychiatry, 36*(Suppl. 10), 69S–84S.

Bernstein, G. A., Warren, S. L., Massie, E. D., & Thuras, P. D. (1999). Family dimensions in anxious-depressed school refusers. *Journal of Anxiety Disorders, 13*(5), 513–528.

Birmaher, B. (1998). Should we use antidepressant medications for children and adolescents with depressive disorders? *Psychopharmacology Bulletin, 34*(1), 35–39.

Birmaher, B., Yelovich, A. K., & Renaud, J. (1998). Pharmacologic treatment for children and adolescents with anxiety disorders. *Pediatric Clinics of North America, 45*(5), 1187–1204.

Boyle, M. H., & Jadad, A. R. (1999). Lessons from large trials: The MTA study as a model for evaluating the treatment of childhood psychiatric disorder. *Canadian Journal of Psychiatry, 44*(10), 991–998.

Chambless, D. L., & Ollendick, T. H. (2001). Empirically supported psychological interventions: Controversies and evidence. *Annual Review of Psychology, 52*, 685–716.

Cohen, J. (1977). *Statistical power analyses for the behavioral sciences.* New York: Academic Press.

Conners, C. (1995). *Conners' Rating Scales.* Toronto, CA: Multi-Health Systems.

Conners, C. K., March, J. S., Frances, A., Wells, K. C., & Ross, R. (2001). Expert Consensus Guidelines Series: Treatment of attention-deficit/hyperactivity disorder. *Journal of Attention Disorders, 4*(Suppl. 1), 1–128.

Dunne, J. E. (1997). Introduction: History and development of the practice parameters. *Journal of the American Academy of Child and Adolescent Psychiatry, 36*(Suppl. 10), 1S–3S.

Frances, A., Kahn, D., Carpenter, D., Frances, C., & Docherty, J. (1998). A new method of developing expert consensus practice guidelines [see comments]. *American Journal of Managed Care, 4*(7), 1023–1029.

Franklin, M. E., Kozak, M. J., Cashman, L. A., Coles, M. E., Rheingold, A. A., & Foa, E. B. (1998). Cognitive-behavioral treatment of pediatric obsessive-compulsive disorder: An open clinical trial. *Journal of the American Academy of Child and Adolescent Psychiatry, 37*(4), 412–419.

Furukawa, T. A. (1999). From effect size into number needed to treat. *Lancet, 353*(9165), 1680.

Greenhill, L. L., Abikoff, H. B., Arnold, L. E., Cantwell, D. P., Conners, C. K., Elliott, G., Hechtman, L., et al. (1996). Medication treatment strategies in the MTA Study: Relevance to clinicians and researchers. *Journal of the American Academy of Child and Adolescent Psychiatry, 35*(10), 1304–1313.

Greenhill, L. L., Pine, D., March, J., Birmaher, B., & Riddle, M. (1998). Assessment issues in treatment research of pediatric anxiety disorders: What is working, what is not working, what is missing, and what needs improvement. *Psychopharmacology Bulletin, 34*(2), 155–164.

Greist, J. H., Jefferson, J. W., Kobak, K. A., Katzelnick, D. J., & Serlin, R. C. (1995). Efficacy and tolerability of serotonin transport inhibitors in obsessive-compulsive disorder: A meta-analysis [see comments]. *Archives of General Psychiatry, 52*(1), 53–60.

Guyatt, G. H., Juniper, E. F., Walter, S. D., Griffith, L. E., & Goldstein, R. S. (1998). Interpreting treatment effects in randomised trials. *British Medical Journal, 316*(7132), 690–693.

Guyatt, G. H., & Rennie, D. (1993). Users' guides to the medical literature [editorial]. *Journal of the American Medical Association, 270*(17), 2096–2097.

Guyatt, G. H., Sackett, D. L., & Cook, D. J. (1993). Users' guides to the medical literature: II. How to use an article about therapy or prevention. A. Are the results of the study valid? Evidence-Based Medicine Working Group. *Journal of the American Medical Association, 270*(21), 2598–2601.

Guyatt, G. H., Sackett, D. L., & Cook, D. J. (1994). Users' guides to the medical literature: II. How to use an article about therapy or prevention. B. What were the results and will they help me in caring for my patients? Evidence-Based Medicine Working Group. *Journal of the American Medical Association, 271*(1), 59–63.

Guyatt, G. H., Sinclair, J., Cook, D. J., & Glasziou, P. (1999). Users' guides to the medical literature: XVI. How to use a treatment recommendation. Evidence-Based Medicine Working Group and the Cochrane Applicability Methods Working Group. *Journal of the American Medical Association, 281*(19), 1836–1843.

Hersen, M., & Bellack, A. S. (1999). *Handbook of comparative interventions for adult disorders* (2nd ed.). New York: Wiley.

Hickling, E. J., & Blanchard, E. B. (1997). The private practice psychologist and manual-based treatments: Post-traumatic stress disorder secondary to motor vehicle accidents [see comments]. *Behaviour Research and Therapy, 35*(3), 191–203.

Hinshaw, S., March, J., Abikoff, H., Arnold, L., Cantwell, D., Conners, C., Elliott, G., et al. (1997). Comprehensive assessment of childhood attention-deficit/hyperactivity disorder in the context of a milti-site, multimodal clinical trial. *Journal of Attention Disorders, 1*(4), 217–234.

Hyman, S. E. (2000). The millennium of mind, brain, and behavior. *Archives of General Psychiatry, 57*(1), 88–89.

Jensen, P. S. (1999). Fact versus fancy concerning the multimodal treatment study for attention-deficit hyperactivity disorder. *Canadian Journal of Psychiatry,* *44*(10), 975–980.

Jensen, P. S., Hinshaw, S. P., Swanson, J. M., Greenhill, L. L., Conners, C. K., Arnold, L. E., Abikoff, H. B., et al. (2001). Findings from the NIMH Multimodal Treatment Study of ADHD (MTA): Implications and applications for primary care providers. *Journal of Developmental and Behavioral Pediatrics,* *22*(1), 60–73

Jensen, P. S., Martin, D., & Cantwell, D. P. (1997). Comorbidity in ADHD: Implications for research, practice, and *DSM-V. Journal of the American Academy of Child and Adolescent Psychiatry, 36*(8), 1065–1079.

Kandel, E., & Squire, L. (2000). Neuroscience: Breaking down scientific barriers to the study of brain and mind. *Science, 290,* 1113–1120.

Kazdin, A. E. (1997). A model for developing effective treatments: Progression and interplay of theory, research, and practice. *Journal of Clinical Child Psychology, 26*(2), 114–129.

King, R. A., Leonard, H., & March, J. (1998). Practice parameters for the assessment and treatment of children and adolescents with obsessive-compulsive disorder. *Journal of the American Academy of Child and Adolescent Psychiatry, 37*(10, Suppl).

Kovacs, M. (1985). The Children's Depression Inventory (CDI). *Psychopharmacology Bulletin, 21,* 995–998.

Kratochvil, C., Kutcher, S., Reiter, S., & March, J. (1999). Pharmacotherapy of pediatric anxiety disorders. In S. Russ & T. Ollendick (Eds.), *Handbook of psychotherapies with children and families* (pp. 345–366). New York: Plenum Press.

Leonard, H. L., March, J., Rickler, K. C., & Allen, A. J. (1997). Pharmacology of the selective serotonin reuptake inhibitors in children and adolescents. *Journal of the American Academy of Child and Adolescent Psychiatry, 36*(6), 725–736.

Levine, M., Walter, S., Lee, H., Haines, T., Holbrook, A., & Moyer, V. (1994). Users' guides to the medical literature: IV. How to use an article about harm. Evidence-Based Medicine Working Group. *Journal of the American Medical Association, 271*(20), 1615–1619.

Ludwig, A. M., & Othmer, K. (1977). The medical basis of psychiatry. *American Journal of Psychiatry, 134*(10), 1087–1092.

March, J. (1998a). Cognitive behavioral psychotherapy for pediatric OCD. In M. Jenike & L. Baer & Minichello (Eds.), *Obsessive-compulsive disorders* (3rd ed., pp. 400–420). Philadelphia: Mosby.

March, J. (1998b). *Manual for the Multidimensional Anxiety Scale for Children (MASC).* Toronto: Multi-Health Systems.

March, J. (1999). Current status of pharmacotherapy for pediatric anxiety disorders. In D. Beidel (Ed.), *Treating anxiety disorders in youth: Current problems and future solutions* (pp. 42–62). Washington, DC: National Institute of Mental Health/Anxiety Disorders Association of America.

March, J. (2000). Child psychiatry: Cognitive and behavior therapies. In B. Sadock & V. Sadock (Eds.), *Kaplan & Sadock's comprehensive textbook of psychiatry* (7th ed., pp. 2806–2812). New York: Williams and Wilkins.

March, J. S. (2002). Combining medication and psychosocial treatments: An evidence-based medicine approach. *International Review of Psychiatry, 14*(2), 155–163.

March, J., Frances, A., Kahn, D., & Carpenter, D. (1997). Expert Consensus

Guidelines Series: Treatment of obsessive-compulsive disorder. *Journal of Clinical Psychiatry, 58*(Suppl. 4), 1–72.

March, J., Mulle, K., & Herbel, B. (1994). Behavioral psychotherapy for children and adolescents with obsessive-compulsive disorder: An open trial of a new protocol-driven treatment package. *Journal of the American Academy of Child and Adolescent Psychiatry, 33*(3), 333–341.

March, J., Mulle, K., Stallings, P., Erhardt, D., & Conners, C. (1995). Organizing an anxiety disorders clinic. In J. March (Ed.), *Anxiety disorders in children and adolescents* (pp. 420–435). New York: Guilford Press.

March, J. S., Biederman, J., Wolkow, R., Safferman, A., Mardekian, J., Cook, E. H., Cutler, N. R., et al. (1998). Sertraline in children and adolescents with obsessive-compulsive disorder: A multicenter randomized controlled trial [see comments]. *Journal of the American Medical Association, 280*(20), 1752–1756.

March, J. S., & Curry, J. F. (1998). Predicting the outcome of treatment. *Journal of Abnormal Child Psychology, 26*(1), 39–51.

March, J. S., & Leonard, H. L. (1998). OCD in children: Research and treatment. In R. Swinson, J. Rachman, M. Antony, & M. Richter (Eds.), *Obsessive-compulsive disorder: Theory, research, and treatment* (pp. 367–394). New York: Guilford.

March, J. S., Swanson, J. M., Arnold, L. E., Hoza, B., Conners, C. K., Hinshaw, S. P., Hechtman, L., et al. (2000). Anxiety as a predictor and outcome variable in the multimodal treatment study of children with ADHD (MTA) [In-process citation]. *J Abnorm Child Psychol, 28*(6), 527–541.

MTA Cooperative Group (1999a). A 14–month randomized clinical trial of treatment strategies for attention-deficit/hyperactivity disorder: Multimodal treatment study of children with ADHD [In-process citation]. *Archives of General Psychiatry, 56*(12), 1073–1086.

MTA Cooperative Group (1999b). Moderators and mediators of treatment response for children with attention-deficit/hyperactivity disorder: the multimodal treatment study of children with attention-deficit/hyperactivity disorder. *Archives of General Psychiatry, 56*(12), 1088–1096.

Norquist, G. S., & Magruder, K. M. (1998). Views from funding agencies. *National Institute of Mental Health, Med Care, 36*(9), 1306–1308.

Ollendick, T. H. (1983). Reliability and validity of the Revised Fear Survey Schedule for Children (FSSC-R). *Behaviour Research and Therapy, 21*, 685–692.

Ollendick, T. H., & Cerny, J. A. (1981). *Clinical behavior therapy with children.* New York: Plenum Press.

Ollendick, T. H., Grills, A. E., & King, N. J. (2001). Applying developmental theory to the assessment and treatment of childhood disorders: Does it make a difference? *Clinical Psychology and Psychotherapy, 8*, 304–314.

Ollendick, T. H., & King, N. J. (2000). Empirically supported treatments for children and adolescents. In P. C. Kendall (Ed.), *Child and adolescent therapy* (2nd ed.). New York: Guilford Press.

Ollendick, T. H., & Seligman, L D. (2000). Cognitive-behaviour therapy. *Recent Advances in Paediatrics, 52*, 135–150.

Ollendick, T. H., & Vasey, M. W. (1999). Developmental theory and the practice of clinical child psychology. *Journal of Clinical Child Psychology, 28*, 457–466.

Pliszka, S. (1998). Comorbidity of attention-deficit/hyperactivity disorder with psychiatric disorder: An overview. *Journal of Clinical Psychiatry, 59*(Suppl 7), 50–58.

Pliszka, S. R., Greenhill, L. L., Crismon, M. L., Sedillo, A., Carlson, C., Conners, C. K., McCracken, J. T., et al. (2000a). The Texas Children's Medication Algorithm Project: Report of the Texas Consensus Conference Panel on Medication Treatment of Childhood Attention-Deficit/Hyperactivity Disorder: Part I. Attention-deficit/hyperactivity disorder. *Journal of the American Academy of Child and Adolescent Psychiatry, 39*(7), 908–919.

Pliszka, S. R., Greenhill, L. L., Crismon, M. L., Sedillo, A., Carlson, C., Conners, C. K., McCracken, J. T., et al. (2000b). The Texas Children's Medication Algorithm Project: Report of the Texas Consensus Conference Panel on Medication Treatment of Childhood Attention-Deficit/Hyperactivity Disorder: Part II. Tactics: Attention-deficit/hyperactivity disorder. *Journal of the American Academy of Child and Adolescent Psychiatry, 39*(7), 920–927.

Pollack, M. H., Otto, M. W., & Rosenbaum, J. F. (1996). *Challenges in clinical practice: Pharmacologic and psychosocial strategies.* New York: Guilford Press.

Research Unit on Pediatric Psychopharmacology Anxiety Study Group. (2001). Fluvoxamine for the treatment of anxiety disorders in children and adolescents. *New England Journal of Medicine, 344*(17), 1279–1285.

Sackett, D., Richardson, W., Rosenberg, W., & Haynes, B. (1997). *Evidence-based medicine.* London: Churchill Livingston.

Sackett, D., Richardson, W., Rosenberg, W., & Haynes, B. (2000). *Evidence-based medicine* (2nd ed.). London: Churchill Livingston.

Scahill, L., Riddle, M. A., McSwiggin-Hardin, M., Ort, S. I., King, R. A., Goodman, W. K., Cicchetti, D., et al. (1997). Children's Yale-Brown Obsessive-Compulsive Scale: Reliability and validity. *Journal of the American Academy of Child and Adolescent Psychiatry, 36*(6), 844–852.

Silverman, W., & Kurtines, W. (1996). *Anxiety and phobic disorders: A pragmatic approach.* New York: Plenum.

Swanson, J. (1993). Effect of stimulant medication on hyperactive children: A review of reviews. *Exceptional Child, 60,* 154–162.

Turner, S., & Heiser, N. (1999). Current status of psychological interventions for childhood anxiety disorders. In D. Beidel (Ed.), *Treating anxiety disorders in youth: Current Problems and future solutions* (pp. 63–76). Washington, DC: National Institute of Mental Health/Anxiety Disorders Association of America.

Van Hasselt, V. B., & Hersen, M. (1993). *Handbook of behavior therapy and pharmacotherapy for children: A comparative analysis.* Boston: Allyn & Bacon.

Weisz, J. R. (2000). Agenda for child and adolescent psychotherapy research: On the need to put science into practice [see comments]. *Archives of General Psychiatry, 57*(9), 837–838.

Weisz, J. R., & Hawley, K. M. (1998). Finding, evaluating, refining, and applying empirically supported treatments for children and adolescents [see comments]. *Journal of Clinical Child Psychology, 27*(2), 206–216.

Wells, K. (1995). Family therapy. In J. March (Ed.), *Anxiety disorders in children and adolescents* (pp. 401–419). New York: Guilford Press.

Wells, K. (2001). Comprehensive vs. matched psychosocial treatment in the MTA study: Conceptual and empirical issues. *Journal of Clinical Child Psychology, 30*(1), 131–135.

Wells, K. C., Pelham, W. E., Jr., Kotkin, R. A., Hoza, B., Abikoff, H. B., Abramowitz, A., Arnold, L. E., et al. (2000). Psychosocial treatment strategies in the MTA study: rationale, methods, and critical issues in design and implementation [In-process citation]. *Journal of Abnormal Child Psychology, 28*(6), 483–505.

II

ASSESSMENT AND TREATMENT OF SPECIFIC DISORDERS

7

SPECIFIC PHOBIA

GOLDA S. GINSBURG & JOHN T. WALKUP

Sometimes a fear is simply a fear, but at other times, a specific fear is just the tip of the anxiety iceberg. The majority of children with specific phobias also have another anxiety disorder. In this chapter, we discuss specific phobia (SP) as both a solitary phenomenon and a symptom of another, more globally impairing, anxiety disorder. This distinction is of particular significance when assessing SP, evaluating the role of comorbid conditions, creating a hierarchy for treatment, and evaluating partial and nonresponders to treatment.

Our goal is to review what is currently known about SP in youth. Readers should be cognizant that several methodological flaws plague this literature. Most problematic is that few studies of SP have effectively ruled out other psychiatric disorders as a cause of the observed fearfulness and avoidance. Not applying the appropriate exclusion criteria in studies of SP is most common prior to publication of *DSM-III-R* in 1987. Sadly, some studies subsequent to 1987 have not identified whether the circumscribed fear and avoidance behavior is truly specific or whether it is the most obvious manifestation of another condition. This fundamental problem in the assessment of SP for research studies makes it very difficult to evaluate the literature to date. Despite this limitation, a growing body of research indicates that promising assessment and treatment strategies exist for SP. It is unclear, however, if these straightforward treatment strategies will generalize to other anxiety symptoms in those with comorbid anxiety disorders.

CLINICAL MANIFESTATIONS

Fearfulness is a universal human experience, and descriptions of its phenomenology have a long and rich history in literature, cinema, and science. In the scientific realm, researchers have documented that mild fears occur as part of children's normal development (Morris & Kratochwill, 1983). In contrast, estimates of clinically impairing fears, referred to as simple phobias in older versions of the *DSM*, occur in 2% to 9% of youth (e.g., Anderson, Williams, McGee, & Silva, 1987; Bird et al., 1988; Costello & Borkovec, 1993; Costello et al., 1988; Essau, Conradt, & Petermann, 2000; Kashani & Orvaschel, 1990). There are several hallmark differences between mild or common fears and SPs. Specifically, unlike common fears, SPs are associated with severe distress, usually lead to avoidance of the fear-provoking object or situation, do not remit with reassurance or information, and result in significant impairment in the daily functioning of children and their families.

The clinical manifestations of SP are best represented by the three-response system—behavioral, cognitive, and physiological—proposed by Lang (1977; see King, Hamilton, & Ollendick, 1988, for review). The primary behavioral manifestation is avoidance of the feared object or situation. For example, children with an SP of insects may not leave their home or may avoid entering certain rooms in their homes (e.g., the basement or garage) to avoid a possible encounter with a bug. Children with an SP of choking may refuse to eat, and children with an SP of medical procedures (such as injections) may refuse to go to doctors' appointments or to hospitals. When confronted with the feared object or situation, children with SPs may suffer quietly but may also tantrum, cry, or even become aggressive to escape the situation.

In terms of the cognitive system, children often report catastrophic beliefs or negative expectancies that involve physical or personal injury (e.g., "The bug will bite me," "I'll choke and die"). Last, children with SP often show physiological responses in the presence of, or in anticipation of, the feared object or situation, such as accelerated heart rate, sweating, shakiness, physical complaints, muscle tension, and vasovagal fainting associated with blood/injection/injury (American Psychiatric Association [APA], 1994; Last, 1991; Page, 1994).

Few studies have systematically examined the clinical manifestations of SP across gender or racial/ethnic groups. With respect to gender, there is a growing literature indicating that girls have higher rates of SP, report more mild fears, and are perceived by others as more fearful than boys in both frequency and intensity (e.g., Anderson et al., 1987; Croake, 1969; Graziano & de Giovanni, 1979; Ollendick, 1983; Ollendick & King, 1994; Ollendick, Yang, Dong, Xia, & Lin, 1995; Ollendick, Yule, & Ollier, 1991; Silverman & Nelles, 1988b). Although few studies have explored the reasons for these differences, biological and psychosocial factors have been implicated. Further research is needed, however, to fully understand the gender differences in the clinical phenomenology of SP.

With respect to ethnic/racial variations, existing research among clinical populations of anxious youth suggest that there are more similarities than differences in the clinical manifestations of SP. For instance, Ginsburg and Silverman (1996) and Last and Perrin (1993) found no differences in rates of SP and levels of fearfulness between white and Hispanic and white and African American children who presented at pediatric anxiety clinics. Among community samples, comparisons of self-reported fears across various ethnic/racial groups in the United States and between the United States and other countries show differences in the content of some fears but also a great deal of similarity, with 5 of the most common 10 fears endorsed being the same across most countries examined (Ollendick, Yang, King, Dong, & Akande, 1996; see Fonseca, Yule, & Erol, 1994, for a review).

DIAGNOSIS AND CLASSIFICATION

According to the *DSM-IV* (APA, 1994), an SP is a persistent and excessive fear in the presence of, or in anticipation of, a circumscribed object or event. Based on this classification system, there are five subtypes of SPs: animal (e.g., cats, dogs, insects), natural environment (e.g., storms, heights, water), blood/injection/injury (e.g., seeing blood, needles), situational (e.g., public transportation, elevators, flying), and other (e.g., loud noises, costume characters). To receive the diagnosis, children must display a persistent, recurrent, or excessive fear reaction toward an object or situation (or all of these). Crying, having tantrums, freezing, or clinging is often a manifestation of this fear reaction. Generally, the phobic situation is avoided or is experienced with severe distress. Children's symptoms must be continuous for 6 months and must significantly impair functioning (at school, home or with peers).

Children should only be given a diagnosis of SP when other anxiety conditions have been ruled out. Specifically, a diagnosis of SP is unwarranted if the child's fear is restricted to situations that involve separation (as in separation anxiety disorder, or SAD), social evaluation and embarrassment (as in social phobia, or SOP), dirt/contamination (as in obsessive-compulsive disorder, or OCD), fears of having a panic attack and being unable to escape or both (as in panic with or without agoraphobia) or part of a larger reaction to a traumatic event (as in posttraumatic stress disorder), or a pervasive pattern of worrying (as in generalized anxiety disorder).

Comorbidity

Several studies have examined the types of comorbid disorders present in clinic-referred children with SP (e.g., Last, Strauss, & Francis, 1987; Last, Perrin, Hersen, & Kazdin, 1992; Silverman & Hammond-Laurence, 1997; Strauss & Last, 1993). Taken together, these studies suggest that over 60% of children with SP have some type of comorbid psychiatric disorder. Among children with SP who also have a comorbid disorder, 50% to 75% have another anxiety disorder (present or lifetime), with SAD being the most frequently occurring comorbid disorder. Other disorders found to be commonly comorbid with SP in clinic samples include depressive disorders and disruptive disorders (Last et al., 1992; Last et al., 1987; Strauss & Last, 1993).

In contrast to the above studies, early findings from nonclinical samples suggested that SP tended to occur alone (Anderson et al., 1987). However, more recent evidence suggests that SP may indeed co-occur with other disorders. For instance, in a recent epidemiological study of adolescents with SP, Essau et al. (2000), found that the most common comorbid disorder was another anxiety disorder (47%), followed by depressive disorders (36%) and somatoform disorders (33%).

Differential Diagnosis

In light of the high rates of comorbidity, it is likely that many children will present with an SP that is part of a complex psychiatric picture. As noted earlier, other anxiety disorders or medical conditions must be ruled out prior to assigning a diagnosis of SP. School refusal, often labeled school phobia, has historically been considered a type of SP. However, children refuse school for myriad reasons (Bernstein & Garfinkel, 1986; Burke & Silverman, 1987; Kearney & Silverman, 1997) that may or may not be related to SP. For instance, children may refuse to attend school because they fear speaking in class and social humiliation (SOP), being away from a parent (SAD), hearing the bell ring (SP, situational subtype), contamination (i.e., OCD), or because they are withdrawing from social interactions (i.e., major depression). Thus, to determine the diagnosis for children who present with school refusal, it is important to carefully assess the specific reasons for the school refusal.

DEVELOPMENTAL COURSE

Because children experience mild fears as part of normal development, determining the developmental course of SP has been difficult. Three sources of information help to inform our understanding of the developmental course of this disorder: (1) adult retrospective studies that provide information about the age of onset, (2) cross-sectional studies that assess fears of children at different ages, and (3) prospective studies examining the stability of SP over time. Retrospective studies of adults with SP indicate that the onset of most SPs occur during childhood or adolescence (e.g., Marks & Gelder, 1966; Ost, 1985, 1987; Ost & Hugdahl, 1983; Sheehan, Sheehan, & Minichiello, 1981; Thyer, Parrish, Curtis, Nesse, & Cameron, 1985). Specifically, phobias of darkness, animals, insects, and blood/injury have been found to begin before age 7, whereas the onset of dental and thunderstorm phobias appears to occur between 11 and 12 years of age.

Last and colleagues (Last et al., 1992; Strauss & Last, 1993) examined the sociodemographic and clinical characteristics, including age of onset, in a large sample of clinic-referred youth (over 200, ages 6 to 18) with primary *DSM-III-R* anxiety diagnoses. The average age of onset for children with a primary diagnosis of SP was 8 years old, whereas the average age at intake for this group was 12.1 years.

An examination of developmental patterns of SP also suggests that the content of children's fears may differ with age in both nonclinical and clinical samples (e.g., Bauer, 1976; Bell-Dolan, Last, & Strauss, 1990; McGee, Feehan, Williams, & Anderson, 1992; Ollendick, King, & Frary, 1989). Earlier reviews of developmental patterns in nonclinical fears indicated that infants and preschoolers are more likely to express fears related to loss of support, loud noises, and unfamiliar people; children in middle school years show fears of imaginary creatures, small animals, and the dark; and early and late adolescents report fears of achievement/performance, social evaluation, and bodily injury (e.g., Morris & Kratochwill, 1983; Ollendick & Francis, 1988). A study of community children ($N = 925$) assessed at age 11 and again at age 15 (using structured diagnostic interview and parent ratings), found that, at age 11, children's fears were likely to be of the dark, heights, or animals, whereas at age 15, the fears were likely to be of social and agoraphobic situations (McGee et al., 1992). Similar patterns have also been found in clinic samples of children who present with anxiety disorders. Last and colleagues found that children with a primary diagnosis of social phobia (SOP; social evaluation/performance fears) tend to be older than children with a primary diagnosis of SAD or SP (animals, the dark; e.g., Last et al., 1992; Strauss & Last, 1993).

Few prospective studies have examined the stability of SP. One exception, conducted by Milne et al. (1995), examined the frequency of clinical phobias (SP, SOP, and agoraphobia combined) and subclinical fears in a community sample of youth over a 3-year period. Of 112 youth assessed at both time periods, 11% (with any type of phobia; $n = 12$) continued to meet diagnostic criteria for that same type of phobia 1 year later. However, a majority (56%) of youth with SP at Time 1 remained symptomatic, presenting with subsyndromal fears (i.e., less impairment) at Time 2. These findings are consistent with one of the classic prospective studies of phobia conducted by Agras, Chapin, and Oliveau (1972). These investigators followed a community sample of 30 untreated phobic individuals (10 children under the age of 20 years, and 20 adults) over a 5-year period. After 5 years, 100% of the children were viewed as "improved," compared with 43% of the adults. Although the conclusion drawn by Agras et al. was that many phobic conditions improve without treatment, particularly in children, a reinterpretation of these data (Ollendick, 1979) revealed that the improved children were not symptom-free, and most continued to exhibit symptoms. Thus, fear and disability associated with SP are likely to persist over time, to some degree, for a proportion of youngsters.

ASSESSMENT

The most comprehensive approach to the assessment of SP involves a complete diagnostic assessment for all conditions and from multiple perspectives (child, parent, teacher, and clinician). In addition, examining the multiple domains of anxiety described earlier (i.e., cognitive, behavioral, physiological) insures that all possible anxiety diagnoses will be assessed. However, as Ronan (1996) and others have suggested, the selection of assessment instruments should also be driven by the goal of the assessment (e.g., screening, diagnosis, monitoring of treatment). At a minimum, a diagnostic interview (for differential diagnosis), a quantitative measure of fearfulness (e.g., fear rating scale), and a measure of impairment are critical. These instruments can be used to identify comorbid conditions as well as to monitor treatment gains. The most common approaches to assessment, namely diagnostic interviews, fear rating scales, and self-monitoring procedures, are briefly described in the following sections.

Diagnostic Interviews

Because of problems with the reliability of diagnoses derived from unstructured clinical interviews (Edelbrock & Costello, 1984), the use of structured and semistructured interview schedules has increased through the years. Of the structured interviews available to assess psychiatric disorders in children (e.g., the Schedule for Affective Disorders and Schizophrenia in School-Age Children [K-SADS]—Puig-Antich & Chambers, 1978; the Diagnostic Interview for Children and Adolescents [DICA]—Herjanic & Reich, 1982; the Diagnostic Interview Schedule for Children [DISC]—Shaffer, Fisher, Lucas, Dulcan, & Schwab-Stone, 2000), only the Anxiety Disorders Interview Schedule for *DSM-IV*, Child and Parent Versions (ADIS-C/P; Silverman & Albano, 1996; Silverman & Nelles, 1988a) was specifically designed to assess SP and other anxiety disorders in children. Its utility for diagnosing anxiety disorders in youth has been extensively studied (Rapee, Barrett, Dadds, & Evans, 1994; Silverman & Eisen, 1992; Silverman & Nelles, 1988a; Silverman & Rabian, 1995; Silverman, Saavedra, & Pina, 2001), and has yielded excellent reliability coefficients (kappa coefficients ranging from .84 to 1.0, depending on the reliability paradigm used (i.e., interrater, test-retest).

To assess the presence of SP, children and parents are read a list of objects/events (e.g., the dark, dogs, needles) and asked to indicate (via yes/no) whether the child feels excessive fear (i.e., greater than most children their own age). For those items to which the child's fear is excessive, a rating (between 0 and 8) of the degree of fear and avoidance is obtained using a feelings thermometer. The feelings thermometer is useful in that it simplifies the rating task for children and removes some of the variability attributed to language skills that occur when young children respond to questionnaires (Barrios, Hartmann, & Shigetomi, 1981).

In addition to fear/avoidance ratings, the ADIS-C/P provides for an assessment of degree of interference by obtaining similar ratings from the child and parent alike using a modified Feelings Thermometer. Additional sections of the ADIS-C/P contain questions addressing onset, course, and etiology of each SP.

Fear Rating Scales

A frequently used method for assessing SP in children is fear rating scales. These instruments generally ask children (or others) to rate the degree of fear experienced in a variety of situations. The most widely used scale for assessing fears in children is the Revised Fear Survey Schedule for Children (FSSC-R; Ollendick, 1983). This measure provides information on the number, severity, and types of fears that children experience in 80 different situations. Factor analysis has revealed five factors, including (1) fear of the unknown, (2) fear of failure and criticism, (3) fear of minor injury and small animals, (4) fear of danger and death, and (5) medical fears (Ollendick, 1983). Other self-rating scales have also been developed to assess a broad range of children's fears, including the Louisville Fear Survey (Miller, Barrett, Hampe, & Noble, 1972) and the Children's Fear Survey Schedule (Ryall & Dietiker, 1979). In addition, self-rating scales have been developed to assess children's specific fears, such as fears of dental procedures (Children's Fear Survey Schedule; Melamed & Lumley, 1988), darkness (Nighttime Coping Response Inventory and Nighttime Fear Inventory; Mooney, 1985), medical procedures/hospital (Fears Schedule; Bradlyn, 1982), snakes (Snake Attitude Measure; Kornhaber & Schroeder, 1975) and tests (Test Anxiety Scale for Children; Sarason, Davidson, Lighthall, Waite, & Ruebush, 1960).

Clinically, these scales are useful for measuring change in levels of fearfulness from pre- to posttreatment. They also provide information about the range of situations in which a child may experience fear, as well as the severity of fearfulness associated with each situation or object. This information can assist the clinician in prioritizing target fears in treatment. Moreover, these instruments are easy to administer and score, have acceptable reliability (test-retest and internal consistency), and can differentiate normal from anxious youth (Beidel & Turner, 1988; Ollendick, 1983). However, fear rating scales are not useful for determining diagnoses, and their validity, particularly discriminant validity among children with psychiatric disorders, remains to be determined (Last, Francis, & Strauss, 1989). For instance, Perrin and Last (1992) examined the discriminant validity of the FSSC-R, as well as other self-report measures of anxiety, using a sample of 213 boys (ages 5–17): 105 with primary diagnoses of anxiety disorders (22 with SP), 56 with primary diagnoses of attention-deficit/hyperactivity disorder (ADHD), and 49 with no psychiatric diagnoses. With respect to children's fears, there were no differences among the three groups on the total or five subscale scores of the FSSC-R.

A more recent study (Weems, Silverman, Saavedra, Pina, & Lumpkin, 1999), however, suggests that such rating scales may be useful in differentiating among children with different subtypes of phobias. In their study, 120 children with phobias of the dark, animals, shots/doctors, or social phobia were compared on the five factors as well as on individual items of the child- and parent-completed FSSC-R. Specific factors and individual items successfully discriminated among the phobic subtypes. (Weems et al., 1999).

Self-Monitoring

Another method of assessing children's fears is via self-monitoring procedures. Although self-monitoring procedures vary along several dimensions (e.g., what behaviors get monitored and whether the procedure is structured or unstructured), they generally require that children (or parents and teachers) observe and systematically record the occurrence of their fearful thoughts and behaviors. Self-monitoring data can also provide information about the antecedents and consequences of fearful reactions as well as the severity and frequency of these reactions. One approach to self-monitoring is via a daily diary. The daily diary requires children to keep a record of the situations in which fear/anxiety was experienced, whether they confronted or avoided the situation, accompanying cognitions, and a rating of fear severity. Clinically, this method is particularly useful because it requires the child to record important aspects of the fear that can then be addressed in treatment. With respect to psychometric properties, structured approaches have more psychometric support (e.g., Beidel, Neal, & Lederer, 1991), but compliance, accuracy, reactivity effects, and whether self-monitoring data are sensitive in showing clinical change from pre- to posttreatment warrant additional investigation.

TREATMENT

Treatments for SP date back to Freud's (1909/1955) description of Little Hans and Watson and Raynor's (1920) fear conditioning and treatment of Little Albert. Since these early reports, a variety of treatments for SP have appeared in the literature, including cognitive and behavioral procedures, emotive imagery, play therapy, family therapy, past-life hypnotic regression, eye movement desensitization and reprocessing, and various pharmacological agents. Among these procedures, cognitive-behavioral therapies have received the most empirical support and are thus the focus of this chapter.

Cognitive and Behavioral Treatments

The most common cognitive and behavioral procedures used to treat child SP include: exposure, systematic desensitization, flooding, modeling, contingency management, relaxation training, and self-control. Cognitive-behavioral therapy (CBT) interventions are generally short term (from 1 to 12 sessions), have been used with children as young as 3 years of age, and can be administered in both group and individual formats. The therapist's stance is active and directive, present oriented, and problem focused. Each of the CBT strategies, alone or in combination, has been used to treat children who display a wide range of fears, including those related to nighttime (Graziano & Mooney, 1980; Graziano, Mooney, Huber, & Ignasiak, 1979; King, Cranstoun, & Josephs, 1989), darkness (Giebenhain & O'Dell, 1984; Heard, Dadds, & Conrad, 1992; Jackson & King, 1981; Kanfer, Karoly, & Newman, 1975), loud noises (Tasto, 1969; Wish, Hasazi, & Jurgela, 1973; Yule, Sacks, & Hersov, 1974), public speaking (Cradock, Cotler, & Jason, 1978; Fox & Houston, 1981), heights (Croghan & Musante, 1975; Holmes, 1936; Ritter, 1968), animals (Bandura, Blanchard, & Ritter, 1969; Glasscock & MacLean, 1990; Obler & Terwilliger, 1970; Sreenivasan, Manocha, & Jain, 1979), water (Lewis, 1974; Menzies & Clarke, 1993; Ultee, Griffioen, & Schellekens, 1982), menstruation (Shaw, 1990), telephones (Babbitt & Parrish, 1991), newspapers (Goldberg & Weisenberg, 1992), bowel movements (Eisen & Silverman, 1991), needles (Rainwater et al., 1988), medical procedures (Heard et al., 1992; Peterson & Shigetomi, 1981), dental procedures (Krochak, Slovin, Rubin, & Kaplan, 1988; Siegel & Peterson, 1980), traveling in cars (Stedman & Murphey, 1984; Thankachan, Mishra, & Kumaraiah, 1992), and illness/diseases (Hagopian, Weist, & Ollendick, 1990).

Despite the large quantity of studies examining CBT strategies, methodological shortcomings limit conclusions about the effectiveness of individual CBT strategies. Specifically, many of these studies were not experimental, did not use multimethod assessment procedures, and have minimal systematic follow-ups. In addition, many of these studies have been conducted with children who had mild fears rather than clinically impairing SP. Finally, there is an absence of research comparing the relative efficacy of one treatment strategy over another (e.g., cognitive-behavioral versus play therapy) and little information about predictors of treatment outcome (e.g., comorbidity, parental anxiety symptoms, treatment duration). With these limitations in mind, a brief description of each of these strategies, and the associated empirical evidence, is presented below (for more detailed descriptions see King & Ollendick, 1997; Ollendick & King, 1998; Silverman & Eisen, 1993). In describing the empirical support for each of these strategies, we were guided by a recent comprehensive review by Ollendick and King (1998), who classified each CBT strategy according to guidelines originally proposed by the American Psychological Association's Division 12 Task Force on Promotion and Dissemination of Psychological Procedures (Chambless, Steketee, Tran, Worden, & Gillis, 1996) and adapted by the Division of Clinical Child Psychology Task Force for empirically supported interventions in children (Lonigan, Elbert, & Bennett-Johnson, 1998). Classifications include *well established*, *probably efficacious*, and *experimental*.

Systematic Desensitization (SD)

Based on the principles of classical conditioning, SD generally involves the imaginal or in-vivo pairing (or both) of an incompatible-fear response (usually relaxation response) with items on a fear hierarchy. The pairing progresses from the least to the most fear provoking item on the hierarchy. The pairing of an incompatible response, such as relaxation, positive imagery, games, or fun activities, is thought to inhibit fear via the process of counterconditioning responses.

Based on controlled and uncontrolled studies of SD for SP, Ollendick & King (1998) concluded that SD (and its variants) met criteria for *probably efficacious*. Across these studies, SD was consistently found to be more effective than no treatment or wait-list control conditions. Several studies have compared forms of SD with each other (e.g., imaginal versus in-vivo SD) and/or other techniques (Bandura et al., 1969; Kondas, 1967; Mann & Rosenthal, 1969; Miller et al., 1972; Ultee et al., 1982). Taken together, these studies suggest that (a) in-vivo SD is more effective than imaginal SD, (b) imaginal SD is more effective than relaxation alone but equal to live modeling and individual psychotherapy, and (c) imaginal SD is less effective than participant modeling. In addition, relaxation and imaginal approaches appear to work better with adolescents compared to young children.

Contingency Management (CM)

CM is based on the principles of operant conditioning and relies on the therapist and parent to ensure that positive consequences follow the child's exposure to the fearful stimulus, and to ensure that positive consequences (e.g., attention) do not follow avoidant/fearful behavior. Several key procedures are used in CM, including shaping, reinforced practice, extinction, and contingency contracting. CM procedures generally require children (and their parents) to devise a list of rewards, which are administered to the child (by parents, therapist, or both) contingent on completion of approach or exposure to the fearful object or situation. In constructing successful contingency contracts, it is critical that the terms on the contract are explicit and specific as to what both parent and child are expected to do.

Empirically, CM procedures meet the criteria for *well-established* interventions for SP (Ollendick & King, 1998), and they have been found to be more effective for reducing excessive fear, when compared with no treatment control conditions (Leitenberg & Callahan, 1973; Obler & Terwilliger, 1970). Studies comparing CM with other strategies suggest that CM is more effective than verbal coping skills (Sheslow, Bondy, & Nelson, 1983) and live adult modeling (Menzies & Clarke, 1993).

Modeling

Based on principles of vicarious conditioning and social learning, modeling involves the child's learning to be less fearful by observing others' handling the fearful object or event. The models observed by the child may be actual (live) models (adult or child), or they may be observed on films or videotapes (symbolic models). A variant of this procedure is when children are assisted in approaching the feared object, referred to as participant modeling.

Empirical support for modeling procedures is considered *well established* for participant modeling and *probably efficacious* for filmed and live modeling (Ollendick & King, 1998). Specifically, controlled experimental studies examining the efficacy of participant modeling have found it to be superior to no treatment/wait-list conditions (Blanchard, 1970; Murphy & Bootzin, 1973) and superior to filmed modeling (Bandura et al., 1969; Lewis, 1974; Ritter, 1968). In contrast, live modeling has been found superior to no treatment control conditions (Bandura, Grusec, & Menlove, 1967; Mann & Rosenthal, 1969), and filmed modeling appears superior only to no treatment comparison conditions (e.g., Bandura & Menlove, 1968; Hill, 1968).

Cognitive/Self-Control

Cognitive/self-control procedures are based on principles of cognitive therapy and the assumption that maladaptive thoughts and beliefs underlie fear and avoidant behavior. Cognitive interventions involve teaching children how to identify and then alter maladaptive thoughts when confronted with the fearful stimulus in order to regulate their anxious and avoidant behavior. These strategies include engaging in positive self-statements (e.g., "I am brave"), cognitive restructuring (e.g., evaluating evidence for and against unrealistic thinking), coping statements, self-evaluation, and self-reward.

Empirical support for cognitive-behavioral procedures is considered *probably efficacious* (Ollendick & King, 1998). Specifically, controlled experimental studies examining the efficacy of CBT have found it to be superior to no treatment/wait-list conditions (Graziano & Mooney, 1980) and superior to stimulus or neutral self-statements (Kanfer, Karoly, & Newman, 1975).

A recent study by Silverman and colleagues (Silverman et al., 1999) compared the relative effectiveness of an exposure-based CM program, an exposure-based self-control (SC) treatment, and an education support (ES) condition in which exposure was discussed but was not directly prescribed (such as through CM or SC procedures). A total of 99 children (aged 6 to 16 years; mean age 9.9 years) and their parents participated in the study. Of the total, 52 were boys and 47 were girls. All children met criteria for a primary *DSM-III-R* diagnosis for phobic disorder, including SP ($n = 82$), social phobia ($n = 10$), or agoraphobia ($n = 7$), based on a structured interview administered separately to the child and parent.

Each of the 99 children and their parents were randomly assigned to one of the three conditions. There were 37 children in the CM condition, 40 in the SC condition, and 22 in ES. Each condition was a 10-week treat-

ment program in which the children and parents were seen in separate treatment sessions with the therapist, followed by a brief conjoint meeting.
Results indicated that all of the procedures that were used to facilitate the
occurrence of exposure—the CM condition and the SC condition, as well
as the ES condition—produced effective therapeutic change on all of the
main outcome measures (child, parent, and clinicians), including the indices of clinically significant change (e.g., return to normative scores on the
Child Behavior Checklist [Achenbach, 1991]). On one outcome measure,
the fear rating during a behavioral approach task, a significantly higher percentage of children in CM (80%) and SC (80%) conditions were more likely
to report little or no fear relative to children in ES (25%) at posttreatment.
Impressively, treatment gains for all conditions were maintained at 3-, 6-,
and 12-month follow-up.

Given the nearly unanimous consensus regarding the efficacy of
cognitive-behavioral interventions for pediatric SP, important next-step
questions include determining the adequate "dosage" of CBT needed for
treatment success as well as identifying which treatment ingredients are
essential. Toward this end, Ost, Svensson, Hellstrom, and Lindwall (2001)
evaluated the efficacy of a one-session exposure-only treatment. Children
(ages 7–17) were randomly assigned to one of three treatment conditions:
one session, child alone (n = 21); one session with child and parent (n =
20); or a wait-list control (n = 19). Children met *DSM–IV* criteria for a
broad range of SPs (over half were phobias of animals or insects), and 42%
of the sample had comorbid psychiatric disorders. Pre- to posttreatment
assessments of anxiety and fear included self-, parent, and clinician reports;
independent evaluators (IE); and behavioral tasks. Results indicated that,
on some measures (e.g., IE ratings of phobic severity) but not others (e.g.,
self-reports of anxiety), children in the two active treatments made significantly greater improvements in anxiety and fear than those on the wait list.
Improvements among children in the active treatments were generally similar. Findings from this study suggest that SPs may be effectively treated with
brief (3-hour) interventions. A larger randomized clinical trial evaluating
one-session treatments is currently underway (T. Ollendick, personal communication, May 6, 2002).

Pharmacological Treatments

Pharmacological treatment trials are few and far between. The lack of pharmacological treatment studies relates to the common misconception of
specific fears as a normal experience and not a condition associated with
impairment or in need of pharmacological intervention. In this section, we
review the literature that does exist regarding pharmacological treatments
of SP.

Approaches to pharmacological treatment of anxiety disorders have
shifted over the past 10 years. Treatment trials for adult anxiety disorders
suggest that the selective serotonin reuptake inhibitors (SSRIs) are the

medications of choice for most anxiety disorders, including SP (Uhlenhuth, Balter, Ban, & Yang, 1999), rather than benzodiazepines and tricyclic anti-depressants. Despite this shift, there is little empirical evidence of the efficacy of the SSRIs for SP in adults or children. Only in the past few years have there been published reports of a controlled trial for SP (e.g., Benjamin, Ben-Zion, Karbofsky, & Dannon, 2000) and a handful of case reports and letters to the editors of various journals (Abene & Hamilton, 1998; Balon, 1999; Viswanathan & Paradis, 1991) suggesting that pharmacological approaches are effective and may need to be considered more seriously for severe and impairing SP in adults.

Two pharmacological treatment trials for SP require special mention. Benjamin and colleagues (2000) completed a small ($N = 11$), 4-week, double-blind, placebo-controlled trial of paroxetine (up to 20 mg per day) for adults ages 53 ± 13 years with SP. The patients had been ill for some time—10.9 ± 14 years—and only one had been offered a medication intervention in the past. Baseline severity on a 10-point severity scale was in the moderate to severe range; Hamilton Anxiety Rating Scale scores were in the mild range. Patients with symptom reduction greater than 50% at end point were considered responders. Of subjects on placebo, 1 out of 6 was considered a responder and 3 out of 6 were considered responders to paroxetine. The authors noted that it was quite difficult to recruit for this study due to the lack of individuals with SP only, in their clinic population. In addition, the authors considered the subject population unusual because of the age of the subjects and severity of the anxiety disorder.

Fairbanks and colleagues (1997) completed a 9-week open trial of fluoxetine in children ages 9 to 18 years with mixed anxiety disorders ($N = 16$). After not responding to brief psychotherapy, subjects were started on low-dose fluoxetine (5 mg per day), which was then increased weekly until side effects or improvement occurred, to a maximum of 40 mg per day (children) and 80 mg per day (adolescents). Of the 16 patients enrolled, 6 had SPs and 4 of those 6 responded to fluoxetine. The medication was well tolerated.

Long-term pharmacological treatment trials for SP are even less common. One long-term follow-up study of adults with SP suggests that only 55% of responders to either pharmacotherapy or psychotherapy were considered to maintain their response at very long-term follow-up (10–16 years; Lipsitz, Markowitz, Cherry, & Fyer, 1999). The other 45% experienced significant symptomatology, as did the adults considered nonresponders in the original study.

Stages of Treatment for Children With Specific Phobia

STAGE 1: SELECTION OF INITIAL TREATMENT   Selecting initial treatments in general, and for SP in particular, begins with identifying interventions that are empirically supported, pose the fewest risks and greatest benefits, and are the most cost effective. In light of the evidence just noted for the treatment of SP, the initial treatment of choice is CBT. This treatment begins with providing information about SP as well as the CBT treatment model and process (e.g., the information that SP is an anxiety disorder whose etiology is multidetermined, and information about the interactions between thoughts, behavior, and affective/physiological manifestations of fear). The importance of exposure or facing fears is emphasized, as is the notion that in order for treatment to work, the children and parents must practice what they learn regularly—just as they would any other skill, such as basketball or playing the piano. In this context, out-of-session activities are often assigned for children to practice newly acquired skills.

STAGE 2: MANAGEMENT OF PARTIAL RESPONSE   Despite the empirical evidence supporting CBT strategies, a significant number of children will only experience a partial response. In evaluating how to manage partial responders, decisions about the reasons for partial response must be considered. First, clinicians should evaluate whether the initial dose of CBT was adequate. If the initial dose of treatment was not adequate, increasing the frequency or intensity of treatment, or both, should be considered first. Second, specific obstacles to treatment success should be examined and addressed. For instance, were the child and family adequately prepared for exposures? Are the items on the fear hierarchy correct? Is there some benefit for the child (or parent) in maintaining the anxiety and avoidance? Third, clinicians should reconsider whether the initial diagnosis continues to best explain the fear, or whether the fear is a manifestation of another anxiety disorder or is not the most important target of treatment. If so, additional treatments, both CBT and medication, may be required. Finally, partial responders may have other, nonanxiety, comorbid disorders (e.g., ADHD, oppositional defiant disorder) that compromise treatment response. In this case, appropriate treatments, based on the empirical literature, would be added to target these conditions.

STAGE 3: TREATMENT OF REFRACTORY SP   The patient with refractory SP is one who is accurately evaluated and has failed to respond to adequate trials of CBT, medication, or their combination and has had a second evaluation for diagnosis and treatment adequacy. Patients cannot truly be considered to have refractory SPs unless they have failed CBT that included in-vivo exposure, family involvement, and consideration of whether group or individual treatment is the best vehicle for treatment. In addition, to be considered to have treatment-refractory SP, a child should have undergone medication trials that target not only the SP, but also comorbid anxiety disorders (e.g., SSRIs for SP with OCD) or other comorbid conditions (e.g., SSRIs plus stimulants). Last, SP can be considered refractory only if the combination of these strategies has been done with special emphasis on coordinating the treatment modalities with each other. For refractory SPs, other interventions or combinations of interventions that are less well studied may need to be implemented. If subjects continue to be refractory to treatment, an additional consultation may be required, with both a CBT expert and a psychopharmacologist.

STAGE 4: CONTINUATION AND MAINTENANCE TREATMENT   Continuation treatment is designed to prevent relapse of an ongoing disorder. Maintenance treatment is designed to prevent the recurrence of another episode of disorder. During continuation treatment, clinicians should consider the appropriate dose required to prevent relapse of the episode under treatment. In CBT, continuation treatment generally falls under the rubric of relapse prevention. Relapse prevention is based on the premise that progress observed during acute treatment may not automatically be maintained and therefore must be explicitly programmed and structured into treatment. Thus, during this treatment stage, information about the typical course of treatment (i.e., that all youth tend to have temporary setbacks or slips, and specific strategies for anticipating and reacting to these slips) are particularly helpful. More specifically, it is helpful to explain that a slip does not mean that the child is back at square one and that the child will still remember all the skills learned. It is even more critical to review these points with the parents, because parental reactions to slips will significantly affect children's reactions. Thus, if a parent feels and expresses the view that the slip is merely a temporary setback that can be overcome, then the child is likely to feel the same. Another key component of relapse prevention is the continued practice of skills learned in treatment, particularly exposure. Regular practice (e.g., exposure, nonnegative thinking) will make slips less likely to occur. Thus, it is helpful to provide guidelines for the amount of exposures the children should engage in after treatment termination to help maintain treatment gains. The children are also told that this amount should increase if fear and avoidance increase. In addition, continuation treatment should include instructions in how to generalize the skills learned by applying them to other fears or anxiety-provoking situations. This can be especially helpful when anticipating future stressful events that may trigger a slip.

The differentiation between continuation and maintenance treatment is a subtle one, but it suggests that at some point the patient's disorder has truly remitted and that subsequent problems are new episodes. Similar strategies for preventing relapse are likely to be useful for preventing recurrences of SP.

Continuation trials for medication treatment for SP have not been done. There have been a number of continuation trials of adult depression and one child study for depression (Emslie et al., 2001). These studies suggest that discontinuing medication shortly after response may be associated with an acute relapse of depressive symptoms for most children. For depression in adults, it is unclear whether medication treatment past 9- to 12-month duration is associated with a higher relapse rate than might be expected for patients who experience a recurrence of depression off medication. There are no long-term maintenance studies for SP.

SUMMARY AND CONCLUSIONS

For uncomplicated SP, assessment strategies are straightforward, and treatments are empirically supported. However, the majority of children with SP have comorbid conditions that may require specific assessment strategies and treatment planning to meet their needs. Given our current diagnostic classification system, it is difficult to identify the relationships between SP and comorbid conditions and to base treatment decisions on this relationship. Moreover, many questions remain unanswered. For example, are some SPs more common in children with SAD or GAD? If so, what is the best treatment approach—to target the SP or the SAD or GAD? In addition, is SP with generalized avoidance behavior different from SP with more specific avoidance behavior, an issue similar to that confronted when social phobia has either generalized or more specific avoidance? What is the relationship between SP and other anxiety disorders (e.g., agoraphobia), depressive disorders, and other behaviors such as fainting (why does fainting occur with blood/injury phobia and not with exposure to animals?), and disgust sensitivity?

Although the treatment of choice for SP is cognitive and behavioral strategies, it is likely that patients with either more severe symptoms or complex comorbidity, or those who are refractory to CBT, may benefit from medication interventions. Given the broad spectrum of activity of the SSRIs, it is likely that these would be more effective than benzodiazepines or other alternatives. Empirical trials are necessary.

REFERENCES

Abene, M. V., & Hamilton, J. D. (1988). Resolution of fear of flying with fluoxetine treatment. *Journal of Anxiety Disorders 12,* 599–603.

Achenbach, T. M. (1991). *Manual for the Child Behavior Checklist: 4–18 and 1991 profile.* Burlington: University of Vermont Department of Psychiatry.

Agras, W. S., Chapin, H. N., & Oliveau, D. C. (1972). The natural history of phobia. *Archives of General Psychiatry, 26,* 315–317.

American Psychiatric Association. (1987). *Diagnostic and statistical manual of mental disorders* (3rd ed., rev.). Washington, DC: Author.

American Psychiatric Association. (1994). *Diagnostic and statistical manual of mental disorders: DSM-IV* (4th ed.). Washington, DC: Author.

Anderson, J. (1994). Epidemiological issues. In T. H. Ollendick, N. J. King, & W. Yule (Eds.), *International handbook of phobic and anxiety disorders in children and adolescents* (pp. 43–66). New York: Plenum Press.

Anderson, J. C., Williams, S., McGee, R., & Silva, P. A. (1987). *DSM-III* disorders in preadolescent children: Prevalence in a large sample from the general population. *Archives of General Psychiatry, 44,* 69–77.

Babbitt, R. L., & Parrish, J. M. (1991). Phone phobia, phact or phantasy? An operant approach to a child's disruptive behavior induced by telephone usage. *Journal of Behavior Therapy and Experimental Psychiatry, 22,* 123–129.

Balon, R. (1999). Fluvoxamine for phobia of storms. *Acta Psychiatrica Scandinavica, 100*(3), 244–246.

Bandura, A., Blanchard, E. B., & Ritter, B. (1969). Relative efficacy of desensitization and modeling approaches for inducing behavioral affective and attitudinal changes. *Journal of Personality and Social Psychology, 13,* 179–199.

Bandura, A., Grusec, J. E., & Menlove, F. L. (1967). Vicarious extinction of avoidance behavior. *Journal of Personality and Social Psychology, 5,* 16–23.

Bandura, A., & Menlove, F. L. (1968). Factors determining vicarious extinction of avoidance behavior through symbolic modeling. *Journal of Personality and Social Psychology, 8,* 99–108.

Barrios, B. A., Hartmann, D. P., & Shigetomi, C. (1981). Fears and anxieties in children. In E. J. Mash & L. G. Terdal (Eds.), *Behavioral assessment of childhood disorders* (pp. 259–304). New York: Guilford Press.

Bauer, D. H. (1976). An exploratory study of developmental changes in children's fears. *Journal of Child Psychology and Psychiatry, 17,* 69–74.

Beidel, D. C., Neal, A. M., & Lederer, A. S. (1991). The feasibility and validity of a daily diary for the assessment of anxiety in children. *Behavior Therapy, 22,* 505–517.

Beidel, D. C., & Turner, S. M. (1988). What are the adult consequences of childhood shyness? *Harvard Mental Health Letter, 15,* 8.

Bell-Dolan, D. J., Last, C. G., & Strauss, C. C. (1990). Symptoms of anxiety disorders in normal children. *Journal of the American Academy of Child and Adolescent Psychiatry, 29,* 759–765.

Benjamin, J., Ben-Zion, I. Z., Karbofsky, E., & Dannon, P. (2000). Double-blind placebo-controlled pilot study of paroxetine for specific phobia. *Journal of Psychopharmacology, 149,* 194–196.

Bernstein, G. A., & Garfinkel, B. D. (1986). School phobia: The overlap of affective and anxiety disorders. *Journal of the American Academy of Child and Adolescent Psychiatry, 25,* 235–241.

Bird, H. R., Canino, G., Rubio-Stipec, M., Gould, M. S., Ribera, J., Sesman, M., Woodbury, M., et al. (1988). Estimates of the prevalence of childhood maladjustment in a community survey in Puerto Rico. *Archives of General Psychiatry, 45,* 1120–1126.

Blanchard, E. B. (1970). Relative contributions of modeling, informational influences, and physical contact in extinction of phobic behavior. *Journal of Abnormal Psychology, 76*(1), 55–61.

Bradlyn, A. S. (1982). *The effects of a videotape preparation package in reducing children's arousal and increasing cooperation during cardiac catheterization.* Unpublished doctoral dissertation, University of Mississippi.

Burke, A. E., & Silverman, W. K. (1987). The prescriptive treatment of school refusal. *Clinical Psychology Review, 7,* 353–362.

Chambless, D. L., Steketee, G., Tran, G. Q., Worden, H., & Gillis, M. M. (1996). Behavioral avoidance test for obsessive-compulsive disorder. *Behavioral Research Therapy, 34,* 73–83.

Costello, E., & Borkovec, T. D. (1993). Efficacy of applied relaxation and cognitive behavioral therapy in the treatment of generalized anxiety disorder. *Journal of Consultation Clinical Psychology, 61,* 611–619.

Costello, E. J., Costello, A. J., Edelbrock, C. S., Burns, B. J., Dulcan, M. J., Brent, D., & Janiszewski, S. (1988). Psychiatric disorders in pediatric primary care: Prevalence and risk factors. *Archives of General Psychology, 45,* 1107–1116.

Cradock, C., Cotler, S., & Jason, L. A. (1978). Primary prevention: Immunization of children for speech anxiety. *Cognitive Therapy and Research, 2,* 389–396.

Croake, J. W. (1969). Fears of children. *Human Development, 12,* 239–247.

Croghan, L. M., & Musante, G. J. (1975). The elimination of a boy's high building phobia by in vivo desensitization and game playing. *Journal of Behavior Therapy and Experimental Psychiatry, 6,* 87–88.

Edelbrock, C., & Costello, A. (1984). Structured psychiatric interviews for children and adolescents. In G. Goldstein & M. Hersen, M. (Eds.), *Handbook of psychological assessment,* (pp. 276–290). New York: Pergamon Press.

Eisen, A. R., & Silverman, W. K. (1991). Treatment of an adolescent with bowel movement phobia using self-control therapy. *Journal of Behavior Therapy and Experimental Psychiatry, 22,* 45–51.

Emslie, G. J., Heiligenstein, J. H., Hoog, S. L., Findling, R. L., Wagner, K. D., Ernest, D. E., VanHoy, B., Nilsson, M., Babcock, S., & Jacobson, J. G. (2001). Fluoxetine for maintenance of recovery from depression in children and adolescents: A placebo-controlled randomized clinical trial. Paper presented at 48th Annual Meeting, American Academy of Child and Adolescent Psychiatry, Honolulu.

Essau, C. A., Conradt, J., & Petermann, F. (2000). Frequency, comorbidity, and psychosocial impairment of specific phobia in adolescents. *Journal of Clinical Child Psychology, 29,* 221–231.

Fairbanks, J. M., Pine, D. S., Tancer, N. K., Dummit, E. S., III, Kentgen, L. M., Martin, J., Asche, B. K., et al. (1997). Open fluoxetine treatment of mixed anxiety disorders in children and adolescents. *Journal of Child and Adolescent Psychopharmacology, 7,* 17–29.

Fonseca, A. C., Yule, W., & Erol, N. (1994). Cross-cultural issues. In T. H. Ollendick, N. J. King, & W. Yule (Eds.), *International handbook of phobic and anxiety disorders in children and adolescents* (pp. 67–84). New York: Plenum Press.

Fox, J. E., & Houston, B. K. (1981). Efficacy of self-instructional training for reducing children's anxiety in any evaluative situation. *Behaviour Research and Therapy, 19,* 509– 515.

Freud, S. (1955). Analysis of a phobia in a five-year-old boy. In J. Strachey (Ed. and Trans.), *Standard edition of the complete psychological works of Sigmund Freud* (Vol. 10, pp. 3–149). London: Hogarth Press. (Original work published 1909)

Giebenhain, J. E., & O'Dell, S. L. (1984). Evaluation of a parent-training manual for reducing children's fear of the dark. *Journal of Applied Behavioral Analysis, 17,* 121–125.

Ginsburg, G. S., & Silverman, W. K. (1996). Phobic and anxiety disorders in Hispanic and Caucasian youth. *Journal of Anxiety Disorders, 10,* 517–528.

Glasscock, S. E., & MacLean, W. E. (1990). Use of contact desensitization and shaping in the treatment of dog phobia and generalized fear of the outdoors. *Journal of Clinical Child Psychology, 19,* 169–172.

Goldberg, J., & Weisenberg, M. (1992). The case of a newspaper phobia in a 9-year-old child. *Journal of Behavior Therapy and Experimental Psychiatry, 23,* 125–131.

Graziano, A. M., & de Giovanni, I. S. (1979). The clinical significance of childhood phobias: A note on the proportion of child-clinical referrals for the treatment of children's fears. *Behaviour Research and Therapy, 17,* 161–162.

Graziano, A. M., & Mooney, K. C. (1980). Family self-control instruction for children's nighttime fear reduction. *Journal of Consulting and Clinical Psychology, 48,* 206–213.

Graziano, A. M., & Mooney, K. C., Huber, C., & Ignasiak, D. (1979). Self-control instructions for children's fear-reduction. *Journal of Behavior Therapy and Experimental Psychiatry, 10,* 221–227.

Hagopian, L. P., Weist, M. D., & Ollendick, T. H. (1990). Cognitive-behavior therapy with an 11-year-old girl fearful of AIDS infection, other diseases, and poisoning: A case study. *Journal of Anxiety Disorders, 4,* 257–265.

Heard, P. M., Dadds, M. R., & Conrad, P. (1992). Assessment and treatment of simple phobias in children: Effects on family and marital relationships. *Behaviour Change, 9,* 73–82.

Herjanic, B., & Reich, W. (1982). Development of a structured psychiatric interview for children: Agreement between child and parent on individual symptoms. *Journal of Abnormal Child Psychiatry, 10,* 307–324.

Hill, L. (1968). New challenges to medical education. *Alabama Journal of Medical Science, 5,* 477–480.

Holmes, F. B. (1936). An experimental investigation of a method of overcoming children's fears. *Child Development, 7,* 6–30.

Jackson, H. J., & King, N. J. (1981). The emotive imagery treatment of a child's trauma-induced phobia. *Journal of Behavior Therapy and Experimental Psychiatry, 12,* 325–328.

Kanfer, F. H., Karoly, P., & Newman, A. (1975). Reduction of children's fear of the dark by confidence-related and situation threat-related verbal cues. *Journal of Consulting and Clinical Psychology, 43,* 251–258.

Kashani, J. H., & Orvaschel, H. (1990). A community study of anxiety in children and adolescents. *American Journal of Psychiatry, 147*(3), 313–318.

Kearney, C. A., & Silverman, W. K. (1997). The evolution and reconciliation of taxonomic strategies for school refusal behavior. *Clinical Psychology: Science and Practice, 3,* 339–354.

King, N. J., Cranstoun, F., & Josephs, A. (1989). Emotive imagery and children's night-time fears: A multiple baseline design evaluation. *Journal of Behavior Therapy and Experimental Psychiatry, 20,* 125–135.

King, N. J., Hamilton, D. I., & Ollendick, T. H. (1988). *Children's phobias: A behavioral perspective.* New York: Wiley.

King, N. J., & Ollendick, T. H. (1997). Treatment of childhood phobias. *Journal of Child Psychology and Psychiatry, 38,* 389–400.

Kondas, O. (1967). Reduction of examination anxiety and "stage-fright" by group desensitization and relaxation. *Behavioral Research Therapy, 5,* 275–281.

Kornhaber, R. C., & Schroeder, H. E. (1975). Importance of model similarity on extinction of avoidance behavior in children. *Journal of Consulting and Clinical Psychology, 43,* 601–607.

Krochak, M., Slovin, M., Rubin, J. G., & Kaplan, A. (1988). Treatment of dental phobia: A report of two cases. *Phobia Practice and Research Journal, 1,* 64–72.

Lang, P. J. (1977). Imagery in therapy: An information processing analysis of fear. *Behavior Therapy, 8,* 862–886.

Last, C. G. (1991). Somatic complaints in anxiety disordered children. *Journal of Anxiety Disorders, 5,* 125–138.

Last, C. G., Francis, G., & Strauss, C. C. (1989). Assessing fears in anxiety-disordered children with the Revised Fear Survey Schedule for Children (FSSC-R). *Journal of Clinical Child Psychology, 18,* 137.

Last, C. G., & Perrin, S. (1993). Anxiety disorders in African-American and White children. *Journal of Abnormal Child Psychology, 2,* 153–164.

194   ASSESSMENT AND TREATMENT

Last, G. C., Perrin, S., Hersen, M., & Kazdin, A. E. (1992). *DSM-III-R* anxiety disorders in children: Sociodemographic and clinical characteristics. *Journal of the American Academy of Child and Adolescent Psychiatry, 31*, 1070–1076.

Last, C. G., Strauss, C. C., & Francis, G. (1987). Comorbidity among childhood anxiety disorders. *Journal of Nervous and Mental Disease, 175*, 726–730.

Leitenberg, H., & Calahan, E. (1973). Reinforced practice and reduction of different kinds of fears in adults and children. *Behaviour Research and Therapy, 11*, 19–30.

Lewis, S. (1974). A comparison of behavior therapy techniques in the reduction of fearful avoidant behavior. *Behavior Therapy, 5*, 648–655.

Lipsitz, J. D., Markowitz, J. C., Cherry, S., & Fyer, A. J. (1999). Open trial of interpersonal psychotherapy for the treatment of social phobia. *American Journal of Psychiatry, 156*, 1814–1816.

Lonigan, Anthony, J. L., & Shannon, M. P. (1998). Diagnostic efficacy of posttraumatic symptoms in children exposed to disaster. *Journal of Clinical Child Psychology, 27*(3), 255–267.

Lonigan, C. J., Elbert, J. C., and Bennett Johnson, S. (1998). Empirically supported psychosocial interventions for children: An overview. *Journal of Clinical Child Psychology, 27*, 138–145.

Mann, J., & Rosenthal, T. L. (1969). Vicarious and direct counterconditioning of test anxiety through individual and group desensitization. *Behaviour Research and Therapy, 7*(4), 359–367.

Marks, I. M., & Gelder, M. G. (1966). Different onset ages in varieties of phobia. *American Journal of Psychiatry, 123*, 218–221.

McGee, R., Feehan, M., Williams, S., & Anderson, J. (1992). *DSM-III* disorders from age 11 to age 15 years. *Journal of the American Academy of Child and Adolescent Psychiatry, 31*, 50–59.

Melamed, B. G., & Lumley, M. A. (1988). Dental subscale of the Children's Fear Survey Schedule. In M. Hersen & A. S. Bellack (Eds.), *Dictionary of behavioral assessment techniques* (p. 171). Oxford, UK: Pergamon Press.

Menzies, R. G., & Clarke, J. C. (1993). A comparison of in vivo and vicarious exposure in the treatment of childhood water phobia. *Behaviour Research and Therapy, 31*, 9–15.

Miller, L. C., Barrett, C. L., Hampe, E., & Noble, H. (1972). Comparison of reciprocal inhibition, psychotherapy, and waiting list control for phobic children. *Journal of Abnormal Psychology, 79*, 269–279.

Milne, J. M., Garrison, C. Z., Addy, C. L., McKeown, R. E., Jackson, K. L., Cuffe, S. P., & Waller, J. L. (1995). Frequency of phobic disorder in a community sample of young adolescents. *Journal of the American Academy of Child and Adolescent Psychiatry, 34*, 1202–1211.

Mooney, K. C. (1985). Children's nighttime fears: Ratings of content and coping behaviors. *Cognitive Therapy and Research, 9*, 309–319.

Morris, R. J. & Kratochwill, T. R. (1983). *Treating children's fears and phobias: A behavioral approach.* New York: Pergamon Press.

Murphy, C. M., & Blootzin, R. R. (1973). Active and passive participation in the contact desensitization of snake fear in children. *Behavior Therapy, 4*, 203–211.

Obler, M., & Terwilliger, R. F. (1970). Pilot study on the effectiveness of systematic desensitization with neurologically impaired children with phobic disorders. *Journal of Consulting and Clinical Psychology, 2*, 314–318.

Ollendick, T. H. (1979). Fear reduction techniques with children. In M. Hersen, R. M. Eisler, & P. M. Miller (Eds.), *Progress in behavior modification* (Vol. 8, pp. 127–168). New York: Academic Press.

Ollendick, T. H. (1983). Reliability and validity of the Revised Fear Survey Schedule for Children (FSSC-R). *Behaviour Research and Therapy, 21,* 395–399.

Ollendick, T. H., & Francis, G. (1988). Behavioral assessment and treatment of childhood phobias. *Behavior Modification, 12,* 165–204.

Ollendick, T. H., & King, N. J. (1994). Diagnosis, assessment, and treatment of internalizing problems in children: The role of longitudinal data. *Journal of Consulting and Clinical Psychology, 62,* 918–927.

Ollendick, T. H., & King, N. J. (1998). Empirically supported treatments for children with phobic and anxiety disorders: Current status. *Journal of Clinical Child Psychology, 27,* 156–167.

Ollendick, T. H., King, N. J., & Frary, R. B. (1989). Fears in children and adolescents: Reliability and generalizability across gender, age and nationality. *Behaviour Research and Therapy, 27,* 19–26.

Ollendick, T. H., Yang, B., Dong, Q., Xia, Y., & Lin, L. (1995). Perceptions of fear in other children and adolescents: The role of gender and friendship status. *Journal of Abnormal Child Psychology, 23,* 439–452.

Ollendick, T. H., Yang, B., King, N. J., Dong, Q., & Akande, A. (1996). Fears in American, Australian, Chinese, and Nigerian children and adolescents: A cross-cultural study. *Journal of Child Psychology and Psychiatry and Allied Disciplines, 37,* 213–220.

Ollendick, T. H., Yule, W., & Ollier, K. (1991). Fears in British children and their relationship to manifest anxiety and depression. *Journal of Child Psychology and Psychiatry and Allied Disciplines, 32,* 321–331.

Ost, L. G. (1985). Ways of acquiring phobias and outcome of behavioral treatments. *Behaviour Research and Therapy, 23,* 683–689.

Ost, L. G. (1987). Age of onset in different phobias. *Journal of Abnormal Psychology, 96*(3), 223–229.

Ost, L. G., & Hugdahl, K. (1983). Acquisition of agoraphobia, mode of onset and anxiety response patterns. *Behaviour Research and Therapy, 21,* 623–631.

Ost, L. G., Svensson, L., Hellerstrom, K., & Lindwall, R. (2001). One-session treatment of specific phobias in youths: A randomized clinical trial. *Journal of Consulting and Clinical Psychology, 69,* 814–824.

Page, A. C. (1994). Blood-injury phobia. *Clinical Psychology Review, 14,* 443–461.

Perrin, S., & Last, C. G. (1992). Do childhood anxiety measures measure anxiety? *Journal of Abnormal Child Psychology, 20,* 567–578.

Peterson, L., & Shigetomi, C. (1981). The use of coping techniques to minimize anxiety in hospitalized children. *Behavior Therapy, 12,* 1–14.

Puig-Antich, J., & Chambers, W. (1978). *The Schedule for Affective Disorders and Schizophrenia for School-Age Children.* New York: New York State Psychiatric Institute.

Rainwater, N., Sweet, A. A., Elliott, L, Bowers, M., McNeil, J., & Stump, N. (1988). Systematic desensitization in the treatment of needle phobias for children with diabetes. *Child and Family Behavior Therapy, 10,* 19–31.

Rapee, R. M., Barrett, P. M., Dadds, M. R., & Evans, L. (1994). Reliability of the *DSM-III-R* childhood anxiety disorders using structured interview: Interrater and parent-child agreement. *Journal of the American Academy of Child and Adolescent Psychiatry, 33,* 984–992.

Ritter, B. (1968). The group desensitization of children's snake phobias using vicarious and contact desensitization procedures. *Behaviour Research and Therapy, 6,* 1–6.

Ronan, K. (1996). Building a reasonable bridge in childhood anxiety assessment: A practitioner's resource guide. *Cognitive Behavior Practice, 3,* 63–90.

Ryall, M. R., & Dietiker, K. E. (1979). Reliability and clinical validity of the Children's Fear Survey Schedule. *Journal of Behavior Therapy and Experimental Psychiatry, 19,* 303– 310.

Sarason, S. B., Davidson, K. S., Lighthall, F. F., Waite, R. R., & Ruebush, B. K. (1960). *Anxiety in elementary school children.* New York: Wiley.

Shaffer, D., Fisher, P., Lucas, C. P., Dulcan, M. K., & Schwab-Stone, M. E. (2000). NIMH Diagnostic Interview Schedule for Children Version IV (NIMH DISC-IV): Description, differences from previous versions, and reliability of some common diagnoses. *Journal of the American Academy of Child and Adolescent Psyshiatry, 39*(1), 28–38.

Shaw, J. (1990). Menstruation phobia treated by cognitive correction: A case report. *Journal of Behavior Therapy and Experimental Psychiatry, 21,* 49–51.

Sheehan, D. V., Sheehan, K. E., & Minichiello, W. E. (1981). Age of onset of phobic disorders: A reevaluation. *Comprehensive Psychiatry, 22,* 544–553.

Sheslow, D., Bondy, A. S., & Nelson, R. O. (1983). A comparison of graduated exposure, verbal coping skills, and their combination in the treatment of children's fears of the dark. *Child and Family Behavior Therapy, 4,* 33–45.

Siegel, L. J., & Peterson, L. (1980). Stress reduction in young dental patients through coping skills and sensory information. *Journal of Consulting and Clinical Psychology, 48,* 785–787.

Silverman, W. K., & Albano, A. M. (1996). *The Anxiety Disorders Interview Schedule for DSM-IV: Child and Parent Versions.* San Antonio, TX: Graywind Publications.

Silverman, W. K., & Eisen, A. R. (1992). Age differences in the reliability of parent and child reports of child anxious symptomatology using a structured interview. *Journal of American Academy of Child and Adolescent Psychiatry, 31,* 117–124.

Silverman, W. K., & Eisen, A. R. (1993). Phobic disorders. In R. T. Ammerman, C. G. Last, & M. Hersen (Eds.), *Handbook of prescriptive treatments for children and adolescents* (pp. 17–197). Boston: Allyn & Bacon.

Silverman, W. K., Kurtines, W. M., Ginsburg, G. S., Weems, C. F., Rabian, B. & Serafini, L. T. (1999). Contingency management, self-control, and education support in the treatment of childhood phobic disorders: A randomized clinical trial. *Journal of Consulting and Clinical Psychology, 67,* 675–687.

Silverman, W. K., & Nelles, W. B. (1988a). The Anxiety Disorders Interview Schedule for Children. *Journal of the American Academy of Child and Adolescent Psychiatry, 27,* 772–778.

Silverman, W. K., & Nelles, W. B. (1988b). The influence of gender on children's ratings of fear in self and same-aged peers. *Journal of Genetic Psychology, 149,* 17–22.

Silverman, W. K., & Rabian, B. (1995). Test-retest reliability of the *DSM-III-R* anxiety childhood disorders symptoms using the Anxiety Disorders Interview Schedule for Children. *Journal of Anxiety Disorders, 9,* 1–12.

Silverman, W. K., Saavedra, L. M., & Pina, A. A. (2001). Test-retest reliability of anxiety symptoms and diagnoses with anxiety disorders interview schedule for *DSM-IV*: Child and parent versions. *Journal of the American Academy of Child and Adolescent Psychiatry, 40,* 937–944.

Sreenivasan, V., Manocha, S. N., & Jain, V. K. (1979). Treatment of severe dog phobia in childhood by flooding: A case report. *Journal of Child Psychology and Psychiatry, 20,* 255–260.

Stedman, J. M., & Murphey, J. (1984). Dealing with specific child phobias during the course of family therapy: An alternative to systematic desensitization. *Family Therapy, 11,* 55–60.

Strauss, C. C., & Last, C. G. (1993). Social and simple phobias in children. *Journal of Anxiety Disorders, 2,* 141–152.

Tasto, D. L. (1969). Systematic desensitization, muscle relaxation and visual imagery in the counterconditioning of a four-year-old phobic child. *Behaviour Research and Therapy, 7,* 409–411.

Thankachan, M. V., Mishra, H., & Kumaraiah, V. (1992). Behavioral intervention with phobic children. *Nimhans Journal, 10,* 95–99.

Thyer, B. A., Parrish, R. T., Curtis, G. C., Nesse, R. M., & Cameron, O. G. (1985). Ages of onset of *DSM-III* anxiety disorders. *Comprehensive Psychiatry, 26,* 113–122.

Uhlenhuth, E. H., Balter, M. B., Ban, T. A., & Yang, K. (1999). Trends in recommendations for the pharmacotherapy of anxiety disorders by an international expert panel. *European Neuropsychopharmacology, 9*(Suppl. 6), S393–S398.

Ultee, C. A., Griffioen, D., & Schellekens, J. (1982). The reduction of anxiety in children: A comparison of the effects of systematic desensitization in vitro and systematic desensitization in vivo. *Behaviour Research and Therapy, 20,* 61–67.

Viswanathan, R., & Paradis, C. (1991). Treatment of cancer phobia with fluoxetine. *American Journal of Psychiatry, 148,* 1090.

Watson, J. B., & Rayner, R. (1920). Conditioned emotional reactions. *Journal of Experimental Psychology, 3,* 1–14.

Weems, C. F., Silverman, W. K., Saavedra, L. S., Pina, A. A, & Lumpkin, P. W. (1999). The discrimination of children's phobias using the Revised Fear Survey Schedule for Children. *Journal of Child Psychology and Psychiatry and Allied Disciplines, 40,* 941–952.

Wish, P. A., Hasazi, J. E., & Jurgela, A. R. (1973). Automated direct deconditioning of a childhood phobia. *Journal of Behavior Therapy and Experimental Psychiatry, 4,* 279–283.

Yule, W., Sacks, B., & Hersov, L. (1974). Successful flooding treatment of nose phobia in an eleven-year-old boy. *Journal of Behavior Therapy and Experimental Psychiatry, 5,* 209–211.

8

SOCIAL ANXIETY DISORDER

ANNE MARIE ALBANO & CHRIS HAYWARD

In this chapter, we describe a framework for understanding social anxiety disorder, otherwise called social phobia, that is developmental, multifactorial, and transactional. Implied in this frame of reference is the view that (a) manifestations of social anxiety disorder vary depending on developmental stage, (b) there are continuities and discontinuities in the expression of social anxiety disorder and its precursors, (c) multiple factors from different domains contribute to the risk of or protection from the development of social anxiety disorder, and (d) interactions between contributory factors may be bidirectional. For example, the influence of the temperamentally socially withdrawn child on a parent may in turn influence parenting behavior that either exaggerates or mitigates social withdrawal. In describing a template for understanding social anxiety disorder that is multidimensional, it follows that both assessment and treatment of social anxiety disorder should be multimodal.

This framework for understanding and treating social anxiety disorder is informed by elements of developmental psychopathology (Cicchetti & Cohen, 1995; Ollendick & Hirshfeld-Becker, 2002). Developmental psychopathology is concerned with the complex course and developmental patterns of behavior over time, taking into account developmental transitions; changes in physical, cognitive, and social emotional development; and interactions between the individual and his or her environment. Implicit in a developmental psychopathology model is the view that there are multiple pathways to develop a particular disorder and that outcomes result from transactions between an individual and his or her environment, which can be both protective and risk enhancing.

The *Diagnostic and Statistical Manual of Mental Disorders: DSM-IV* (American Psychiatric Association, 1994) defines the key feature of social anxiety disorder as a marked and persistent fear of situations in which the person feels that he or she is the focus of attention or evaluation by others. Moreover, in youth, the disorder may manifest as an excessive shrinking away from unfamiliar people (cf. stranger anxiety). To meet the diagnostic criteria, the anxiety and impairment in functioning associated with the disorder must occur stably for a minimum of 6 months. Social anxiety disorder was first introduced into the U.S. psychiatric nomenclature in 1980, resulting in a surge of studies investigating the phenomenology and treatment of the disorder in adults (Heimberg, Hope, Leibowitz, & Schneier, 1995). Investigations into the phenomenology of the disorder in youth were soon to follow (see Beidel & Turner, 1999; March, 1995), however the increased attention that childhood social anxiety disorder has recently received is in part related to a growing body of research identifying promising pharmacological (Compton et al., 2001; Research Unit on Pediatric Psychopharmacology [RUPP] Anxiety Study Group, 2001; Van Ameringen, Mancini, Farvolden, & Oakman, 1999) and cognitive-behavioral treatment modalities (Beidel, Turner, & Morris, 2000; Hayward et al., 2000; Spence, Donovan, & Brechman-Toussaint, 2000). As in many areas of psychopathology, research blossoms when effective treatments become available. Although much of the outcomes research on social anxiety disorder has occurred in adult populations, it is a disorder that frequently has its precursors in childhood, and the most common age of onset is during adolescence (Davidson, Hughes, George, & Blazer, 1993; Last, Perrin, Hersen, & Kazdin, 1992; Schneier, Johnson, Horing, Liebowitz, & Weissman, 1992; Wittchen, Stein, & Kessler, 1999). For this reason, we believe that more focus is needed on the phenomenology, assessment, and treatment of social anxiety disorder in the first 2 decades of life.

DEVELOPMENTAL STAGE-RELATED VARIATIONS IN THE MANIFESTATIONS OF SOCIAL ANXIETY DISORDER

Withdrawn, avoidant, shy, and more recently, behaviorally inhibited temperaments have been described for many years (Kagan, Reznick, & Snidman, 1988). Although the temperamental traits of shyness and behavioral inhibition are often described as possible early manifestations of social anxiety disorder, in fact, most children with shy or behaviorally inhibited temperaments do not go on to develop clinically significant social anxiety disorder (Hayward, Killen, Kraemer, & Taylor, 1998; Schwartz, Snidman, & Kagan, 1999). However, as will be discussed in more detail later in the chapter, children with a behaviorally inhibited temperament appear to be at increased risk for developing social anxiety disorder by adolescence, compared with those without such a temperament. Thus, behavioral inhibition (BI) appears to be a predisposing, vulnerability characteristic or risk factor for the development of social anxiety disorder, rather than an early manifestation of the illness. Ultimately, determining whether behavioral inhibition is a risk factor or an early manifestation of the illness will require better understanding of the etiology and pathophysiology of social anxiety disorder.

Considering only *DSM*-defined social anxiety disorder, and not related traits such as shyness, it is nevertheless the case that the presentation of social anxiety disorder is *stage dependent*. For example, social anxiety disorder in young children may be characterized by somatic complaints, clinging, crying, and whining (Albano, Chorpita, & Barlow, 2003). School refusal may be an early manifestation of childhood social anxiety disorder (Kearney, 2001; Last & Strauss, 1990). Young children with social anxiety disorder may even appear oppositional in their resistance to engage in social activities (Beidel, Turner, & Morris, 1999).

In latency, children with social anxiety disorder may exhibit more typical fears and avoidant behavior seen in adolescents. In one series of 50 children with social anxiety disorder (mean age 10, age range of 7 to 13), Beidel et al. (1999) described five of the most frequently endorsed feared situations. In order of frequency, they were as follows: (a) reading in front of the class, (b) musical or athletic performance, (c) joining in on a conversation, (d) speaking to adults, and (e) starting a conversation. Of note, the children in this study were also suffering considerable social impairment: 75% of the sample reported no or few friends, 50% were not involved in any extracurricular or peer activities, and 50% reported that they did not like school.

Adolescence marks the period of highest risk for onset of social anxiety disorder (Wittchen et al., 1999). In considering the developmental tasks associated with adolescence, this is not surprising. In early adolescence, roughly ages 12 to 14, gender differences in reported self-consciousness emerge, with girls reporting greater levels than boys (La Greca & Lopez, 1998). Adolescents identify their most common anxieties to be their relationships with peers of the opposite sex, peer rejection, public speaking, blushing, self-consciousness, and excessive worry about past behavior (Bell-Dolan, Last, & Strauss, 1990). La Greca and Lopez (1998) examined 250 high school students (mean age 17, range 15 to 18 years) with a self-report measure of social anxiety. Increasing levels of social anxiety were associated with feeling less accepted and supported by peers, less romantically attracted to others, and fewer close friends. Moreover, girls in particular reported having friendships that were less intimate and less satisfying than their non-socially-anxious peers.

Adolescents with social anxiety disorder have poor social networks, underachieve in school and work, and exhibit poor social skills (Albano, 1995). Their avoidance behavior is consistent with their developmental stage, for example, avoidance of school dances, gym, taking tests, and eating in the cafeteria, as well as interacting with peers. Adolescents with social anxiety disorder may also avoid attending parties, using the telephone, meeting new people, attending family functions, using public restrooms, or eating in public (Albano, 1995). These avoidance behaviors during adolescence portend the avoidance behavior of adult social anxiety disorder, for example, avoidance of work-related functions and difficulties meeting members of the opposite sex, as well as difficulty using public restrooms, eating in public, or using the telephone. In fact, in a study examining the situational domains of adolescents with social phobia, Hofmann and colleagues (1999) examined in a clinical sample the most common situations reported as provoking social anxiety. Younger adolescents (ages 13 to 14) reported more anxiety in unstructured social situations such as being in the school hallways or cafeteria, joining in on conversations, and attending parties. In contrast, older adolescents (ages 15 to 17) reported higher anxiety for structured or compulsory social situations such as public speaking or speaking to authority figures. Thus, a transition may occur during adolescence, in which those with social anxiety learn that certain situations can be avoided (e.g., choosing to avoid going to a party or enter the cafeteria), whereas others cannot due to required responsibilities (e.g., giving the oral report results in a certain grade, similar to receiving a paycheck for doing one's job).

Implications for understanding the stage-dependent presentation of social anxiety disorder indicate that assessment, treatment, and prevention efforts must be carefully chosen and adjusted to fit the developmental stage of the child. Furthermore, the early onset and significant impairment associated with social anxiety disorder suggests a need for intervention at a young age, because social anxiety disorder is associated with later psychopathology and problems in living (Albano et al., 2003; Masia, Klein, Storch, & Corda, 2001). For example, untreated adolescents with social anxiety disorder have alarmingly high rates of onset of major depression (Hayward et al., 2000).

HOMOTYPIC AND HETEROTYPIC CONTINUITY

The high rate of major depression among those with social anxiety disorder (Hayward et al., 2000; Schatzberg, Samson, Rothschild, Bond, & Regier, 1998; Stein et al., 2001) is related to the constructs of homotypic and heterotypic continuity—concepts also derived from developmental psychopathology. Homotypic continuity refers to continuity (the presence of the illness over time) within one disorder. Heterotypic continuity refers to continuity across diagnoses (having an illness over time, but the illness varies across time points).

There is evidence for considerable discontinuity (low homotypic continuity) in youth with social anxiety disorder. In one study, the majority of youth (age range 5 to 18) with social anxiety disorder did not have the disorder 3 to 4 years later (Last, Perrin, Hersen, & Kazdin, 1996). Similarly, most adolescents with social anxiety disorder do not have the disorder as young adults (Pine, Cohen, Gurley, Brook, & Ma, 1998). Furthermore, most infants with behavioral inhibition at infancy are not characterized as behaviorally inhibited at age 7.5 (Kagan & Snidman, 1999). This low homotypic continuity among those with either behavioral inhibition or social anxiety disorder is in contrast to high rates of heterotypic continuity observed for social anxiety. For example, in the Dunedin Study, approximately 80% of those with social anxiety disorder as young adults had either an affective disorder or an anxiety disorder as adolescents (Newman et al., 1996). Pine (1999) argues for the need to identify factors that contribute to persistent emotional problems and suggests that biological factors might best predict the persistence of illness over time. Understanding the factors that contribute to homotypic and heterotypic continuity as well as discontinuity in social anxiety disorder remains a fundamental research question, one that requires longitudinal study designs.

EVIDENCE THAT THE DEVELOPMENT OF SOCIAL ANXIETY DISORDER IS MULTIFACTORIAL

The premise that social anxiety disorder is multifactorial is based on the likelihood that the development of most common psychiatric disorders is probabilistic in nature. Furthermore, the probability of developing a disorder is constantly changing as life experiences interact with predispositions. In this model, the risk of developing social anxiety disorder for any given individual is determined by the contribution of multiple factors acting additively or synergistically.

Is there evidence that the etiology of social anxiety disorder, in particular, is multifactorial in origin? Perhaps the best evidence comes from two domains which have received considerable attention in recent years: genetic studies and studies of temperament. In each case, review of the literature shows that there appears to be a role for genetic influences as well as temperamental influences in the development of social anxiety disorder. Equally important, however, is the observation that neither genetic influences alone nor temperamental factors alone account for the majority of cases of social anxiety disorder. In fact, it is likely that no one factor will be found necessary or sufficient to develop social anxiety disorder, in most cases; rather, it is probably a confluence of factors over time that determine the probability for developing social anxiety disorder.

In the case of the genetic contribution to the risk for social anxiety disorder, the best estimate of heritability comes from Kendler et al. (1999). In a study using the Virginia Twin Registry, measurement errors associated with unreliability and instability of diagnoses were reduced by obtaining two assessments of lifetime history of social anxiety disorder 8 years apart. Heritability for social anxiety was estimated to be 51%, the highest estimate of any study estimating heritability of social anxiety disorder (reviewed by Saudino, 2001). Estimates of heritability, of course, can vary depending on environmental context. In one environment, heritability can appear high and, in a different environment, variance accounted for by heritable factors can be quite low (Rutter, 2002). Nevertheless, twin studies appear to substantiate that genetic influences are important but do not explain the majority of cases of social anxiety disorder. The way in which genetic and environmental factors interact over time to enhance or reduce risk for the development of social anxiety disorder has not been well characterized.

Genetic variation in risk for either social anxiety as a trait or social anxiety as a disorder may manifest early in life as temperamental variability (Stein et al., 2001). Research in the area of temperament in relationship to social anxiety has become the focus of increasing attention among researchers. Much of this work owes its beginnings to the longitudinal studies of behaviorally inhibited children carried out by Kagan and colleagues (for review, see Kagan & Snidman, 1999). Behavioral inhibition is a temperamental characteristic defined by a constellation of behaviors including withdrawal, shyness, avoidance, and fear of unfamiliar people and objects (Kagan, Reznick, & Snidman, 1988). The construct has been developed in laboratory settings and has both a behavioral component (social withdrawal) and a physiological component (increased salivary cortisol and high stable heart rates; Kagan et al., 1988). Behavioral inhibition manifests as irritability in infants, shyness and fearful behavior in toddlers, and social withdrawal in school-age children (Kagan et al., 1988).

As previously discussed, there have been attempts to identify the risk of social anxiety disorder in those with histories of behavioral inhibition. In one prospective study, Hayward and colleagues (1998) utilized a community-based sample of 2,242 high school-aged adolescents assessed over 4 years. Among those free from social anxiety disorder at the study baseline assessment, retrospective self-reported behavioral inhibition in elementary school increased the risk for the onset of adolescent social anxiety disorder during the course of the study.

A second prospective study (Schwartz et al., 1999) evaluated adolescents who were part of the original cohort of behaviorally inhibited children defined as having BI by Kagan's group. Eleven years after the assessment of BI, these children were assessed at age 13 with a structured diagnostic interview. Generalized social anxiety disorder was three times more common in those adolescents identified as inhibited children compared to the uninhibited children. This finding was specific for generalized social anxiety and did not apply to circumscribed performance anxiety.

A third study (Prior, Smart, Sanson, & Oberklaid, 2000) assessed the relationship between a shy-inhibited temperament in childhood and anxiety symptoms in adolescence. A large nonclinical sample of children was followed for 13 years. Shyness was assessed on eight different occasions, from infancy through age 13, with a parent questionnaire. Anxiety symptoms in adolescence were measured using a self-report questionnaire. The authors describe results indicating a modest relationship between a shy temperament in childhood and anxiety problems in early adolescence. The strength of the association increased with shorter intervals between the assessment of shyness and the measurement of adolescent anxiety symptoms, and also increased with the more times a child was rated as being shy.

Of equal importance is the observation that, in the two studies that used a population-based design, most of those with adolescent anxiety symptoms or adolescent social anxiety disorder did not have a history of shyness or an inhibited temperament (Hayward et al., 1998; Prior et al., 2000). Measurement error in characterizing temperament or false positive diagnoses of social anxiety disorder could also lead to this finding. However, the consistency across both studies suggests that there are other important explanatory variables contributing to the onset of social anxiety disorder during adolescence.

The role of other explanatory variables becomes more apparent when the clinical significance of the association between behavioral inhibition and social anxiety disorder is examined by calculating the attributable risk. The attributable risk for the population is used to describe the clinical significance of a risk factor by numerically determining the maximal proportion of disease in the population that is attributable to a risk factor. This is important because measurements of potency—in these studies, for example, hazard ratios (Hayward et al., 1998), chi-squares (Schwartz et al., 1999), and odds ratios (Prior et al., 2000—do not directly translate into clinical significance (Kraemer et al., 1999). A risk factor can be potent but account for very few cases if the risk factor is rare—for example, pulmonary exposure to asbestos and the risk of lung cancer. Conversely, high base rates of a risk factor can yield very clinically meaningful results even with a lower potency for the association—for example, smoking and heart disease. Attributable risk for the population increases as both the base rate and potency of the risk factor increase. In the case of behavioral inhibition, the higher estimates for the base rate are approximately 20% (Kagan & Snidman, 1999). Taking the low (1.4) and high (4.9) estimates of potency (risk ratios) for the association between an inhibited temperament (or shyness, for Prior et al., 2000) and adolescent social anxiety disorder (or anxiety problems, for Prior et al.), the estimated attributable risk for the population ranges from 7% to 44%. For comparison, the attributable risk for the population for smoking in middle-aged men leading to a first coronary event is estimated at 32% (Kelsey, Thompson, & Evans, 1986). One interpretation of this range of possible attributable risks is that temperament may be minimally or quite important, but in either case, we are still missing a big piece of the explanatory pie.

Further evidence that the development of social anxiety disorder is multifactorial comes from the same longitudinal prospective study of high school students reviewed previously in this chapter (Hayward et al., 1998; Hayward et al., 2000). In this study, a number of factors were shown to increase the risk for development of social anxiety disorder during high school, including self-reported behavioral inhibition as a child, a history of parental separation and divorce, early pubertal maturation in females, and minority status (membership in an ethnic group other than one of the three most prevalent ethnic groups: white, Hispanic, and Asian). Figure 8.1 shows the cumulative effect of multiple risk factors for the onset of social anxiety disorder during high school in females. One third of those with three or more risk factors develop social phobia during high school, compared with less than 5% without any of these risk factors.

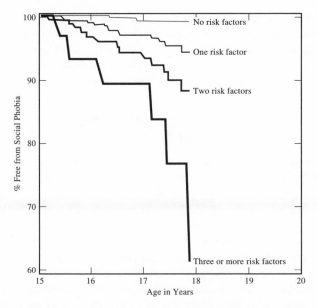

Figure 8.1. Percentage of adolescent females free from social phobia.
Note: Survival curves demonstrate the risk of onset of social phobia in adolescent females ($N = 1,072$) among those free from disorder at study entry. Risk factors include selfreported childhood behavioral inhibition, parental history of separation or divorce, early pubertal maturation, and ethnic minority status (membership in one of the least represented ethnic groups—i.e., not Caucasian, Asian, or Hispanic).

Similarly, in a community-based sample of Canadian youth evaluated in the Ontario Health Survey, there was also evidence that multiple risk factors are associated with a history of social phobia (Chartier, Walker, & Stein, 2001). For subjects between the ages of 15 and 64, associations were observed for (a) lack of a close relationship with an adult, (b) not being the firstborn (males only), (c) marital conflict in the family of origin, (d) parental history of mental disorder, (e) moving more than three times as a child, (f) juvenile justice and child welfare involvement, (g) running away from home, (h) childhood physical and sexual abuse, (i) failing a grade, (j) requirement of special education before age 9, and (k) dropping out of school. These studies provide some empirical support for a multifactorial etiology of social anxiety disorder. The present challenge is to test multiple risk factors in a single study design to establish the relative contribution of each, as well as their interactions at different stages of the life cycle.

As one example, Lieb et al. (2000) report that the association between parental rejection and adolescent social anxiety disorder is greater in the presence of parental psychopathology. There are, of course, many other possible factors associated with risk for social anxiety disorder, such as conditioning events or cognitive factors (see Albano et al., 2003; Ollendick & Hirshfeld-Becker, 2002; and Velting & Albano, 2001, for reviews). As mentioned, overprotective, rejecting, and anxious parenting styles have also been examined as risk factors or factors that maintain social anxiety disorder (see Velting & Albano, 2001, for a review). The work in parenting styles illustrates another important tenet of developmental psychopathology—the transactional or bidirectional nature of many predisposing factors.

TRANSACTION BETWEEN CHILDHOOD DISPOSITION AND PARENTING STYLES

Evidence from developmental studies of parent-child dyads indicates that children's behavior and temperament impact or affect parental response differentially. Parents may adopt different parenting styles, depending on the characteristics of the child. Preliminary evidence suggests that this is the case for children with behavioral inhibition or social withdrawal. Pioneering work by Rubin, Nelson, Hastings, and Asendorpf (1999) indicates that childhood inhibition and associated parental beliefs may reinforce the development of social withdrawal. For example, Rubin and Stewart (1996) proposed that early social withdrawal might elicit parenting responses of overprotection and overcontrol. These parenting styles may reinforce social withdrawal, resulting in a bidirectional family system that increases the probability of developing social anxiety disorder. In essence, a self-defeating and self-perpetuating cycle develops (*self*, in this case, refers to the family system as a whole) whereby the child-withdrawal and parent overprotection interact to prevent the child from gaining experience with mastery over his or her environment and anxiety reactions (cf. Albano et al., 2003; Barlow, 2002). Other support for the relationship between child fearfulness and parental overcontrol comes from Belsky, Putnam, and Crnic, 1997; LaFreniere and Doumas, 1992; Rubin, Hastings, Stewart, Henderson, and Chen, 1997; and Rubin and Mills, 1990.

Rubin et al. (1999) have further shown that it is the parental perception of the child's characteristics that best predicts child-rearing practices by the parent. If a parent perceives the child as socially withdrawn or shy, even if there is objective evidence to the contrary, the parent may be more likely to respond with a parenting style that is overprotective. Although these findings are preliminary, they provide some evidence for the bidirectional nature of transactions between parent and child that may increase the risk for social anxiety disorder.

Although studies of this sort are difficult to carry out, they highlight the importance of considering interactions between individuals and their environments in considering the risk for developing social anxiety disorder. In this scenario, for example, one could imagine socially withdrawn children and adolescents having few friends and having social interactions characterized by considerable behavioral avoidance. This behavioral avoidance, in turn, creates a response from peers that is neglecting and distancing. Note our use of the term *neglecting* as opposed to *rejecting*. Many investigators in this arena have documented peer *neglect* as the failure to consider the inclusion of certain peers in social activities, as opposed to the conscious rejection of peers who may be considered noxious for some reason (e.g., bullies; Christoff & Myatt, 1987; Rubin, LeMare, & Lollis, 1990). Due to the cognitive nature of social anxiety, however, this peer neglect is interpreted as peer rejection by the youth with social anxiety disorder. Socially anxious children and adolescents may be greatly affected by this neglect (perceived rejection), which then leads them to further social withdrawal. We suggest that testing bidirectional, transactional models will better facilitate an understanding of the development of social anxiety disorder.

One other study which is of particular interest with respect to social anxiety disorder when considering the transactional relationship between individuals and their social environment is a study of Chinese youth (Chen, Rubin, Li, & Li, 1999). This study showed that, unlike their counterparts in the United States, Chinese youth who scored high on a measure of social anxiety were socially valued by their peer group. In China, social withdrawal and social reticence are considered positive attributes. In other words, the relationship of social anxiety to psychiatric morbidity may be context dependent. In cultures where introversion is highly valued the embarrassment and shame associated with social anxiety in Western societies may be absent. The data from China raises the possibility that the characteristics of social anxiety and even the clinical course of those with extreme social anxiety may vary according to the cultural value placed on the trait.

In summary, social anxiety must be approached with a multifactorial and transactional model, whereby biological vulnerability interacts with and is shaped by contexts such as parenting style, peer relations, school settings, and culture. To fully understand and effectively treat youth with social anxiety disorder the fluidity of person-environment interactions must be uncovered through appropriate assessment and intervention strategies.

MULTIMODAL ASSESSMENT OF SOCIAL ANXIETY DISORDER

Assessment should always guide treatment, both at its onset as the treatment plan is formulated and as an integrated part of the treatment process, to inform clinical decisions such as addressing patient goals, titration of medication, or frequency and intensity of psychosocial interventions, and defining termination and relapse prevention strategies. A template for understanding normative social anxiety reactions is necessary but not sufficient for the assessment of social anxiety disorder in youth. As noted earlier in this chapter, research in the broad arena of child development has provided a guide for understanding expected age-related increases in anxiety, including those triggered by social and evaluative situations (cf. Albano, Causey, & Carter, 2001; King, Hamilton, & Ollendick, 1988). The *DSM* system defines certain time parameters for the presence of a minimum number of symptoms and level of impairment in order to assign an anxiety diagnosis to a child or adolescent. For social anxiety disorder, these symptoms and associated impairments must be present and relatively stable for at least 6 months. This time frame is theoretically (not empirically) derived to allow for the waxing and waning of social anxiety at the various ages or developmental stages discussed previously and summarized in Table 8.1. As noted in the table, certain developmental tasks or situations provide cues for heightened social anxiety.

The child or adolescent will experience a rise in anxiety, as a normative state, on confronting the trigger in certain contexts. However, the anxiety should be relatively brief and not impair functioning or result in avoidance to any significant degree. Over time, with repeated experience with the trigger and context, the anxiety response should attenuate and dissipate more quickly or not occur at all (cf. Albano et al., 2003; Barrios & O'Dell, 1998; Ollendick, Matson, & Helsel, 1985). Thus, problematic social anxiety must be assessed in a developmental context. The anxiety of a child at age 7 who is afraid to order for himself at a McDonald's is not the same as that of the 14-year-old who is likewise too anxious to order food in a restaurant. In the former, the child is likely experiencing normative levels of stranger anxiety and task unfamiliarity, whereas ordering food should be common to all adolescents and completed with ease. Thus, the assessment of social anxiety disorder must involve understanding the normative developmental variations of social anxiety along with specific age and stage-related tasks of development.

In the remainder of this section, we outline the assessment of social anxiety disorder, involving multiple methods and multiple informants, to capture historical, developmental, and current factors impacting the child or adolescent's functioning and experience of social anxiety. Our focus in this section is on the process and variables we consider necessary in assessing social anxiety disorder, rather than recommending and reviewing specific assessment scales and forms. However, we provide a summary of measures to assess social anxiety and related constructs in Appendix A. The reader interested in a detailed analysis of the various available instruments and forms is referred to reviews such as March and Albano's (1998), or books such as Mash and Terdal's (1997).

Diagnostic Evaluation and Developmental Assessment

To answer the question "Is this child or adolescent experiencing normative levels of social anxiety, or is this social anxiety disorder?" a careful diagnostic evaluation forms the foundation from which the assessment, and ultimately the treatment process, will emerge. The diagnostic evaluation should involve the differential assessment of symptoms and associated functional impairments for the range of anxiety, mood, and behavioral disorders of youth. Information should be gathered through direct interview of the child or adolescent, separate interview with the parents, and a process of combining the information, using clinical judgment regarding the reliability of the report and knowledge of psychopathology and development.

Table 8.1. Ages and Specific Contexts Associated With Expression of Normative Social Anxiety

Age/Developmental Level	Focus of Social Anxiety	Implied Trigger for Social Anxiety	Contexts
2–4 years/toddler	Stranger anxiety	Interactions with unfamiliar persons (including same-age peers)	Play situations, family events, preschool or daycare, and social events such as parties
5–8 years/early childhood	Stranger anxiety; task unfamiliarity/evaluation anxiety	Interactions with same-age peers, adults (e.g., teachers, sitters) and introduction to academic and social evaluative situations	Play situations; school situations including meeting teachers, peers, and their parents; evaluations
9–12 years/late childhood	Evaluation anxiety; rejection sensitivity	Homework, exams, oral reports, other methods of evaluation; Potential for exclusion from peer events such as parties and clubs	Academic tasks designed for evaluation, peer activities such as invited events, clubs, performance-based activities
13–15 years/Adolescence	Social anxiety including evaluation (real or perceived); rejection sensitivity; heightened self-consciousness	Academic tasks, peer relationships, teasing, intimacy and romantic relationships, social skill, performance-based activities	Academic tasks, peer group approval or disapproval, access and readiness to enter peer situations, self-perception of physical attractiveness and/or adeptness, inclusion in a peer group, establishing close friendships
16 years and older/late adolescence and into emerging adulthood	Social anxiety including evaluation fears; rejection sensitivity; heightened self-consciousness	Academic tasks, completion of basic educational requirements, formation of long-term goals, establishment of a romantic partner, greater call for self-reliance, formation of self-identify	Academic tasks including college admission tests, applications, and interviews; job interviews; peer situations involving greater levels of intimacy and trust; situations calling for independent functioning

Structured or semistructured diagnostic interview methods have high utility in providing reliable differential diagnoses for the trained, competent clinician (March & Albano, 1998) but can be cumbersome in clinical practice settings where the time burden may preclude their use. However, familiarity with a structured interview format, such as the Anxiety Disorders Interview Schedule for *DSM-IV*, Child Version (Silverman & Albano, 1996), may serve as a useful resource when differential diagnostic quandaries present themselves.

A common problem in making the diagnosis of social anxiety disorder in youth is confusion with other anxiety disorders such as generalized anxiety disorder (GAD). In GAD, the cardinal feature is persistent worry about any number of situations, including social and academic functioning, in which the child feels that the worry is difficult to control. Although not carefully delineated in the *DSM-IV* criteria, social anxiety disorder may be distinguished from GAD on the basis of the cognitions associated with the anxiety (Albano & Hack, in press; Kendall, Krain, & Treadwell, 1999). In social anxiety disorder, the anxiety stems from the fear of negative evaluation or rejection by others, or humiliating oneself in front of others. In contrast, the worry about social and academic tasks in GAD typically involves a fear of failing oneself by not reaching some internal, self-generated goal or standard. For example, the fear of receiving less than adequate grades, for the child with social anxiety disorder, is linked to what the teacher or other students will think ("They will think I'm stupid"), whereas the child with GAD may be fearful of not passing the course, making good enough grades for college, and ultimately having a miserable future due to poor school performance.

Interwoven into the diagnostic evaluation are assessments of the child's psychiatric history, medical history, and an understanding of normative developmental processes and age-appropriate functioning. The psychiatric history involves probing for past disorders such as separation anxiety disorder, selective mutism, attention deficit/hyperactivity disorder, and other psychiatric conditions that may have predated the social anxiety disorder. In addition to establishing any history of a prior condition, the clinician should assess the course of the disorder, response to any interventions, and factors that may have precipitated the prior disorder and any present conditions. A developmental history is also taken to gather information concerning the child's age at meeting developmental milestones, assess the child's temperament during early development, and note any prior delays or present behavioral deficits or excesses. In addition, the presence of certain chronic developmental conditions should be evaluated, as these may impact the prognosis and may dictate a different or modified treatment plan. For example, youth with pervasive developmental disorder (PDD) are oftentimes inappropriately referred to groups targeting social anxiety disorder for treatment (Albano, 1995). The referral source is hoping for a social skills training experience for the child with PDD; however, the nature of social skills deficits in the two disorders is different in both etiology and malleability. Youth with PDD present with varying degrees of neuropsychiatric impairment in the ability to develop and refine both concrete and higher order social skills, from basic conversational skills to the more abstract skills necessary to decode nonverbal and otherwise ambiguous communications (see Volkmar, 1998). The child with social anxiety disorder, barring any independent and significant learning disability, will have the necessary cognitive information-processing capacity to learn and refine social skills but may be delayed or arrested in skill development due to the anxiety. Addressing the anxiety should free the child to progress in social skill development without hitting a predetermined ceiling, as will likely happen to the child with PDD.

In addition to the assessment of developmental milestones and disorders, a developmental assessment also provides a basis for understanding the child's social behavior, friendship patterns, and degree of independent functioning at various stages. These areas should be of specific interest to the clinician working with socially anxious youth because the parents of these children typically take on too much responsibility for managing these areas for the child, as compared with parents of nonanxious children (cf. Barrett, Dadds, Rapee, & Ryan, 1994; Chorpita, Albano, & Barlow, 1996). The child's social anxiety may interact with parental rearing styles and parenting behavior in a negative feedback loop in which the child is too anxious to approach/invite other children to play, whereas the parent feels compelled to protect the child from the anxiety or perceived social injustices (such as neglect, isolation) and so becomes overly involved in managing the child's social interactions (arranges play dates, negotiates peer conflicts). This results in the child's not gaining important and normative social experience with managing uncomfortable and challenging social interactions. Hence, the anxiety and avoidance is maintained in the child, and the compensatory parenting behaviors likewise persist in this vicious cycle. Of course, this is a chicken-and-egg scenario, as we cannot identify what came first, the child's anxiety or the parental rearing style, and in fact, as noted earlier in the chapter, there are multiple pathways to the social anxiety disorder. It is possible that a child's temperament and higher levels of social anxiety work to modify the parents' behavior to be overprotective and accommodating (Rubin et al., 1999; Logsden-Conradsen, 1997). Ultimately, certain interpersonal skills such as initiating friendships, conflict resolution, and assertiveness can be absent or underdeveloped in the child with social anxiety disorder. A careful developmental assessment will determine whether these deficits exist, as well as any associated reciprocal or compensatory behavior on the part of the parents. These skills and interaction patterns can then become a focus of the treatment plan. The developmental assessment may complement or take place during the course of a complete medical history and examination, which is necessary to rule out a physical basis for the anxiety disorder.

Family and School History Evaluations

Prior to the age of majority, children and adolescents spend their time largely in two contexts, the home and school environments. The influence of the family on the development and maintenance of social anxiety disorder may in fact begin prior to the conception of the child. A comprehensive history of first- and second-degree relatives can uncover heritable risks for psychopathology in general or social anxiety disorder in particular, although probably more relevant to treatment planning is the nature of the child's interactions with any affected family members (affected by any type of psychopathology). If a child is at risk due to genetic or temperamental factors, the nature of the family environment can set the stage for the realization of psychological vulnerabilities. Parental overprotection; parental psychopathology, economic, and employment problems; and parental marital discord are among family variables identified as increasing stress on the child and contributors to childhood disorders (see Vasey & Dadds, 2001), whether or not there exists an endogenous risk factor such as inhibited temperament. The evaluation of family relationships and environment, such as whether the family encourages interaction and communication, degree of warmth, level of and methods for resolving conflict, discipline practices, and expectations for responsibility (e.g., chores, independent functioning) should be examined in formulating proposed etiological pathways and also when considering treatment options. Moreover, the parents' understanding of normative development and their expectations for the child or adolescent's social functioning at a given age may also interact with the child in a transactional manner. Thus, evaluation of family history should also involve assessing the parents' expectations and understanding of the child's functioning and capabilities.

Examination of the child's school history and records, including teacher reports, will provide the clinician with invaluable information about the child's cognitive and social development. Anxiety may manifest early in the school years and exert a negative impact on academic functioning over time. For example, research by Ialongo, Edelsohn, Werthamer-Larsson, Crockett, and Kellam (1994, 1995) demonstrated that the presence of anxiety symptoms at 5 years of age predicted children's adaptive functioning 4 years later. After controlling for level of adaptive functioning, Ialongo and colleagues found that children evidencing the top third of anxious symptoms during first grade were 10 times more likely to be in the bottom third for academic achievement in fifth grade.

For youth with social anxiety disorder, uneven academic achievement patterns may indicate real or perceived difficulty with certain school factors or contexts, such as teacher personalities and teaching styles, demands for class participation, class size, or assignment of group projects. In such cases, academic decline may indicate the child's struggle to manage anxiety in the classroom. Functional impairment in academic tasks can be attributed to anxiety symptoms such as impaired attention and concentration, avoiding class participation or activities garnering the focus of others' attention, and preoccupation with self-defeating thoughts. Narrative summaries of the child's school progress by teachers can provide invaluable information concerning the child's level of participation in class activities, initiative, assertiveness, response to criticism and feedback, and social relationships with peers. Teachers' comments may contain information not readily apparent as suggestive of social anxiety disorder, such as "He is so quiet and compliant. What a pleasure, I don't even know he's there!" or "Rather than go out on the playground, Erin prefers to read in the classroom during recess." These common observations are not necessarily innocuous but instead may portend the emergence of intense fears of negative evaluation. The school history evaluation is easily accomplished through a review of academic reports and parent recall of teacher conferences but may be greatly enhanced by speaking directly to the teacher and by the use of standardized teacher rating scales such as the Achenbach Child Behavior Checklist and Teacher Report Form (Achenbach, 1991).

One area that is often overlooked in the assessment of family and school functioning is the effect of environmental context on the child or adolescent's level of anxiety. That is, the clinician must ascertain the nature of the environments in which the child lives and attends school. Questions should address whether the environments are safe and nurturing or potentially dangerous. Youth living in an abusive home or a high-crime community may have difficulty with anxiety in general, but with regard to social anxiety, there may be valid reasons for a lack of social interaction or opportunities to interact freely with peers. A school that has been plagued by violence or crime may not offer activities outside the structured classroom experience. Also, in some cases it may not be logistically feasible for the youth to interact with peers on a regular basis.

For example, if the child lives a distance from the school or peer group (such as a child who lives in a rural setting or one who travels to school outside the home community), gatherings or extracurricular activities can be rendered difficult and rare due to travel constraints. Similarly, the child who has recently relocated or started attending a new school may evidence an exacerbation of social anxiety symptoms. Finally, the clinician must make a careful assessment of when certain environmental issues interact with the social anxiety to make it easier to avoid social or evaluative situations. If the setting is innocuous but logistically challenging, the social anxiety disorder may make it easier for the youth to make excuses to avoid social interactions. "It's too far for me to travel." "No one stays after school for clubs or sports." "It's too much trouble for my parents to drive me to the party." Thoughts such as these can be uncovered and addressed in the context of treatment, as they serve to maintain the social anxiety disorder.

Self-Report and Behavioral Assessment

A plethora of self-report scales exists for accessing child and parent reports for the constructs discussed throughout this chapter, such as anxiety, social anxiety, fears, family history, family environment, temperament, avoidance behavior, self-image, friendship patterns, loneliness, depression, worry, physical sensations of anxiety, cognitive processes, assertiveness, school environment, perceived stress, psychosocial stressors, and pubertal status. In fact, the list of standardized questionnaires to assess the range of constructs and contexts mentioned in this chapter fill volumes. In the multimodal assessment approach, self-report scales provide the child or adolescent with an alternative way of expressing thoughts, feelings, and behaviors. In some cases, the paper-and-pencil method serves to free the child from the social desirability that may accompany an interview format, and thus a greater degree of symptomatology is endorsed. In others, the youth may feel constrained or deny the anxiety on paper and in the absence of probing and more direct questioning. A self-report measure may contain a lie scale to assess the degree of responding in a socially desirable manner and raise doubts about the validity of the report. In fact, one study revealed that the Lie scale of the Revised Children's Manifest Anxiety Scale (RCMAS) did in fact predict adolescents' diagnosis of social phobia (DiBartolo, Albano, Heimberg, & Barlow, 1998). Reading level must always be considered when administering self-report scales, as most require at least third-grade reading and reading-comprehension levels for completion. Questionnaires are also administered to parents and teachers, as noted above. Overall, paper-and-pencil measures are relatively easy and quick to administer and score and can be used to assess social anxiety and related constructs. These measures provide screening information or additional information to that accessed through interviews but do not allow for the differential diagnosis of any disorder.

Behavioral assessment involves assessing the behavioral limits of the child when stressed by a social anxiety-provoking stimulus (Barrios & Hartmann, 1988). Although standardized behavioral assessment techniques exist to assess specific child or adolescent characteristics (e.g., social skill) or for use in research studies (see Albano & Barlow, 1996), most common in the assessment of social anxiety disorder are individualized, clinician-driven challenges for the patient. For example, reading aloud, having a conversation with an unfamiliar person, ordering food, and asking an unfamiliar person for directions are typical scenarios constructed by the therapist to evaluate the behavioral limits of a patient with social anxiety. Known as the behavioral approach task (BAT), the BAT provides information related to whether the child can initiate the task, how long the client can stay in the situation, the level of anxiety reached during the task, and whether the child escapes or actively refuses to try the task. The presence or absence of parents during the task also provides information relating to whether the child feels comforted and able to perform (or whether, conversely, the situation is made worse) and also allows for the parents' response to the child to be observed. Administering the BAT pre- and posttreatment provides a method of assessing overt behavior and can be augmented by having the child list any thoughts that occurred during the task, along with rating his or her level of anxiety—for example, from 0 (none at all) to 100 (extreme). Table 8.2 presents an overall summary of assessment strategies.

TREATMENT OF SOCIAL ANXIETY DISORDER IN YOUTH

Assessment guides treatment, and on receiving the diagnosis of social anxiety disorder, the next question posed by parents and youth is typically, "Well, now what do we do?" This question is generally followed by a series of related questions concerning the types and appropriateness of available treatments for the disorder. The general consensus in the scientific community is that cognitive-behavioral treatment (CBT), as a psychosocial modality, and pharmacotherapy with a selective serotonin reuptake inhibitor (SSRI) show the most promise as efficacious treatments for anxiety disorders in youth, including social anxiety disorder (American Academy of Child and Adolescent Psychiatry [AACAP], 1997; Kazdin & Weisz, 1998; Leonard, March, Rickler, & Allen, 1997; March, 1999; Ollendick & King, 1998). A number of trials have evaluated the efficacy of nonspecific CBT protocols for youth with social anxiety disorder, separation anxiety disorder, or generalized anxiety disorder (Barrett, Dadds, & Rapee, 1996; Kendall, 1994; Kendall & Southam-Gerow, 1996; Mendlowitz et al., 1999; Silverman, Kurtines, Ginsburg, Weems, Lumpkin, et al., 1999; Silverman, Kurtines, Ginsburg, Weems, Rabian, et al., 1999). These trials enrolled youth with any of the three disorders (or combination of disorders); the primary outcomes focused on a decrease in the disorder of worst severity at intake.

Other CBT protocols have been developed specifically for the treatment of social anxiety disorder in youth and tested in controlled trials and smaller open trials (Albano, Marten, Holt, Heimberg, & Barlow, 1995; Beidel et al., 2000; Hayward et al., 2000; Spence, Donovan, & Brechman-Toussaint, 2000). Of note is that all of these CBT trials used specific treatment manuals designed to address the social anxiety disorder through the delivery of a combination of cognitive-behavioral procedures. These manuals typically incorporated psychoeducation, cognitive restructuring, somatic management, and behavioral exposures, in either group or individual format, but differed on the emphasis given to specific procedures. Moreover, the manuals and studies differed in the age of the participants and the degree to which parents were involved in the protocols. For example, the Spence et al. trial compared parent involvement to no involvement for children with social anxiety and found relatively little additional benefit to involving parents in treatment. Overall, CBT has been found to be efficacious for 50% to 74% of youth affected with anxiety disorders, including social anxiety disorder.

There is a fairly extensive literature substantiating the efficacy of pharmacologic agents in the treatment of social anxiety disorder in adults (Tancer & Uhde, 1995). Adults who suffer from the disorder may opt for treatment with a monoamine oxidase inhibitor (MAOI; e.g., Liebowitz et al., 1992), benzodiazepine (Gelernter et al., 1991) or a selective serotonin

Table 8.2. Guide to Integrated, Developmentally Sensitive, and Multimodal Assessment for Social Anxiety Disorder

Target of Assessment	Method of Assessment	Informant(s) and Source of Information	Comments
Diagnostic evaluation	Structured interview and mental status exam	Parents, child (or adolescent)	Systematically evaluate symptoms, diagnostic conditions, and associated impairments as experienced by the child and observed by parents
Child/adolescent's developmental history	Clinical interview, including develop-mental assessment from prenatal period through present day	Parents, child or adolescent, and compilation of information gathered from teachers, medical and mental health professionals; historical data from medical file and school records	Gather data to examine developmental mile-stones, social behavior, onset and course of any problems such as developmental delays, areas of strengths and weaknesses
Child/adolescent's psychiatric history	Clinical interview (including lifetime diagnoses)	Parents, child or adolescent, former diagnosticians and therapists, archival reports, and chart reviews	Examine onset, severity, and course of disorder; type of and response to any treatment
Medical history and evaluation	Physical exam, chart review	Parents, pediatrician	Evaluate current status in development including pubertal status; identify any physical limitations or conditions that may precipitate or exacerbate anxiety
Family history	Clinical interview, questionnaire methods	Parents or primary caretakers	Use as a context for understanding the risks (genetic, environmental) and protective factors inherent in the child's family and environment; evaluate family relationships and interaction patterns
School history	Clinical interview and psychoeducational assessments	Parents, child or adolescent, former and present teachers; historical data from school records	Track any changes in academic performance, examine class teachers' comments regarding class participation and other overt social behaviors
Self-reports	Paper-and-pencil standardized questionnaires	Parents, child, or adolescent	Use as an alternative method for accessing information on targeted syndromes, associated conditions, and a range of functional domains
Behavioral assessment	Observation (either structured or unstructured) of the child or adolescent in various social contexts	Independent observer such as teacher, parent, or clinical assistant	May involve contrived social situations, whereas unstructured observation involves observing the child in his or her natural surroundings (e.g., school playground)

reuptake inhibitor (SSRI; Stein et al., 1998), in addition to having other classes of medications as choices. In contrast, there are very few controlled trials examining the efficacy of medications in the treatment of social anxiety disorder in youth. In part, the hesitancy of physicians and parents to treat a child with medications bearing certain side effect profiles, such as the MAOIs or benzodiazepines, may have restricted both their evaluation and off-label use. In contrast, the SSRIs are receiving wider attention and evaluation, probably owing to their demonstrated short-term safety and tolerability in children and adolescents. An early study demonstrated good efficacy of the SSRIs in the treatment of selective (elective) mutism (Black & Uhde, 1994), a childhood disorder thought to be a variant of social anxiety disorder (Black & Uhde, 1992).

More recently, the SSRIs have been studied in youth diagnosed with social anxiety disorder, separation anxiety disorder, or GAD (Birmaher et al., 1994; RUPP Anxiety Study Group, 2001). Similar to outcomes for the nonspecific cognitive-behavioral treatment packages, the outcomes reported by these studies showed that the SSRIs were superior to pill placebo in controlled, randomized trials involving children with varying types of anxiety disorders. Also, one large randomized trial (Compton et al., 2001) and a smaller open case series (Mancini, Van Ameringen, Oakman, & Farvolden, 1999) found the SSRIs effective in targeting social anxiety disorder in youth. Response rates of up to 76% for treated youth versus 29% for placebo have been reported (RUPP Anxiety Study Group, 2001) and appear quite promising. However, results of medication trials are generally reported for short-term, acute treatment (e.g., 8 to 12 weeks), with the long-term safety and efficacy of the SSRIs unknown.

Whether concerning CBT or medication, the research has often been criticized for a variety of methodological flaws including but not limited to idiosyncratic definitions for responder status, length of follow-up (medication), inadequate control conditions (CBT), and self-selection biases in the study sample. Owing to the respective criticisms is the absence of any well-controlled studies examining the treatment of social anxiety disorder in the same population of youth, using randomized, controlled procedures, and offering CBT, medication, their combination, and a credible placebo condition. Beyond the criticisms that behavioral scientists may employ when evaluating the extant literature, the average parent with a child or adolescent disabled by social anxiety disorder will likely be interested in what works, in the immediate sense and over the long term, and—statistical significance aside—what makes sense clinically to offer any individual youth in need.

DEVELOPING AN INTEGRATED TREATMENT PLAN

The child or adolescent's clinical presentation, along with the evaluation of developmental and contextual factors, will guide the practitioner in developing a coherent treatment plan that (a) is minimally invasive and (b) has the potential to be maximally beneficial. By *minimally invasive*, we refer to methods that will be the least burdensome to the youth and family members in terms of the efforts necessary to comply with treatment, as well as time and cost burdens. In addition, AACAP (1997) recommends that medications be used judiciously in the treatment of anxious youth. Hence, youth with relatively mild levels of social anxiety disorder should be offered the least burdensome and invasive treatments, with more aggressive treatment regimes (e.g., combined approaches) reserved for those who are more severely disabled. In response to marketing of medications for social anxiety disorder, negative publicity in the popular press has warned of the "pathologizing of shyness." Parents and youth may also be wary of both psychosocial and pharmacological interventions, with a lack of understanding of the differences between being shy or being hesitant to be the center of attention and having pathological levels of anxiety that dictate one's response and prevent one from engaging in various social activities. Thus, whether moving forward with CBT, medication, or their combination, psychoeducation must always be the common element in all treatment plans for social anxiety disorder. Families must receive education about the nature of social anxiety, pathways to its expression, familial and contextual factors that become intertwined with the anxiety, and developmental tasks and factors that should be taken into account for a child of any given age.

In deciding on a course of treatment for a child or adolescent, we make great use of the information gained through our integrated developmental/diagnostic assessment. Children and adolescents in our programs typically receive the diagnosis of social anxiety disorder on the basis of the Anxiety Disorders Interview Schedule for *DSM-IV*, Child Version (Silverman & Albano, 1996). Following the completion of the interviews (a separate interview with the child and parent, with decision rules for combining their information), a clinician severity rating (CSR) is assigned to the diagnosis on a 0 to 8 scale, with increasing levels suggesting higher levels of symptom severity, increased disturbance and disability. Each successive CSR subsumes the behavioral descriptors of the previous level. Thus, youth with a CSR of 6 will likely evidence some or all of the symptoms and disability associated with a CSR of 4, but at a greater intensity, frequency, and degree of disability. In Table 8.3, we provide a rough outline, based on our clinical experience, of the symptoms and presentation of socially anxious youth at various levels of the CSR. The CSR then directs us towards a recommended treatment plan, with psychoeducation as the basic intervention for mild symptoms that may be developmentally appropriate, CBT as the first-line treatment for youth who meet full diagnostic criteria and moderate levels of social anxiety disorder, and a combination of CBT plus medication with an SSRI for those youth with more severe and disabling levels of social anxiety disorder.

Our CBT approach is typically group format with other socially anxious youth; however, access to groups is often difficult in community settings. Hence, individual CBT is often the starting point, with an emphasis on between-session exposures to enhance treatment effects. Our general

Table 8.3. Treatment Recommendations for Youth With Social Anxiety Disorder at Increasing Levels of Severity

---

CSR Rating = 0

Absence of symptoms/No disturbance in functioning/No disability

---

The child or teen may express (verbally or noted via observation by others) developmentally appropriate levels of social anxiety that are circumscribed to specific events/ interactions and brief in duration (*for the most part, the anxiety dissipates spontaneously during the course of the social situation*). The youth does not avoid the social stimulus or situation and is able to function well in all areas (social, academic, family, self-care) with no disruption or disability.

Recommendation: Basic psychoeducation about social anxiety and development.

CSR Rating = 2

Mild symptoms/Slight disturbance in functioning/Not really disabling

---

Child or teen exhibits (verbal statements or via observation by others) developmentally appropriate levels of social anxiety. This anxiety is circumscribed to specific events or social interactions, and the anxiety is relatively brief in duration. *The anxiety may not dissipate during the course of the first several social encounters or situations; however, the youth **does not avoid** the social event and is able to function in all areas (social, academic, family, self-care) with very minor disruption but no disability.* The youth may take several days to a week, or need several experiences with the social situation before the anxiety habituation occurs.

Recommendation: Basic psychoeducation about social anxiety and development. Reevaluate in 6 months to track child or teen's progress.

CSR Rating = 4

Moderate symptoms/Definite disturbance in functioning/Disabling

---

Youth meets full criteria for social anxiety disorder (minimum number of required symptoms) plus evident impairment in one or more contexts. The child or adolescent may or may not be able to acknowledge the presence of symptoms or disability, but parents' or others (e.g., teachers) may note overt behavioral avoidance of, or anxiety related to, age-appropriate activities and tasks. The youth's anxiety remains constant for a period of at least six months, with no true abatement of symptoms or disability. That is, despite ongoing opportunities to engage in various social evaluative tasks, the youth remains anxious (does not habituate to the task) and may engage in active avoidance of these situations. Moreover, there is evidence for disruption in functioning, such as having fewer friendships than same-age peers or an inability to initiate and/or maintain friends, academic problems, and/or family conflict secondary to the anxiety.

Recommendation: Begin cognitive behavioral treatment for social anxiety. Involvement of parents will depend upon the degree to which they are involved in the anxiety process, level of impairment for the child or teen, and cognitive/developmental factors. Set specific goals for 4, 8, and 12 weeks of treatment, but expect treatment to continue upward of 16 to 20 weeks. Consider appropriate adjunctive therapy (family, medication) if progress is not evident, symptoms persist or worsen, and/or contextual and family variables impede progress. Following adequate recovery, taper the CBT sessions and then provide booster CBT during times of high stress or developmental changes (e.g., transition from elementary to high school).

(*continued*)

Table 8.3. (*continued*)

CSR = 6

Severe symptoms/Marked disturbance in functioning/Markedly disabling

The child or teen meets full criteria for social anxiety disorder (minimum number of required symptoms) plus *marked impairment* in a variety of contexts. The child or adolescent may or may not be able to acknowledge the presence of symptoms or disability. Parents report noticing the child/adolescent's discomfort regarding social situations and can identify overt behavioral avoidance of, or anxiety related to, age-appropriate activities and tasks. The anxiety is stable for at least 6 months and there is no evidence that it will remit without intervention. The youth engages in active avoidance of social and evaluative situations. There is evidence of considerable disruption in functioning, such as having few or no friendships or an inability to initiate and/or maintain friends, academic problems, and/or family conflict secondary to the anxiety.

Recommendation: Offer CBT and medication as concurrent options. May begin with CBT alone, with interim goals specified for 4 and 8 weeks of treatment. If medication treatment is not initiated and progress is not evident at point of interim goals, medication should be reconsidered. Adjunctive treatments for family, school, or contextual issues that impede progress should be considered. Following adequate recovery and tapering of treatment, provide booster CBT during times of high stress or developmental changes.

CSR = 8

Very severe symptoms/Very severe disturbance in functioning/Very severely disabling

The child or teen meets full criteria for social anxiety disorder (minimum number of required symptoms) plus *extreme impairment* in *most* areas of funcitioning. This child or adolescent is at a level of severity that may warrant intensive intervention. The child or adolescent may or may not acknowledge the presence of symptoms or disability however these symptoms are readily apparent to others just by observation. The anxiety has likely been evident and stable for most of the child's time in school and it will not remit without intervention. The youth actively avoids most social and evaluative situations. Disruption in functioning is evident as the child may have no friendships or an inability to initiate and/or maintain friends, academic problems, and/or family conflict secondary to the anxiety.

Recommendation: Begin combined course of treatment of CBT plus medication. CBT may be more intensive (twice weekly) initially, with tapering to weekly sessions as improvement becomes evident. Set interim goals for 4, 8, and 12 weeks of treatment. Treatment with CBT may be extended to 6 months or more and may involve both individual CBT and group treatment for socially anxious youth. May need to involve adjunctive services to promote school attendance, address comorbidity such as depression, and more actively involve parents in the treatment process. Maintain medication through one full year of adequate improvement and functioning. Provide booster CBT sessions throughout the course of medication taper, and also during times of high stress or developmental changes (e.g., transition from elementary to high school).

guideline for parent involvement is that greater involvement occurs when the child is younger, more severely disabled, has higher comorbidity patterns (especially with externalizing disorders), and the anxiety is actively entwined with family interactions and functioning. We suggest less parent involvement for adolescents who must meet the developmental tasks of individuation and independence (see Albano, 1995; Albano & Barlow, 1996), as the responsibility for change should be gently fostered in the adolescent. Also, we rely on less involvement of the parents when there is a high level of parent conflict (e.g., marital distress), presence of parental psychopathology that could impede progress, or other family factors that may serve to hinder the progress of therapy. Thus, the assessment of the child's family environment and supports is essential to decisions on when or how to involve parents in treatment. Similarly, we may involve teachers as needed, and we conduct exposure sessions is the settings where the anxiety is most likely to occur (e.g., in the school, parks, restaurants) whenever feasible and appropriate. In this way, we attempt to address contextual cues through direct exposure for habituation to the anxiety, to allow practice of the CBT skills in an applied sense, and to foster generalization of gains outside the safety of the therapy room.

Finally, the decisions on when and how to stop treatment also rest with assessment. Throughout the course of the child or adolescent's treatment program, repeated assessment through the use of standardized questionnaires, informal interview with the patient and parents, or ideographic methods (e.g., "my top ten social anxiety fears") will provide information on severity of illness and improvement. As the child progresses and meets the goals outlined in the treatment plan, a tapering of CBT sessions occurs, and greater responsibility is placed on the youth for challenging anxiety-provoking situations. Various relapse prevention plans include creating written action plans for future events, role reversal (in which the child or teen serves as therapist to demonstrate acquisition and knowledge of CBT principles), and creating a video commercial of the key strategies learned for mastering anxiety (see Kendall et al., 1999). If medication has been a part of the treatment plan, we recommend that the medication regime be maintained for 6 months to a year beyond the point of stopping CBT and having achieved good functioning. Then, CBT sessions should be restarted at the initiation of the medication taper and continue through the discontinuation. The main focus of the CBT is to reinforce the child or adolescent's coping with anxiety-provoking situations, to normalize the experience of anxiety, and to assist (when necessary) the patient's taking responsibility for his or her gains as opposed to owing any positive changes to the medication or to the clinician.

SUMMARY AND CONCLUSIONS

In conclusion, social anxiety disorder is more than mere shyness; it presents through a multidetermined process of endogenous and exogenous factors;

and it is expressed differently at various ages and stages of development and in concert with environmental and contextual factors. Although research indicates that cognitive-behavioral and pharmacological treatments of social anxiety disorder are promising as monotherapies, there has been an absence of research addressing their combined effects, in addition to the field's being limited in providing scientifically sound guidelines for the management of this disorder in clinical settings. Thus, we offer not only that a comprehensive assessment is necessary to accurately identify the disorder in youth, but also that assessment must continue throughout the course of treatment to inform decisions such as modality, involvement of parents, and discontinuation. A clinically derived guide for when to begin with CBT or the combination of CBT and medication is offered; however, empirical testing of these recommendations is needed. Overall, social anxiety disorder is a complex and multidetermined condition that is amenable to intervention delivered in a developmentally sensitive manner.

APPENDIX A: ASSESSMENT METHODS FOR SOCIAL ANXIETY DISORDER

Diagnostic Interview and Clinician-Administered Assessments

The Anxiety Disorders Interview Schedule for DSM-IV, Parent and Child Versions (ADIS-P; ADIS-C; Silverman & Albano, 1996) provides direct coverage of a broad range of anxiety, mood, and externalizing behavior disorders in youth and screens for the presence of several additional disorders, including developmental, psychotic, and somatoform disorders. The ADIS also addresses age of onset, impairment, and avoidance and has been described as the premier instrument for assessing anxiety disorders in youth (Stallings & March, 1995). Impairment ratings are generated for each diagnosis via the Clinician Severity Rating (CSR; range = 0 to 8) with a rating greater than 4 required to assign a diagnosis. Earlier versions possess the best psychometric profile for the diagnostic assessment of childhood anxiety disorders of available diagnostic measures (Silverman & Eisen, 1992; Silverman & Nelles, 1988). The interview has good interrater reliability (r = 0.98 for the parent interview and r = 0.93 for the child interview; Silverman & Nelles, 1988) and test-retest reliability (e.g., k = 0.76 for the parent interview; Silverman & Eisen, 1992) and has shown sensitivity to treatment effects in studies of youth with anxiety disorders (e.g., Dadds et al., 1992; Kendall et al., 1997). Psychometric studies of the DSM-IV version of the instrument are excellent (Silverman et al., 2001; Piacentini et al., 2002).

The Pediatric Anxiety Rating Scale (PARS; Walkup & Davies, 1999) is a clinician-rated anxiety severity rating scale for children and adolescents and includes a 50-item anxiety symptom checklist and 7 anxiety severity ratings specifically addressing the combined severity of symptoms of separation anxiety disorder (SAD), social phobia (SOP), and generalized anxiety disorder (GAD). The PARS requires approximately 30 minutes to complete. It has excellent inter-rater reliability (> 0.97) across anxiety severity (Walkup & Davies, 1999).

The Global Assessment Scale for Children (C-GAS; Shaffer et al., 1983) provides a measure of global impairment and functioning over the previous month. The scale ranges from 1 (lowest) to 100 (highest) functioning. Green et al. (1994) provide evidence for the psychometric soundness of the C-GAS and suggest that ratings obtained in clinical contexts may reflect evaluations of functional competence rather than symptom severity.

Background and Screening Measures

Demographics/History   The ADIS contains sections to collect information on each patient and his or her family regarding demographic status, medical history, past history of mental health (including anxiety) treatment, and family history of psychiatric disorders.

Medical Examination   Medical examinations should include history and physical exam and urine screens for pregnancy (females of child-bearing age) and use of illicit substances.

Measures of Social Anxiety

The Social Phobia and Anxiety Inventory for Children (SPAI-C; Beidel, Turner, & Morris, 1995) is a 26-item inventory assessing social anxiety in a variety of settings. A youth self-report form is available, with the parent report form under development. Separate items measure the cognitive, somatic, and behavioral components of social anxiety. The SPAI-C demonstrates excellent psychometric properties (Beidel & Turner, 1998).

The Social Anxiety Scale for Children (and Adolescents)–Revised (SASC-R; La Greca, 1998; La Greca & Stone, 1993) is comprised of 22 items assessing three specific factors: fear of negative evaluation, social avoidance and distress in new situations, and social avoidance and distress in general and is available in a child, adolescent, and parent version. The authors report excellent internal consistency and test-retest reliability in several studies.

Anxiety Symptom Self-Report Measures

The Multidimensional Anxiety Scale for Children (MASC; March, Parker, Sullivan, Stallings, & Conners, 1997) is a 39-item, four-point Likert self-report rating scale that has shown robust psychometric properties in clinical, epidemiological, and treatment studies. It includes four factors: physical symptoms (tense/restless and somatic/autonomic subfactors), social anxiety (humiliation/rejection and public performance subfactors), harm avoidance (anxious coping and perfectionism subfactors), and separation/panic anxiety. Three-week test-retest reliability for the MASC is .79 in clinical (March et al., 1997) and .88 in school-based samples (March & Sullivan, 1999).

The Screen for Child Anxiety Related Emotional Disorders (SCARED; Birmaher et al., 1997, 1999) is a 41-item child and parent self-report instrument that asses *DSM-IV* symptoms of panic disorder, SAD, SOC, GAD, and school refusal. The SCARED has shown very good psychometric properties in two different large clinical samples (Birmaher et al., 1997, 1999) and in a community sample (Muris et al., 1998). The SCARED has both a child and a parent form.

The Fear Survey Schedule for Children-Revised (FSSC-R; Ollendick, 1987) assesses phobic symptoms, including fear of failure and criticism, fear of the unknown, fear of injury and small animals, fear of danger and death, and medical fears. A parent version of the scale can be administered to assess the parents' perception of their child's number and level of specific fears. The FSSC-R has demonstrated excellent psychometric properties and is widely used across cultures and settings.

The Children's Negative Affectivity Self-Statement Questionnaire (NASSQ; Ronan, Kendall, & Rowe, 1994) provides a measure of specific self-statements (cognitions) associated with negative affect. This measure contains a series of self-statements that are rated by children on a five-point scale in terms of frequency of occurrence. The NASSQ consists of separate items for younger and older children. The measure possesses good test-retest and internal reliability and is sensitive to CBT treatment (Kendall et al., 1997).

Parent and Teacher Report Forms

The Child Behavior Checklist Parent Form and Teacher Report Form (Achenbach, 1991) are 118-item self-report scales assessing behavioral problems and social and academic competence. The CBCL is one of the most extensively tested rating scales available and possesses excellent psychometrics.

Functional Status

Information regarding the impact of treatment for social anxiety on the social and academic functioning of subjects may be collected from the "Interpersonal Relationships" section of the ADIS (e.g., questions regarding friends, activities), the "School History" and "School Refusal" sections of the ADIS (e.g., questions regarding school grades and attendance patterns), and the competency subscale of the CBCL (e.g., number of friends, preferred activities).

The Social Adjustment Scale–Self-Report (SAS-SR; Weissman et al., 1978; Weissman et al., 1980) is a self-report measure assessing social adjustment across four major role areas (school behavior, spare time, peer relations, and family behavior). Youngsters rate 21 items on a five-point scale, with higher scores reflecting greater impairment. A total adjustment score and separate role area scores are computed. Two additional items on dating are only administered to children over age 12. The SAS-SR-C possesses acceptable psychometric properties.

The School Refusal Assessment Scale (SRAS; Kearney & Silverman, 1993) assesses the conditions maintaining school refusal behavior. The SRAS is administered to the child and separately to each parent. Escape from social anxiety has been identified as a principal motivating condition for youth who refuse school (Kearney, 2001).

Environments

The Family History Screen for Epidemiologic Studies (FHE; Lish et al., 1995) asks a primary informant (e.g., mother, father, guardian) to report on prevalence of psychiatric disorder in first- and second-degree relatives. The FHE screens for 15 *DSM-IV* psychiatric diagnoses and possesses adequate psychometric properties for this purpose.

The Brief Symptom Inventory (BSI; Derogatis, 1993) is a 56-item, widely used measure that provides an efficient dimensional measure of parental psychopathology. The BSI, which is a psychometrically valid shortened version of the SCL-90, is independently completed by mothers and fathers about themselves. The BSI measures nine dimensions of distress: somatization, obsessive-compulsive, interpersonal sensitivity, depression, anxiety, hostility, phobic anxiety, paranoid ideation, and psychoticism. Both convergent and construct validity with other measures of psychopathology have been demonstrated for this scale.

The Self-Report Measure of Family Functioning Scale (SRMFF; Bloom, 1985) provides a reliable and valid measure of three general dimensions of family function (relationship, value, system maintenance). A 65-item, 13-factor version of this scale has been used to reliably characterize family functioning in children with anxiety disorders and to discriminate between children with anxiety disorders and youngsters with depression and other psychiatric diagnoses (Stark et al., 1990, 1993).

REFERENCES

Achenbach, T. M. (1991). *Manual for the Child Behavior Checklist: 4–18 and 1991 profile*. Burlington: University of Vermont Department of Psychiatry.

Albano, A. M. (1995). Treatment of social anxiety in adolescents. *Cognitive and Behavioral Practice, 2,* 271–298.

Albano, A. M., & Barlow, D. H. (1996). Breaking the vicious cycle: Cognitive behavioral group treatment for socially anxious youth. In E. D. Hibbs & P. S. Jensen (Eds.), *Psychosocial treatments for child and adolescent disorders: Empirically based strategies for clinical practice* (pp. 43–62). Washington, DC: American Psychological Association.

Albano, A. M., & Hack, S. (in press). Generalized anxiety disorder in children and adolescents. In R. G. Heimberg, D. Mennin, & C. Turk (Eds.), *Generalized anxiety disorder: Diagnosis, assessment and treatment*. New York: Guilford Press.

Albano, A. M., Causey, D., & Carter, B. (2001). Fear and anxiety in children. In C. E. Walker & M. C. Roberts (Eds.), *Handbook of clinical child psychology* (3rd ed., pp. 291–316). New York: Wiley.

Albano, A. M., Chorpita, B. F., & Barlow, D. H. (2003). Anxiety disorders. In E. J. Mash & R. A. Barkley (Eds.), *Child psychopathology* (2nd ed.). New York: Guilford Press.

Albano, A. M., Marten, P. A., Holt, C. S., Heimberg, R. G., & Barlow, D. H. (1995). Cognitive-behavioral group treatment for social phobia in adolescents: A preliminary study. *Journal of Nervous and Mental Disease, 183,* 685–692.

American Academy of Child and Adolescent Psychiatry. (1997). Practice parameters for the assessment and treatment of children and adolescents with anxiety disorders. *Journal of the American Academy of Child and Adolescent Psychiatry, 36,* 69–84.

American Psychiatric Association. (1994). *Diagnostic and statistical manual of mental disorders: DSM-IV* (4th ed.). Washington, DC: Author.

Amies, P., Gelder, M., & Shaw, P. (1983). Social phobia: A comparative clinical study. *British Journal of Psychiatry, 142,* 174–179.

Asendorpf, J. (1994). The malleability of behavioral inhibition: A study of individual developmental function. *Developmental Psychology, 30,* 912–919.

Barlow, D. H. (2002). *Anxiety and its disorders* (2nd ed.). New York: Guilford Press.

Barrett, P. M., Rapee, R. M., Dadds, M. M., & Ryan, S. M. (1994). Family enhancement of cognitive style in anxious and aggressive children. *Journal of Abnormal Child Psychology, 24,* 187–203.

Barrett, P., Dadds, M., Rapee, R. (1996). Family treatment of childhood anxiety: A controlled trial. *Journal of Consulting and Clinical Psychology, 64,* 333–342.

Barrett, P., Rapee, R., Dadds, M., & Ryan, A. (1996). Family enhancement of cognitive style in anxious and aggressive children. *Journal of Abnormal Child Psychology, 24,* 187–203.

Barrios, B. A., & Hartmann, D. B. (1988). Fears and anxieties. In E. J. Mash & L. G. Terdal (Eds.) *Behavioral assessment of childhood disorders* (2nd ed., pp. 196–264). New York: Guilford Press.

Barrios, B. A., & Hartmann, D. P. (1997). Fears and anxieties. In E. J. Mash & L. G. Terdal (Eds.), *Behavioral assessment of childhood disorders* (3rd ed., pp. 230–327). New York: Guilford Press.

Barrios, B. A., & O'Dell, S. L. (1998). Fears and anxieties. In E. J. Mash & R. A. Barkley (Eds.), *Treatment of childhood disorders* (2nd ed., pp. 249–337). New York: Guilford Press.

Beidel, B. C., & Turner, T. M. (1999). The natural course of shyness and related syndromes. In L.A. Schmidt & J. Schulkin (Eds.). *Extreme fear, shyness, and social phobia* (pp. 203–223). New York: Oxford University Press.

Beidel, D. C., & Turner, S. M. (1998). *Shy children, phobic adults: Nature and treatment of social phobia.* Washington, DC: American Psychological Association.

Beidel, D. C., Turner, S. M., & Morris, T. L. (1995). A new inventory to assess childhood social anxiety and phobia: The social phobia and anxiety inventory for children. *Psychological Assessment, 7,* 73–79.

Beidel, D. C., Turner, S. M., & Morris, T. L. (1999). Psychopathology of childhood social phobia. *Journal of the American Academy of Child and Adolescent Psychiatry, 38*(6), 643–650.

Beidel, D. C., Turner, S. M., & Morris, T. L. (2000). Behavioral treatment of childhood social phobia. *Journal of Consulting and Clinical Psychology, 68,* 1072–1080.

Bell-Dolan, D., Last, C. G., & Strauss, C. C. (1990). Symptoms of anxiety disorders in normal children. *Journal of the American Academy of Child and Adolescent Psychiatry, 29,* 759–765.

Belsky, J., Putnam, S., & Crnic, K. (1997). Coparenting, parenting, and early emotional development. *New Directions in Child Development, 74,* 45–56.

Birmaher, B., Brent, D. A., Chiappetta, L., Bridge, J., Monga, S., & Baugher, M. (1999). Psychometric properties of the Screen for Child Anxiety Related Emotional Disorders (SCARED): A replication study. *Journal of the American Academy of Child and Adolescent Psychiatry, 38*(10), 1230–1236.

Birmaher, B., Khetarpal, S., Brent, D., Cully, M., Balach, L., Kaufman, J., & McKenzie Neer, S. (1997). The Screen for Child Anxiety Related Emotional Disorders (SCARED): Scale construction and psychometric characteristics. *Journal of the American Academy of Child and Adolescent Psychiatry, 36,* 545–553.

Birmaher, B., Waterman, G. S., Ryan, N., Cully, M., Balach, L., Ingram, J., & Brodsky, M. (1994). Fluoxetine for childhood anxiety disorders. *Journal of the American Academy of Child and Adolescent Psychiatry, 33,* 993–999.

Black, B., & Uhde, T. W. (1992). Elective mutism as a variant of social phobia. *Journal of the American Academy of Child and Adolescent Psychiatry, 31,* 1090–1094.

Black, B., & Uhde, T. W. (1994). Treatment of elective mutism with fluoxetine: A double-blind, placebo-controlled study. *Journal of the American Academy of Child and Adolescent Psychiatry, 33,* 1000–1006.

Black, B., & Uhde, T. W. (1996). Psychiatric characteristics of children with selective mutism: A pilot study. *Journal of the American Academy of Child and Adolescent Psychiatry, 35,* 1000–1006.

Bloom, B. L. (1985). A factor analysis of self-report measures of family functioning. *Family Process, 24*(2), 225–239.

Chartier, M. J., Walker, J. R., & Stein, M. B. (2001). Social phobia and potential childhood risk factors in a community sample. *Psychological Medicine, 31*(2), 307–315.

Chen, X., Rubin, K. H., Li, B., & Li, Z. (1999). Adolescent outcomes of social functioning in Chinese children. *International Journal of Behavioral Development, 23*(1), 199–223.

Chorpita, B. F., Albano, A. M., & Barlow, D. H. (1996). Cognitive processing in children: Relation to anxiety and family influences. *Journal of Clinical Child Psychology, 25,* 170–176.

Christoff, K. A., & Myatt, R. J. (1987). Social isolation. In M. Hersen & V. B. Van Hasselt (Eds.), Behavior therapy with children and adolescents: A clinical approach (pp. 512–535). New York: Wiley.

Cicchetti, D., Cohen, D. J. (Eds.). (1995). *Developmental psychopathology: Vol. 1. Theory and methods.* New York: Wiley.

Compton, S. N., Grant, P. J., Chrisman, A. K., Gammon, P. J., Brown, V. L., &

March, J. S. (2001). Sertraline in children and adolescents with social anxiety disorder: An open trial. *Journal of the American Academy of Child and Adolescent Psychiatry, 40,* 564–571.

Dadds, M. R., Sanders, M. R., Morrison, M., & Rebgetz, M. (1992). Childhood depression and conduct disorder II: An analysis of family interaction patterns in the home. *Journal of Abnormal Psychology, 101*(3), 505 -513.

Dadds, M. R., & Sanders, M. R. (1992). Family interaction and child psychopathology: A comparison of two observation strategies. *Journal of Child and Family Studies, 4,* 371 -391.

Davidson, J. R. T., Hughes, D. L., George, L. K., & Blazer, D. G. (1993). The epidemiology of social phobia: Findings from the Duke Epidemiological Catchment Area Study. *Psychological Medicine, 23,* 709–718.

Derogatis, L. R. (1993). *The Brief Symptom Inventory* (2nd ed.). Riderwood, MD: Clinical Psychometric Research.

DiBartolo, P. M., Albano, A. M., Barlow, D. H, & Heimberg, R. G. (1997, March). Clinical issues in the treatment of social phobia in youth. In C. L. Masia & T. L. Morris (Chairs), *Treating anxiety disorders in children and adolescents: Cost-effective interventions and clinical considerations.* Symposium presented at the Anxiety Disorders Association of America Meeting, New Orleans, LA.

DiBartolo, P. M., Albano, A. M., Barlow, D. H., & Heimberg, R. G. (1998). Cross-informant agreement in the assessment of social phobia in youth. *Journal of Abnormal Child Psychology, 26,* 213–220.

Flannery-Schroeder, E., & Kendall, P. C. (2000). Group and individual cognitive-behavioral treatments for youth with anxiety disorders: A randomized clinical trial. *Cognitive Therapy and Research, 24,* 251–278.

Gelernter, C. S., Uhde, T. W., Cimbolic, P., Arnkoff, D. A., Vittone, B. J., Tancer, M. E., & Bartko, J. J. (1991). Cognitive behavioral and pharmacological treatments of social phobia: A controlled study. *Archives of General Psychiatry, 48,* 938–945.

Green, B. L., Grace, M. C., Vary, M. G., Kramer, T. L., Gleser, G. C., & Leonard, A. C. (1994). Children of disaster in the second decade: A 17-year follow-up of the Buffalo Creek survivors. *Journal of the American Academy of Child and Adolescent Psychiatry, 33,* 71–79.

Hayward, C., Killen, J. D., Kraemer, H. C., & Taylor, C. B. (1998). Linking self-reported childhood behavioral inhibition to adolescent social phobia. *Journal of the American Academy of Child and Adolescent Psychiatry, 37*(12), 1308–1316.

Hayward, C., Varady, S., Albano, A. M., Thieneman, M., Henderson, L., & Schatzberg, A. F. (2000). Cognitive-behavioral group therapy for female socially phobic adolescents: Results of a pilot study. *Journal of the American Academy of Child and Adolescent Psychiatry, 39,* 721–726.

Heimberg, R. G., Liebowitz, M., Hope, D., & Schneier, F. (Eds.) (1995). *Social phobia: Diagnosis, assessment, and treatment.* New York: Guilford Press.

Heimberg, R. G., Salzman, D. G., Holt, C. S., & Blendell, K. A. (1993). Cognitive-behavioral group treatment for social phobia: Effectiveness at five-year follow-up. *Cognitive Therapy and Research, 17,* 325–329.

Hofmann, S., Albano, A. M., Heimberg, R. G., Tracey, S., Chorpita, B. F., & Barlow, D. H. (1999). Subtypes of social phobia in adolescents. *Depression and Anxiety, 9,* 8–15.

Ialongo, N., Edelsohn, G., Werthamer-Larsson, L., Crockett, L., & Kellam, S. (1994). The significance of self-reported anxious symptoms in first-grade children. *Journal of Abnormal Child Psychology, 22,* 441–455.

Ialongo, N., Edelsohn, G., Werthamer-Larsson, L., Crockett, L., & Kellam, S. (1995). The significance of self-reported anxious symptoms in first-grade children: Prediction to anxious symptoms and adaptive functioning in fifth grade. *Journal of Child Psychology & Psychiatry & Allied Disciplines, 36,* 427–437.

Kagan, J. (1997). Temperament and the reactions to unfamiliarity. *Child Development* 68(1): 139–143.

Kagan, J., & Snidman, N. (1999). Early childhood predictors of adult anxiety disorders. *Biological Psychiatry, 46*(11), 1536–1541.

Kagan, J., Reznick, J. S., & Snidman, N. (1988). Biological bases of childhood shyness. *Science, 240,* 167–171.

Kazdin, A. E., & Weisz, J. R. (1998). Identifying and developing empirically supported child and adolescent treatments. *Journal of Consulting and Clinical Psychology, 66,* 19–36.

Kearney, C. A. (2001). *School refusal behavior in youth: A functional approach to assessment and treatment.* Washington, DC: American Psychological Association.

Kearney, C. A., & Silverman, W. K. (1993). Measuring the function of school refusal behavior: The School Refusal Assessment scale. *Journal of Clinical Child Psychology, 22,* 85–96.

Kelsey, J., Thompson, W. D., & Evans, A. S. (1986). *Methods in observational epidemiology.* New York: Oxford University Press.

Kendall, P. C. (1994). Treating anxiety disorders in children: Results of a randomized clinical trial. *Journal of Consulting and Clinical Psychology, 62,* 100–110.

Kendall, P. C., & Southam-Gerow, M. A. (1996). Long-term follow-up of a cognitive-behavioral therapy for anxiety disordered youth. *Journal Consultation of Clinical Psychology, 4,* 37–62.

Kendall, P. C., Flannery-Schroeder, E., Panichelli-Mindel, S. M., Southam-Gerow, M. A., Henin, A., &Warman, M. (1997). Therapy for youths with anxiety disorders: A second randomized clinical trial. *Journal of Consulting and Clinical Psychology, 65,* 366–380.

Kendall, P. C., Krain, A., & Treadwell, K. R. (1999). Generalized anxiety disorders. In R. T. Ammerman, M. Hersen, & C. G. Last (Eds.), *Handbook of prescriptive treatments for children and adolescents* (2nd ed., pp. 155–171). Needham Heights, MA: Allyn & Bacon.

Kendler, K. S., & Prescott, C. A. (1999). A population-based twin study of lifetime major depression in men and women. *Archives of General Psychiatry, 56*(1), 39–44.

Kendler, K. S., Gardner, C. O, & Prescott, C. A. (1999). Clinical characteristics of major depression that predict risk of depression in relatives. *Archives of General Psychiatry, 56*(4), 322–327.

Kendler, K. S., Karkowski, L. M., & Prescott, C. A. (1999). Fears and phobias: reliability and heritability. Psychological Medicine, *29*(3), 539–553.

Kendler, K. S., Karkowski, L. M., & Prescott, C. A. (1999). The assessment of dependence in the study of stressful life events: Validation using a twin design. *Psychological Medicine, 29*(6), 1455–1460.

Kendler, K. S., Karkowski, L. M., Corey, L. A., Prescott, C. A., & Neale, M. C. (1999). Genetic and environmental risk factors in the aetiology of illicit drug initiation and subsequent misuse in women. *British Journal of Psychiatry, 175,* 351–356.

Kendler, K. S., Neale, M. C., Kessler, R. C., Heath, A. C., & Eaves, L. J. (1992). The genetic epidemiology of phobias in women: The interrelationship of agoraphobia, social phobia, situational phobia, and simple phobia. *Archives of General Psychiatry, 49*(4), 273–281.

Kendler, K. S., Neale, M. C., Sullivan, P., Corey, L. A., Gardner, C. O., & Prescott, C. A. (1999). A population-based twin study in women of smoking initiation and nicotine dependence. *Psychological Medicine, 29*(2), 299–308.

King, N. J., Hamilton, D. I., & Ollendick, T. H. (1988). *Children's fears and phobias: A behavioural perspective.* Chichester, UK: Wiley.

Klimes-Dougan, B., Free, K., Ronsaville, D., Stilwell, J., Welsh, C. J., & Radke-Yarrow, M. (1999). Suicidal ideation and attempts: A longitudinal investigation of children of depressed and well mothers. *Journal of the American Academy of Child and Adolescent Psychiatry, 38*(6), 651–659.

Kraemer, H. C., Kazdin, A. E., Offord, D. R., Kessler, R. C., Jensen, P. S., & Kupfer, D. J. (1999). Measuring the potency risk of factors for clinical or policy significance. *Psychological Methods, 4,* 257–271.

La Greca, A. M. (1998). It's "all in the family": Responsibility for diabetes care. *Journal of Pediatric Endocrinology and Metabolism, 11*(Suppl. 2), 379–385.

La Greca, A. M. (2001). Friends or foes? Peer influences on anxiety among children and adolescents. In W. K. Silverman & P. Treffers (Eds.), *Anxiety disorders in children and adolescents* (pp. 159–186). New York: Cambridge University Press.

La Greca, A. M., & Lopez, N. (1998). Social anxiety among adolescents: Linkages with peer relations and friendships. *Journal of Abnormal Child Psychology, 26,* 83–94.

La Greca, A. M., & Stone, W. L. (1993). Social Anxiety Scale for Children–Revised: Factor structure and concurrent validity. *Journal of Clinical Child Psychology, 22,* 17–27.

La Greca, A. M., Silverman, W. K., & Wasserstein, S. B. (1998). Children's pre-disaster functioning as a predictor of posttraumatic stress following Hurricane Andrew. *Journal of Consulting and Clinical Psychology, 66*(6), 883–892.

LaFreniere, P. J., & Dumas, J. E. (1992). A transactional analysis of early childhood anxiety and social withdrawal. *Development and Psychopathology, 4,* 385–402.

Last, C. G., & Strauss, C. C. (1990). School refusal in anxiety-disordered children and adolescents. *Journal of the Academy of Child and Adolescent Psychiatry, 29*(1), 31–35.

Last, C. G., Perrin, S., Hersen, M., & Kazdin, A. E. (1992). *DSM-III-R* anxiety disorders in children: Sociodemographic and clinical characteristics. *Journal of the American Academy of Child and Adolescent Psychiatry, 31*(6), 1070–1076.

Last, C. G., Perrin, S., Hersen, M., & Kazdin, A. E. (1996). A prospective study of childhood anxiety disorders. *Journal of the American Academy of Child and Adolescent Psychiatry, 35*(11), 1502–1510.

Leonard, H., March, J., Rickler, K., & Allen, A. (1997). Pharmacology of the selective serotonin reuptake inhibitors in children and adolescents. *Journal of the American Academy of Child and Adolescent Psychiatry, 36,* 725–736.

Lieb, R., Wittchen, H. U., Höfler, M., Fuetsch, M., Stein, M. B., & Merikangas, K. R. (2000). *Archives of General Psychiatry, 56,* 859–866.

Liebowitz, M. R., Schneier, F., Campeas, R., Hollander, E., Hatterer, J., Fyer, A., Gorman, J., et al. (1992). Phenelzine vs. atenolol in social phobia: a placebo-controlled comparison. *Archives of General Psychiatry, 49,* 290–300.

Lish, J. D., Weissman, M. M., Adams, P. B., Hoven, C. W., & Bird, H. (1995). Family psychiatric screening instruments for epidemiologic studies: Pilot testing and validation. *Psychiatry Research, 57(2),* 169–180.

Logsden-Conradsen, S. (1998). *Family interaction patterns in adolescents with social phobia.* Unpublished doctoral dissertation. University of Louisville, KY.

Mancini, C., Van Ameringen, M., Oakman, J., & Farvolden, P. (1999). Serotonergic agents in the treatment of social phobia in children and adolescents: A case series. *Depression and Anxiety, 10,* 33–39.

March, J. (1999). Pharmacotherapy of pediatric anxiety disorders: A critical review. In D. Beidel (Ed.), *Treating anxiety disorders in youth: Current problems and future solutions* (pp. 42–62). Washington, DC: Anxiety Disorders Association of America.

March, J. S. (1995). *Anxiety disorders in children and adolescents.* New York: Guilford Press.

March, J. S. (1995). Cognitive-behavioral psychotherapy for children and adolescents with OCD: A review and recommendations for treatment. *Journal of the American Academy of Child and Adolescent Psychiatry, 34,* 7–18.

March, J. S., & Albano, A. M. (1998). Advances in the assessment of pediatric anxiety disorders. *Advances in Clinical Child Psychology, 20,* 213–241.

March, J., & Sullivan, K. (1999). Test-retest reliability of the Multidimensional Anxiety Scale for Children. *Journal of Anxiety Disorders, 13,* 349–358.

March, J., Parker, J. D., Sullivan, K., Stallings, P., & Conners, C. K. (1997). The Multidimensional Anxiety Scale for Children (MASC): Factor structure, reliability, and validity. *Journal of the American Academy of Child and Adolescent Psychiatry, 36,* 554–565.

Mash, E. J., & Terdal, L. G. (Eds.). (1997). *Behavioral assessment of childhood disorders* (3rd ed.). New York: Guilford Press.

Masia, C. L., Klein, R. G., Storch, E. A., & Corda, B. (2001). School-based behavioral treatment for social anxiety disorder in adolescents: Results of a pilot study. *Journal of the American Academy of Child and Adolescent Psychiatry, 40(7),* 780–786.

Mendlowitz, S. L., Manassis, K., Bradley, S., Scapillato, D., Miezitis, S., & Shaw, B. F. (1999). Cognitive-behavioral group treatments in childhood anxiety disorders: The role of parental involvement. *Journal of the American Academy of Child and Adolescent Psychiatry, 38,* 1223–1229.

Muris, P., Meesters, C., Merckelbach, H., Sermon, A., & Zwakhalen, S. (1998). Worry in normal children. *Journal of the American Academy of Child and Adolescent Psychiatry, 37(7),* 703–710.

Muris, P., Merckelbach, H., Mayer, B., & Meesters, C. (1998). Common fears and their relationship to anxiety disorders symptomatology in normal children. *Personality and Individual Differences, 24(4),* 575–578.

Muris, P., Merckelbach, H., Mayer, B., van Brakel, A., Thissen, S., Moulaert, V., & Gadet, B. (1998). The Screen for Child Anxiety Related Emotional Disorders (SCARED) and traditional childhood anxiety measures. *Journal of Behavior Therapy and Experimental Psychiatry, 29(4),* 327–339.

Muris, P., Merckelbach, H., Schmidt, H., & Mayer, B. (1998). The revised version of the Screen for Child Anxiety Related Emotional Disorders

(SCARED-R): Factor structure in normal children. *Personality and Individual Differences, 26,* 99–112.

Muris, P., Merckelbach, H., van Brakel, A., Mayer, B., & van Dongen, L. (1998). The Screen for Child Anxiety Related Emotional Disorders (SCARED): Relationship with anxiety and depression in normal children. *Personality and Individual Differences, 24*(4), 451–456.

Newman, D. L., Moffitt, T. E., Caspi, A., Magdol, L., Silva, P. A., & Stanton, W. R. (1996). Psychiatric disorder in a birth cohort of young adults: Prevalence, comorbidity, clinical significance, and new case incidence from ages 11 to 21. *Journal of Consulting and Clinical Psychology, 64*(3), 552–562.

Ollendick, T. H., & Hirshfeld-Becker, D. R. (2002). The developmental psychopathology of social anxiety disorder. *Biological Psychiatry, 51*(1), 44–58.

Ollendick, T. H., & King, N. J. (1998). Empirically supported treatments for children with phobic and anxiety disorders. *Journal of Clinical Child Psychology, 27,* 156–167.

Ollendick, T. H., King, N. J., & Frary, R. B. (1989). Fears in children and adolescents: Reliability and generalizability across gender, age and nationality. *Behaviour Research and Therapy, 27,* 19–26.

Ollendick, T. H., Matson, J. L., & Helsel, W. J. (1985). Fears in children and adolescents: Normative data. *Behavior Research and Therapy, 23,* 465–467.

Piacentini, J., & Roblek, T. (2002). Recognizing and treating childhood anxiety disorders. *Western Journal of Medicine, 176*(3), 149–151.

Piacentini, J., Bergman, R. L., Jacobs, C., McCracken, J. T., & Kretchman, J. (2002). Open trial of cognitive behavior therapy for childhood obsessive-compulsive disorder. *Journal of Anxiety Disorders, 16*(2), 207–219.

Pine, D. S. (1999). Pathophysiology of childhood anxiety disorders. *Biological Psychiatry, 46*(11), 1555–1566.

Pine, D. S., Cohen, P., Gurley, D., Brook, J., & Ma, Y. (1998). The risk for early-adulthood anxiety and depressive disorders in adolescents with anxiety and depressive disorders. *Archives of General Psychiatry, 55,* 56–64.

Prior, M., Smart, D., Sanson, A., & Oberklaid, F. (2000). Does shy-inhibited temperament in childhood lead to problems in adolescence? *Journal of the American Academy of Child and Adolescent Psychiatry, 39,* 461–468.

Research Unit on Pediatric Psychopharmacology Anxiety Study Group. (2001). Fluvoxamine for the treatment of anxiety disorders in children and adolescents. *New England Journal of Medicine, 344,* 1279–1285.

Reznick, J. S., Hegeman, I. M., Kaufman, E. R., Woods, S. W., & Jacobs, M. (1992). Retrospective and concurrent self-report of behavioral inhibition and their relation to adult mental health. *Development and Psychopathology, 4*(2), 301–321.

Ronan, K., Kendall, P. C, & Rowe, M. (1994). Negative affectivity in children: Development and validation of a self-statement questionnaire. *Cognitive Therapy and Research, 18,* 509–528.

Rosenberg, E. J., & Dohrenwend, B. S. (1975). Effects of experience and ethnicity on ratings of life events as stressors. *Journal of Health and Social Behavior, 16*(1), 127–129.

Rubin, K. H., & Mills, R. S. (1990). Maternal beliefs about adaptive and maladaptive social behaviors in normal, aggressive, and withdrawn preschoolers. *Journal of Abnormal Child Psychology, 18*(4), 419–435.

Rubin, K. H., & Stewart, S. L. (1996). Social withdrawal in childhood. In E. J.

Mash & R. A. Barkley (Eds.), *Child psychopathology* (pp. 277–307). New York: Guilford Press.

Rubin, K. H., Hastings, P. D., Stewart, S. L, Henderson, H. A., & Chen, X. (1997). The consistency and concomitants of inhibition: Some of the children, all of the time. *Child Development, 68*(3), 467–483.

Rubin, K. H., LeMare, L. J., & Lollis, S. (1990). Social withdrawal in childhood: Developmental pathways to peer rejection. In S. R. Asher & J. D. Coie (Eds.), Peer rejection in childhood (pp. 217–249). Cambridge, UK: Cambridge University Press.

Rubin, K. H., Nelson, L. J., Hastings, P., & Asendorpf, J. (1999). The transaction between parents' perceptions of their children's shyness and their parenting styles. *International Journal of Behavioral Development, 23*(4), 937–958.

Rutter, M. (2002). Nature, nurture, and development: From evangelism through science toward policy and practice. *Child Development, 73*(1), 1–21.

Sanson, A., Smart, D. F., Prior, M., & Oberklaid, F. (1993). *Interactions between parenting and temperament among 3- to 7-year-old children.* Unpublished manuscript.

Saudino, K. (2001). Behavioral genetics, social phobia, social fears, and related temperaments. *Theoretical Perspectives.*

Schatzberg, A. F., Samson, J. A., Rothschild, A. J., Bond, T. C., & Regier, D. A. (1998). McLean Hospital depression research facility: Early-onset phobic disorders and adult-onset major depression. *British Journal of Psychiatry Supplement,* 29–34.

Schneier, F. R., Johnson, J., Horing, C. D., Liebowitz, M. R., & Weissman, M. M. (1992). Social phobia: Comorbidity and morbidity in an epidemiological sample. *Archives of General Psychiatry, 49,* 282–288.

Schwartz, C. E., Snidman, N., & Kagan, J. (1999). Adolescent social anxiety as an outcome of inhibited temperament in childhood. *Journal of the American Academy of Child and Adolescent Psychiatry, 38*(8), 1008–1015.

Shaffer, D., Gould, M. S., Brasic, J., Ambrosini, P., Fisher, P., Bird, H., & Aluwahlia, S. (1983). A children's global assessment scale (C-GAS). *Archives of General Psychiatry, 40,* 1228–1231.

Silverman, W. K., & Albano, A. M. (1996). *The Anxiety Disorders Interview Schedule for DSM-IV–Child and Parent Versions.* San Antonio, TX: Graywind Publications/Psychological Corporation.

Silverman, W. K., & Berman, S. L. (2001). Psychosocial interventions for anxiety disorders in children: Status and future directions. In W. K. Silverman & P. D. A. Treffers (Eds.), *Anxiety disorders in children and adolescents: Research, assessment and intervention* (pp. 313–334). Cambridge, UK: Cambridge University Press.

Silverman, W. K., & Eisen, A. R. (1992). Age differences in the reliability of parent and child reports of child anxious symptomatology using a structured interview. *Journal of the American Academy of Child and Adolescent Psychiatry, 31,* 117–124.

Silverman, W. K., & Nelles, W. B. (1988). The Anxiety Disorders Interview Schedule for Children. *Journal of the American Academy of Child and Adolescent Psychiatry, 27*(6), 772–778.

Silverman, W. K., & Nelles, W. B. (1988). The influence of gender on children's ratings of fear in self and same-aged peers. *Journal of Genetic Psychology, 149,* 17–22.

Silverman, W. K., & Treffers, P. D. A. (Eds.). (2001). *Anxiety disorders in children and adolescents: Research, assessment and intervention.* Cambridge, UK: Cambridge University Press.

Silverman, W. K., Kurtines, W. M., Ginsburg, G. S., Weems, C. F., Lumpkin, P., White, C., & Hicks, D. (1999). Treating anxiety disorders in children with group cognitive-behavioral therapy: A randomized clinical trial. *Journal of Consulting and Clinical Psychology, 67,* 995–1003.

Silverman, W. K., Kurtines, W. M., Ginsburg, G. S., Weems, C. F., Rabian, B., & Serafini, L. T. (1999). Contingency management, self-control, and education support in the treatment of childhood phobic disorders: A randomized clinical trial. *Journal of Consulting and Clinical Psychology, 67,* 675–687.

Silverman, W. K., Saavedra, L. M., & Pina, A. A. (2001). Test-retest reliability of anxiety symptoms and diagnoses with anxiety disorders interview schedule for *DSM-IV*: Child and parent versions. *Journal of the American Academy of Child and Adolescent Psychiatry, 40,* 937–944.

Spence, S. H., Donovan, C., & Brechman-Toussaint, M. (2000). The treatment of childhood social phobia: The effectiveness of a social skills training-based cognitive-behavioral intervention with and without parental involvement. *Journal of Child Psychology and Psychiatry, and Allied Disciplines, 41,* 713–726.

Stallings, P., & March, J. S. (1995). Assessment. In J. S. March (Ed.), *Anxiety disorders in children and adolescents* (pp. 125–147). New York: Guilford Press.

Stark, K. D., Humphrey, L. L., Crook, K., & Lewis, K. (1990). Perceived family environments of depressed and anxious children: Child's and maternal figure's perspectives. *Journal of Abnormal Child Psychology, 18(5),* 527–47.

Stark, K. D., Humphrey, L. L., Laurent, J., Livingston, R., & Christopher, J. (1993). Cognitive, behavioral, and family factors in the differentiation of depressive and anxiety disorders during childhood. *Journal of Consulting and Clinical Psychology, 61(5),* 878–886.

Stein, M. B., Fuetsch, M., Müller, N., Höfler, M., Lieb, R., & Wittchen, H. U. (2001). Social anxiety disorder and the risk of depression. *Archives of General Psychiatry, 58,* 251–256.

Stein, M. B., Liebowitz, M. R., Lydiard, R. B., Pitts, C. D., Bushnell, W., & Gergel, I. (1998). Paroxetine treatment of generalized social phobia: a randomized controlled trial. *Journal of the American Medical Association, 280,* 708–713.

Tancer, M. E., & Uhde, T. W. (1995). Social phobia: a review of pharmacological treatment. *CNS Drugs, 3,* 267–278.

Van Ameringen, M., Mancini, C., Farvolden, P., & Oakman, J. (1999). Pharmacotherapy for social phobia: What works, what might work , and what does not work at all. *CNS Spectrums, 4,* 61–68.

Vasey, M. W., & Dadds, M. R. (Eds.). (2001). *The developmental psychopathology of anxiety.* New York: Oxford University Press.Volkmar, F. R. (Ed.). (1998). *Autism and pervasive developmental disorders.* Cambridge, UK: Cambridge University Press.

Velting, O. N., & Albano, A. M. (2001). Current trends in the understanding and treatment of social phobia in youth. *Journal of Child Psychology and Psychiatry, 42(1),* 127–140.

Walkup, J., & Davies, M. (1999, October). The Pediatric Anxiety Rating Scale (PARS): A reliability study. *Scientific Proceedings of the 46th Annual Meeting of the American Academy of Child and Adolescent Psychiatry*, Chicago, p. 107 [abstract].

Wittchen, H. U., Stein, M. B., & Kessler, R. C. (1999). Social fears and social phobia in a community sample of adolescents and young adults: Prevalence, risk factors and co-morbidity. *Psychological Monitor, 29*, 309–323.

9

SCHOOL REFUSAL

David Heyne, Neville J. King, & Bruce Tonge

Debates continue on the definition and conceptualization of school non-attendance problems (Kearney, 2001; N. J. King & Bernstein, 2001). Some authors use the term *school-refusal behavior* to describe cases of "child-motivated refusal to attend school or difficulties remaining in classes for an entire day" (Kearney & Silverman, 1996, p. 345), including problems of *truancy*. We prefer to use the term *school refusal* to refer to cases in which difficulty attending school is associated with emotional distress (e.g., Granell de Aldaz, Vivas, Gelfand, & Feldman, 1984; N. J. King & Bernstein, 2001; Martin, Cabrol, Bouvard, Lepine, & Mouren-Simeoni, 1999; Okuyama, Okada, Kuribayashi, & Kaneko, 1999) and is not associated with serious antisocial behavior (e.g., Hansen, Sanders, Massaro, & Last, 1998; Heyne, King, et al., 2002; McShane, Walter, & Rey, 2001), as a way of distinguishing it from truancy. In this way, school refusal and truancy are regarded as two reasonably distinct types of attendance problems requiring different approaches to intervention. A third type of attendance problem, *school withdrawal*, is associated with parental ambivalence or opposition toward the child attending school regularly (Kahn & Nursten, 1962).

The criteria provided by Berg and colleagues (Berg, 1996, 1997; Berg, Nichols, & Pritchard, 1969; Bools, Foster, Brown, & Berg, 1990) are helpful in identifying school refusal and distinguishing it from truancy and school withdrawal. In effect, school refusal is defined by (a) reluctance or refusal to attend school, often leading to prolonged absence; (b) the child's usually remaining at home during school hours, rather than concealing the problem from parents; (c) displays of emotional upset at the prospect of attending school, which may be reflected in excessive fearfulness, temper tantrums, misery, or possibly in unexplained physical symptoms; (d) an absence of severe antisocial tendencies, beyond the child's resistance to parental attempts to get him or her to school; and (e) reasonable parental efforts to secure the child's attendance at school at some stage in the history of the problem.

CLINICAL MANIFESTATION

Typically, parents report a wide range of anxiety symptoms associated with a child's difficulty attending school. When pressured to attend, the young person's anxiety may be manifest as resistive behaviors such as refusing to get out of bed or to get ready for school, complaints about school, whining, crying, temper tantrums, and refusing to get into the car to travel to school or to get out of the car on arrival at school. Some young people threaten to run away or to harm themselves (Blagg, 1987). Other overt signs of fearfulness may include trembling, shaking, and agitation.

Somatic symptoms are commonly experienced by school refusers. Documented symptoms that appear to be due to the child's anxiety about attending school include abdominal pain, nausea, vomiting, headaches, sweating, diarrhea, dizziness, pallor, sore throat, fever, and frequent urination. These symptoms occur with high frequency relative to non-school-refusing children (Thyer & Sowers-Hoag, 1986), and medical examinations fail to reveal any obvious cause for them (Flakierska, Lindstrom, & Gillberg, 1988). The more common physiological symptoms appear to be headaches and stomachaches (Berg, 1980; Torma & Halsti, 1975).

The cognitive component of school refusal involves irrational fears and dysfunctional thoughts associated with school attendance. Hersov (1985) observed that "many children insist that they want to go to school and prepare to do so but cannot manage it when the time comes" (p. 384). In these situations, young people may, for example, overestimate the likelihood of anxiety-provoking situations occurring at school or harm befalling their parents, underestimate their own ability to cope with anxiety-provoking situations, or magnify the unpleasant aspects of school attendance.

Although many children refuse to leave home for school, some set out for school but rush home in a state of anxiety before arriving at school or before entering the school building. Others telephone home and request to be retrieved from school, and yet others appear to behave normally after arriving at school, their fear seeming to have rapidly dissipated, only to recur the next day when it is time for school again (Berg, 1996). There may be little evidence of anxiety when the pressure to attend school is removed or on weekends and during school holidays. In other cases, school refusers display more pervasive emotional disturbance (Bools et al., 1990).

In the clinical presentation of school refusal, we see children and adolescents with a range of maladaptive fears and excessive anxiety (N. J. King, Ollendick, & Tonge, 1995). Some have exaggerated fears of specific situations such as being bullied by peers or punished by teachers, whereas some are afraid of separation from their parents (usually the mother). Other young people have extreme fears of taking tests and performing other evaluative tasks in the classroom. Fear of entering a new school, fear of vomiting, fear of interpersonal interaction, and fear of undressing in the gym dressing room are also evinced in some school-refusal cases. Young people refusing to attend often display multiple and diffuse fears in relation to home, school settings, or both.

School refusers may also present with depressive features including dysphoria, irritability, tearfulness, withdrawal, difficulty concentrating, and sleep disturbance (Kearney, 1993). Although certainly not true in all cases, relationships with classmates or teachers can also be impaired, and some children are described as loners or poor mixers. By definition, pervasive conduct problems are not characteristic of school refusal. However, children and adolescents presenting with school refusal may become stubborn, argumentative, and may display aggressive behaviors when parents attempt to get them to school (Hersov, 1985; Hoshino et al., 1987; N. J. King & Ollendick, 1989b). As well as being an expression of a young person's anxiety, such behaviors may represent an exaggeration of distress to induce parental guilt and acquiescence, with the aim of avoiding anxiety-provoking situations (Kearney, 2001). In all, the clinical presentation of school refusal is heterogeneous, with considerable variation in symptomatology from case to case (Kearney & Beasley, 1994). Certainly, one would be mistaken to view school refusal as a unitary syndrome or well-defined set of symptoms.

DIAGNOSIS AND CLASSIFICATION

Perhaps reflecting historical influences that emphasized mother-child relationships in school refusal, an overly common assumption even today is that school refusal is caused by separation anxiety (Pilkington & Piersel, 1991). This situation is complicated further because one of the criteria for separation anxiety disorder in the Diagnostic and Statistical Manual of Mental Disorders (*DSM-IV*; American Psychiatric Association [APA], 1994) is "persistent reluctance or refusal to go to school or elsewhere because of fear of separation" (p. 113). Given the variable clinical presentation of school refusal, however, many potential diagnostic categories are of relevance.

Last and Strauss (1990) reported on 63 school-refusing children and adolescents referred to an outpatient anxiety disorder clinic. Using *DSM-III-R* (APA, 1987) criteria, the most common primary diagnoses included separation anxiety disorder (38%), social phobia (30%), and simple phobia (22%). In Bernstein, Warren, Massie, and Thuras's (1999) sample of 46 anxious-depressed school refusers, *DSM-III-R* anxiety disorders included overanxious disorder (91%), simple phobia (89%), social phobia (71%), avoidant disorder (52%), agoraphobia (39%), separation anxiety disorder (30%), obsessions (20%), compulsions (13%), panic disorder (7%), and posttraumatic stress disorder (7%). The primary *DSM-IV* diagnoses in Heyne, King, et al.'s (2002) sample of 61 anxiety-disordered school refusers included adjustment disorder with anxiety (39%), anxiety disorder not other-wise specified (15%), separation anxiety disorder (10%), social phobia (10%), generalized anxiety disorder (3%), specific phobia (3%), obsessive-compulsive disorder (2%), agoraphobia without history of panic disorder (2%), and panic disorder with agoraphobia (2%).

Multiple diagnoses are frequently indicated for school-refusing youth, and a proportion have comorbid anxiety and depressive disorders. Diagnostically, Bernstein and Garfinkel (1986) reported that as many as 69% of "school phobics" met DSM-III (APA, 1980) criteria for depression, and 50% met criteria for concurrent depressive and anxiety disorders. These figures may be confounded by the fact that the sample seemed to contain both school refusers and truants. Using a semistructured diagnostic interview schedule (the Kiddie Schedule for Affective Disorders and Schizophrenia [K-SADS]; Puig-Antich & Ryan, 1986), Last and Strauss (1990) found that 13% of a clinically referred sample of school refusers received a *DSM-III-R* diagnosis of major depression, and in almost every case the principal diagnosis was an anxiety disorder. More recently, Martin et al. (1999) reported depression in 31% of a sample of 51 school refusers, also using the K-SADS and the DSM classification system. In a study of 61 school-refusing children and adolescents with anxiety disorders, Heyne, King, et al. (2002) found comorbid mood disorders in 15% of cases.

Young people with comorbid anxiety and depressive disorders present a special challenge in assessment and treatment. Indeed, a recent study suggested that school-refusing adolescents with comorbid anxiety and depressive disorders might be far less responsive to treatment than those with anxiety disorders only (Bernstein et al., 2000). Oppositional defiant disorder has also been reported in approximately one quarter (McShane et al., 2001), one fifth (Heyne, King, et al., 2002), and one tenth (Hansen et al., 1998) of clinical samples of school refusers. In all, we see considerable heterogeneity in the diagnostic profile of school-refusing children.

Although relations between school refusal and psychiatric disorders have been extensively investigated, the role of learning difficulties and communication problems has received scant attention. This is surprising, because such problems cause significant challenges in the school setting and may predispose the vulnerable child or youth to school refusal. Naylor, Staskowski, Kenney, and King (1994), for example, found that school-refusing depressed adolescents on an inpatient unit had significantly more learning disabilities and language impairments than matched psychiatric controls. They concluded that "academic and communicative frustration and the adolescent's resulting inability to meet the academic and social demands in the school environment may play a role in the etiology of school refusal" (p. 1331).

DEVELOPMENTAL COURSE

The developmental course of school refusal has not been sufficiently re-searched. Certainly, school refusal can occur throughout the entire range of school years, and several reports suggest that there are major referral-related peaks at certain ages and transition points in the young person's life. Hersov's (1985) review suggested that it is more prevalent between 5 and 7 years of age, at 11 years of age, and at 14 years of age and older, roughly corresponding to early schooling, change of school, and nearing the end of compulsory education. In a study of 63 school refusers, Last and Strauss (1990) observed that school refusal was prevalent in children of all ages, but that the peak age range for referral was from 13 to 15 years, with some elevation also noted at 10 years of age. Although their clinic accepted referrals for young people from 5 years of age, the vast majority (92%) of referred school refusers were aged 10 and older. Other authors have similarly suggested that school refusal has a higher prevalence in preadolescence and adolescence than in early or middle childhood (e.g., Kearney, Eisen, & Silverman, 1995; Last, 1992).

An important consideration with respect to age-related trends is the distinction between the age at onset of the first episode of school refusal and the young person's age when he or she is ultimately referred for help. In a review of the case files of 63 school refusers assessed at the Maudsley Hospital in the United Kingdom, Smith (1970) observed two peaks for age at onset: 5 to 6 years and 11 to 12 years. It will be recognized that these two peaks coincide with school entry and major school transitions. In a large Australian sample of clinic-referred school refusers aged 10 to 17 years (N = 192), the majority (78%) first exhibited school refusal in the first or second year of secondary school, with a mean age of onset of 12.3 years (SD = 2.6; McShane et al., 2001). Notwithstanding methodological problems such as the possibility of biased referral practices, these studies highlight the importance of programs to help in curbing or preventing school-refusal problems during school transitions.

There are suggestions that the development, clinical presentation, and severity of school refusal also vary according to age. According to Hersov (1985), acute onset is more typical of younger school refusers, whereas older refusers are more likely to display an insidious onset. For children whose school refusal begins in primary school, the clinical presentation is suggested to be very different from that of children whose school refusal commences at puberty or in early adolescence (Atkinson, Quarrington, & Cyr, 1985). As an example, Last and Strauss (1990) found that separation anxiety symptomatology was frequently associated with young school refusers, whereas social phobic behavior and specific phobic behavior appeared to be more typical of older school refusers. Regarding severity of the problem, Eisenberg (1959) observed that the adolescent school refuser is far more disturbed than the younger school refuser, and this impression has received empirical support (see review by Atkinson et al., 1985). In a similar vein, Hansen et al. (1998) found that increased age was predictive of more severe school refusal as measured by greater levels of absenteeism. No relationship was found between severity and the length of the problem or the occurrence of a prior episode of school refusal.

Despite the obvious importance of longitudinal data, few follow-up studies of children with school refusal have been reported. Relying mainly on register data, Flakierska and her colleagues (Flakierska et al., 1988; Flakierska-Praquin, Lindstrom, & Gillberg, 1997) conducted two controlled follow-up investigations of the same sample of school refusers who received inpatient or outpatient treatment in Sweden. In the second study, the follow-up interval was 20 to 29 years, with all individuals being older than 30 years at the time of follow-up. The original sample was confined to school refusers seen at ages 7 to 12 years, whose chart histories met *DSM-III* criteria for separation anxiety disorder (n = 35). These children were compared with age- and sex-matched non-school-refusal child psychiatric patients (n = 35) and a sample of children from the general population (n = 35). The investigation revealed that the original school-refusal group received more psychiatric consultations and continued to live with their parents more often than the general population group, and they had fewer children than both comparison groups. These findings suggest that many separation-anxious school refusers may continue to have problems with independence as adults.

ASSESSMENT

School-refusing children vary widely regarding etiological history, clinical presentation, school functioning, family dynamics, and overall strengths and difficulties. In order to best understand each case and appropriately plan for treatment, we recommend that assessment be multimethod and multi-informant (Ollendick & King, 1998). Assessment of school refusal typically involves clinical-behavioral interviews, diagnostic interviews, self-report measures, self-monitoring, parent- and teacher-completed measures, a review of the child's attendance record, and a functional analysis assessment.

The assessment follows an initial screening to identify those young people meeting the criteria for school refusal (as previously described), as distinct from cases obviously involving truancy or school withdrawal. Having school systems in place to facilitate early identification and referral for evidence-based treatments is important (Stickney & Miltenberger, 1998). During screening or in the early stages of assessment, the family doctor is also consulted. Because school attendance problems often arise following periods of absenteeism due to genuine physical illness (e.g., viral infection) and often are associated with somatic complaints, it is important to establish the young person's current health status prior to implementing a treatment plan.

Clinical-Behavioral Interviews

Of the many assessment procedures that are employed, the clinical interview is the most widely used and indispensable part of assessment (Mash & Terdal, 1997). Clinical interviews are usually structured to obtain detailed information about target behaviors and their controlling variables, to begin the formulation of specific treatment plans, and to develop a relationship with the young person and his or her family. The young person and parents often have different perspectives on the school-refusal problem, so conducting separate interviews with them allows each the opportunity to freely discuss their views (Blagg, 1987). This may be achieved via a dual clinical model, with one clinician working closely with the young person and another with the parents (Heyne & Rollings, 2002). The clinical interview also informs the selection of additional assessment methods required to explore areas such as learning difficulties.

Blagg's (1987) guidelines for conducting behavioral interviews with school-refusing children, their parents, and school staff provide an efficient way to obtain pertinent information and to develop an invaluable aide mémoire. His record form includes specific areas related to the child (e.g., attendance patterns and history, associated symptoms, out-of-school activities, attitudes toward school refusal, intellectual functioning, peer relationships), the family (e.g., its structure and relationships, familial sources of stress and anxiety, the costs and benefits of the school-refusal behavior, the implicit and explicit patterns of influence and control), and the school itself (e.g., schooling history, school-related anxieties, staff attitudes and flexibility). Such a comprehensive view helps us to become aware of familial, social, and setting events that may occasion and maintain behaviors related to school refusal.

Our team (Heyne & Rollings, 2002) has also prepared interview schedules for use with school refusers and their parents. In addition to questioning about central areas (e.g., history of school refusal, home and school stressors, attitudes toward the problem, prior efforts to address the school refusal), these interviews encourage close inquiry regarding the household routine on school mornings, the child's activities when not at school, the child's social involvement, the experience of school transitions, and attributions regarding the maintenance of school refusal. We conduct self-statement assessments (drawing on the work of Mansdorf and Lukens, 1987) with school refusers and their parents to supplement the information gained through the clinical-behavioral interviews (see Heyne & Rollings, 2002). The self-statement assessments help us to systematically identify child and parent cognitions that may be associated with the development and maintenance of the school-refusal problem, and that may warrant attention during intervention.

Although we conduct the clinical-behavioral interviews in our outpatient clinic, they may be conducted at school in those cases in which young people are not phobic of the school setting per se. When feasible, direct observations of the young person and parents are conducted in the home and school settings, providing a source of detailed information about the antecedents and consequences of the young person's reluctance and resistance. When this is not feasible, parents and school staff are supported in the process of making and recording behavioral observations, using tailored monitoring diaries. (See Kearney, 2001, for a discussion of direct behavioral observations.)

We also visit the school to interview relevant staff about the young person's social, emotional, behavioral, and academic functioning at school, with a particular focus on the manifestation of anxious and depressive symptomatology. This interview provides an opportunity to start building a good working relationship with school staff in preparation for the treatment phase.

Diagnostic Interviews

Diagnostic interviews assist in developing a diagnostic profile of the young person's functioning. Silverman and Albano's (1996) Anxiety Disorders Interview Schedule for Children permits differential diagnosis among major *DSM-IV* disorders. Separate interview schedules are available for use with the child (ADIS-C) and with the parents (ADIS-P), and composite diagnoses are developed on the basis of the reports of both parties. Although other diagnostic interviews are available (see Kearney, 2001), the ADIS-C and ADIS-P are the only interviews specifically designed for the diagnosis of anxiety-related disorders in children and adolescents. They help to clarify the nature and severity of anxiety problems potentially associated with the young person's school refusal, and they are extensive in their coverage, incorporating mood disorders and behavior disorders, together with sections specifically addressing the history and behaviors associated with school refusal. The ADIS-C and ADIS-P are superior to clinical judgment alone, because they increase diagnostic reliability by reducing clinician bias during the diagnostic process and by ensuring that all major diagnoses are explored (cf. Last, 1992). They have demonstrated adequate interrater reliability (Rapee, Barrett, Dadds, & Evans, 1994) and satisfactory test-retest reliability at the symptom (Silverman & Rabian, 1995) and disorder (Silverman & Eisen, 1992) levels.

Self-Report Measures

There is now a plethora of psychometrically sound self-report measures that may be used to efficiently assess levels of fear, anxiety, and depression in the school-refusing child or adolescent, relative to other children and adolescents. Commonly employed measures include the Fear Survey Schedule for Children-Revised (FSSC-R; Ollendick, 1983), the Revised-Children's Manifest Anxiety Scale (RCMAS; Reynolds & Richmond, 1978), and the Children's Depression Inventory (CDI; Kovacs, 1992). Newer psychometrically sound self-report measures for the assessment of fear and anxiety include, for example, the Fear Survey Schedule for Children-II (FSSC-II; Gullone & King, 1992) and the Spence Children's Anxiety Scale (SCAS; Spence, 1998). More focused measures might be employed during assessment, such as the Social Anxiety Scale for Children-Revised (SASC-R; La Greca & Stone, 1993).

A recently developed self-report measure focuses on the cognitions of school refusers. Heyne et al. (1998) reported on the development and psychometric evaluation of the Self-Efficacy Questionnaire for School Situations (SEQ-SS). This measure is the first to provide a standardized assessment of the efficacy expectations of young people regarding their ability to cope with potential anxiety-provoking situations such as doing school work, handling peers' questions about absence from school, and being separated from parents during school time. Factor analysis yielded two factors labeled *academic/ social stress* and *separation/discipline stress*. Recent reviews provide more detailed discussion of these and other self-report measures in relation to the assessment of school refusers (see Kearney, 2001; Ollendick & King, 1998).

Self-Monitoring

Self-monitoring facilitates a more focused assessment of the school refuser's functioning, with the young person reporting on clinically relevant target behaviors at the time of their occurrence. In our work with school-refusing children, we frequently ask young persons to monitor their emotional distress on successive school mornings (Ollendick & King, 1998). The young person is given an index card titled "Feelings about going to school" and is asked to circle a number from 1 to 5 regarding his or her feelings:

1—*I feel happy and good about going to school.*

2—*I'm a little nervous and upset today, but I can still go to school.*

3—*I'm nervous and upset and I'm not sure if I can go to school today.*

4—*I'm very nervous and upset and I don't think I can go to school today.*

5—*I'm so nervous and upset that I know I cannot go to school today.*

The children are also asked to complete a similar rating on how sick they feel. At the end of the school day, they are asked to complete another section of the card that asks them to indicate (a) whether they went to school, (b) whether they stayed in school all day, and (c) what the day in school was like. Depending on the young person's age and compliance, self-monitoring procedures can be used to help identify antecedents and consequences that maintain school refusal (Ollendick & King, 1998). For example, diaries might be tailored to specific experiences such as attending certain classes or being in the schoolyard. Beidel, Neal, and Lederer (1991) developed a daily diary for the assessment of anxiety in school children, and this may also be usefully employed with school refusers.

Parent- and Teacher-Completed Measures

Corresponding with self-monitoring by the young person, parents are provided with diaries which allow them to rate the young person's attendance and emotional distress and his or her levels of cooperation and resistance in getting ready for school, on the way to school, and when being dropped off at school. Parents may also be asked to record vital clinical information on levels of partner support, parental responses to the young person's emotional distress and noncompliance, and levels of stress experienced by the family (Kearney & Albano, 2000a, 2000b).

At a more general level, a variety of parent- and teacher-completed measures have been used in the assessment of school-refusing children and adolescents. Perhaps the most popular of these is the Child Behavior Checklist (CBCL; Achenbach, 1991a). The CBCL assesses the competencies and behavior problems of children aged 4 to 18 years from the perspective of the parent. There are corresponding measures for gaining the perspective of school staff (Teacher's Report Form [TRF]; Achenbach, 1991b) and the perspective of youth aged 11 to 18 years (Youth Self-Report Form [TSR]; Achenbach, 1991c).

Each of these measures yields scores for two broadband behavioral dimensions (internalizing and externalizing), together with scores for subscales including withdrawal, social problems, anxiety/depression, somatic complaints, attention problems, aggressive behaviors, and delinquent behaviors. The internalizing subscales are particularly relevant in the assessment of school refusal, but useful information can be gained from the externalizing subscales as well. Information derived from the TRF can be compared and contrasted with the parents' reports on the CBCL, to develop a fuller understanding of the child's behavior across settings. There is much research support for the psychometric properties of these measures (Daugherty & Shapiro, 1994), and their clinical utility is enhanced by the extensive normative data for boys and girls of varying ages (N. J. King & Ollendick, 1989a).

Measures of parent and family functioning are also important in gaining a fuller understanding of the situation surrounding the young person's school refusal (cf. Kearney, 2001). To this end, we ask parents to complete the Beck Depression Inventory (Beck, Steer, & Brown, 1996), the Brief Symptom Inventory (Derogatis, 1993), and the Abbreviated Dyadic Adjustment Scale (Sharpley & Rogers, 1984). Parents and adolescent school refusers are also asked to complete the general functioning subscale of the McMaster Family Assessment Device (Epstein, Baldwin, & Bishop, 1983; see Kearney, 2001, for a review of parent and family measures that might be employed in cases of school refusal).

Review of Attendance Record

When daily school records are available, a review of the record can provide useful information about the extent and pattern of the young person's nonattendance. Regular absences associated with certain school activities (e.g., school excursions), classes (e.g., physical education classes or language classes), or days of the week (e.g., following overnight visits with the noncustodial parent) may help to shed light on factors maintaining the attendance problem.

Systematic Functional Analysis

A self-report measure and an associated parent-completed measure warrant specific attention. Developed by Kearney and Silverman (1993), the child and parent versions of the School Refusal Assessment Scale (SRAS) were designed to facilitate a systematic functional analysis for school-refusal behavior (i.e., school refusal and truancy). The 16 items in the child and parent questionnaires assess four functions hypothesized to maintain school-refusal behavior. The four functions are represented in subscales labeled (1) avoidance of stimuli that provoke a sense of general negative affectivity, (2) escape from aversive social or evaluative situations, (3) attention-seeking behavior, and (4) pursuit of tangible reinforcement outside school. Each question is rated on a Likert-type scale from 0 (*never*) to 6 (*always*). Item means for the four functional conditions are computed and compared with each other. The functional condition in which the young person attains the highest score is deemed to be the primary maintaining variable of the school-refusal behavior.

Prescribed treatments are indicated for each of the functional conditions identified by the SRAS (see Kearney & Albano, 2000a, 2000b). For example, systematic desensitization is recommended for young people motivated by a desire to avoid anxiety and other negative affectivity, as in the first functional category. To determine the most appropriate form of treatment, initial hypotheses arising from the SRAS functional analysis system need to be further developed in the light of other information gathered during the assessment (cf. Kearney, 2001; Meyer, Hagopian, & Paclawskyj, 1999). The SRAS has variable psychometric qualities and is most likely beneficial as a useful decision aid in developing a treatment plan (Daleiden, Chorpita, Kollins, & Drabman, 1999).

Integration of Assessment Information

In our experience, the foregoing assessment information is often gathered in two 1.5-hour sessions with the child, two 1.5-hour sessions with the parents, a 1-hour visit to the school, and several phone conversations with other professionals such as the family doctor. This includes the time spent developing a therapeutic relationship with the child and parents. Abbreviated assessments may be possible, but elongated assessments are sometimes required, for example, when an assessment of learning difficulties is indicated and when more time is required to build a working relationship, especially with some adolescent school refusers (Heyne & Rollings, 2002).

If a dual-clinician model has been employed during assessment, the practitioners meet to develop a composite diagnostic profile and arrive at a shared case formulation. These are based on the information gathered from the clinical-behavioral interviews, diagnostic interviews, behavioral observations, review of the attendance record, and the administration of self-report measures, parent- and teacher-completed measures, self-monitoring devices, and systematic functional analyses. In part, the various sources of information are used to confirm or disconfirm components of the diagnostic profile arising from the diagnostic interviews. Discrepant information (e.g., disparate child and parent reports on the SRAS regarding the function of the school refusal) is evaluated in reference to other sources of information and according to clinical judgment about the reliability of informant reports (cf. Kearney, 2001). As well as being used to develop the diagnostic profile, the assessment information is used to build a case formulation incorporating the predisposing, precipitating, perpetuating, and protective factors associated with the school refusal (Heyne & King, in press).

PSYCHOSOCIAL TREATMENTS

A range of psychosocial treatment approaches (e.g., play therapy, psychodynamic psychotherapy, family therapy, cognitive-behavioral therapy) has been used with school refusers, but nearly all are of unknown efficacy and acceptability (Blagg, 1987; Gullone & King, 1991). Only cognitive-behavioral therapy (CBT) has been subjected to rigorous evaluation in randomized controlled clinical trials. Empirical support for CBT is drawn from two randomized clinical trials (N. J. King, Tonge, et al., 1998; Last, Hansen, & Franco, 1998) and from a study comparing the efficacy of CBT treatment components (Heyne, King, et al., 2002).

The N. J. King, Tonge, et al. (1998) trial involved 34 school refusers, aged 5 to 15 years, who experienced persistent school attendance problems and emotional distress. Diagnostic examination revealed that most (79%) experienced a principal diagnosis associated with anxiety or phobia. Families were randomly assigned to either a 4–week cognitive-behavioral intervention (six sessions with the child, five with the parents, and one with the teacher) or a wait-list control condition. The manual-based intervention emphasized coping skills training, exposure/return to school, and contingency management at home and at school.

Relative to wait-list controls, more of the children who received therapy exhibited a clinically significant improvement in school attendance—nearly all (15 of 17) were attending school at least 90% of the time. Treated children also showed improvement on self-reports of fear (FSSC-II), anxiety (RCMAS), and depression (CDI). At the same time, the children developed confidence in their ability to cope with anxiety-provoking situations as measured by the SEQ-SS. A parent-completed measure (CBCL) provided further confirmation of the beneficial effects of treatment, with reports of significant reductions in internalizing problems. The maintenance of therapeutic gains was demonstrated at 3-month follow-up. A recent report suggested that, for 13 of the 16 treated young people who could be located, improvements in school attendance were maintained from 3 to

5 years after intervention, and no new psychological problems were evidenced (N. J. King, Tonge, et al., 2001). Given that the methodology involved telephone interviews, claims for the long-term efficacy of CBT need to be supported by more rigorous follow-up investigations.

An important clinical and research question is the extent to which treatment improvements might be due to nonspecific aspects of intervention such as expectations of improvement and having a supportive clinician. In the study by Last et al. (1998), school refusers aged 6 to 17 years were randomly assigned to 12 weekly sessions of CBT or educational support therapy (EST). Children were included if they had an anxiety disorder diagnosis, no diagnosis of major depression, and at least 10% absenteeism from the regular classroom situation, although many were absent much more of the time. The two major components of CBT with the child consisted of graduated in-vivo exposure and coping self-statement training. The EST condition controlled for the nonspecific effects of treatment, incorporating educational presentations, encouragement for children to talk about their fears, and a daily diary for recording feared situations and associated thoughts and feelings. There were 20 completers in the CBT condition and 21 in the EST condition.

Both the CBT and EST groups displayed improvements in attendance and self-reports of fear (FSSC-R), anxiety (Modified State-Trait Anxiety Inventory for Children; Fox & Houston, 1983), and depression (CDI). At posttreatment, 65% of the CBT group and 50% of the EST group no longer met criteria for their primary anxiety disorder, although this difference was not significant. Last and colleagues (1998) concluded that the structured CBT approach may not be superior to the less structured treatment method encompassed in EST. At the same time, in the details of the study, Last and colleagues reported disparate nonresponse rates at 4–week follow-up: The school attendance of 40% of the EST group had not improved, compared with 14% of the CBT group. Moreover, the CBT group experienced a significantly greater reduction in depression relative to the EST group. Although the EST group showed a greater decrease in somatic anxiety, school refusers in this group reported significantly higher somatic anxiety at pretreatment, and this does not appear to have been accounted for in the pretreatment-posttreatment analyses.

On the basis of Last and colleagues' (1998) study, it may be premature to argue that a less structured approach is equally effective as CBT for school refusal, particularly in view of possible overlap between the two approaches used in this study. That is, the EST condition included self-monitoring of thoughts and feelings and a focus on maladaptive thinking. Clearly, we still have much to learn about the modus operandi or crucial mechanisms in CBT for school refusal. (For a discussion of future research directions, see N. J. King, Tonge, Heyne, & Ollendick, 2000.)

Heyne, King, and colleagues (2002) evaluated the relative efficacy of the two major components of the N. J. King, Tonge, et al. (1998) CBT program for school refusal. Eight sessions of child therapy were compared with eight sessions of parent therapy and teacher training, and with a combination of child therapy and parent/teacher training. By 4.5-month follow-up, all three CBT approaches were found to be effective in increasing school attendance and self-efficacy (SEQ-SS) and in reducing the school refusers' fear (FSSC-II), anxiety (RCMAS), and depression (CDI); no between-group differences were observed. Although the design of this component analysis study did not include a control group, the results are supportive of the use of CBT in the treatment of school refusal.

The results pertaining to depression are of particular interest to the development of a *stages of treatment model* for the treatment of school refusal. Heyne, King, et al. (2002) reported significant reductions in young people's depressive symptomatology following treatment, even though the CBT programs focused on anxiety-based school refusal were not designed to address depression in particular. Specifically, 71.4% of the young people with clinical levels of depressive symptomatology at pretreatment reported nonclinical levels at 4.5-month follow-up. Related unpublished data (Heyne, 1999) indicate that only one child warranted a *DSM-IV* diagnosis of mood disorder at follow-up, and there were no new cases of mood disorder. At pretreatment, nine young people had mood disorders, and four more had adjustment disorders with mixed anxiety and depressed mood. That is, 13 young people (21.3%) had pretreatment diagnoses marked by mood-related problems.

When Kendall (1994) found a reduction in depressive symptomatology in children who had received anxiety-focused treatment, he proposed that the alleviation of anxious emotional distress had the correlated effect on dysphoric mood because of the high incidence of comorbid anxiety and depression in children. Another explanation for our results (Heyne, 1999; Heyne, King, et al., 2002) is that the return to regular schooling facilitated a reduction in depression. With a return to regular schooling, children were likely to have become more active and to have had the opportunity to enjoy greater social involvement. Moreover, they had overcome their problems, and they could "be like all the other kids again," a report that was sometimes made by children at the follow-up assessments.

Post hoc analyses were conducted on the Heyne, King, et al. (2002) data to further explore the relationship between school attendance and depression. Children were divided into two groups on the basis of their level of attendance at follow-up; those with attendance of 90% or greater (*success; n = 35*) and those with less than 90% attendance (*nonsuccess; n = 24*). At pretreatment, posttreatment, and follow-up, *t*-tests were conducted comparing CDI scores for the success and nonsuccess cases. There was no significant difference between the success group (mean CDI score = 13.86) and the nonsuccess group (mean = 14.13) at pretreatment. At posttreatment, depression for the success group (mean = 5.37) was significantly less than that for the nonsuccess group (mean = 11.48), $p < .01$. A significant difference in depressive symptomatology was also found between the success group (mean = 3.60) and the nonsuccess group (mean = 10.61) at follow-up, $p < .001$.

These results suggest that successful attendance at follow-up was not related to a difference in depressive symptomatology at pretreatment. That is, it cannot be argued that those who were attending school successfully at follow-up were able to do so because they were less depressed at pretreatment. In fact, it appears that a high level of depression at pretreatment was not necessarily a hindrance to successful school attendance after treatment. For the successful cases, mean depression scores decreased during the course of treatment (i.e., by posttreatment) and continued to decrease at follow-up. It is possible that reductions in depression led to a greater likelihood of successful attendance at follow-up, but given that the treatment program was not focused on depression, it may be that the experience of increased attendance facilitated a reduction in depressive symptomatology. Future research might further explore the relationship between depression and attendance over time.

We now outline our empirically supported CBT program for school refusers and their caregivers (Heyne, King, et al., 2002; N. J. King, Tonge, et al., 1998). In the conceptualization of such intervention, it is useful to differentiate between child therapy and parent/teacher training. Child therapy involves the use of behavioral and cognitive procedures directly with the young person. This level of intervention aims to help the child acquire and employ skills and strategies for coping with the stressors associated with school return and regular attendance. Parent/teacher training focuses on the role that parents and teachers can play in managing environmental contingencies at home and school—contingencies that are maintaining the school-refusal problem and those that facilitate the young person's regular and voluntary school attendance.

Intervention is often conducted across 4 weeks, including between six and eight sessions with the young person, five and eight sessions with the parents, and one consultation and regular telephone contact with school staff. The young persons and their parents are encouraged to engage in specially tailored between-session practice tasks to reinforce and generalize skills beyond the clinical setting and to effect change in the young persons' behavior in the home and school environments.

The child-, parent-, and school-based interventions involve the judicious selection of and emphasis on intervention components. This individualized approach rests on the complex array of possible etiological and maintenance factors, together with the need to be sensitive to the individuality of each child, family, and school situation (cf. Barrett, Dadds, & Rapee, 1996; Kendall, 1994). The child's developmental level will have a large bearing on the manner in which intervention components are implemented.

Child Therapy

Four major components of CBT with school-refusing children and adolescents include relaxation training, enhancement of social competence, cognitive therapy, and exposure. Clinically based indications for the use of each component are addressed in turn.

RELAXATION TRAINING The purpose of relaxation training is to provide young people with a means of countering feelings of physiological arousal associated with school attendance (e.g., approaching the school grounds on the day of their return; giving class talks). In learning to manage discomforting feelings, young people are better placed to confront challenging situations and to employ other skills and strategies in the process of coping with school attendance. Indications for relaxation training might include elevated scores on the subscales of selected measures (e.g., the physiological subscale of the RCMAS and the somatic complaints subscales of the CBCL and TRF), together with reports of somatic complaints during clinical-behavioral and diagnostic interviews. Relaxation training may also occur in preparation for systematic desensitization procedures to be employed with the young person (discussed later).

Several scripts have been developed for conducting progressive muscle relaxation training with children of different ages (e.g., Koeppen, 1974; Ollendick & Cerny, 1981). Obviously, the clinician must be creative in teaching relaxation to young people, aiming to engage them sufficiently to ensure that some form of cue-controlled relaxation is ultimately acquired. Alternative forms of relaxation training that may be used with school refusers are presented in Heyne, King, Tonge, and Cooper (2001).

ENHANCEMENT OF SOCIAL COMPETENCE Enhancing social competence via social skills training is indicated in two predominant situations. First, many school refusers report anxiety about facing questions from peers or teachers regarding their absence from school. Such reports are elicited via the SEQ-SS or arise through the clinical interview. Second, some children's skills in making and maintaining friendships or handling teasing and bullying may be underdeveloped, leaving them vulnerable to isolation and seeking to avoid the school situation. Social competencies, social withdrawal, and social problems are assessed via subscales on the CBCL, TRF, and SRAS, through interviews with parents, children, and school staff and to a lesser extent through observation in the clinical setting. Moreover, self-reported social concerns are assessed in the RCMAS and in more specific measures such as the SASC-R.

Typically, the enhancement of social competence relies on the clinician's modeling desired social behaviors and having the young person rehearse the behaviors through role plays. The young person receives reinforcing and corrective feedback from the clinician. We aim to have the young person experience increasing degrees of pressure or social threat during the training sessions. This is in keeping with the range of social reactions that can be experienced by the young person outside the clinic. The young person's success in responding to more challenging role-play situations can strengthen his or her sense of self-efficacy in readiness for facing real-life social situations.

COGNITIVE THERAPY In our experience, a vital aspect of school-refusal intervention is a focus on the young person's cognitions. Emotionally distressed school refusers may process information in a distorted manner (e.g., "John didn't ask me to his party—he hates me!"), engage in anxiety provoking and depressogenic (cf. Seligman et al., 1984) self-talk (e.g., "I'll probably make a fool of myself during drama class"; "Why would anybody want to be my friend?"), and harbor negative expectations in relation to school attendance (e.g., "Other kids will make fun of me"), perpetuating their distress (cf. Mansdorf & Lukens, 1987). During assessment, indicators of the importance of cognitive therapy during intervention may come from the clinical-behavioral interview with the child (including the adjunctive self-statement assessment), the diagnostic interview (particularly questions associated with generalized anxiety disorder), self-efficacy expectations assessed via the SEQ-SS, the worry/oversensitivity subscale of the RCMAS, and items in the CDI. Of course, many more indications will arise through the course of intervention with the young person, especially during the process of detecting and evaluating the young person's cognitions.

The aim of cognitive therapy is to effect a change in the young persons' emotions and behavior, mobilizing them toward school attendance, by modifying maladaptive cognitions. The seven *D*s list is an aid in the process of conducting cognitive therapy, emphasizing key components involved in *d*escribing the cognitive therapy model, *d*etecting cognitions, *d*etermining maladaptive cognitions, *d*isputing maladaptive cognitions, *d*iscovering adaptive cognitions, *d*oing a home task, and *d*iscussing the outcome of the home task (Heyne & Rollings, 2002). Cartoon materials are often useful in helping younger children understand the connection between thoughts, feelings, and actions, and in engaging them in the process of detecting their maladaptive cognitions and discovering more adaptive cognitions (e.g., Kendall, 1992; Kendall et al., 1992). Disputational procedures more suited to adolescent school refusers with a greater capacity for examining their thoughts are presented elsewhere (e.g., Beck, 1995; Wilkes, Belsher, Rush, & Frank, 1994; Zarb, 1992).

EXPOSURE   In conjunction with the above preparatory strategies, school-return arrangements must be negotiated with the child, parents, and school staff. For young people who have been fully absent from school (as opposed to attending sporadically), we aim for school return to occur midway through the intervention. This allows sufficient time for the young person to develop the previously mentioned coping skills, as well as opportunities to collaboratively troubleshoot difficulties that arise during the return to school.

For many school refusers exhibiting high levels of anxiety, a graduated return to school is usually negotiated, similar to in-vivo desensitization (Wolpe, 1958). This involves a step-by-step approach to conquering the anxiety elicited by school return (e.g., attending one class on the first day, two classes the next day, etc.), with the child drawing on relaxation skills to manage the associated anxiety. We sometimes find the last class of the school day to be a good starting point in school return (cf. Ayllon, Smith, & Rogers, 1970), although the young person's input into the development of a plan for graded return is ultimately important. When the child's anxiety is very high, imaginal desensitization can occur prior to planned school return, perhaps incorporating emotive imagery with younger children (cf. N. J. King et al., 1995; N. J. King, Heyne, Gullone, & Molloy, 2001; for a discussion of attendance hierarchies or attendance plans, see Heyne & Rollings, 2002).

On the other hand, some young people and their families prefer a rapid return to school. Usually more stressful than a graduated return to school, rapid school return involves immediate and full-time school attendance (i.e., flooding). Rapid return programs attempt to prevent or minimize the complications of prolonged absence from school, including the embarrassment for young people of having to explain why they are leaving school partway through the day. We believe that rapid school return is probably more appropriate for young children with mild or acute school refusal.

Parent/Teacher Training

As noted, the cognitive-behavioral treatment of school refusal typically involves parents and school staff. Following the work of Forehand and McMahon (1981), parents might receive training in command-giving, with emphasis on gaining the young person's attention and using clear and specific instructions. This is particularly important for those parents who give vague and imprecise instructions about school-related issues.

Consistent with operant principles, parents and teachers are instructed in the recognition and reinforcement of the young person's appropriate coping behaviors and school attendance and the planned ignoring of inappropriate behaviors such as tantrums, arguments, and somatic complaints without known organic cause (Blagg, 1987; Kearney & Roblek, 1998). The clinician also helps parents to plan and institute smooth morning routines pertinent to the young person (e.g., waking up, getting showered and dressed), and to manage the young person's access to reinforcing events and experiences when at home during school hours. This serves to reduce the secondary gain that may otherwise strengthen the child's resolve not to attend school. Assessment of secondary gain occurs through clinical interviews and, to a lesser extent, via Subscale 4 on the SRAS.

During the child therapy and caregiver training, if the child does not come to the point of attending school voluntarily, parents are advised to be firmer with the child. Having issued clear expectations and instructions regarding attendance, parents may be required to physically escort the child to school, a role that necessitates good planning and support (Kearney & Roblek, 1998; Kennedy, 1965). This process of "professionally informed parental pressure" (Gittelman-Klein & Klein, 1971) is an important aspect of treatment, allowing parents to deal with a young person's entrenched avoidance of school. Parents will often benefit from cognitive and behavioral strategies aimed at helping them remain calm and committed during management of the child's nonattendance (Kearney & Roblek, 1998).

Working with school staff (e.g., classroom teachers, homeroom teachers, and counselors) is vital to ensure the integration of the young person into the classroom as well as the schoolwide system. To achieve this goal, it is often helpful to have the child or school staff select one or two children to act as buddies and provide peer support during the early stages of school reentry (Blagg, 1987). Depending on the young person's preference, classmates may be advised of the school return and encouraged to be supportive and to refrain from probing about nonattendance. A supportive teacher or counselor may also be identified, to help the young person settle in on arrival at school and to familiarize the young person with the routine for the day.

Engineering positive experiences for the child such as special classroom responsibilities or lunchtime privileges can help to make the school environment a more reinforcing place to be. The clinician and school staff can also explore special arrangements to temporarily or permanently accommodate the young person's special needs (e.g., reduced homework requirements, academic remediation, change of classroom). In general, we have found that parents and teachers are cooperative regarding the behavior management strategies covered in the program, and they rate the acceptability of the intervention highly (Heyne, 1999; N. J. King, Tonge, et al., 1998).

PHARMACOLOGICAL TREATMENTS

Pharmacological treatments are commonly employed in cases of school refusal (N. J. King et al., 1995), despite the lack of unequivocal evidence that they are effective. Commonly considered pharmacological treatments include tricyclic anti-depressants (TCAs), selective serotonin reuptake inhibitors (SSRIs), and benzodiazepines. However, only the TCAs have been investigated in randomized placebo-controlled trials of pharmacological treatments for school refusal.

Tricyclic Antidepressants

In an early randomized double-blind placebo-controlled trial, school refusers and their families received behaviorally oriented standard clinical practice (SCP), and children also received either the TCA imipramine or a placebo (Gittelman-Klein & Klein, 1971), over a period of 6 weeks. Superior outcomes were identified for the children in the imipramine-plus-SCP group relative to the placebo-plus-SCP group, with respect to school return and global improvement as rated by children, mothers, and clinicians. Three subsequent studies failed to demonstrate that TCAs (either imipramine or clomipramine) were superior to placebos in the treatment of school refusal

(Berney et al., 1981; Bernstein, Garfinkel, & Borchardt, 1990) or in the treatment of children with separation anxiety disorder, the majority of whom also resisted school attendance (Klein, Koplewicz, & Kanner, 1992). The inconclusive findings are attributed to small sample sizes, differences in comorbidity patterns, lack of control for adjunct therapies, and differences in medication dosages (N. J. King & Bernstein, 2001).

More recently, Bernstein and colleagues (2000) reported a randomized double-blind placebo-controlled trial of imipramine in 63 school-refusing adolescents (mean age 13.9 ± 3.6 years) with comorbid anxiety and major depressive disorders. Both the imipramine and placebo conditions were combined with CBT. After the 8-week treatment, those in the imipramine-plus-CBT group displayed significantly improved attendance and a significantly faster rate of improvement relative to the placebo-plus-CBT group. Both groups displayed significantly reduced anxiety and depression, but depression decreased significantly faster for those receiving imipramine and CBT. The authors concluded that imipramine plus CBT was more efficacious than placebo plus CBT for the group of adolescent school refusers with comorbid anxiety and depression.

At the same time, almost half (45.8%) of the adolescents in the imipramine-plus-CBT group were still not able to attend school at least 75% of the time (this study's definition of remission). It thus appears that the presence of comorbid major depression in anxious school refusers may limit the effectiveness of high-strength interventions (i.e., imipramine plus cognitive-behavioral therapy). In a 1-year naturalistic follow-up study (Bernstein, Hektner, Borchardt, & McMillan, 2001), the imipramine-plus-CBT group and the placebo-plus-CBT group were found to be similar with respect to prevalence rates of anxiety and depressive disorders. Across the whole group, almost two thirds (64.1%) continued to meet criteria for an anxiety disorder and one third (33.3%) continued to meet criteria for a depressive disorder. Unfortunately, rates of school attendance were not reported at the follow-up. Bernstein et al. (2001) concluded that aggressive treatments are important in the treatment of school refusal associated with comorbid anxiety and depressive disorders, and that the optimal duration of acute and maintenance treatments for this group needs to be determined.

Selective Serotonin Reuptake Inhibitors

The increasing use of SSRIs in the treatment of anxiety disorders in young people exhibiting school refusal is largely based on the broad, powerful anxiolytic effects evidenced in adult studies (Labellarte, Ginsburg, Walkup, & Riddle, 1999), and on clinical experience. There are no studies specifically investigating SSRIs in a population of children exhibiting school refusal.

There is strong evidence of the efficacy of SSRIs in the treatment of obsessive-compulsive disorder in children and adolescents (e.g., March et al., 1998; Riddle et al., 2001). With respect to the broader range of anxiety-related disorders (e.g., overanxious disorder, social phobia, separation anxiety disorder, selective mutism), there are three open-label studies (Birmaher et al., 1994; Dummit, Klein, Tancer, Asche, & Martin, 1996; Fairbanks et al., 1997) and a small double-blind, placebo-controlled study (Black & Uhde, 1994) that suggest that fluoxetine is beneficial in children and adolescents.

In a larger randomized placebo-controlled trial ($N = 128$), fluvoxamine was found to be beneficial for children and adolescents with anxiety disorders (Research Units of Pediatric Psychopharmacology Anxiety Study Group, 2000). Of the fluvoxamine group, 76% had a Clinical Global Impressions score of much improved or better, compared with just 29% of the placebo group. Limited improvements were sustained in the subsequent 6- to 8-month open-label extension, as measured via the Pediatric Anxiety Rating Scale and the Clinician Global Improvement Rating Scale (Greenhill, Pine, Walkup, Riddle, & Vitiello, 2000).

Given the heterogeneity of school refusal, research on the efficacy of SSRIs in the treatment of depression in young people is also of importance. There is some, albeit less impressive, evidence of the efficacy of SSRIs in treating depressed young people. For instance, Emslie and colleagues (1997) conducted a randomized, double-blind study in which 8 weeks of fluoxetine was found to be more efficacious than 8 weeks of placebo in the treatment of 96 children and adolescents with major depressive disorder. There were significant improvements in the fluoxetine group, compared with the placebo group, in clinician-rated depression scores and in one of the measures of global improvement. However, there was no significant difference between the groups with respect to self-reported depression or an alternate global rating scale. (For a review of pharmacological treatment with depressed children and adolescents, see Emslie & Mayes, 2001.)

Other Pharmacological Treatments

Some early uncontrolled trials suggested that benzodiazepines might have a role in the treatment of school refusal (e.g., D'Amato, 1962; Kraft, Ardali, Duffy, Hart, & Pearce, 1965). Likewise, case reports and open-label studies (e.g., Biederman, 1987; Pfefferbaum et al., 1987) indicated effectiveness in reducing anxiety in young people. However, the findings from double-blind placebo-controlled trials have failed to clearly demonstrate the efficacy of benzodiazepines with young people displaying school refusal (Bernstein et al., 1990) or anxiety disorders (Siméon et al., 1992). It has been suggested that benzodiazepines may be employed on a very short-term basis in cases of "overwhelming anxiety associated with school refusal" (Tonge, 1998) and cases of "severe school refusal" (N. J. King & Bernstein, 2001). King and Bernstein (2001) suggested that benzodiazepines may be combined with an SSRI or TCA, to alleviate acute anxiety symptoms until the effects of the antidepressant are experienced.

Adverse Effects of Pharmacological Treatments

The use of TCAs is problematic, because of their tendency to produce troublesome adverse effects and their toxicity. Commonly reported adverse effects include dry mouth, constipation, nausea, dizziness and postural hypotension, blurred vision, sedation or insomnia, and weight loss or weight gain (Velosa & Riddle, 2000). Less common adverse effects include behavioral disturbances such as agitation or irritability, or neurological disturbances including tics or epilepsy. Cardiac adverse effects are of the greatest concern, and sudden death has been reported in two young people taking imipramine and six young people taking desipramine, an active metabolite of imipramine (Popper & Ziminitzky, 1995; Riddle, Geller, & Ryan, 1993; Riddle et al., 1991; Saraf, Klein, Gittelman-Klein, & Groff, 1974; Varley & McClellan, 1997). Although we lack an understanding of whether or how TCAs contributed to the deaths of these children (Varley & McClellan, 1997), it is evident that a child with a positive family history of heart disease or sudden death should have a thorough cardiovascular assessment before a TCA is used (Gutgesell et al., 1999). Desipramine has been reported to be more toxic in overdose than other TCAs (Popper & Elliot, 1993), and Riddle et al. (1991) suggested that its use in children should be avoided.

The SSRIs are associated with significantly fewer unpleasant adverse effects in adults than tricyclic antidepressants (Montgomery et al., 1994). There is less information regarding SSRI adverse effects for young people, but Tonge (1998) identified case reports of hypomania, memory impairment, and galactorrhea and hyperprolactinemia. In the previously discussed studies of fluoxetine for anxiety disorders (Birmaher et al., 1994; Black & Uhde, 1994; Dummit et al., 1996; Fairbanks et al., 1997), most children and adolescents experienced no adverse effects or minimal adverse effects of a transitory nature.

The Emslie et al. (1997) study just mentioned found that about 8% of those receiving fluoxetine for depression discontinued treatment due to adverse effects, which included manic excitement in 6% and severe rashes in 2%. In the Greenhill et al. (2000) study of fluvoxamine for anxiety disorders in young people, headaches and increased irritability were the most common adverse effects. Less commonly, the young people reported apathy and indifference, insomnia, and nausea. There have been some case reports of increased suicidal ideation with fluoxetine use in young people (R. A. King et al., 1991), but others have not identified this as a problem (Boulos, Cutcher, Gardner, & Young, 1992). Although the reported suicidal behavior may have been unrelated to fluoxetine, it highlights the need for caution in the prescription of this drug for young people (Tonge, 1998).

The more commonly experienced adverse effects of benzodiazepine use in children and adolescents include drowsiness, irritability, oppositional behavior, headache, nausea, and fatigue, whereas paradoxical effects may include irritability, tantrums, overexcitement, hyperactivity, and angry outbursts (Velosa & Riddle, 2000). Data relating to child and adolescent dependence on benzodiazepines is lacking (Velosa & Riddle, 2000), but in light of the likelihood of dependence, they should be used for several weeks instead of months (Riddle et al., 1999). There are also concerns about difficulty with discontinuation and about abuse potential (Labellarte et al., 1999), and unprescribed use for self-medication and intoxication has been reported in adolescents (Pedersen & Lavik, 1991). In their review of pharmacological treatment of anxiety disorders in children and adolescents, Velosa and Riddle (2000) suggested that benzodiazepines, like TCAs, should only be considered when SSRIs have been ineffective or have produced adverse effects outweighing their benefits.

STAGES OF TREATMENT

The value of designing treatments around the specific needs of each school refuser was emphasized by Burke and Silverman (1987). Subsequently, Kearney and Silverman (1990, 1993, 1999) advanced the differential application of treatments according to functional analysis, and empirical support for this approach is still in its infancy. An alternative, albeit imperfect, approach to treatment planning is to utilize diagnostic information to develop a stagewise approach to treatment.

We propose that the development of a treatment plan be informed by a thorough assessment yielding diagnostic information (principal diagnosis, comorbid diagnoses, and severity), together with information on parental and family functioning. The more robust treatment outcome studies for school refusal (i.e., Bernstein et al., 2000; Heyne, King, et al., 2002; N. J. King, Tonge, et al., 1998; Last et al., 1998) have included diagnostic assessment of the respective school-refusing samples, and the findings of these studies inform the diagnostically driven *stages of treatment* model we propose. This model also draws on our own clinical experience and the clinical experience of other authors in the field, and it will undergo modification and refinement as the empirically based knowledge of school-refusal treatments grows.

The following treatment model assumes that the school attendance problem is associated with emotional distress (often manifest as varying levels of anxiety and depression) and is not associated with comorbid conduct disorder (mostly associated with truancy). It is important to recall that school refusal is marked by its heterogeneity, with multiple causes, varied manifestations, and a broad range of applicable diagnoses. Thus, any model for determining treatment will not identify appropriate treatment pathways for all possible cases. At the same time, the following model can be expected to support the clinician in making treatment decisions pertinent to many of the school refusers and families seen.

Stage 1: Selection of Initial Treatment

Based on the studies by N. J. King, Tonge, et al. (1998), Last et al. (1998), and Heyne, King, et al. (2002), the first line of treatment for school refusers diagnosed with a principal anxiety disorder should be CBT. Although the empirical support for CBT in the treatment of school refusal might still be considered sparse (N. J. King & Bernstein, 2001), this form of treatment has encouraging empirical support, and our recommendation is cognizant of the brevity and clinical utility of CBT, as well as the acceptability of this approach on the part of families and school staff (Gullone & King, 1991; Heyne, 1999; Kearney & Beasley, 1994; N. J. King, Ollendick, Murphy, & Molloy, 1998; N. J. King, Tonge, et al., 1998).

CBT equips the child, parents and school staff with strategies for managing current and future difficulties, and it eliminates the potential issues of adverse effects and dependence that can be associated with pharmacological treatments. As suggested by Klein et al. (1992), it is desirable to avoid first-stage pharmacological treatments if children may derive satisfactory benefit from psychosocial treatments, especially when the psychosocial treatments are brief enough so as not to unduly delay other interventions if the psychosocial treatments are ineffective. In all, the strategy of employing psychosocial interventions as a first stage of treatment matches Labellarte and colleagues' (1999) conservative algorithm for treating anxiety disorders in children.

The study by Heyne, King, et al. (2002) explored the relative efficacy of two predominant components of CBT for school refusal—child therapy and parent/teacher training. In the absence of evidence for the superior effectiveness of combined child therapy and parent/teacher training, Heyne and colleagues suggested that the more economical approach of working solely with parents may be sufficient when the child is younger and displays minimal emotional distress. Subsyndromal anxiety or mild fears may exist for these young people, and these may be satisfactorily addressed through caregiver training on the management of behaviors associated with school refusal. Children with more disturbed behavioral and emotional functioning are more likely to benefit from direct clinical work.

Clearly, treatment planning also needs to include consideration of the presence and severity of depressive symptomatology (cf. Kearney, 1993). Again, insufficient clinical research attention has been given to the outcomes of psychosocial interventions for depressed children exhibiting school refusal (N. J. King et al., 2000). Although there are many reports of depression associated with school refusal, no treatment studies have specifically examined outcome according to the presence versus absence of mood disorders at pretreatment. Moreover, one of the key studies (Last et al., 1998) excluded cases with comorbid depression, and another (N. J. King, Tonge, et al., 1998) had very few cases with comorbid depression.

At a general level, pharmacological treatments have been advocated for school refusers displaying comorbid anxiety and depressive disorders

(N. J. King & Bernstein, 2001). This is based on the notion that symptomatology is severe and typically unresponsive to psychosocial interventions alone. In a *stages of treatment* model, a more sophisticated but as-yet-untested approach is to make decisions about concurrent psychosocial and pharmacological treatments on the basis of the severity of the depression.

For cases involving mild or moderate depression, initial CBT as outlined previously may be sufficient to help a child return to school and to reduce emotional distress, including depressive symptomatology, as suggested by the findings of our group (Heyne, 1999; Heyne, King, et al., 2002). CBT might be adapted to the specific needs of the depressed young person (Kearney, 1993), including greater attention to depressogenic cognitions, facilitation of social involvement, and the inclusion of pleasant events scheduling. These additional targets for treatment with the depressed school refuser would probably require additional sessions over a longer time (Kearney, 1993).

There are a few circumstances in which clinicians may consider implementing a second-stage treatment plan from the outset. These include the presence of severe depression for the young person, and the family's strong preference for an integrated treatment plan.

Stage 2: Management of Partial Response

Although many school-refusing children and adolescents fully respond to CBT, some exhibit minimal or no response, even with the most competent and sensitive of clinicians. This may be particularly likely with school-refusing youth suffering from both anxiety disorders and depression (Bernstein et al., 2000; 2001). From the perspective of the integrated psychosocial and pharmacological treatment (IPPT) model developed in chapter 6 of this volume, the clinician managing a partial response should consider combining CBT with pharmacological treatment.

The current state of knowledge suggests that medications should be used concomitantly with CBT, and not in place of CBT (American Academy of Child and Adolescent Psychiatry, 1997; Tonge, 1998). Although controlled trials of combined medication and CBT for school refusal have been confined to imipramine (Bernstein et al., 2000), we recommend that an SSRI be the first-line medication to be employed in tandem with CBT. On balance, it is likely that the SSRIs have fewer problematic adverse effects in young people and are safer than TCAs (Tonge, 1998). Furthermore, SSRIs are emerging as the initial choice for pharmacological treatment of anxiety disorders in children and adolescents (Velosa & Riddle, 2000), and there is emerging evidence for their effectiveness in the treatment of depression in young people. If, during the integrated use of psychosocial and pharmacological treatments, the combination of an SSRI and CBT is less than optimal at sufficient dosage, TCAs may be tried, in combination with CBT.

Extrapolating from Bernstein and colleagues' (2000, 2001) work with anxious and depressed school-refusing adolescents, we propose that young

people who are more severely distressed (as indicated by a diagnosis of severe depression) may benefit from the combined use of psychosocial and
pharmacological treatments as a first-stage treatment. More severe disturbance in the form of severe depression is likely to prolong the treatment
process and impede early return to school, a key factor in the successful
management of school refusal (Blagg, 1987; Kennedy, 1965).

Another option as a second stage of treatment is to consider an extended
trial of CBT. This is especially pertinent when outcomes of the initial treatment lead to a reformulation of the function of the young person's refusal
to attend school. For example, it may only be during the attempted school
return for a young person with an initial diagnosis of separation anxiety
disorder that the young person's social anxiety becomes apparent. In some
cases, a greater focus may need to be paid to conducting CBT directly with
the child, if CBT with parents and school staff was the initial focus of treatment. Extended CBT may also be pertinent when families are disinclined
toward the use of medication, although it is important to be mindful of
Klein and colleagues' (1992) notion that the undue delay of an alternative
and potentially effective treatment (in this case, combined CBT and medication) may be problematical. When medication seems indicated, treatment
adherence may be improved by involving the child in the decision to include pharmacological treatment, and by helping him or her to understand
the nature of any adverse effects that may occur (Tonge, 1998).

Stage 3: The Treatment-Refractory Patient

Unfortunately, there will always be young people and families who do not
appear to benefit at all from treatment, even in the case of a high-strength
IPPT program involving CBT and medication. Following reasonable trials
(in delivery, duration, and dose) of CBT and routinely employed pharmacological treatments (e.g., SSRIs, TCAs), alternatives need to be considered. Sometimes we are able to help the treatment-refractory patient through
a refocusing of the IPPT program. At other times, newer or less mainstream
treatments are tried.

Refocusing of the IPPT program may involve greater emphasis on
parent and family functioning (cf. Kearney & Roblek, 1998). CBT strategies employed to address parental anxiety, depression, and marital distress
may place parents in a better position to manage their own distress and to
more effectively employ behavioral strategies helpful in supporting the
young person's return to school. Although this could well be considered
important during the development of the initial treatment plan, there are
as yet no treatment outcome studies that indicate how important such adjunct treatment is or in which cases it is most warranted.

School-refusing children and their families may benefit from alternate
psychosocial approaches, such as psychodynamic psychotherapy or family
therapy. For example, Kearney and Albano (2000b) suggested that family
therapy may be necessary to address those family dynamics that reduce

motivation for participation in behaviorally orientated programs. Bernstein and colleagues (1999) suggested that, for some families, family therapy may help to reduce the severity and attenuate the course of school refusal. Perhaps this is especially true for the families of the anxious-depressed adolescent school refusers with whom they worked. Alternate pharmacological treatments may also be considered. The reader is directed to Tonge's (1998) review of pharmacological treatments for school refusal, including treatments that are regarded as experimental (e.g., serotonin/norepinephrine reuptake inhibitors, serotonin antagonist/reuptake inhibitors, beta blockers).

Stage 4: Treatment Maintenance

The effectiveness of school-refusal treatments is often conceptualized in terms of the young person's level of school attendance. *Successful attendance* or *remission* has been variously defined as 95% attendance (Last et al., 1998), 90% attendance (Heyne, King, et al., 2002; Kearney & Silverman, 1990; N. J. King, Tonge, et al., 1998; N. J. King, Tonge, et al., 2001) and 75% attendance (Bernstein et al., 2000). Clinical improvement has also been measured with respect to reductions in emotional distress (e.g., CDI score less than 13) and the absence of a *DSM* diagnosis (Heyne, King, et al., 2002).

The 3- to 5-year follow-up study by N. J. King, Tonge, and colleagues (2001) provides tentative support for the longer-term effectiveness of a 4-week CBT treatment program with school refusers and their parents. On the other hand, the 1-year follow-up of anxious-depressed school-refusing adolescents (Bernstein et al., 2001) emphasized the need to determine the optimal type and duration of acute and maintenance treatments, to develop treatments with long-lasting effectiveness. Last et al. (1998) also emphasized the need for optimal maintenance treatments to be addressed by future research. On the basis of their clinical experience, Last and colleagues suggested that booster treatment sessions conducted before and during the new school year are helpful in preventing relapse associated with school reentry.

Based on their research on the functioning in families of school refusers, Bernstein and Borchardt (1996) speculated that treatment adherence may differ according to family type (i.e., single-parent families versus intact families). Furthermore, they speculated that response to pharmacological or psychosocial interventions, or both, may also vary according to family constellation. In the absence of applicable data to guide our thinking, we propose that extra support during longer psychosocial interventions may need to be provided to single parents. Because of the complex family dynamics that may be more likely to evolve in such families (e.g., the parent relating to the child more as a peer than as a parent; the child becoming oppositional and controlling), it may be harder for single parents to remedy school refusal (Bernstein & Borchardt, 1996).

CONCLUSIONS

School refusal is a serious problem characterized by a variable and complex clinical presentation, necessitating a robust and flexible approach to assessment and treatment. Clearly, the clinician is presented with an array of options in planning treatment with school-refusing children and adolescents, their families, and school staff. Although the status of treatment outcome data does not allow for definitive recommendations, decisions about the various stages of treatment may be guided by currently available data and accumulated clinical wisdom.

Presently, CBT is the only intervention to have sufficient empirical support to be considered a first-line treatment approach. However, treatment research is not sufficiently advanced to offer comment on underlying mechanisms or the most crucial components of CBT. Treatment may begin with CBT, either alone or in combination with medication, depending on the severity of the young person's emotional distress. If CBT alone is ineffective, medication may be added, or CBT alone may be continued in modified form. Particular emphasis may need to be given to parental psychopathology and to broader family problems. Alternative psychosocial treatments may also need to be tried.

Future school-refusal research would ideally compare CBT, pharmacological treatment, and their combination (Bernstein et al., 2000). It should also explore the causal relationship between depression and school refusal (Kearney, 1993). By stratifying random assignment to treatment conditions according to the presence and severity of comorbid depression, we could better understand the impact of depression on treatment outcome, and thus determine the need to adapt school-refusal treatments to target depressive symptomatology. Further research along the lines of Kearney and Silverman's (1993) functional classification system will also help in making decisions about which components of CBT may be more helpful for different groups of school refusers.

The optimal duration of acute and maintenance treatments is also a key research priority. A range of factors could be explored in relation to optimal treatment duration, including the chronicity and severity of the young person's nonattendance, the lack of volition to attend, and personality (Okuyama et al., 1999). Treatment duration will also be influenced by its intensity, for example, by the need to address the young person's distress at the same time as parental psychopathology and broader family functioning are addressed. An enhanced capacity to predict optimal treatment intensity may prevent situations in which a family's experience of an unsuccessful treatment of lesser intensity discourages their participation in a subsequent, more intensive treatment program.

REFERENCES

Achenbach, T. M. (1991a). *Manual for the Child Behavior Checklist: 4–18 and 1991 profile*. Burlington: University of Vermont Department of Psychiatry.

Achenbach, T. M. (1991b). *Manual for the Teacher's Report Form and 1991 profile.* Burlington: University of Vermont Department of Psychiatry.

Achenbach, T. M. (1991c). *Manual for the Youth Self-Report and 1991 profile.* Burlington: University of Vermont Department of Psychiatry.

American Academy of Child and Adolescent Psychiatry. (1997). Practice parameters for the assessment and treatment of children and adolescents with anxiety disorders. *Journal of the American Academy of Child and Adolescent Psychiatry, 36*(Suppl.), 69S–84S.

American Psychiatric Association. (1980). *Diagnostic and statistical manual of mental disorders* (3rd ed.). Washington, DC: Author.

American Psychiatric Association. (1987). *Diagnostic and statistical manual of mental disorders: DSM-III-R* (3rd ed., rev.). Washington, DC: Author.

American Psychiatric Association. (1994). *Diagnostic and statistical manual of mental disorders: DSM-IV* (4th ed.). Washington, DC: Author.

Atkinson, L., Quarrington, B., & Cyr, J. J. (1985). School refusal: The heterogeneity of a concept. *American Journal of Orthopsychiatry, 55,* 83–101.

Ayllon, T., Smith, D., & Rogers, M. (1970). Behavioral management of school phobia. *Journal of Behavior Therapy and Experimental Psychiatry, 1,* 125–138.

Barrett, P. M., Dadds, M. R., & Rapee, R. M. (1996). Family treatment of childhood anxiety disorders: A controlled trial. *Journal of Consulting and Clinical Psychology, 64,* 333–342.

Beck, A. T., Steer, R. A., & Brown, G. K. (1996). *Beck Depression Inventory* (2nd ed.). New York: Psychological Corporation.

Beck, J. (1995). *Cognitive therapy: Basics and beyond.* New York: Guilford Press.

Beidel, D. C., Neal, A. M., & Lederer, A. S. (1991). The feasibility and validity of a daily diary for the assessment of anxiety in children. *Behavior Therapy, 22,* 505–517.

Berg, I. (1980). School refusal in early adolescence. In L. Hersov & I. Berg (Eds.), *Out of school: Modern perspectives* (pp. 231–249). Chichester, UK: Wiley.

Berg, I. (1996). School avoidance, school phobia, and truancy. In M. Lewis (Ed.), *Child and adolescent psychiatry: A comprehensive textbook* (2nd ed., pp. 1104–1110). Sydney, Australia: Williams & Wilkins.

Berg, I. (1997). School refusal and truancy. *Archives of Disease in Childhood, 76,* 90–91.

Berg, I., Nichols, K., & Pritchard, C. (1969). School phobia: Its classification and relationship to dependency. *Journal of Child Psychology and Psychiatry, 10,* 123–141.

Berney, T., Kolvin, I., Bhate, S. R., Garside, R. F., Jeans, J., Kay, B., & Scarth, L. (1981). School phobia: A therapeutic trial with clomipramine and short-term outcome. *British Journal of Psychiatry, 138,* 110–118.

Bernstein, G. A., & Borchardt, C. M. (1996). School refusal: Family constellation and family functioning. *Journal of Anxiety Disorders, 10,* 1–19.

Bernstein, G. A., Borchardt, C. M., Perwien, A. R., Crosby, R. D., Kushner, M. G., Thuras, P. D., & Last, C. G. (2000). Imipramine plus cognitive-behavioral therapy in the treatment of school refusal. *Journal of the American Academy of Child and Adolescent Psychiatry, 39,* 276–283.

Bernstein, G. A., & Garfinkel, B. D. (1986). School phobia: The overlap of affective and anxiety disorders. *Journal of the American Academy of Child and Adolescent Psychiatry, 25,* 235–241.

Bernstein, G. A., Garfinkel, B. D., & Borchardt, C. M. (1990). Comparative studies of pharmacotherapy for school refusal. *Journal of the American Academy of Child and Adolescent Psychiatry, 29,* 773–781.

Bernstein, G. A., Hektner, J. M., Borchardt, C. M., & McMillan, M. H. (2001). Treatment of school refusal: One-year follow-up. *Journal of the American Academy Child and Adolescent Psychiatry, 40,* 206–213.

Bernstein, G. A., Warren, S. L., Massie, E. D., & Thuras, P. D. (1999). Family dimensions in anxious-depressed school refusers. *Journal of Anxiety Disorders, 13,* 513–528.

Biederman, J. (1987). Clonazepam in the treatment of prepubertal children with panic-like symptoms. *Journal of Clinical Psychiatry, 48*(Suppl.), 38–41.

Birmaher, B., Waterman, G. S., Ryan, N., Cully, M., Balach, L., Ingram, J., & Brodsky, M. (1994). Fluoxetine for childhood anxiety disorders. *Journal of the American Academy of Child and Adolescent Psychiatry, 33,* 993–999.

Black, B., & Uhde, T. W. (1994). Treatment of elective mutism with fluoxetine: A double-blind, placebo-controlled study. *Journal of the American Academy of Child and Adolescent Psychiatry, 33,* 1000–1006.

Blagg, N. (1987). *School phobia and its treatment.* New York: Croom Helm.

Bools, C., Foster, J., Brown, I., & Berg, I. (1990). The identification of psychiatric disorders in children who fail to attend school: A cluster analysis of a non-clinical population. *Psychological Medicine, 20,* 171–181.

Boulos, C., Cutcher, S., Gardner, D., & Young, E. (1992). An open naturalistic trial of fluoxetine in adolescents and young adults with treatment resistant major depression. *Journal of Child and Adolescent Psychopharmacology, 2,* 103–111.

Burke, A. E., & Silverman, W. K. (1987). The prescriptive treatment of school refusal. *Clinical Psychology Review, 7,* 353–362.

Daleiden, E. L., Chorpita, B. F., Kollins, S. H., & Drabman, R. S. (1999). Factors affecting the reliability of clinical judgments about the function of children's school-refusal behavior. *Journal of Clinical Child Psychology, 28,* 396–406.

D'Amato, G. (1962). Chlordiazepoxide in management of school phobia. *Diseases of the Nervous System, 23,* 292–295.

Daugherty, T. K., & Shapiro, S. K. (1994). Behavior checklists and rating forms. In T. H. Ollendick, N. J. King, & W. R. Yule (Eds.), *International handbook of phobic and anxiety disorders in children and adolescents* (pp. 331–346). New York: Plenum Press.

Derogatis, L. R. (1993). *The Brief Symptom Inventory* (2nd ed.). Riderwood, MD: Clinical Psychometric Research.

Dummit, E. S., Klein, R. G., Tancer, N. K., Asche, B., & Martin, J. (1996). Fluoxetine treatment of children with selective mutism: An open trial. *Journal of the American Academy of Child and Adolescent Psychiatry, 35,* 615–621.

Eisenberg, L. (1959). The pediatric management of school phobia. *Journal of Pediatrics, 55,* 758–766.

Emslie, G. J., & Mayes, T. L. (2001). Mood disorders in children and adolescents: Psychopharmacological treatment. *Biological Psychiatry, 49,* 1082–1090.

Emslie, G. J., Rush, A. J., Weinberg, W. A., Kowatch, R. A., Hughes, C. W., Carmody, T., & Rintelmann, J. (1997). A double-blind, randomized, placebo-controlled trial of fluoxetine in children and adolescents with depression. *Archives of General Psychiatry, 54,* 1031–1037.

Epstein, N. B., Baldwin, L. M., & Bishop, D. S. (1983). The McMaster Family Assessment Device. *Journal of Marital and Family Therapy, 9,* 171–180.

Fairbanks, J. M., Pine, D. S., Tancer, N. K., Dummit, E. S., III, Kentgen, L. M., Martin, J., Asche, B. K., et al. (1997). Open fluoxetine treatment of mixed anxiety disorders in children and adolescents. *Journal of Child and Adolescent Psychopharmacology, 7,* 17–29.

Flakierska, N., Lindstrom, N., & Gillberg, C. (1988). School refusal: A 15–20-year follow-up study of 35 Swedish urban children. *British Journal of Psychiatry, 152,* 834–837.

Flakierska-Praquin, N., Lindstrom, M., & Gillberg, C. (1997). School phobia with separation anxiety disorder: A comparative 20- to 29-year follow-up study of 35 school refusers. *Comprehensive Psychiatry, 38,* 17–22.

Forehand, R. L., & McMahon, R. J. (1981). *Helping the noncompliant child: A clinician's guide to parent training.* New York: Guilford Press.

Fox, J. E., & Houston, B. K. (1983). Distinguishing between cognitive and somatic trait and state anxiety in children. *Journal of Personality and Social Psychology, 45,* 862–870.

Gittelman-Klein, R., & Klein, D. F. (1971). Controlled imipramine treatment of school phobia. *Archives of General Psychiatry, 25,* 204–207.

Granell de Aldaz, E., Vivas, E., Gelfand, D. M., & Feldman, L. (1984). Estimating the prevalence of school refusal and school-related fears: A Venezuelan sample. *Journal of Nervous and Mental Disease, 172,* 722–729.

Greenhill, L. L., Pine, D., Walkup, J., Riddle, M., & Vitiello, B. (2000, October 24–29). A randomized clinical trial of fluvoxamine for anxiety disorder. Presented at the 47th Annual Meeting of the American Academy of Child and Adolescent Psychiatry, New York.

Gullone, E., & King, N. J. (1991). Acceptability of alternative treatments for school refusal: Evaluations by students, caregivers and professionals. *British Journal of Educational Psychology, 61,* 346–354.

Gullone, E., & King, N. J. (1992). Psychometric evaluation of a revised fear survey schedule for children and adolescents. *Journal of Child Psychology and Psychiatry, 33,* 987–998.

Gutgesell, H., Atkins, D., Barst, R., Buck, M., Franklin, W., Humes, R., Ringel, R., Shaddy, R., & Taubert, K. A. (1999). AHA scientific statement: Cardiovascular monitoring of children and adolescents receiving psychotropic drugs. *Journal of the American Academy of Child and Adolescent Psychiatry, 38,* 1047–1050.

Hansen, C., Sanders, S. L., Massaro, S., & Last, C. G. (1998). Predictors of severity of absenteeism in children with anxiety-based school refusal. *Journal of Clinical Child Psychology, 27,* 246–254.

Hersov, L. (1985), School refusal. In M. Rutter & L. Hersov (Eds.), *Child and adolescent psychiatry: Modern approaches,* (2nd ed., pp. 382–399). Oxford, UK: Blackwell Scientific Publications.

Heyne, D. (1999). *Evaluation of child therapy and caregiver training in the treatment of school refusal.* Unpublished doctoral dissertation, Monash University, Melbourne, Australia.

Heyne, D., & King, N. (in press). Treatment of school refusal. In P. Barrett & T. Ollendick (Eds.), *Handbook of interventions that work with children and adolescents: Prevention and treatment.* New York: Wiley.

Heyne, D., King, N., Tonge, B., & Cooper, H. (2001). School refusal: Epidemiology and management. *Paediatric Drugs, 3,* 719–732.

Heyne, D., King, N. J., Tonge, B., Rollings, S., Pritchard, M., Young, D., & Myerson, N. (1998). The Self-Efficacy Questionnaire for School Situations: Development and psychometric evaluation. *Behaviour Change, 15,* 31–40.

Heyne, D., King, N. J., Tonge, B. J., Rollings, S., Young, D., Pritchard, M., & Ollendick, T. H. (2002). Evaluation of child therapy and caregiver training in the treatment of school refusal. *Journal of the American Academy of Child and Adolescent Psychiatry, 41*(6), 687–695.

Heyne, D., & Rollings, S. (with King, N. J., & Tonge, B. J.). (2002). *School refusal.* Oxford, UK: Blackwell.

Hoshino, Y., Nikkuni, S., Kaneko, M., Endo, M., Yashima, Y., & Kumashiro, H. (1987). The application of *DSM-III* diagnostic criteria to school refusal. *The Japanese Journal of Psychiatry and Neurology, 41,* 1–7.

Kahn, J. H., & Nursten, J. P. (1962). School refusal: A comprehensive view of school phobia and other failures of school attendance. *American Journal of Orthopsychiatry, 32,* 707–718.

Kearney, C. A. (1993). Depression and school refusal behavior: A review with comments on classification and treatment. *Journal of School Psychology, 31,* 267–279.

Kearney, C. A. (2001). *School refusal behavior in youth: A functional approach to assessment and treatment.* Washington, DC: American Psychological Association.

Kearney, C. A., & Albano, A. M. (2000a). *When children refuse school: A cognitive-behavioral therapy approach—Parent workbook.* San Antonio, TX: Graywind Publications.

Kearney, C. A., & Albano, A. M. (2000b). *When children refuse school: A cognitive-behavioral therapy approach—Therapist guide.* San Antonio, TX: Graywind Publications.

Kearney, C. A., & Beasley, J. F. (1994). The clinical treatment of school refusal behavior: A survey of referral and practice characteristics. *Psychology in the Schools, 31,* 128–132.

Kearney, C. A., Eisen, A. R., & Silverman, W. K. (1995). The legend and myth of school phobia. *School Psychology Quarterly, 10,* 65–85.

Kearney, C. A., & Roblek, T. L. (1998). Parent training in the treatment of school refusal behavior. In J. M. Briesmeister & C. E. Schaefer (Eds.), *Handbook of parent training: Parents as co-therapists for children's behavior problems* (pp. 225–256). New York: Wiley.

Kearney, C. A., & Silverman, W. K. (1990). A preliminary analysis of a functional model of assessment and treatment for school refusal behavior. *Behavior Modification, 14,* 340–366.

Kearney, C. A., & Silverman, W. K. (1993). Measuring the function of school refusal behavior: The School Refusal Assessment Scale. *Journal of Clinical Child Psychology, 22,* 85–96.

Kearney, C. A., & Silverman, W. K. (1996). The evolution and reconciliation of taxonomic strategies for school refusal behavior. *Clinical Psychology: Science and Practice, 3,* 339–354.

Kearney, C. A., & Silverman, W. K. (1999). Functionally based prescriptive and nonprescriptive treatment for children and adolescents with school refusal behavior. *Behavior Therapy, 30,* 673–696.

Kendall, P. C. (1992). Childhood coping: Avoiding a lifetime of anxiety. *Behaviour Change, 9,* 229–237.

Kendall, P. C. (1994). Treating anxiety disorders in children: Results of a randomized clinical trial. *Journal of Consulting and Clinical Psychology, 62,* 100–110.

Kendall, P. C., Chansky, T. E., Kane, M. T., Kim, R. S., Kortlander, E., Ronan, K. R., Sessa, F. M., et al. (1992). *Anxiety disorders in youth: Cognitive-behavioral interventions.* Boston: Allyn & Bacon.

Kennedy, W. A. (1965). School phobia: Rapid treatment of fifty cases. *Journal of Abnormal Psychology, 70,* 285–289.

King, N. J., & Bernstein, G. A. (2001). School refusal in children and adolescents: A review of the past ten years. *Journal of the American Academy of Child and Adolescent Psychiatry, 40,* 197–205.

King, N. J., Heyne, D., Gullone, E., & Molloy, G. N. (2001). Usefulness of emotive imagery in the treatment of childhood phobias: Clinical guidelines, case examples and issues. *Counselling Psychology Quarterly, 14,* 95–101.

King, N. J., & Ollendick, T. H. (1989a). Children's anxiety and phobic disorders in school settings: Classification, assessment, and intervention issues. *Review of Educational Research, 59,* 431–470.

King, N. J., & Ollendick, T. H. (1989b). School refusal: Graduated and rapid behavioural treatment strategies. *Australian and New Zealand Journal of Psychiatry, 23,* 213–223.

King, N. J., Ollendick, T. H., Murphy, G. H., & Molloy, G. N (1998). Utility of relaxation training in school settings: A plea for realistic goal setting and evaluation. *British Journal of Educational Psychology, 68,* 53–66.

King, N. J., Ollendick, T. H., & Tonge, B. J. (1995). *School refusal: Assessment and treatment.* Boston: Allyn & Bacon.

King, N. J., Tonge, B. J., Heyne, D., & Ollendick, T. H. (2000). Research on the cognitive-behavioral treatment of school refusal: A review and recommendations. *Clinical Psychology Review, 20,* 495–507.

King, N. J., Tonge, B. J., Heyne, D., Pritchard, M., Rollings, S., Young, D., Myerson, N., et al. (1998). Cognitive-behavioral treatment of school-refusing children: A controlled evaluation. *Journal of the American Academy of Child and Adolescent Psychiatry, 37,* 375–403.

King, N. J., Tonge, B. J., Heyne, D., Turner, S., Pritchard, M., Young, D., Rollings, S., et al. (2001). Cognitive-behavioral treatment of school-refusing children: Maintenance of improvements at 3- to 5-year follow-up. *Scandinavian Journal of Behaviour Therapy, 30,* 85–89.

King, R. A., Riddle, M. A., Chappell, P. B., Hardin, M. T., Anderson, G. M., Lombroso, P., & Scahill, L. (1991). Emergence of self-destructive phenomena in children and adolescents during fluoxetine treatment. *Journal of the American Academy of Child and Adolescent Psychiatry, 30,* 179–186.

Klein, R. G., Koplewicz, H. S., & Kanner, A. (1992). Imipramine treatment of children with separation anxiety disorder. *Journal of the American Academy of Child and Adolescent Psychiatry, 31,* 21–28.

Koeppen, A. S. (1974). Relaxation training for children. *Elementary School Guidance and Counseling,* 14–21.

Kovacs, M. (1992). *Children's Depression Inventory.* New York: Multi-Health Systems.

Kraft, I. A., Ardali, C., Duffy, J. H., Hart, J. T., & Pearce, P. (1965). A clinical study of chloridazepoxide used in psychiatric disorders of children. *International Journal of Neuropsychiatry, 1,* 433–437.

Labellarte, M. J., Ginsburg, G. S., Walkup, J. T., & Riddle, M. A. (1999). The treatment of anxiety disorders in children and adolescents. *Biological Psychiatry, 46,* 1567–1578.

La Greca, A. M., & Stone, W. L. (1993). Social Anxiety Scale for Children–Revised: Factor structure and concurrent validity. *Journal of Clinical Child Psychology, 22,* 17–27.

Last, C. G. (1992). Anxiety disorders in childhood and adolescence. In W. M. Reynolds (Ed.), *Internalizing disorders in children and adolescents* (pp. 61–106). New York: Wiley.

Last, C. G., Hansen, C., & Franco, N. (1998). Cognitive-behavioral treatment of school phobia. *Journal of the American Academy of Child and Adolescent Psychiatry, 37,* 404–411.

Last, C. G., & Strauss, C. C. (1990). School refusal in anxiety-disordered children and adolescents. *Journal of the American Academy of Child and Adolescent Psychiatry, 29,* 31–35.

Mansdorf, I. J., & Lukens, E. (1987). Cognitive-behavioral psychotherapy for separation anxious children exhibiting school phobia. *Journal of the American Academy of Child and Adolescent Psychiatry, 26,* 222–225.

March, J. S., Biederman, J., Wolkow, R., Safferman, A., Mardekian, J., Cook, E. H., Cutler, N. R., et. al. (1998). Sertraline in children and adolescents with obsessive-compulsive disorder: A multicenter randomized controlled trial. *Journal of the American Medical Association, 280,* 1752–1756.

Martin, C., Cabrol, S., Bouvard, M. P., Lepine, J. P., & Mouren-Simeoni, M. C. (1999). Anxiety and depressive disorders in fathers and mothers of anxious school-refusing children. *Journal of the American Academy of Child and Adolescent Psychiatry, 38,* 916–922.

Mash, E. J., & Terdal, L. G. (1997). Assessment of child and family disturbance: A behavioral-systems approach. In E. J. Mash & L. G. Terdal (Eds.), *Assessment of childhood disorders* (3rd ed., pp. 3–68). New York: Guilford Press.

McShane, G., Walter, G., & Rey, J. M. (2001). Characteristics of adolescents with school refusal. *Australian and New Zealand Journal of Psychiatry, 35,* 822–826.

Meyer, E. A., Hagopian, L. P., & Paclawskyj, T. R. (1999). A function-based treatment for school refusal behavior using shaping and fading. *Research in Developmental Disabilities, 20,* 401–410.

Montgomery, S. A., Henry, J., McDonald, G., Dinnan, T., Lader, M., Hinmarch, I., Clare, A., et al. (1994). Selective serotonin reuptake inhibitors: Meta-analysis of discontinuation rates. *International Journal of Clinical Psychopharmacology, 9,* 47–53.

Naylor, M. W., Staskowski, M., Kenney, M. C., & King, C. A. (1994). Language disorders and learning disabilities in school-refusing adolescents. *Journal of the American Academy of Child and Adolescent Psychiatry, 33,* 1331–1337.

Okuyama, M., Okada, M., Kuribayashi, M., & Kaneko, S. (1999). Factors responsible for the prolongation of school refusal. *Psychiatry and Clinical Neurosciences, 53,* 461–469.

Ollendick, T. H. (1983). Reliability and validity of the Revised Fear Survey Schedule for Children (FSSC-R). *Behaviour Research and Therapy, 21,* 685–692.

Ollendick, T. H., & Cerny, J. A. (1981). *Clinical behavior therapy with children.* New York: Plenum Press.

Ollendick, T. H., & King, N. J. (1998). Assessment practices and issues with school-refusing children. *Behaviour Change, 15,* 16–30.

Pedersen, W., & Lavik, N. J. (1991). Adolescents and benzodiazepines: Prescribed use, self-medication and intoxication. *Acta Psychiatrica Scandinavica, 84*, 94–98.

Pfefferbaum, B., Overall, J. E., Boren, H. A., Frankel, L. S., Sullivan, M. P., & Johnson, K. (1987). Alprazolam in the treatment of anticipatory and acute situational anxiety in children with cancer. *Journal of the American Academy of Child and Adolescent Psychiatry, 26*, 532–535.

Pilkington, C. L., & Piersel, W. C. (1991). School phobia: A critical analysis of the separation anxiety theory and an alternative conceptualization. *Psychology in the Schools, 28*, 290–303.

Popper, C. W., & Elliot, G. R. (1993). Postmortem pharmacokinetics of tricyclics: Are some deaths during treatment misattributed to overdose? *Journal of Child and Adolescent Psychopharmacology, 3*, x–xii.

Popper, C. W., & Ziminitzky, B. (1995). Sudden death putatively related to desipramine treatment in youth: A fifth case and a review of speculative mechanisms. *Journal of Child and Adolescent Psychopharmacology, 5*, 283–300.

Puig-Antich, J., & Ryan, N. D. (1986). *Schedule for Affective Disorders and Schizophrenia for School-Age Children (6–16) (K-SADS-P)*. [Fourth working draft].

Rapee, R. M., Barrett, P. M., Dadds, M. R., & Evans, L. (1994). Reliability of the *DSM-III-R* childhood anxiety disorders using structured interview: Interrater and parent-child agreement. *Journal of the American Academy of Child and Adolescent Psychiatry, 33*, 984–992.

Research Units of Pediatric Psychopharmacology Anxiety Study Group. (2000, May 30–June 2). A multi-site double-blind placebo-controlled trial of fluvoxamine for children and adolescents with anxiety disorders. Presented at the 40th New Clinical Drug Evaluation Unit Annual Meeting, Boca Raton, Florida.

Reynolds, C. R., & Richmond, B. O. (1978). What I think and feel: A revised measure of children's manifest anxiety. *Journal of Abnormal Child Psychology, 6*, 271–280.

Riddle, M. A., Bernstein, G. A., Cook, E. H., Leonard, H. L., March, J. S., & Swanson, J. M. (1999). Anxiolytics, adrenergic agents, and naltrexone. *Journal of the American Academy of Child and Adolescent Psychiatry, 38*, 546–556.

Riddle, M. A., Geller, B., & Ryan, N. (1993). Case study: Another sudden death in a child treated with desipramine. *Journal of the American Academy of Child and Adolescent Psychiatry, 32*, 792–797.

Riddle, M. A., Nelson, J. C., Kleinman, C. S., Rasmusson, A., Leckman, J. F., King, R. A., & Cohen, D. J. (1991). Sudden death in children receiving Norpramin: A review of three reported cases and commentary. *Journal of the American Academy of Child and Adolescent Psychiatry, 30*, 104–108.

Riddle, M. A., Reeve, E. A., Yaryura-Tobias, J. A., Yang, H. M., Claghorn, J. L., Gaffney, G., Greist, J. H., et al. (2001). Fluvoxamine for children and adolescents with obsessive-compulsive disorder: A randomized, controlled, multicenter trial. *Journal of the American Academy of Child and Adolescent Psychiatry, 40*, 222–229.

Saraf, K., Klein, D., Gittelman-Klein, R., Groff, S. (1974). Imipramine side effects in children. *Psychopharmacologia, 37*, 265–274.

Seligman, M. E. P., Peterson, C., Kaslow, N. J., Tanenbaum, R. L., Alloy, L. B., & Abramson, L. Y. (1984). Attributional style and depressive symptoms among children. *Journal of Abnormal Psychology, 93*, 235–238.

Sharpley, C. F., & Rogers, H. J. (1984). Preliminary validation of the abbreviated Spanier Dyadic Adjustment Scale: Some psychometric data regarding a screening test of marital adjustment. *Educational and Psychological Measurement, 44,* 1045–1050.

Silverman, W. K., & Albano, A. M. (1996). *Anxiety Disorders Interview Schedule for DSM-1V: Child and parent versions.* San Antonio, TX: Psychological Corporation.

Silverman, W. K., & Eisen, A. R. (1992). Age differences in the reliability of parent and child reports of child anxious symptomatology using a structured interview. *Journal of the American Academy of Child and Adolescent Psychiatry, 31,* 117–124.

Silverman, W. K., & Rabian, B. (1995). Test-retest reliability of the *DSM-III-R* childhood anxiety disorder symptoms using the Anxiety Disorders Interview Schedule for Children. *Journal of Anxiety Disorders, 9,* 139–150.

Siméon, J. G., Ferguson, H. B., Knott, V., Roberts, N., Gauthier, B., Dubois, B. A., & Wiggins, D. (1992). Clinical, cognitive, and neurophysiological effects of alprazolam in children and adolescents with overanxious and avoidant disorders. *Journal of the American Academy of Child and Adolescent Psychiatry, 31,* 29–33.

Smith, S. L. (1970). School refusal with anxiety: A review of sixty-three cases. *Canadian Psychiatric Association Journal, 15,* 257–264.

Spence, S. H. (1998). A measure of anxiety symptoms among children. *Behaviour Research and Therapy, 36,* 545–566.

Stickney, M. I., & Miltenberger, R. G. (1998). School refusal behavior: Prevalence, characteristics, and the schools' response. *Education and Treatment of Children, 21,* 160–170.

Thyer, B. A., & Sowers-Hoag, K. M. (1986). The etiology of school phobia: A behavioral approach. *School Social Work Journal, 10,* 86–98.

Tonge, B. (1998). Pharmacotherapy of school refusal. *Behaviour Change, 15,* 98–106.

Torma, S., & Halsti, A. (1975). Factors contributing to school phobia and truancy. *Psychiatria Fennica,* 209–220.

Varley, C. K., & McClellan, J. (1997). Case study: Two additional sudden deaths with tricyclic antidepressants. *Journal of the American Academy of Child and Adolescent Psychiatry, 36,* 390–394.

Velosa, J. F., & Riddle, M. A. (2000). Pharmacologic treatment of anxiety disorders in children and adolescents. *Child and Adolescent Psychiatric Clinics of North America, 9,* 119–133.

Wilkes, T. C. R., Belsher, G., Rush, A. J., & Frank, E. (1994). *Cognitive therapy for depressed adolescents.* New York: Guilford Press.

Wolpe, J. (1958). *Psychotherapy by reciprocal inhibition.* Stanford, CA: Stanford University Press.

Zarb, J. (1992). *Cognitive-behavioral assessment and therapy with adolescents.* New York: Bruner/Mazel.

10

SEPARATION ANXIETY DISORDER

Amy R. Perwien & Gail A. Bernstein

OVERVIEW OF SEPARATION ANXIETY DISORDER

Clinical Manifestations of Separation Anxiety Disorder

Separation anxiety disorder (SAD) was fully described in the third edition of the *Diagnostic and Statistical Manual of Mental Disorders* (*DSM-III*; American Psychiatric Association [APA], 1980, 2000) and it has been included in subsequent editions of *DSM* (APA, 1987, 1994). Over the most recent three editions of the diagnostic manual, the symptoms of SAD have remained relatively consistent. SAD is the only anxiety disorder included in the *DSM-IV* section of "other disorders of infancy, childhood or adolescence" (APA, 1994, p. 110). The hallmark of SAD is centered on fears related to being apart from home or attachment figure(s) that are beyond what would be expected given a child's developmental level. The cluster of SAD symptoms (which include distress prior to and during times of separation, anxiety about being separated from attachment figures, school refusal, clinging to attachment figures, difficulty sleeping alone, nightmares, and somatic complaints) must be present for a minimum of 4 weeks, according to *DSM-IV*. Even though the manual also specifies that the presentation of the disorder must occur prior to age 18, a diagnosis may be made in adults who have a history of onset before age 18. Consistent with the diagnostic criteria for other anxiety disorders, SAD must cause "clinically significant distress or impairment in social, academic (occupational), or other important areas of functioning" (APA, 1994, p. 113). Early onset may be specified for children who present with the disorder prior to age 6.

In order to make an accurate diagnosis of SAD, the clinician or researcher must consider normal development while ruling out other psychiatric disorders that have symptoms in common with SAD. In the following sections, we discuss normal manifestations of anxiety and clinical disorders that overlap with SAD.

Separation Anxiety Symptoms in Children and Adolescents

Determining what constitutes an anxiety disorder versus normal anxiety is a challenging issue for both clinicians and researchers. Bell-Dolan, Last, and Strauss (1990) examined symptoms of anxiety disorders, including SAD, in a sample of never psychiatrically ill children. Although symptoms of overanxious and phobic disorders were among the most frequently endorsed, just over 16% of the children reported subclinical fears related to harm befalling an attachment figure. More recent studies by Muris and colleagues in the Netherlands (Muris, Meesters, Merckelbach, Sermon, & Zwakhalen, 1998; Muris, Merckelbach, Gadet, & Moulaert, 2000; Muris, Merckelbach, Mayer, & Prins, 2000) suggest that worries in normal children are relatively common. Although symptoms of SAD were not specifically examined in these studies, the researchers found that nearly 70% of a nonclinical sample of children worried "every now and then." Worries related to dying, illness of others, and health were among the most frequently reported intense worries (Muris, Merckelbach, Mayer, & Meesters, 1998). A later study by the same research group (Muris, Merckelbach, Mayer, et al., 2000) found that nearly 15% of a sample of schoolchildren reported subclinical symptoms of SAD, and 4.8% fulfilled criteria for SAD on the basis of structured interviews. Regarding nightmares involving themes of separation, Muris, Merckelbach, Gadet, et al. (2000) provided some information about the frequency of these dreams in school-aged children, with 17.3% of the sample reporting dreams of harm to self or others, 14.7% experiencing dreams of kidnapping, 6.8% dreaming of dying or death of others, and 2.1% reporting dreams involving separation from parents. Although it is unknown what percentage of the children experienced nightmares repeatedly and met criteria for SAD, the data suggest that nightmares involving separation themes are not uncommon in children.

Developmental Considerations in the Diagnosis
of Separation Anxiety Disorder

During the preschool years, symptoms of separation anxiety may be present, but a distinction between symptoms appropriate to the developmental stage and the disorder must be made (Rapoport & Ismond, 1996). For example, preschool children may manifest symptoms of separation anxiety when confronted with new circumstances involving separations (e.g., being brought to daycare for the first time). Likewise, school-age children may manifest separation difficulties in particular situations such as going to a sleep-away camp, staying over at a peer's house for the first time, or returning to school after an extended illness or vacation. Although separation anxiety problems are thought to occur more frequently in children (Last, Hersen, Kazdin, Finkelstein, & Strauss, 1987), adolescents may also manifest these difficulties when adjusting to stressful situations (e.g., difficulties at school or with peers). At any age, symptoms of separation anxiety may be developmentally normal, subclinical, or clinical in nature depending on the type of symptoms experienced, the severity of the symptoms, the duration of the symptoms, and how much of an impact the symptoms have on the child's functioning. In addition, the factors surrounding the onset of the symptoms should be considered to rule out the possibility of an adjustment disorder with anxious features.

Prevalence

Several studies within both community and primary care settings have estimated the prevalence of SAD in nonreferred children. Variability in methodologies likely contributes to the different prevalence estimates. In a population-based study of psychiatric disorders based on *DSM-III-R* criteria, SAD was the most frequently occurring anxiety disorder in preadolescent children, with an estimated prevalence of 3.5% (Anderson, Williams, McGee, & Silva, 1987). A slightly lower estimate (2.4% prevalence rate) was found in a community epidemiological study of adolescents (Bowen, Offord, & Boyle, 1990). The Great Smoky Mountains Study, which used a screening-stratified sampling design, estimated that the 3-month prevalence of SAD was 3.5%, with a higher rate in females (4.3%) than in males (2.7%) (Costello et al., 1996). Although a study by Kashani and Orvaschel (1990) found much higher estimates of SAD in a community population of school-age children (13% prevalence), this is likely an overestimate given the consensus in findings from other studies. The prevalence rate of SAD in primary care settings is of particular interest because children with symptoms of separation anxiety may initially present to their pediatrician rather than to a mental health professional. The rate of SAD in a pediatric primary care sample of children revealed a 1-year prevalence of 4.1% when diagnoses obtained from parents and children were combined (Benjamin, Costello, & Warren, 1990). It is of interest that estimated rates for SAD based solely on parent report were lower than rates based on child report, suggesting the importance of using multiple informants in the assessment of SAD. A more recent study found a prevalence of 3.6% based on parental interviews (Briggs-Gowan, Horwitz, Schwab-Stone, Leventhal, & Leaf, 2000). To summarize findings from epidemiological studies, SAD likely occurs in 3% to 4% of children and is slightly less frequent in adolescents. However, rates within community care settings may be higher.

Associated Characteristics

Although girls appear more likely to have SAD than boys (Francis, Last, & Strauss, 1987; Kashani & Orvaschel, 1990; Last et al., 1987), some studies have found similar rates between boys and girls (Anderson et al., 1987). A recent study by Compton, Nelson, and March (2000) examined symptoms of separation anxiety and social phobia in community and clinical samples using a self-report measure of anxiety. In the community sample, females reported a higher rate of symptoms of separation anxiety than males. However, in the clinical sample, males were more likely to report symptoms of separation anxiety than females. The authors interpreted this finding as possibly due to a difference in mental health service utilization and referral patterns. Specifically, males experiencing symptoms of separation anxiety may be more likely than females to be referred for help and to receive mental health attention.

It has been suggested that symptom presentation varies between children and adolescents, with younger children expressing amorphous fears of separation and older children reporting more specific separation fears (Fischer, Himle, & Thyer, 1999). In addition to reporting different symptom constellations, younger children with SAD tend to report more symptoms than older children with the disorder (Francis et al., 1987). Regarding age at onset, children with SAD tend to be younger than children diagnosed with other anxiety disorders (Last et al., 1987; Last, Perrin, Hersen, & Kazdin, 1992). Westenberg, Siebelink, Warmenhoven, and Treffers (1999) noted that, although children with SAD tend to be younger than those diagnosed with overanxious disorder, the presence of a particular anxiety disorder appears to be related more to psychosocial maturity than to chronological age per se.

Although few studies have examined the relations between SAD and cognitive functioning in children, a study conducted by Toren, Sadeh, et al. (2000) attempted to look at neuropsychological features of children with SAD, overanxious disorder, or both. The children with anxiety disorders had more difficulty with verbal learning and memory skills than the children without anxiety. In comparison, anxiety did not appear to be associated with nonverbal processing or memory skills. Even though the study sample size was relatively small (19 children with anxiety and 14 control children), the findings highlight the importance of examining how separation anxiety and other related anxiety disorders impact cognitive functioning.

Course

Based on prospective research, Last, Perrin, Hersen, and Kazdin (1996) suggested that clinically referred children and adolescents with anxiety disorders tend to have generally favorable outcomes, with the majority free of their original anxiety disorders at 3- to 4-year follow-up. Of the anxiety disorders examined, SAD had the highest rate of recovery (95.7%) and one of the lowest rates related to the development of a new anxiety disorder (8.3%). Compared with children with other anxiety disorders, however, children with SAD were generally at equal risk for developing a new psychiatric disorder. Although a longitudinal study conducted by Ialongo and colleagues (Ialongo, Edelsohn, Werthamer-Larsson, Crockett, & Kellam, 1995) did not focus specifically on SAD, findings suggested that symptoms of anxiety identified in first grade were predictive of later anxiety symptoms and adaptive functioning as measured by standardized achievement test scores.

Several retrospective studies examining the connection between SAD and adult anxiety disorders have noted that early SAD may be linked to panic disorder in adulthood (Battaglia et al., 1995; Silove et al., 1995; Silove & Manicavasagar, 1993); however, other studies have not documented the relation between the two disorders (Manicavasagar, Silove, & Hadzi-Pavlovic, 1998). In fact, some have proposed that SAD may pose a risk for developing several of the adult anxiety disorders rather than panic disorder specifically (Lipsitz et al., 1994). Other researchers have suggested that SAD in childhood may progress into a poorly recognized adult form of the disorder labeled as adult SAD (Manicavasagar, Silove, Curtis, & Wagner, 2000).

ASSESSMENT OF SEPARATION ANXIETY DISORDER

Completion of a thorough initial assessment is important not only to document the presence of symptoms and disorders, but also to assist in the development of an appropriate treatment plan. Follow-up assessments can be used to examine the course of symptoms and disorders and to evaluate the effectiveness of treatments. Real-life constraints (e.g., clinician time, resources available to the clinician, and family time) must also be taken into account when considering particular assessment strategies. For SAD, several assessment methods are available, including clinical interviews, self-report scales, parent report measures, and observational methods. These methods are discussed in the following sections, with a critique of their strengths and weaknesses. At the end of the section, recommendations for the selection of assessment strategies are provided.

Diagnostic Interviews

Clinical interviews, conducted by clinicians familiar with the *DSM-IV* criteria for SAD as well as other child and adolescent disorders, are perhaps the most common assessment strategy (Fischer et al., 1999). A number of structured, semistructured, and pictorial clinical interviews have been developed for children and adolescents. Structured interviews are highly specific in their wording of questions, criteria for assessing responses, and instructions for conducting them. In comparison, semistructured interviews generally provide questions but do not require that questions be asked exactly as they are written (Teare, Fristad, Weller, Weller, & Salmon, 1998). Pictorial interviews are a relatively new interview method that rely on drawings to illustrate psychological symptoms. Brief descriptions of several clinical interviews and specific information about the available psychometric properties related to SAD are presented in the section that follows. Psychometric studies of diagnostic interviews generally include information about the test-retest reliability and the diagnostic agreement between clinicians and respondents. For a more thorough review of the clinical interviews described in the following sections, the reader is referred to a series of articles appearing in the January 2000 issue of the *Journal of the American Academy of Child and Adolescent Psychiatry*. In general, these interviews were developed and are appropriate for use in children and adolescents 6 to 18 years of age. One interview, the Preschool-Age Psychiatric Assessment (PAPA; Angold & Costello, 2000) was developed for 3- to 6-year-olds. Although most psychiatric interviews have child, adolescent, and parent versions available, the researcher or clinician should carefully consider which respondent(s) to use when incorporating data from structured psychiatric interviews. In assessing SAD, it is often helpful to include information from both parent and child interviews.

STRUCTURED AND SEMISTRUCTURED DIAGNOSTIC INTERVIEWS The Schedule for Affective Disorders and Schizophrenia for School-Age Children (K-SADS) a semistructured interview, was originally developed to assess both lifetime and current episodes of psychopathology by trained clinicians (Ambrosini, 2000). The most recent K-SADS was updated to be compatible with both *DSM-III-R* and *DSM-IV* and includes several versions: present state (K-SADS-P), epidemiologic (K-SADS-E), lifetime (K-SADS-L), and present/lifetime (K-SADS-PL). Ambrosini (2000) reported generally adequate test-retest reliability for separation anxiety with the present, epidemiologic, and present/lifetime versions of the K-SADS (kappa range $[k]$ = 0.24 to 0.85).

The most recent version of the Diagnostic Interview Schedule for Children (DISC-IV) is a highly structured interview that is based on *DSM-IV* and *ICD-10* (Shaffer, Fisher, Lucas, Dulcan, & Schwab-Stone, 2000). Both the youth and parent versions of the DISC are available in English and Spanish. The DISC-IV assesses for disorders in the past 12 months and the past 4 weeks, and has an optional whole-life module that assesses for diagnoses occurring after age 5 and prior to the previous 12 months. In psychometric studies of the DISC, test-retest reliability for SAD was generally adequate for parent and youth versions in both community (k = .46 to .58) and clinical samples (k = .25 to .54) (Jensen et al., 1995; Schwab-Stone et al., 1996). Agreement between DISC diagnoses of SAD and clinician ratings were moderate for the child report (k = .59) and combined parent/child report (k = .40), but low for parent report (k = .29; Schwab-Stone et al., 1996).

Although the Diagnostic Interview for Children and Adolescents (DICA) was once considered a structured interview, it can be used in a semistructured format (Reich, 2000). The DICA assesses for lifetime diagnoses using *DSM-III-R* and *DSM-IV* criteria (interviewer-based version) or *DSM-IV* criteria only (computer-based version). Adequate test-retest reliability (0.75) was found in a study of children and adolescents (Reich, 2000). Agreement between DICA and discharge diagnoses of SAD was in the low to moderate range for child and parent respondents (k = .15 and k = .50, respectively; Carlson, Kashani, de Fatima Thomas, Vaidya, & Daniel, 1987). Diagnostic agreement between parents and children/adolescents was examined using a Spanish version of the DICA in Barcelona (Ezpeleta et al., 1997). Diagnostic agreement for SAD was calculated between clinicians and children/adolescents, between clinicians and parents, and between parents and children/adolescents and found to be in the low to moderate range. Agreement between all combinations of respondents was better for children (k = .27 to .61) than for adolescents (k = .05 to .21).

The Child and Adolescent Psychiatric Assessment (CAPA) is an interviewer-based structured interview, allowing the interviewer to make diagnostic decisions based on information gathered from the respondent (Angold & Costello, 2000). The CAPA focuses on the preceding 3-month time period, although information on infrequent behaviors occurring prior to this period is also obtained. A study by Angold and Costello (1995) examining the reliability of the CAPA found adequate agreement between interviewers (k = .63). Test-retest reliability findings supported the stability of anxiety disorder diagnoses using the CAPA; however, specific data were not reported for SAD.

The Interview Schedule for Children and Adolescents (ISCA) is a symptom-oriented semistructured interview that can be used for intake (ISCA–Current and Lifetime), follow-up interviews during childhood and adolescence (ISCA–Current and Interim), and follow-up interviews during adulthood (FISA–Follow-up Interview Schedule for Adults; Sherrill & Kovacs, 2000). Although SAD is not part of the core instrument, it is included in the addendum. In a longitudinal study of anxiety disorders, test-retest reliability for SAD was found to be high (0.81) on the ISCA over a short time period (Last et al., 1987).

A relatively recently developed clinical interview, the Children's Interview for Psychiatric Symptoms (ChIPS), is highly structured and based on *DSM-IV* criteria. The ChIPS was specifically developed to include simple language and brief sentences (Weller, Weller, Fristad, Rooney, & Schecter, 2000). In a sample of 6- to 18-year-old inpatients, Fristad, Cummins, et al. (1998) found adequate diagnostic agreement for SAD between the ChIPS (child version) and the DICA (k = .58) as well as the ChIPS and clinician diagnoses (k = .69). Findings from community-based samples were relatively consistent (Fristad, Glickman, et al., 1998). Slightly higher agreement was found when comparisons were made between parents' reports on the ChIPS and clinician diagnoses (k = .71) in a sample of 36 children (Fristad, Teare, Weller, Weller, & Salmon, 1998). In this same sample, moderate levels of agreement between the parent and child versions of the ChIPS were found for SAD ($k = .49$).

The Anxiety Disorders Interview Schedule for Children (ADIS) was developed as a semistructured interview to provide information about anxiety symptomatology, etiology, and course (Silverman & Albano, 1996; Silverman & Nelles, 1988). In addition, the ADIS allows the interviewer to rule out alternative diagnoses (e.g., mood disorders) and to obtain a functional analysis of the anxiety disorder. The most recent version of the ADIS is consistent with *DSM-IV* criteria and involves interviewing the child and parent separately to determine a composite diagnosis (March & Albano, 1998). In the initial description of the ADIS, interrater agreement between clinicians was high for both the child and parent versions of the interview (Silverman & Nelles, 1988). Test-retest reliability has been found to be adequate for both the diagnosis of SAD and the majority of separation anxiety symptoms (Silverman & Eisen, 1992; Silverman & Rabian, 1995).

PICTORIAL DIAGNOSTIC INTERVIEWS   The Dominic-R and the Terry are pictorial questionnaires developed to illustrate the *DSM-III-R* emotional and behavioral symptoms for school-aged white and African American children, respectively (Valla, Bergeron, & Smolla, 2000). A computer version of the Dominic-R is based on *DSM-IV* criteria. The Dominic-R is available in English, Spanish, German and French, and the Terry is available in English and French. Studies of the Dominic-R (Valla, Bergeron, Berube, Gaudet, & St-Georges, 1994; Valla, Bergeron, Bidaut-Russell, St-Georges, & Gaudet, 1997) found adequate estimates of internal consistency and test-retest reliability for SAD using the Dominic-R. Support for the validity of the measure was found, with higher rates of SAD in referred children than in nonreferred children (Valla et al., 1994). Furthermore, a comparison of diagnoses generated by the instrument and those of clinicians supported the validity of the measure for assessing SAD. In a small sample of African American boys, mother-child agreement was poor, test-retest reliability for the child interview was adequate, and internal consistency estimates were moderate for SAD on the Terry (Bidaut-Russell, Valla, Thomas, Bergeron, & Lawson, 1998).

Compared with the age range for which the Dominic-R and the Terry were designed, the age range for the Pictorial Instrument for Children and Adolescents (PICA-III-R) is broader (it was developed for children 6 to 16 years of age). The PICA-III-R is a semistructured interview with pictures developed to illustrate emotions, behaviors, thoughts, and vegetative signs relevant to *DSM-III-R* diagnoses (Ernst, Cookus, & Moravec, 2000). The anxiety scale, which includes SAD, was found to be internally consistent, was found to relate moderately well to the depression subscale, and was sensitive to change over time (Ernst, Godfrey, Silva, Pouget, & Welkowitz, 1994).

Critique of Diagnostic Interviews   Structured, semistructured, and pictorial interviews have been primarily used in research settings, including epidemiological, longitudinal, and treatment outcome studies. Using established measures is an important component of the diagnostic and follow-up phases in clinical trials. Clinical interviews have the benefit of covering a wide spectrum of anxiety disorders while also screening for disorders that may coexist with anxiety. An area of concern is the overreliance on *DSM-IV* criteria; for example, children who do not carry a psychiatric diagnosis may still have significant impairment (Angold, Costello, Farmer, Burns, & Erkanli, 1999).

Despite some variability, the interviews discussed in the previous sections have undergone rigorous development procedures and generally have sound psychometric properties in relation to SAD. To make an informed decision about instrument selection, several factors should be considered, including the purpose of the assessment, the resources available to the clinician or researcher, and the population to be assessed. Specific issues may include the following: What disorders are included in the measure? Should separate interviews be conducted with parents and children? How much time does it take to administer the measure? What qualifications and training are necessary for interviewers? Is it possible to obtain severity ratings from the interview? The clinician or researcher must also decide how information obtained from different informants will be used to arrive at a diagnosis (i.e., how the data will be integrated). In reviewing characteristics of the measures, it is also important to carefully examine the psychometric properties in relation to SAD, while acknowledging that varying amounts of information are available for the different measures.

Clinician Rating Scales

The Hamilton Anxiety Rating Scale (HARS; Hamilton, 1959), the Anxiety Rating for Children-Revised (ARC-R; Bernstein, Crosby, Perwien, & Borchardt, 1996), and the Pediatric Anxiety Rating Scale (PARS; Walkup & Davies, 1999) are clinician rating scales that assess overall level of anxiety severity. The 14-item HARS includes items that are related but not specific to separation anxiety (e.g., anxious mood, fear, somatic symptoms). The ARC-R includes an anxiety subscale with five items (anxious mood, cognitive, tension, fears, separation anxiety) and a physiological subscale with six items (muscular, sensory, cardiovascular, respiratory, gastrointestinal, autonomic). The symptoms in the anxiety items are consistent with the HARS but were developed for children and adolescents. Bernstein et al. (1996) found high test-retest reliability and internal consistency in a combined sample of psychiatric outpatients and inpatients. In a nonoverlapping clinic sample of school refusers, internal consistency estimates for the anxiety subscale, physiological subscale, and combined total were adequate. Although data specific to children and adolescents with SAD were not available, the validity of the ARC-R was supported. Specifically, the ARC-R related more strongly to anxiety self-report measures than to depression self-report measures and discriminated between children with and without an anxiety disorder. The PARS is a relatively new clinician rating scale that was successfully used as an outcome measure in a recent multicenter pharmacological treatment study of fluvoxamine for children and adolescents with anxiety disorders (Research Units on Pediatric Psychopharmacology [RUPP] Anxiety Study Group, 2001; Rupp, 2002). This 57-item clinician-rating scale had high interrater reliability in an initial study of its psychometric properties (Walkup & Davies, 1999).

Critique of Clinician Rating Scales   Clinician ratings can be useful in obtaining anxiety severity by incorporating the report of the child with the expertise of the clinician. Because these measures yield overall anxiety scores, they are less able to connect severity and impairment with specific anxiety disorders (e.g., SAD) and symptoms (e.g., worries related to harm befalling an attachment figure). However, the ARC-R provides some information about SAD because it has a separation anxiety item. Included in this item are multiple probes that are generally consistent with *DSM* symptoms for SAD (e.g., "When you're not with your folks, are you afraid or worried about something bad happening to them?"). At the present time, data are not available about how this item specifically relates to SAD. Clinician rating scales may best be used in a complementary fashion with other assessment tools. The diagnostic interview would be included to obtain information about the presence or absence of SAD, and in some cases the duration and onset of symptoms. A clinician rating scale can add to the diagnostic picture by quantifying anxiety severity. For example, a treatment study of school refusal in adolescents (Bernstein et al., 2000) used diagnostic interviews and clinician rating scales for anxiety and depression to determine eligibility for study inclusion (i.e., presence of disorders and severity) and clinician rating scales to assess change in symptom severity over time.

Self-Report Measures of Anxiety

There has been much progress in the measurement of self-reported anxiety in children and adolescents, with several measures recently developed and subjected to rigorous psychometric testing. Self-report measures vary in terms of how anxiety is assessed, with some including general questions about anxiety and others including scales related to specific disorders. However, the current direction of scale development appears to be toward the inclusion of scales that assess for *DSM-IV* symptom constellations. In the discussion that follows, we highlight measures that specifically assess for separation anxiety symptoms. Therefore, traditional anxiety self-report measures such as the Revised Children's Manifest Anxiety Scale (RCMAS; Reynolds & Richmond, 1978) and the State-Trait Anxiety Inventory for Children (STAIC; Spielberger, 1973) are not included in the discussion. The Fear Survey Schedule for Children-Revised (FSSC-R; Ollendick, 1983) and Visual Analogue for Anxiety–Revised (VAA-R; Bernstein & Garfinkel, 1992) are also not discussed because they focus primarily on phobic symptoms and school-associated anxiety, respectively. Table 10.1 presents summary information about both newly developed and traditional self-report measures of anxiety.

March, Parker, Sullivan, Stallings, and Conners (1997) originally developed the Multidimensional Anxiety Scale for Children (MASC) due to their concern about the lack of developmentally appropriate and psychometrically sound self-report measures available for assessment of anxiety in children. The MASC has undergone a rigorous developmental process resulting in a measure with generally sound psychometric properties (March et al., 1997; March & Sullivan, 1999). A factor analysis supported a separate nine-item separation anxiety scale, which was labeled as Separation Anxiety/Panic. The separation anxiety scale of the MASC has been found to be reliable as shown by high internal consistency and 3-week test-retest reliability estimates. Convergent and divergent validity analyses with anxiety and depression self-report measures (RCMAS and Children's Depression Inventory [CDI]) have further supported psychometric properties of the MASC and its separation anxiety scale.

The Screen for Child Anxiety Related Emotional Disorders (SCARED), a 41-item scale, was developed by Birmaher et al. (1997) as a child and parent report measure to screen for children with anxiety disorders. A factor analysis with the SCARED yielded an 8-item separation anxiety scale, which was found to have good internal consistency and test-retest reliability (Birmaher et al., 1999; Birmaher et al., 1997). Regarding discriminant validity, the SCARED and its separation anxiety scale successfully discriminated between children with and without anxiety disorders. Furthermore, children with diagnosed SAD had significantly higher scores on the separation anxiety scale than children with other anxiety disorders, supporting the validity of the scale (Birmaher et al., 1999; Birmaher et al., 1997; Monga et al., 2000). A five-item SCARED for epidemiological screening was developed by selecting one item from each of the scales based on results from discriminant function analysis (Birmaher et al., 1999). The item from the separation anxiety scale is "I'm afraid to be alone in the house." A series of reports by Muris and colleagues in the Netherlands is consistent with the previously reported findings (Muris, Merckelbach, Mayer, van Brakel, et al., 1998; Muris, Merckelbach, Schmidt, & Mayer, 1998; Muris, Merckelbach, van Brakel, Mayer, & van Dongen, 1998). In addition, the Dutch researchers found good convergent validity between the SCARED and other anxiety measures, including the MASC.

In a factor analytic study, Spence (1997) examined how individual anxiety symptoms cluster and found several factors that were generally consistent with the *DSM-IV* classification system. Based on data from this study, the Spence Children's Anxiety Scale (SCAS) was developed, and the psychometric properties of the measure were examined (Spence, 1998). The SCAS includes a six-item SAD scale that was supported through factor analysis. Reliability analysis of the scale indicated adequate internal consistency and 6-month test-retest reliability. The SCAS, including the separa-

Table 10.1. Assessment of Separation Anxiety Using Established Self-Report Measures

Measure	Structure of Measure	Age Range*	Assessment of Separation Anxiety and Other Anxiety Symptoms
Child Anxiety Sensitivity Index (CASI) (Silverman, Fleisig, Rabian, & Peterson, 1991)	18 items	6–17	Purpose of the measure is to assess responsivity of children to various symptoms of anxiety (e.g., "It scares me when my heart beats fast"); may have different scales/factors (physical concerns, mental incapacitation concerns).
Multidimensional Anxiety Scale for Children (MASC) (March, Parker, Sullivan, Stallings, & Conners, 1997)	39 items 4 scales, 6 subscales, anxiety disorder index, inconsistency index	8–19	One scale specifically assesses symptoms of separation anxiety; other scales include physical symptoms, harm avoidance, and social anxiety; 10-item version may be useful for epidemiological studies; inconsistency index examines response patterns.
Revised Children's Manifest Anxiety Scale (RCMAS) (Reynolds & Richmond, 1978)	37 items 3 anxiety subscales, lie subscale	6–19	Does not have a specific separation anxiety scale, and relatively few of the items are specifically relevant to separation anxiety; anxiety subscales included are physiological, worry/oversensitivity, and fear/concentration.
Screen for Child Anxiety Related Emotional Disorders (SCARED) (Birmaher et al., 1997)	41 items 5 scales Parent form available	8–18	Includes separate scales assessing separation anxiety and school phobia; other scales address panic/somatic symptoms, generalized anxiety, and social phobia; reduced 5-item version may be useful for epidemiological studies.
Spence Children's Anxiety Scale (SCAS) (Spence, 1997)	44 items (38 symptoms of anxiety, 6 filler items) 6 scales	8–12	Has a separate scale assessing separation anxiety; other scales include social phobia, obsessive compulsive disorder, panic/agoraphobia, generalized anxiety, and fears of physical illness.
State–Trait Anxiety Inventory for Children (STAIC) (Spielberger, 1973)	40 items 2 scales	8–12	Does not include items specific to separation anxiety; items tend to assess overall anxiety level both in the present (state) and in general (trait); symptoms addressed do not directly correspond to *DSM* symptoms of anxiety.
Visual Analogue Scale for Anxiety–Revised (VAA-R) (Bernstein & Garfinkel, 1992)	11 items	8–18	Does not specifically address separation anxiety symptoms; most items address anxiety associated with specific school situations (e.g., riding the school bus, being called on by the teacher).

*Appropriate age ranges were based on reported normative and psychometric data.

tion anxiety scale, related more strongly to an anxiety measure (RCMAS) than to a measure of depression (CDI). Comparisons between clinically anxious children and nonclinical controls further supported the validity of the SCAS.

Critique   Self-report measures are easy to administer, provide valuable data about anxiety symptoms, and are useful in assessing treatment progress. In addition, they require little clinician time, which is an important feature in this age of managed care. However, there have been concerns related to the ability of these anxiety measures to discriminate between diagnostic groups and to be sensitive to developmental issues (Schniering, Hudson, & Rapee, 2000). Furthermore, children may attempt to present themselves in a favorable light by underreporting symptoms of anxiety. Self-report measures may be most valuable as part of an initial multimethod assessment for SAD and to monitor treatment progress. Clinicians and researchers are fortunate to be able to select from several well-developed measures that include appropriate assessments of separation anxiety.

One difference between the SCARED and the other measures is the availability of a parent-report version. The authors of the SCARED recommend the administration of both the parent and child versions due to differences in parent and child reports of internalizing symptoms (Birmaher et al., 1999). The 5-item version of the SCARED and the 10-item MASC may be most useful for epidemiological studies rather than for clinical evaluations.

Deciding on the Assessment Plan

A multimethod, multi-informant assessment should be conducted, both to document the presence of SAD and to rule out other disorders. The child and at least one caregiver should always be part of the assessment process, and whenever possible, all of the important caregivers should be included in assessment. In addition, teachers and school professionals provide important information about the child's functioning within the school setting. At a minimum, the initial assessment for SAD should include a clinical interview, self-report measures, and parent report measures. Clinician rating scales may provide additional information about overall severity of anxiety. As can be seen from the previous review, many reliable and valid assessment tools are available.

To diagnose SAD while ruling out other disorders, a thorough clinical interview should be conducted. According to practice parameters from the American Academy of Child and Adolescent Psychiatry, or AACAP (1997), information should be obtained from several areas: (a) developmental, psychiatric, medical, school, social, and family history; (b) mental status of the child; (c) current academic functioning; and (d) current medical status (i.e., to rule out physical conditions that mimic SAD). Because of the high rates of comorbidity between SAD and other disorders, a thorough interview should explore other anxiety (e.g., generalized anxiety disorder, phobic disorders, panic disorder) and other mental disorders (e.g., mood disorders, attention-deficit/hyperactivity disorder). Structured, semistructured, and pictorial clinical interviews can standardize the assessment of symptoms and are therefore well suited for research protocols.

Self-report measures often provide good insight into the child's perception of his or her symptoms. An anxiety measure should be included in the assessment as well as other relevant self-report measures (e.g., depression). As with all self-report measures, the clinician must be aware of the potential for the child to underreport symptoms. In terms of anxiety self-report measures, the MASC, SCARED, and SCAS are the most promising because they include specific SAD scales. These measures can also be readministered during and following treatment to assess for change in symptoms.

Although not reviewed in this chapter, parent and teacher report measures such as the Child Behavior Checklist (CBCL; Achenbach, 1991a), Behavior Assessment System for Children (BASC; Reynolds & Kamphaus, 1992), and Teacher Report Form (TRF; Achenbach, 1991b), should be included in the assessment phase. If more than one parent or guardian is available, measures should be completed separately to provide a picture of how the child's symptoms are perceived by both parents or guardians. Teachers offer a unique perspective related to the manifestation of SAD symptoms in the school setting and can provide valuable information about the child's functioning in school, especially related to interference due to SAD symptomatology. In a relatively recent study of preadolescent children, teachers were more likely than parents to observe internalizing and social problems in children with self-reported anxiety (Mesman & Koot, 2000). According to the authors, teachers are in the position to observe certain indicators of internalizing problems (e.g., poor social skills) and are able to compare a child's behavior with that of children in an appropriate peer group.

Throughout the assessment, observations of the behavior of the child and his or her parents can provide useful clinical information relevant to separation issues. Separations from parents should be observed both for the child's reactions (e.g., ease of separating) and the parents' reactions (e.g., reinforcement of SAD behaviors). Other observations of the child may include, but are not limited to, the following: (a) nervous, edgy behavior; (b) clinging behavior (e.g., sitting very close to the parent); (c) need for reassurance from the parent or clinician; (d) initial and later interactions with the clinician; and (e) somatic complaints or behaviors (e.g., complaining of stomachache or clutching stomach).

A routine pediatric examination is also a good idea. This frequently serves to rule out organic etiologies of anxiety (e.g., excessive caffeine use, substance use, hyperthyroidism). Extensive workups are generally not warranted unless specific physical symptoms such as focal neurological signs or thyromegaly (enlarged thyroid gland) are present. If the workup is negative, parents can be informed that the somatic symptoms are likely a manifestation of underlying anxiety, depression, or both. Somatic symptoms,

especially gastrointestinal and autonomic, are common in anxious and depressed youth (Bernstein et al., 1997).

TREATMENT OF SEPARATION ANXIETY DISORDER

Since the mid-1990s, there have been significant advances in the area of
treatment for anxiety disorders in children. Many treatment studies have
been published; however, we have chosen to focus on those that have strong
research methodology and are most relevant to SAD. Summaries of type of
treatment, participants, design, and outcome information from psychosocial and pharmacological treatment studies are presented in Tables 10.2 and
10.3, respectively. Given the frequent comorbidity between the anxiety disorders, it is not surprising that our review of the existing treatment studies
did not yield any studies with a pure separation anxiety sample (i.e., presence of SAD and absence of any other anxiety disorders). In fact, there was
much variability in the percentage of children with SAD included in treatment studies.

In the next sections, we discuss findings from psychosocial, psychopharmacology, and combination treatment studies. Our discussion focuses
on studies that had enough participants for statistical analyses (i.e., we excluded case studies), included at least two different conditions, and had a
substantial proportion of participants with SAD (> 30%). Of the psychosocial treatment studies reviewed and presented in Table 10.2, five had samples
with at least 30% of children diagnosed with SAD. Following a discussion
of the psychosocial studies, psychopharmacology and combination treatment studies are reviewed.

Psychosocial Treatment Studies

As can be seen in Table 10.2, cognitive-behavioral therapy (CBT) was the
most frequently used treatment in psychosocial studies. Specific treatments
examined in these studies included individual CBT (Barrett, Dadds, &
Rapee, 1996; Flannery-Schroeder & Kendall, 2000; Kendall, 1994;
Kendall et al., 1997; King et al., 1998; Last, Hansen, & Franco, 1998),
CBT plus family management (Barrett, 1998; Barrett et al., 1996), group
CBT (Barrett, 1998; Flannery-Schroeder & Kendall, 2000; Mendlowitz
et al., 1999), and educational-support therapy (Last et al., 1998). In addition to incorporating a wait-list control group, several of these studies compared the efficacy of different types of treatments. As previously mentioned,
this chapter describes in more detail those studies that had a substantial proportion of children diagnosed with SAD.

The Australian research group of Barrett and colleagues (1996) examined individual CBT alone and in combination with family management and wait-list control. The 12-session individual CBT used the *Coping
Koala Workbook* (Barrett, Dadds, & Rapee, 1991), which is the Australian adaptation of the *Coping Cat Workbook* designed by Kendall (1990).

This workbook included components related to recognizing anxiety symptoms, cognitive restructuring of anxiety-producing situations, coping self-statements, exposure, performance evaluation, and administering self-reinforcement. The weekly family management, which followed the individual CBT session, was aimed at teaching parents skills in behavioral management strategies, management of their own anxiety, and communication and problem-solving skills. It is notable that therapist contact time was matched for both conditions, with the CBT condition sessions lasting 60 to 80 minutes and the combined condition being split between CBT (30 minutes) and family management (40 minutes). There was a significant difference in outcome between the two active treatment conditions, with 57% of children receiving CBT alone not meeting diagnostic criteria for anxiety disorder and 84% of children receiving CBT plus family management being diagnosis-free. At 6-month and 12-month follow-ups, the proportion of children who were free of anxiety disorders increased for both groups (70% for CBT and 96% for CBT plus family management). Improvements in clinical evaluation scales, self-report measures of anxiety, and parent reports of internalizing symptoms were found for both groups, with some evidence for the added benefit of the combined treatment (CBT plus family management). Regarding diagnostic groups, the authors noted that the success of both treatments and the greater improvements associated with family management applied equally to the specific anxiety groups (SAD, overanxious disorder, and social phobia). Treatment condition, however, interacted with age and gender, with girls and younger children having a better outcome with CBT plus family management.

Building on the previously described treatment study, Barrett (1998) examined the efficacy of group CBT alone and in combination with group family management by using session content similar to that used in the earlier Barrett et al. (1996) study. Both treatment conditions showed significant improvements in anxiety according to self-reports, clinician evaluations, and parent reports, compared with the wait-list control group. In addition, nearly two thirds of the children in active treatment were anxiety-diagnosis free, compared with 25% of the wait-list control children. Improvements were maintained at 12-month follow-up, with 65% of the group CBT children and 85% of the group CBT-plus-family-management children no longer meeting diagnostic criteria. Although both treatment conditions were efficacious, results suggested that there were some added benefits from the family management treatment component.

The efficacies of CBT and educational-support therapy (an attention-placebo control) for anxious children with school phobia were compared in a treatment study conducted by Last et al. (1998). The 12-session CBT treatment focused on graduated in-vivo exposure to anxiety-producing stimuli (i.e., returning to school) and teaching of coping self-statements. Educational-support therapy is aimed at encouraging children to discuss their fears and to learn about fears, anxiety, and phobias. There is no exposure component to this therapy. To accomplish this, educational materials

Table 10.2. Psychosocial Treatment Studies for Children With Anxiety Disorders, Including Separation Anxiety Disorder

Treatments	Participants and Design	Outcome
Individual CBT 16 sessions (Kendall, 1994; Kendall & Southam-Gerow, 1996)	9- to 13-year-olds ($N = 47$) 17% had SAD Randomly assigned to CBT or WLC	Self-reported anxiety (RCMAS and STAIC), depression (CDI), anxious self-talk (NASSQ), and management of anxiety-producing situations improved with treatment; parent-reported internalizing symptoms (CBCL) decreased with treatment; improvements maintained over follow-up (average 3.4 years).
Individual CBT Individual CBT+FAM 12 sessions (Barrett, Dadds, & Rapee, 1996)	7- to 14-year-olds ($N = 79$) 38% had SAD Randomly assigned to CBT, CBT+FAM, or WLC	Most children in both treatment groups no longer met diagnostic criteria by the end of treatment and at follow-up; both treatment groups showed decreased anxiety (FSSC-R and RCMAS) and internalizing symptoms (CBCL); CBT+FAM children generally showed the most improvement.
Cognitive-behavioral family-based group intervention 10 sessions (Dadds et al., 1999; Dadds, Spence, Holland, Barrett, & Laurens, 1997)	7- to 14-year-olds ($N = 128$) > 5% had SAD or SAD features Randomly assigned to intervention or monitoring group	Results from this early intervention and prevention study indicated that both groups showed improvements immediately following the intervention; change was only maintained by the intervention group.
Individual CBT 16–20 sessions (Kendall et al., 1997)	9- to 13-year-olds ($N = 94$) 23% had SAD Randomly assigned to CBT or WLC	Anxiety (RCMAS), negative affectivity self-statements (NASSQ), and coping-with-anxiety situations improved after treatment; anxiety based on parent report (CBCL) improved with treatment; treatment gains were generally maintained over 1-year follow-up.
Group CBT Group CBT+FAM 12 sessions (Barrett, 1998)	7- to 14-year-olds ($N = 60$) 43% had SAD Randomly assigned to group CBT, group CBT+FAM, or WLC	Nearly 65% of actively treated children no longer met criteria for an anxiety disorder, compared with 25% of WLC children; self-reported anxiety (FSSC) and clinician-rated anxiety improved in treated groups; marginal benefits were found from the use of combination treatment, compared with CBT alone; gains were generally maintained (12-month follow-up).
Individual CBT Individual CBT+PAM 10–14 sessions (Cobham, Dadds, & Spence, 1998)	7- to 14-year olds ($N = 67$) 12% had SAD Divided by parental anxiety level, then randomly assigned to treatment condition	Children in all conditions had less self-reported anxiety (RCMAS and STAIC) and fewer parent-reported internalizing symptoms; changes were generally maintained at follow-up; children with and without an anxious parent responded differentially to the treatments (CBT vs. CBT+PAM).

Individual CBT plus parent/teacher training 4-week program (6 sessions) (King et al., 1998)	5- to 15-year-olds ($N = 34$) 24% had SAD with SR Randomly assigned to CBT or WLC	Greater improvements for CBT children, compared with WLC children, were found for anxiety (RCMAS and FSSC-II), depression (CDI), school attendance, perceived ability to manage anxiety-producing school situations, and parent and teacher reported internalizing symptoms, and clinician rating of functioning (GAF).
Individual CBT Educational-support therapy 12 sessions (Last, Hansen, & Franco, 1998)	6- to 17-year-olds ($N = 56$) 32% had SAD with SR Randomly assigned to CBT or educational-support therapy	Both the CBT and educational-support therapy groups improved on self-reported anxiety (FSSC-R and STAIC) and school attendance; CBT children had greater reduction in depression (CDI); attendance treatment gains were maintained over a 4-week follow-up period for both groups.
Parent and child—group CBT Child—group CBT Parent—group CBT 12 sessions (Mendlowitz et al., 1999)	7- to 12-year-olds ($N = 62$) ~33% had SAD Randomly assigned to one of the three treatments	Self-reported anxiety (RCMAS) and depression (CDI) for all 3 groups decreased following treatment; children's adaptive coping strategies (i.e., active coping) improved significantly only in the parent-child condition; parent ratings of child improvement were highest in the parent-child condition posttreatment.
Parent-child group therapy 10 sessions (Toren, Wolmer, et al., 2000)	6- to 13-year-olds ($N = 24$) 52% had SAD 44% had SAD and OAD No control group	Anxiety based on a self-report measure (RCMAS) decreased significantly by end of treatment; most children (70%) did not meet criteria for an anxiety disorder posttreatment; anxiety and depressive (CDI) symptoms further decreased at 1-year follow-up.
Individual CBT Group CBT 18 sessions (Flannery-Schroeder & Kendall, 2000)	8- to 14-year-olds ($N = 25$) 44% had SAD Randomly assigned to individual CBT, group CBT, or WLC	Self- and parent-reported trait anxiety (STAIC) and coping improved by the end of treatment; 73% of children in the individual-CBT condition and 50% in the group-CBT condition did not meet criteria for their primary anxiety diagnosis posttreatment (compared with 8% of WLC children).

Note. CBCL = Child Behavior Checklist; CBT = cognitive-behavioral therapy; CDI = Children's Depression Inventory; FAM = family management; FSSC = Fear Survey Schedule for Children; GAF = Global Assessment of Functioning; OAD = overanxious disorder; PAM = parental anxiety management; RCMAS = Revised Children's Manifest Anxiety Scale; SAD = separation anxiety disorder; SR = school refusal; STAIC = State-Trait Anxiety Inventory for Children; WLC = wait-list control

Table 10.3. Psychopharmacology Treatment Studies for Children With Anxiety Disorders, Including Separation Anxiety Disorder

Active Treatment	Participants and Design	Outcome
Imipramine 6 weeks of medication (Gittelman-Klein & Klein, 1971)	6- to 14-year-olds (N = 35) Majority had separation anxiety Randomized DBPC	Clinicians, mothers, and children reported greater overall improvement for the imipramine group, compared with the placebo group; clinician ratings of symptoms indicated more improvement in the imipramine group; more children in the imipramine group attended school by the end of treatment.
Imipramine Alprazolam 8 weeks of medication (Bernstein, Garfinkel, & Borchardt, 1990)	7- to 17-year-olds (N = 24) with school refusal 58% had SAD or OAD Randomized DBPC	Although the active medication groups had more improvement in clinician-rated anxiety (ARC-R), no significant differences between the groups were found for self-reported or clinician-rated anxiety (ARC-R and RCMAS) or depression (CDI, CDRS-R, CDS), when baseline scores were covaried.
Imipramine 6 weeks of medication (Klein, Koplewicz, & Kanner, 1992)	6- to 15-year-olds (N = 20) All had SAD Randomized DBPC	Global improvement was noted for half the children; no significant improvements based on self-report (RCMAS), clinician report, or parent report (Conners Parent Questionnaire) for either condition; children in the imipramine group reported more side effects than the placebo group.
Fluoxetine Up to 10 months of medication (Birmaher et al., 1994)	11- to 17-year-olds (N = 21) 71% had SAD Open-label trial	Based on clinician ratings (CGI), 95% of children showed some improvement in anxiety, with most having moderate to marked improvement in anxiety (81%); severity of anxiety decreased according to clinician ratings; improvements were generally noted after 6 to 8 weeks of treatment.
Buspirone 4 weeks of medication plus psychotherapy (Simeon et al., 1994)	4- to 14-year-olds (N = 15) 73% had SAD 2-week placebo phase followed by an open-label trial	Decreases in anxiety symptoms over the course of treatment were noted on self-report (RCMAS) and parent-report (CPRS) measures; clinician rating scales (BPRS-C and ARC-R) indicated steady improvement in anxiety and depression; global clinical severity (CGI) decreased by the end of treatment.

Treatment	Sample	Findings
Clonazepam 4 weeks of medication (Graae, Milner, Rizzotto, & Klein, 1994)	7- to 13-year-olds ($N = 12$) 92% had SAD Double-blind crossover design	50% of the children did not meet diagnostic criteria for an anxiety disorder by the end of the study; although most children showed at least some clinical improvement, no statistically significant improvements were found, according to both clinician ratings (CGI) and self-report (BPRS-C).
Fluoxetine 9 weeks of medication (Fairbanks et al., 1997)	9- to 18-year-olds ($N = 16$) 63% had SAD Open-label trial	Global ratings (CGI) indicated improvement in all children at treatment end point, with 60% of SAD children rated as much improved by the end of treatment and 40% viewed as improved; overall impairment (CGAS) decreased by the end of treatment.
Imipramine 8 weeks of imipramine or placebo, both in combination with CBT (Bernstein et al., 2000)	12–18-year-olds ($N = 47$) 33% had SAD Randomized DBPC	Clinician-rated and self-reported anxiety (ARC-R and RCMAS) and depression (CDRS-R and BDI) improved for both groups; clinician-rated depression improved faster in the imipramine plus CBT group; greater and faster improvement in attendance was found for the imipramine plus CBT group, compared with the placebo plus CBT group
Fluvoxamine 8 weeks of medication or placebo, in combination with supportive psychotherapy (Research Unit on Pediatric Psychopharmacology [RUPP] Anxiety Study Group, 2001)	6–17-year-olds ($N = 128$) 59% had SAD Randomized DBPC	Children in the fluvoxamine group had the greatest improvement in clinician-rated anxiety symptoms (PARS); more children in the active treatment group had a positive response to treatment (76%), compared with the placebo group (29%), on global ratings (CGI).

Note. ARC-R = Anxiety Rating for Children–Revised; BDI = Beck Depression Inventory; BPRS-C = Brief Psychiatric Rating Scale for Children; CDI = Children's Depression Inventory; CDRS-R = Children's Depression Rating Scale–Revised; CDS = Children's Depression Scale; CGAS = Children's Global Assessment Scale; CGI = Clinician Global Impressions; CPRS = Conners Parent Rating Scale; DBPC = double-blind placebo controlled; PARS = Pediatric Anxiety Rating Scale.

are presented to the children, and they are given supportive psychotherapy without any specific encouragement or instructions to manage behavioral avoidance of school and anxious thoughts. The researchers found that children in both the CBT and educational-support treatments reported decreased symptoms of anxiety by the end of treatment. Both groups significantly increased their school attendance over the course of treatment, but there were no significant differences between the groups. Later analyses found that, compared with children with other anxiety diagnoses, children with a primary diagnosis of SAD showed more improvement in school attendance by the end of the study, with no differences between the treatment conditions (C. G. Last & C. Hansen, personal communication, October 2000).

Mendlowitz et al. (1999) examined the role of parental involvement in CBT treatment of anxiety disorders by using a 12-session group therapy format. Parent-child dyads were randomly assigned to one of three treatment conditions including parent and child intervention, child-only intervention, and parent-only intervention. The *Coping Bear Workbook* (Scapillato & Mendlowitz, 1993), an adaptation of Kendall's (1990) *Coping Cat Workbook*, was used for the 12-session child treatment program and focused on identification of anxiety symptoms, relaxation training, use of coping self-statements, and self-reinforcement of coping efforts. The parent groups were primarily psychoeducational in nature, focusing on understanding of anxiety, effects of parent anxiety on children, and how to manage an anxious child. Findings showed a decrease in anxiety and depressive symptoms for all treatment groups. Children in the parent-child intervention group used more active coping strategies by the end of treatment and were viewed as more improved overall, according to parent reports. Consistent with findings from the studies conducted by Barrett (1998) and colleagues (Barrett et al., 1996), there appears to be additional benefit from parental involvement in the treatment of childhood anxiety.

Group CBT was also examined in a study conducted by Flannery-Schroeder and Kendall (2000). In this investigation, group CBT and individual CBT were compared with wait-list control in a sample of children 8 to 14 years of age. The 18-week treatment protocol was based on the *Coping Cat Workbook* (Kendall, 1990). At the end of treatment, significantly more children who received individual CBT and group CBT did not meet criteria for their original anxiety disorder (73% and 50%, respectively), compared with wait-list control children (8%). Relative to children in the wait-list condition, those in both CBT conditions experienced greater improvements in self- and parent-reported anxiety and coping. In general, there were no significant differences in improvement between the two treatment groups related to anxious symptomatology or coping.

Overall, the psychosocial treatment studies support the efficacy of CBT for children with anxiety and indicate that there is some additional benefit to including a parental treatment component. In addition, providing therapy in a group format appears to be efficacious and economically advantageous. None of the studies included only youth with SAD, but there is support for the treatment of this disorder using CBT either alone or in combination with a family component (family management, psychoeducation, or both). It should be noted that the majority of treatment studies focused primarily on children and included relatively few adolescents, indicating that future research should examine the efficacy of these treatments with adolescents. Other issues of importance include determining (a) how to best transport empirically validated treatments into community and clinic settings (e.g., training practitioners to deliver empirically-validated treatments); (b) the effectiveness of psychotherapy in cases with coexisting disorders (e.g., comorbid anxiety and depression or comorbid anxiety and attention deficit hyperactivity disorder), complex symptomatology, or both; (c) the components of treatment that are most critical to effect change; (d) the optimal duration of psychotherapy treatment; (e) the added benefit from booster sessions; and (f) the effectiveness of combined treatment modalities (e.g., CBT and medication).

Pharmacotherapy Treatment Studies

Of the nine studies reviewed and described in Table 10.3, the majority contained a substantial proportion of children with SAD. Although open-label and crossover medication studies provide useful information, our discussion focuses on those studies that incorporated double-blind placebo-controlled design. One double-blind placebo-controlled study (Berney et al., 1981) was not included in the table, because the children were described as having school phobia/school refusal without specific diagnoses being provided. (For a more comprehensive review of medication treatment for pediatric anxiety disorders, see Bernstein & Perwien, 1995; Leonard, March, Rickler, & Allen, 1997; Riddle et al., 1999; Velosa & Riddle, 2000.)

Although an initial study with children who had school phobia suggested that imipramine was an efficacious treatment for separation anxiety (Gittelman-Klein & Klein, 1971; Gittelman-Klein & Klein, 1973), a later study by Klein, Koplewicz, and Kanner (1992) did not replicate these findings. In the 1992 study by Klein et al., children with SAD who had not improved following a 4-week behavioral therapy treatment were randomly assigned to either an imipramine or placebo condition (6 weeks of treatment). Although improvement was found in half of the children, there were no group differences based on self-report measures, parent report measures, clinician ratings, or teacher ratings. Furthermore, children with imipramine reported significantly more side effects than those treated with placebo, including behavioral disinhibition in several cases.

Bernstein, Garfinkel, and Borchardt (1990) compared the efficacy of imipramine and alprazolam for the treatment of anxiety in a small sample of school refusers, using a double-blind placebo-controlled design. When controlling for baseline differences in self-reported and clinician-rated anxiety and depression, no significant differences between the treatment and placebo groups were found. In addition, attendance improvements were noted across conditions for the great majority of children in the study. Although more side effects were found in the active medication groups, none of the participants reported any interference from these effects, which were generally reported as being mild.

A study by Bernstein et al. (2000) examined the efficacy of imipramine in combination with CBT for the treatment of coexisting anxiety and major depressive disorders in school-refusing adolescents. The adolescents were randomly assigned to 8 weeks of either imipramine or placebo, each administered in combination with CBT. The CBT was adapted from a 13-session school-refusal treatment protocol developed and used in a psychosocial treatment study that compared CBT and educational support for school refusal (Last et al., 1998). The CBT had several components, including psychoeducation, development of a gradual school reentry plan, identification of anxious thoughts, teaching of coping self-statements, and behavioral contracting. School attendance improved significantly for the imipramine-plus-CBT group but not for the placebo-plus-CBT group; moreover, the imipramine-plus-CBT group improved at a faster rate. At the end of 8 weeks of treatment, the imipramine group was attending school 70% of the time, compared with school attendance 28% of the time for the placebo group. Self-reported and clinician-rated symptoms of anxiety and depression improved for both groups. The only differential effect on anxiety or depression was in the rate of clinician-rated depressive symptoms, which improved faster in the imipramine group than the placebo group.

In open-label studies, selective serotonin reuptake inhibitors (SSRIs) have also been successfully used (Birmaher et al., 1994; Fairbanks et al., 1997), suggesting that this medication class may be a promising treatment for SAD. A study conducted by the RUPP Anxiety Study Group (2001) used a relatively large sample of children and adolescents with SAD, generalized anxiety disorder, social phobia, or more than one of these diagnoses, to examine the efficacy of fluvoxamine by using a double-blind, placebo-controlled design. Of the 128 children participating in the study, 59% had SAD. Prior to the medication trial, children and their families participated in 3 weeks of supportive, psychoeducational therapy. Only those children who were able to attend weekly appointments and continued to have significant symptomatology were randomly assigned to either receive fluvoxamine or placebo. Both were given in combination with supportive psychotherapy. Results indicated that the fluvoxamine group had a greater reduction in clinician-rated anxiety symptoms than the placebo group. In addition, fluvoxamine was generally well tolerated, with the exception of increased abdominal discomfort and greater motor activity level compared with the placebo group. Overall, this study suggests that fluvoxamine is an efficacious treatment for children and adolescents with anxiety disorders, including SAD.

The psychosocial treatment studies have clearly documented the efficacy of CBT in children with anxiety disorders. Although there have been some inconsistent findings from earlier pharmacotherapy studies, recent studies that employed strong methodological designs show that medication may be beneficial in improving anxiety symptoms (RUPP Anxiety Study Group, 2001) and associated symptoms, such as school attendance difficulties and symptoms of depression (Bernstein et al., 2000). Despite the suggestion that medication may improve attendance and internalizing symptoms, only one study (Bernstein et al., 2000) directly compared CBT plus placebo with CBT plus medication. Further studies are needed to answer several important issues about pharmacotherapy in the treatment of childhood anxiety disorders, including (a) whether medications provide additional benefit to psychosocial treatment, (b) whether there are certain characteristics that more clearly benefit from the use of medication (e.g., anxiety co-occurring with depression), (c) the optimal time frame for adding medication to the treatment plan (i.e., whether medication should be used with CBT immediately or added only when CBT alone is not effective), and (d) the optimal duration of pharmacotherapy.

Deciding on the Treatment Plan

When treating a child or adolescent with SAD, the "treatment plan is formulated from the diagnostic evaluation and assessment of impairment. Short-term, intermittent, or long-term treatment and follow-up may be required" (AACAP, 1997, p. 79S). Strong consideration should be given to a multimodal treatment plan (AACAP, 1997). This may consist of education for the parents and child about SAD, consultation (e.g., with school staff or primary care physician), CBT, family interventions (e.g., parent training, family therapy), and medication.

Consultation with school staff may consist of recommending a support person at the school for the child to talk to if he or she becomes extremely anxious about separation; gradual school reentry (exposure) if school refusal is one of the presenting symptoms; limiting visits to the school nurse; and limiting calls home to check on the safety of parents. The school nurse should receive guidance about returning children to the classroom following minor physical complaints. The pediatrician, family practitioner, or nurse practitioner may be advised to avoid writing medical excuses for separation-anxious children to stay home from school for minor physical symptoms. Generally, we recommend that a temperature greater than 100.6 is needed to allow a child to stay home from school.

As discussed in this chapter, a number of well-designed, well-controlled studies support the efficacy of CBT in the treatment of SAD. Both individual (Barrett et al., 1996; Flannery-Schroeder & Kendall, 2000) and group CBT (Flannery-Schroeder & Kendall, 2000; Mendlowitz et al., 1999) are efficacious. Follow-up studies for periods up to 3.5 years demonstrate that benefits from CBT can be lasting (Kendall & Southam-Gerow, 1996). Studies suggest that the addition of a parent or family component to CBT confers additional benefits for the anxious child (Barrett, 1998; Barrett et al., 1996). Therefore, the first step in treatment of SAD is usually individual or group CBT, sometimes with a family or parent training intervention as well. In cases in which a child or adolescent has severe anxiety symptoms, a high level of impairment, or both, a combination of CBT and antianxiety medication may be considered as the initial treatment.

If initial treatment with CBT alone produces only a partial remission of separation-anxiety symptoms, the addition of anxiolytic medication may be beneficial. The first choice is an SSRI, as supported by a multicenter treatment study demonstrating that fluvoxamine is efficacious in the treatment of children and adolescents with anxiety disorders (RUPP Anxiety Study Group, 2001). Overall, the SSRIs are well tolerated, with stomachaches and motor activation occurring more commonly in children receiving fluvoxamine than in those receiving placebo (RUPP Anxiety Study Group, 2001). A second-line medication option is a tricyclic antidepressant (TCA), which has more side effects than an SSRI and requires electrocardiogram and blood-level monitoring. Benzodiazepines can be used on a short-term basis, alone or in combination with an SSRI or TCA while the SSRI or TCA is being titrated to the therapeutic dosage. Although the issue has not yet been studied sufficiently (Velosa & Riddle, 2000), there is the theoretical possibility of dependence in children with benzodiazepines (Riddle et al., 1999). Benzodiazepines should be avoided in youths with a history of drug dependence.

Youth with SAD who do not have remission of symptoms following an optimum course of CBT—and after at least two medication trials of adequate dosage and length, and combinations of medications, as indicated—would be described as treatment resistant (March & Ollendick, chapter 6, this volume). At present, only a small amount of data exists to support medication trials other than SSRIs, TCAs, or benzodiazepines in the treatment of SAD. A few studies support psychosocial trials other than CBT (e.g., Heinicke & Ramsey-Klee, 1986; Target & Fonagy, 1994).

After remission of symptoms, a decision should be made regarding how long to continue treatment. Risks associated with continuation of treatment (e.g., medication side effects) versus risks associated with discontinuation (e.g., relapse of symptoms) need to be taken into consideration. Further research is needed to guide the clinician regarding the duration of acute treatment with CBT, pharmacotherapy, or both and the benefit of CBT booster sessions. When there is a good response to SSRIs or TCAs, pharmacotherapy is usually continued for a number of months, with consideration of tapering at the end of the school year.

Several of the anxiety rating scales described earlier have been shown to be useful in monitoring responses to treatment. For example, the PARS was sensitive to change with treatment in the multicenter fluvoxamine study (RUPP Anxiety Study Group, 2001). Rating scales can be obtained before initiating an intervention and after a trial of CBT, medication, or both to document response to treatment.

Additional research is needed to compare CBT-only, drug-only, and combined treatments. Studies to identify predictors of positive response are warranted. For example, the study by Barrett et al. (1996) indicates that younger children and girls show the most benefit from adding family intervention to CBT for anxious children.

In refractory cases, it is necessary to assess whether there may be confounding variables or extenuating circumstances that are contributing to nonresponse to treatment. Adherence to treatment should be evaluated. Lack of compliance with taking medications or poor attendance and lack of participation in CBT sessions may explain treatment nonresponse. Cultural acceptability of the treatment approaches should also be considered. Family stressors and family dynamics can contribute to poor response to treatment. Some of the factors that may impede treatment success are change in family structure (e.g., separation/divorce), illness of family member(s), poverty, and change of residence.

It is also important to consider whether comorbid disorders may be present that were not initially identified. Comorbid conditions may require an additional form of treatment. Furthermore, antianxiety medications can exacerbate comorbid disorders (e.g., motor activation from SSRIs may serve to increase hyperactivity in a child with attention-deficit/hyperactivity disorder). To avoid relapse in a child who is in remission, both pharmacologic and behavioral treatments should be tapered before discontinuation. The dosage of medication needs to be gradually tapered while the child is observed for reappearance of anxiety symptoms. Similarly, the period of time between CBT sessions or booster sessions can be gradually increased before CBT treatment is terminated, as anxiety symptoms are carefully monitored.

SUMMARY

SAD is one of the most common anxiety disorders in preadolescents. It is important to assess a child or adolescent with SAD from a developmental perspective, using a multi-informant and multimethod approach. There is solid evidence to support the efficacy of individual CBT and of group CBT in the treatment of youth with anxiety disorders, including SAD. Open-label studies and a recent multicenter controlled study support the benefit of SSRIs for anxious children, including those with SAD. It is suggested that future investigations focus on this subset of anxious youth to identify the specific interventions that are efficacious in targeting SAD. Other areas of exploration are highlighted in the chapter.

NOTE

This work was supported in part by a training grant from the National Institutes of Health (T32 HD07524).

REFERENCES

Achenbach, T. M. (1991a). *Manual for the Child Behavior Checklist: 4–18 and 1991 profile*. Burlington: University of Vermont Department of Psychiatry.

Achenbach, T. M. (1991b). *Manual for the Teacher's Report Form and 1991 Profile*. Burlington: University of Vermont Department of Psychiatry.

Ambrosini, P. J. (2000). Historical development and present status of the schedule for affective disorders and schizophrenia for school-age children (K-SADS). *Journal of the American Academy of Child and Adolescent Psychiatry, 39*(1), 49–58.

American Academy of Child and Adolescent Psychiatry. (1997). Practice parameters for the assessment and treatment of children and adolescents with anxiety disorders. *Journal of the American Academy of Child and Adolescent Psychiatry, 36*(Suppl. 10), 69S–84S.

American Psychiatric Association. (1980). *Diagnostic and statistical manual of mental disorders* (3rd ed.). Washington, DC: Author.

American Psychiatric Association. (1987). *Diagnostic and statistical manual of mental disorders: DSM-III-R* (3rd ed., rev.). Washington, DC: Author.

American Psychiatric Association. (1994). *Diagnostic and statistical manual of mental disorders: DSM-IV* (4th ed.). Washington, DC: Author.

Anderson, J. C., Williams, S., McGee, R., & Silva, P. A. (1987). *DSM-III* disorders in preadolescent children: Prevalence in a large sample from the general population. *Archives of General Psychiatry, 44*(1), 69–76.

Angold, A., & Costello, E. J. (1995). A test-retest reliability study of child-reported psychiatric symptoms and diagnoses using the Child and Adolescent Psychiatric Assessment (CAPA-C). *Psychological Medicine, 25*(4), 755–762.

Angold, A., & Costello, E. J. (2000). The Child and Adolescent Psychiatric Assessment (CAPA). *Journal of the American Academy of Child and Adolescent Psychiatry, 39*(1), 39–48.

Angold, A., Costello, E. J., Farmer, E. M., Burns, B. J., & Erkanli, A. (1999). Impaired but undiagnosed. *Journal of the American Academy of Child and Adolescent Psychiatry, 38*(2), 129–137.

Barrett, P. M. (1998). Evaluation of cognitive-behavioral group treatments for childhood anxiety disorders. *Journal of Clinical Child Psychology, 27*(4), 459–468.

Barrett, P. M., Dadds, M. R. & Rapee, R. M. (1991). *Coping koala workbook*. Unpublished manuscript. Nathan, Australia: Griffith University School of Applied Psychology.

Barrett, P. M., Dadds, M. R., & Rapee, R. M. (1996). Family treatment of childhood anxiety: A controlled trial. *Journal of Consulting and Clinical Psychology, 64*(2), 333–342.

Battaglia, M., Bertella, S., Politi, E., Bernardeschi, L., Perna, G., Gabriele, A., & Bellodi, L. (1995). Age at onset of panic disorder: influence of familial liability to the disease and of childhood separation anxiety disorder. *American Journal of Psychiatry, 152*(9), 1362–1364.

Bell-Dolan, D. J., Last, C. G., & Strauss, C. C. (1990). Symptoms of anxiety disorders in normal children. *Journal of the American Academy of Child and Adolescent Psychiatry, 29*(5), 759–765.

Benjamin, R. S., Costello, E. J., & Warren, M. (1990). Anxiety disorders in a pediatric sample. *Journal of Anxiety Disorders, 4,* 293–316.

Berney, T., Kolvin, I., Bhate, S. R., Garside, R. F., Jeans, J., Kay, B., & Scarth, L. (1981). School phobia: A therapeutic trial with clomipramine and short-term outcome. *British Journal of Psychiatry, 138,* 110–118.

Bernstein, G. A., Borchardt, C. M., Perwien, A. R., Crosby, R. D., Kushner, M. G., Thuras, P. D., & Last, C. G. (2000). Imipramine plus cognitive-behavioral therapy in the treatment of school refusal. *Journal of the American Academy of Child and Adolescent Psychiatry, 39*(3), 276–283.

Bernstein, G. A., Crosby, R. D., Perwien, A. R., & Borchardt, C. M. (1996). Anxiety Rating for Children-Revised: Reliability and validity. *Journal of Anxiety Disorders, 10*(2), 97–114.

Bernstein, G. A., & Garfinkel, B. D. (1992). The Visual Analogue Scale for Anxiety–Revised: Psychometric properties. *Journal of Anxiety Disorders, 6*(3), 223–239.

Bernstein, G. A., Garfinkel, B. D., & Borchardt, C. M. (1990). Comparative studies of pharmacotherapy for school refusal. *Journal of the American Academy of Child and Adolescent Psychiatry, 29*(5), 773–781.

Bernstein, G. A., Massie, E. D., Thuras, P. D., Perwien, A. R., Borchardt, C. M., & Crosby, R. D. (1997). Somatic symptoms in anxious-depressed school refusers. *Journal of the American Academy of Child and Adolescent Psychiatry, 36*(5), 661–668.

Bernstein, G. A., & Perwien, A. R. (1995). Anxiety disorders. *Child and Adolescent Psychiatric Clinics of North America, 4*(2), 305–322.

Bidaut-Russell, M., Valla, J. P., Thomas, J. M., Bergeron, L., & Lawson, E. (1998). Reliability of the Terry: A mental health cartoon-like screener for African-American children. *Child Psychiatry and Human Development, 28*(4), 249–263.

Birmaher, B., Brent, D. A., Chiappetta, L., Bridge, J., Monga, S., & Baugher, M. (1999). Psychometric properties of the Screen for Child Anxiety Related Emotional Disorders (SCARED): A replication study. *Journal of the American Academy of Child and Adolescent Psychiatry, 38*(10), 1230–1236.

Birmaher, B., Khetarpal, S., Brent, D., Cully, M., Balach, L., Kaufman, J., & Neer, S. M. (1997). The Screen for Child Anxiety Related Emotional Disorders (SCARED): Scale construction and psychometric characteristics. *Journal of the American Academy of Child and Adolescent Psychiatry, 36*(4), 545–553.

Birmaher, B., Waterman, G. S., Ryan, N., Cully, M., Balach, L., Ingram, J., & Brodsky, M. (1994). Fluoxetine for childhood anxiety disorders. *Journal of the American Academy of Child and Adolescent Psychiatry, 33*(7), 993–999.

Bowen, R. C., Offord, D. R., & Boyle, M. H. (1990). The prevalence of overanxious disorder and separation anxiety disorder: Results from the Ontario Child Health Study. *Journal of the American Academy of Child and Adolescent Psychiatry, 29*(5), 753–758.

Briggs-Gowan, M. J., Horwitz, S. M., Schwab-Stone, M. E., Leventhal, J. M., & Leaf, P. J. (2000). Mental health in pediatric settings: Distribution of disorders and factors related to service use. *Journal of the American Academy of Child and Adolescent Psychiatry, 39*(7), 841–849.

Carlson, G. A., Kashani, J. H., de Fatima Thomas, M., Vaidya, A., & Daniel, A. E. (1987). Comparison of two structured interviews on a psychiatrically hospitalized population of children. *Journal of the American Academy of Child and Adolescent Psychiatry, 26*(5), 645–648.

Cobham, V. E., Dadds, M. R., & Spence, S. H. (1998). The role of parental anxiety in the treatment of childhood anxiety. *Journal of Consulting and Clinical Psychology, 66*(6), 893–905.

Compton, S. N., Nelson, A. H., & March, J. S. (2000). Social phobia and separation anxiety symptoms in community and clinical samples of children and adolescents. *Journal of the American Academy of Child and Adolescent Psychiatry, 39*(8), 1040–1046.

Costello, E. J., Angold, A., Burns, B. J., Stangl, D. K., Tweed, D. L., Erkanli, A., & Worthman, C. M. (1996). The Great Smoky Mountains Study of Youth: Goals, design, methods, and the prevalence of *DSM-III-R* disorders. *Archives of General Psychiatry, 53*(12), 1129–1136.

Dadds, M. R., Holland, D. E., Laurens, K. R., Mullins, M., Barrett, P. M., & Spence, S. H. (1999). Early intervention and prevention of anxiety disorders in children: Results at 2–year follow-up. *Journal of Consulting and Clinical Psychology, 67*(1), 145–150.

Dadds, M. R., Spence, S. H., Holland, D. E., Barrett, P. M., & Laurens, K. R. (1997). Prevention and early intervention for anxiety disorders: a controlled trial. *Journal of Consulting and Clinical Psychology, 65*(4), 627–635.

Ernst, M., Cookus, B. A., & Moravec, B. C. (2000). Pictorial Instrument for Children and Adolescents (PICA-III-R). *Journal of the American Academy of Child and Adolescent Psychiatry, 39*(1), 94–99.

Ernst, M., Godfrey, K. A., Silva, R. R., Pouget, E. R., & Welkowitz, J. (1994). A new pictorial instrument for child and adolescent psychiatry: a pilot study. *Psychiatry Research, 51*(1), 87–104.

Ezpeleta, L., de la Osa, N., Domenech, J. M., Navarro, J. B., Losilla, J. M., & Judez, J. (1997). Diagnostic agreement between clinicians and the Diagnostic Interview for Children and Adolescents—DICA-R—in an outpatient sample. *Journal of Child Psychology and Psychiatry and Allied Disciplines, 38*(4), 431–440.

Fairbanks, J. M., Pine, D. S., Tancer, N. K., Dummit, E. S., III, Kentgen, L. M., Martin, J., Asche, B. K., et al. (1997). Open fluoxetine treatment of mixed anxiety disorders in children and adolescents. *Journal of Child and Adolescent Psychopharmacology, 7*(1), 17–29.

Fischer, D. J., Himle, J. A., & Thyer, B. A. (1999). Separation anxiety disorder. In R. T. Ammerman, M. Hersen, & C. G. Last (Eds.), *Handbook of prescriptive treatments for children and adolescents* (2nd ed., pp. 141–154). Boston: Allyn & Bacon.

Flannery-Schroeder, E. C., & Kendall, P. C. (2000). Group and individual cognitive-behavioral treatments for youth with anxiety disorders: A randomized clinical trial. *Cognitive Therapy and Research, 24*(3), 251–278.

Francis, G., Last, C. G., & Strauss, C. C. (1987). Expression of separation anxiety disorder: The roles of age and gender. *Child Psychiatry and Human Development, 18*(2), 82–89.

Fristad, M. A., Cummins, J., Verducci, J. S., Teare, M., Weller, E. B., & Weller, R. A. (1998). Study IV: Concurrent validity of the *DSM-IV-Revised* Children's Interview for Psychiatric Syndromes (ChIPS). *Journal of Child and Adolescent Psychopharmacology, 8*(4), 227–236.

Fristad, M. A., Glickman, A. R., Verducci, J. S., Teare, M., Weller, E. B., & Weller, R. A. (1998). Study V: Children's Interview for Psychiatric Syndromes (ChIPS): Psychometrics in two community samples. *Journal of Child and Adolescent Psychopharmacology, 8*(4), 237–245.

Fristad, M. A., Teare, M., Weller, E. B., Weller, R. A., & Salmon, P. (1998). Study III: Development and concurrent validity of the Children's Interview for Psychiatric Syndromes–Parent version (P-ChIPS). *Journal of Child and Adolescent Psychopharmacology, 8*(4), 221–226.

Gittelman-Klein, R., & Klein, D. F. (1971). Controlled imipramine treatment of school phobia. *Archives of General Psychiatry, 25,* 204–207.

Gittelman-Klein, R., & Klein, D. F. (1973). School phobia: Diagnostic considerations in the light of imipramine effects. *Journal of Nervous and Mental Disease, 156*(3), 199–215.

Graae, F., Milner, J., Rizzotto, L., & Klein, R. G. (1994). Clonazepam in childhood anxiety disorders. *Journal of the American Academy of Child and Adolescent Psychiatry, 33*(3), 372–376.

Hamilton, M. (1959). The assessment of anxiety states by rating. *British Journal of Medical Psychology, 32*(1), 50–55.

Heinicke, C. M., & Ramsey-Klee, D. M. (1986). Outcome of child psychotherapy as a function of frequency of session. *Journal of the American Academy of Child and Adolescent Psychiatry, 25,* 247–253

Ialongo, N., Edelsohn, G., Werthamer-Larsson, L., Crockett, L., & Kellam, S. (1995). The significance of self-reported anxious symptoms in first-grade children: Prediction to anxious symptoms and adaptive functioning in fifth grade. *Journal of Child Psychology & Psychiatry & Allied Disciplines, 36,* 427–437.

Jensen, P., Roper, M., Fisher, P., Piacentini, J., Canino, G., Richters, J., Rubio-Stipec, M., et al. (1995). Test-retest reliability of the Diagnostic Interview Schedule for Children (DISC-2.1): Parent, child, and combined algorithms. *Archives of General Psychiatry, 52*(1), 61–71.

Kashani, J. H., & Orvaschel, H. (1990). A community study of anxiety in children and adolescents. *American Journal of Psychiatry, 147*(3), 313–318.

Kendall, P. C. (1990). *Coping cat manual.* Ardmore, PA: Workbook Publishing.

Kendall, P. C. (1994). Treating anxiety disorders in children: Results of a randomized clinical trial. *Journal of Consulting and Clinical Psychology, 62*(1), 100–110.

Kendall, P. C., Flannery-Schroeder, E., Panichelli-Mindel, S. M., Southam-Gerow, M., Henin, A., & Warman, M. (1997). Therapy for youths with anxiety disorders: A second randomized clinical trial. *Journal of Consulting and Clinical Psychology, 65*(3), 366–380.

Kendall, P. C., & Southam-Gerow, M. A. (1996). Long-term follow-up of a cognitive-behavioral therapy for anxiety-disordered youth. *Journal of Consulting and Clinical Psychology, 64*(4), 724–730.

King, N. J., Tonge, B. J., Heyne, D., Pritchard, M., Rollings, S., Young, D., Myerson, N., & Ollendick, T. H. (1998). Cognitive-behavioral treatment of school-refusing children: A controlled evaluation. *Journal of the American Academy of Child and Adolescent Psychiatry, 37*(4), 395–403.

Klein, R. G., Koplewicz, H. S., & Kanner, A. (1992). Imipramine treatment of children with separation anxiety disorder. *Journal of the American Academy of Child and Adolescent Psychiatry, 31*(1), 21–28.

Last, C. G., Hansen, C., & Franco, N. (1998). Cognitive-behavioral treatment of school phobia. *Journal of the American Academy of Child and Adolescent Psychiatry, 37*(4), 404–411.

Last, C. G., Hersen, M., Kazdin, A. E., Finkelstein, R., & Strauss, C. C. (1987). Comparison of *DSM-III* separation anxiety and overanxious disorders: Demographic characteristics and patterns of comorbidity. *Journal of the American Academy of Child and Adolescent Psychiatry, 26*(4), 527–531.

Last, C. G., Perrin, S., Hersen, M., & Kazdin, A. E. (1992). *DSM-III-R* anxiety disorders in children: Sociodemographic and clinical characteristics. *Journal of the American Academy of Child and Adolescent Psychiatry, 31*(6), 1070–1076.

Last, C. G., Perrin, S., Hersen, M., & Kazdin, A. E. (1996). A prospective study of childhood anxiety disorders. *Journal of the American Academy of Child and Adolescent Psychiatry, 35*(11), 1502–1510.

Leonard, H. L., March, J., Rickler, K. C., & Allen, A. J. (1997). Pharmacology of the selective serotonin reuptake inhibitors in children and adolescents. *Journal of the American Academy of Child and Adolescent Psychiatry, 36*(6), 725–736.

Lipsitz, J. D., Martin, L. Y., Mannuzza, S., Chapman, T. F., Liebowitz, M. R., Klein, D. F., & Fyer, A. J. (1994). Childhood separation anxiety disorder in patients with adult anxiety disorders. *American Journal of Psychiatry, 151*(6), 927–929.

Manicavasagar, V., Silove, D., Curtis, J., & Wagner, R. (2000). Continuities of separation anxiety from early life into adulthood. *Journal of Anxiety Disorders, 14*(1), 1–18.

Manicavasagar, V., Silove, D., & Hadzi-Pavlovic, D. (1998). Subpopulations of early separation anxiety: Relevance to risk of adult anxiety disorders. *Journal of Affective Disorders, 48*(2–3), 181–190.

March, J. S., & Albano, A. M. (1998). New developments in assessing pediatric anxiety disorders. *Advances in Clinical Child Psychology, 20*, 213–241.

March, J. S., Parker, J. D., Sullivan, K., Stallings, P., & Conners, C. K. (1997). The Multidimensional Anxiety Scale for Children (MASC): Factor structure, reliability, and validity. *Journal of the American Academy of Child and Adolescent Psychiatry, 36*(4), 554–565.

March, J. S., & Sullivan, K. (1999). Test-retest reliability of the Multidimensional Anxiety Scale for Children. *Journal of Anxiety Disorders, 13*(4), 349–358.

Mendlowitz, S. L., Manassis, K., Bradley, S., Scapillato, D., Miezitis, S., & Shaw, B. F. (1999). Cognitive-behavioral group treatments in childhood anxiety disorders: The role of parental involvement. *Journal of the American Academy of Child and Adolescent Psychiatry, 38*(10), 1223–1229.

Mesman, J., & Koot, H. M. (2000). Child-reported depression and anxiety in preadolescence: I. Associations with parent- and teacher-reported problems. *Journal of the American Academy of Child and Adolescent Psychiatry, 39*(11), 1371–1378.

Monga, S., Birmaher, B., Chiappetta, L., Brent, D., Kaufman, J., Bridge, J., & Cully, M. (2000). Screen for Child Anxiety-Related Emotional Disorders (SCARED): Convergent and divergent validity. *Depression and Anxiety, 12*(2), 85–91.

Muris, P., Meesters, C., Merckelbach, H., Sermon, A., & Zwakhalen, S. (1998). Worry in normal children. *Journal of the American Academy of Child and Adolescent Psychiatry, 37*(7), 703–710.

Muris, P., Merckelbach, H., Gadet, B., & Moulaert, V. (2000). Fears, worries, and scary dreams in 4– to 12–year-old children: Their content, developmental pattern, and origins. *Journal of Clinical Child Psychology, 29*(1), 43–52.

Muris, P., Merckelbach, H., Mayer, B., & Meesters, C. (1998). Common fears and their relationship to anxiety disorders symptomatology in normal children. *Personality and Individual Differences, 24*(4), 575–578.

Muris, P., Merckelbach, H., Mayer, B., & Prins, E. (2000). How serious are common childhood fears? *Behaviour Research and Therapy, 38*(3), 217–228.

Muris, P., Merckelbach, H., Mayer, B., van Brakel, A., Thissen, S., Moulaert, V., & Gadet, B. (1998). The Screen for Child Anxiety Related Emotional Disorders (SCARED) and traditional childhood anxiety measures. *Journal of Behavior Therapy and Experimental Psychiatry, 29*(4), 327–339.

Muris, P., Merckelbach, H., Schmidt, H., & Mayer, B. (1998). The revised version of the Screen for Anxiety Related Emotional Disorders (SCARED-R): Factor structure in normal children. *Personality and Individual Differences, 26*, 99–112.

Muris, P., Merckelbach, H., van Brakel, A., Mayer, B., & van Dongen, L. (1998). The Screen for Child Anxiety Related Emotional Disorders (SCARED): Relationship with anxiety and depression in normal children. *Personality and Individual Differences, 24*(4), 451–456.

Ollendick, T. H. (1983). Reliability and validity of the Revised Fear Survey Schedule for Children (FSSC-R). *Behaviour Research and Therapy, 21*(6), 685–692.

Rapoport, J. L., & Ismond, D. R. (1996). *DSM-IV training guide for diagnosis of childhood disorders.* New York: Brunner/Mazel.

Reich, W. (2000). Diagnostic interview for children and adolescents (DICA). *Journal of the American Academy of Child and Adolescent Psychiatry, 39*(1), 59–66.

Research Units on Pediatric Psychopharmacology Anxiety Study Group. (2001). Fluvoxamine for the treatment of anxiety disorders in children and adolescents. *New England Journal of Medicine, 344*(17), 1279–1285.

Research Units on Pediatric Psychopharmacology Anxiety Study Group (2002). The Pediatric Anxiety Rating Scale (PARS): Development and psychomatric properties. *Journal of the American Academy of Child and Adolescent Psychiatry, 41*(9), 1061–1069.

Reynolds, C. R., & Kamphaus, R. (1992). *Behavioral Assessment System for Children.* Circle Pines, MN: American Guidance.

Reynolds, C. R., & Richmond, B. O. (1978). What I think and feel: A revised measure of children's manifest anxiety. *Journal of Abnormal Child Psychology, 6*(2), 271–280.

Riddle, M. A., Bernstein, G. A., Cook, E. H., Leonard, H. L., March, J. S., & Swanson, J. M. (1999). Anxiolytics, adrenergic agents, and naltrexone. *Journal of the American Academy of Child and Adolescent Psychiatry, 38*(5), 546–556.

Scapillato, D., & Mendlowitz, S. L. (1993). *Coping Bear Workbook.* Unpublished manuscript. Toronto, Ontario: Hospital for Sick Children.

Schniering, C. A., Hudson, J. L., & Rapee, R. M. (2000). Issues in the diagnosis and assessment of anxiety disorders in children and adolescents. *Clinical Psychology Review, 20*(4), 453–478.

Schwab-Stone, M. E., Shaffer, D., Dulcan, M. K., Jensen, P. S., Fisher, P., Bird, H. R., Goodman, S. H., et al. (1996). Criterion validity of the NIMH Diagnostic Interview Schedule for Children Version 2.3 (DISC-2.3). *Journal of the American Academy of Child and Adolescent Psychiatry, 35*(7), 878–888.

Shaffer, D., Fisher, P., Lucas, C. P., Dulcan, M. K., & Schwab-Stone, M. E. (2000). NIMH Diagnostic Interview Schedule for Children Version IV (NIMH DISC-IV): Description, differences from previous versions, and reliability of some common diagnoses. *Journal of the American Academy of Child and Adolescent Psychiatry, 39*(1), 28–38.

Sherrill, J. T., & Kovacs, M. (2000). Interview schedule for children and adolescents (ISCA). *Journal of the American Academy of Child and Adolescent Psychiatry, 39*(1), 67–75.

Silove, D., Harris, M., Morgan, A., Boyce, P., Manicavasagar, V., Hadzi-Pavlovic, D., & Wilhelm, K. (1995). Is early separation anxiety a specific precursor of panic disorder-agoraphobia? A community study. *Psychological Medicine, 25*(2), 405–411.

Silove, D., & Manicavasagar, V. (1993). Adults who feared school: Is early separation anxiety specific to the pathogenesis of panic disorder? *Acta Psychiatrica Scandinavica, 88*(6), 385–390.

Silverman, W. K., & Albano, A. M. (1996). *Anxiety Disorders Interview Schedule for DSM-IV, Child and Parent Versions*. San Antonio, TX: Psychological Corporation.

Silverman, W. K., & Eisen, A. R. (1992). Age differences in the reliability of parent and child reports of child anxious symptomatology using a structured interview. *Journal of the American Academy of Child and Adolescent Psychiatry, 31*(1), 117–124.

Silverman, W. K., Fleisig, W., Rabian, B., & Peterson, R. A. (1991). Childhood Anxiety Sensitivity Index. *Journal of Clinical Child Psychology, 20*, 162–168.

Silverman, W. K., & Nelles, W. B. (1988). The Anxiety Disorders Interview Schedule for Children. *Journal of the American Academy of Child and Adolescent Psychiatry, 27*(6), 772–778.

Silverman, W. K., & Rabian, B. (1995). Test-retest reliability of the *DSM-III-R* childhood anxiety disorders symptoms using the Anxiety Disorders Interview Schedule for children. *Journal of Anxiety Disorders, 9*(2), 139–150.

Simeon, J. G., Knott, V. J., Dubois, C., Wiggins, D., Geraets, I., Thatte, S., & Miller, W. (1994). Buspirone therapy of mixed anxiety disorders in childhood and adolescence: A pilot study. *Journal of Child and Adolescent Psychopharmacology, 4*(3), 159–170.

Spence, S. H. (1997). Structure of anxiety symptoms among children: A confirmatory factor-analytic study. *Journal of Abnormal Psychology, 106*(2), 280–297.

Spence, S. H. (1998). A measure of anxiety symptoms among children. *Behaviour Research and Therapy, 36*(5), 545–566.

Spielberger, C. (1973). *Manual for the State-Trait Anxiety Inventory for Children.* Palo Alto, CA: Consulting Psychologists Press.

Target, M., & Fonagy, P. (1994). Efficacy of psychoanalysis for children with emotional disorders. *Journal of the American Academy of Child and Adolescent Psychiatry, 33*, 361–371.

Teare, M., Fristad, M. A., Weller, E. B., Weller, R. A., & Salmon, P. (1998). Study I: Development and criterion validity of the Children's Interview for Psychiatric Syndromes (ChIPS). *Journal of Child and Adolescent Psychopharmacology, 8*(4), 205–211.

Toren, P., Sadeh, M., Wolmer, L., Eldar, S., Koren, S., Weizman, R., & Laor, N. (2000). Neurocognitive correlates of anxiety disorders in children: A preliminary report. *Journal of Anxiety Disorders, 14*(3), 239–247.

Toren, P., Wolmer, L., Rosental, B., Eldar, S., Koren, S., Lask, M., Weizman, R., et al. (2000). Case series: Brief parent-child group therapy for childhood anxiety disorders using a manual-based cognitive-behavioral technique. *Journal of the American Academy of Child and Adolescent Psychiatry, 39*(10), 1309–1312.

Valla, J. P., Bergeron, L., Berube, H., Gaudet, N., & St-Georges, M. (1994). A structured pictorial questionnaire to assess *DSM-III-R*-based diagnoses in children (6–11 years): development, validity, and reliability. *Journal of Abnormal Child Psychology, 22*(4), 403–423.

Valla, J. P., Bergeron, L., Bidaut-Russell, M., St-Georges, M., & Gaudet, N. (1997). Reliability of the Dominic-R: A young child mental health questionnaire combining visual and auditory stimuli. *Journal of Child Psychology and Psychiatry and Allied Disciplines, 38*(6), 717–724.

Valla, J. P., Bergeron, L., & Smolla, N. (2000). The Dominic-R: A pictorial interview for 6- to 11–year-old children. *Journal of the American Academy of Child and Adolescent Psychiatry, 39*(1), 85–93.

Velosa, J. F., & Riddle, M. A. (2000). Pharmacologic treatment of anxiety disorders in children and adolescents. *Child and Adolescent Psychiatric Clinics of North America, 9*(1), 119–133.

Walkup, J., & Davies, M. (1999, October). The Pediatric Anxiety Rating Scale (PARS): A reliability study. *Scientific Proceedings of the 46th Annual Meeting of the American Academy of Child and Adolescent Psychiatry*, Chicago, p. 107 [abstract].

Weller, E. B., Weller, R. A., Fristad, M. A., Rooney, M. T., & Schecter, J. (2000). Children's Interview for Psychiatric Syndromes (ChIPS). *Journal of the American Academy of Child and Adolescent Psychiatry, 39*(1), 76–84.

Westenberg, P. M., Siebelink, B. M., Warmenhoven, N. J., & Treffers, P. D. (1999). Separation anxiety and overanxious disorders: Relations to age and level of psychosocial maturity. *Journal of the American Academy of Child and Adolescent Psychiatry, 38*(8), 1000–1007.

11

CHILDHOOD-ONSET
PANIC DISORDER

BORIS BIRMAHER & THOMAS H. OLLENDICK

The prevalence of panic disorder (PD) in child and adolescent community samples has been reported to range between 0.5% and 5.0% (e.g., Essau, Conradt, & Petermann, 1999; Hayward, Killen, Kraemer, & Taylor, 2000; Hayward et al., 1997; Macaulay & Kleinknecht, 1989; Moreau & Follet, 1993), and in pediatric psychiatric clinics from 0.2% to 10% (Biederman et al., 1997; Birmaher, personal communication, July 2000; Kearney, Albano, Eisen, Allan, & Barlow, 1997; Last & Strauss, 1989), with most cases occurring in female adolescents. Retrospective investigations in adults have found that up to 40% of patients with PD report that their disorders began before they were 20 years old (Moreau & Follet, 1993). The peak onset of PD in these studies has been reported to be between 15 and 19 years of age, with 10% to 18% of the youths experiencing their first panic attack (PA) before they were 10 years old (Thyer, Parrish, Curtis, Nesse, & Cameron, 1985; Von Korff, Eaton, & Keyl, 1985). These prevalence rates, together with preliminary evidence that there is a decrease in age of onset of PD in successive generations (Battaglia, Bertella, Bajo, Binaghi, & Bellodi, 1998), indicate the need to study the clinical characteristics, course, and treatment of PD in children and adolescents.

PD is usually a disabling condition accompanied by psychosocial, family, peer, and academic difficulties (Moreau & Weissman, 1992; Ollendick, Mattis, & King, 1994). Moreover, PD is associated with increased risk for major depressive disorder (MDD), substance abuse, and perhaps suicide (Moreau & Weissman, 1992; Ollendick et al., 1994; Strauss et al., 2000). Such adverse outcomes are more prevalent in persons whose PD started early in life (≤ 17 years of age; see Weissman et al., 1997). Despite this, it takes an average of 12.7 years from the onset of symptoms to initiate treatment (Moreau & Follet, 1993) and, unfortunately, it appears that very few youngsters with PD seek help (Essau et al., 1999, 2000; King, Gullone, Tonge, & Ollendick, 1993; Ollendick, 1995).

Early recognition and intervention for children and adolescents with PD may reduce the just-noted complications and, perhaps, alter the long-term course of anxiety in adulthood (Ollendick & King, 1994; Pine, Cohen, Gurley, Brook, & Ma, 1998; Pollack et al., 1996). However, in contrast with the adult literature (e.g., American Psychiatric Association [APA], 1998), there are few investigations on childhood-onset PD.

In this chapter, we review the current literature on the clinical characteristics, diagnosis, longitudinal course, assessment, treatment, and prevention of childhood-onset PD. In addition, we emphasize the limitations of these studies and highlight directions for future research and clinical practice.

CLINICAL MANIFESTATION

In order to meet diagnostic criteria for PD, it is necessary to experience recurrent PAs. Therefore, we first describe the clinical manifestations of PAs and then the characteristics of PD in children and adolescents.

Panic Attacks

A PA is an acute temporal anxiety episode in which the person, in the absence of real danger, experiences emotional, cognitive, and somatic symptoms similar to those triggered by actual threatening situations. Specifically, the person experiences intense fear and at least 4 of the 13 symptoms described in the *Diagnostic and Statistical Manual of Mental Disorders: DSM-IV* (APA, 1994) for PAs (see Table 11.1). Often the PA peaks in intensity within 5 to 10 minutes before gradually subsiding. The person feels that something is wrong or that something bad is going to happen but does not know what is going to happen, when it will happen, where it will happen, and (perhaps most important) why it will happen. As a consequence, the person may believe that he or she is about to go crazy, lose control, faint, have a severe illness (e.g., a heart attack), or die. The symptoms, by themselves, can increase the person's level of anxiety and create a vicious circle, which worsens and maintains PA frequency, intensity, and duration (APA, 1998; Ollendick, 1998).

There are three types of PAs: (1) *uncued* (unexpected, spontaneous, out of the blue), (2) *cued* (situationally bound), and (3) *situationally predisposed* (likely to occur in certain situations but not necessarily so). Situationally bound PAs almost always occur immediately on exposure to, or in anticipation of, a triggering event (e.g., the presence of a phobic object). Situationally predisposed PAs are also triggered by certain situations (e.g., a threatening or embarrassing situation); however, the attacks do not

Table 11.1. *DSM-IV* Criteria for Panic Attack (American Psychiatric Association, 1994)

A discrete period of intense fear or discomfort, in which four (or more) of the following symptoms developed abruptly and reached a peak within 10 minutes:

- Palpitations, pounding heart, or accelerated heart rate
- Sweating
- Trembling or shaking
- Sensations of shortness of breath or smothering
- Feeling of choking
- Chest pain or discomfort
- Nausea or abdominal distress
- Feeling dizzy, unsteady, lightheaded, or faint
- Derealization (feelings of unreality) or depersonalization (being detached from oneself)
- Fear of losing control or going crazy
- Fear of dying
- Paresthesia (numbness or tingling sensations)
- Chills or hot flushes

always occur immediately after exposure to the external trigger (APA, 1998). For example, an adolescent may experience an attack at a theater or shopping mall but does not always do so. It is important to note that a PA may initially be uncued but, over time, may become paired with specific stimuli (e.g., elevator, shopping center, being in a crowed place), thus resulting in situationally bound or situationally predisposed attacks. Frequently, regardless of the type of PA, avoidance behaviors follow.

Community studies using structured psychiatric interviews have found that 2% to 18% of adolescents have experienced at least one four-symptom PA during their lives (Essau et al., 1999; Hayward et al., 2000; Hayward et al., 1997). Although studies using self-report questionnaires have reported much higher prevalence rates (43% to 60%; King et al., 1993; King, Ollendick, Mattis, Yang, & Tonge, 1997; Lau, Calamari, & Waraczynski, 1996; Macaulay & Kleinknecht, 1989), reliance on questionnaires alone tends to increase the rate of false-positive cases (Hayward et al., 1997). That is, many of these cases turn out not to be true cases of PA. PAs are equally prevalent in males and females (Essau et al., 1999; Hayward et al., 2000; King et al., 1993), but severe PAs tend to be more frequent in females (Hayward et al., 2000; Hayward, Killen, & Taylor, 1989; King, Ollendick, Mattis, et al., 1997; Macaulay & Kleinknecht, 1989). PAs can and do occur in children but are much less prevalent than in adolescents (Hayward et al., 1989; King, Ollendick, Mattis, et al., 1997; Ollendick et al., 1994).

In community samples, approximately 20% to 50% of the PAs are reported to be uncued (Essau et al., 1999; King, Ollendick, Mattis, et al., 1997; Macaulay & Kleinknecht, 1989). Female and male adolescents usually experience palpitations, trembling/shaking, nausea, abdominal distress, chills, hot flushes, sweating, and dizziness (Essau et al., 1999; Macaulay &

Kleinknecht, 1989), which are similar to symptoms reported in adult studies. However, cognitive symptoms (e.g., fear of losing control) are less frequently reported than somatic symptoms (Ollendick et al., 1994).

Among youngsters with PA, 10% to 30% develop moderate to severe avoidance behaviors (e.g., agoraphobia) of specific situations (schools, restaurants, crowds) for fear of having another attack (Essau et al., 1999; Hayward et al., 2000; King et al., 1993). Similar to adults (APA, 1998), youths with PAs—in particular, those with more severe symptoms—may experience other anxiety and depressive symptoms or disorders (Essau et al., 1999; Hayward et al., 2000; Hayward et al., 1989; King et al., 1993; Macaulay & Kleinknecht, 1989). Youngsters with severe PAs have reported less social support from family members and more family-related psychosocial stressors (King et al., 1993; King, Ollendick, Mattis, et al., 1997; Macaulay & Kleinknecht, 1989). PAs can also affect the well-being and self-esteem of these children and adolescents, because they may see the PAs as a sign of emotional weakness or presume that these are an indicator of a life-threatening illness or possibly even death. In addition, PAs may increase the risk of developing MDD during adulthood (Pine et al., 1998).

Panic Disorder

PD is characterized by recurrent *uncued* PAs that last at least 1 month, persistent concern about having another PA (anticipatory anxiety), worry about the implications and consequences of the PA, and impairment in functioning (APA, 1994, 1998). In addition, to diagnose PD, the PA should not be accounted for primarily by other physical or psychiatric illnesses. The *International Statistical Classification of Diseases* manual (*ICD-10*; World Health Organization, 1992–1994) includes similar diagnostic criteria.

Clinical studies (Alessi & Magen, 1988; Alessi, Robbins, & Dilsaver, 1988; Biederman et al., 1997; Birmaher, 2002; Kearney et al., 1997; Last & Strauss, 1989; Moreau & Follet, 1993) have shown that most PD pediatric patients seen in clinics are older adolescents, Caucasian, female, and middle class. However, these results need to be viewed with caution, because the demographics of the patients included in these studies reflect the socioeconomic status, geographical areas, and settings where the studies took place. Similar to the adult literature, pediatric studies report that more than half of the patients have palpitations, tremor, dizziness, shortness of breath, faintness, sweating, chest pressure/pain, and fear of dying.

Although PD has been reported in children, it appears that this disorder is less frequent in this age range. It has been suggested that children have less PD because they do not have the cognitive ability to make internal, catastrophic misinterpretations of the somatic symptoms associated with PD (e.g., thoughts of losing control, going crazy, or dying in response to the somatic symptoms; see Nelles & Barlow, 1988). However, these notions have not been supported empirically. On the contrary, although children of varying ages do tend to make noncatastrophic interpretations of these symptoms (e.g., "I am catching a cold or the flu"), they are *capable* of making internal, catastrophic cognitions (e.g., "I must be dying like my grandfather"; see Mattis & Ollendick, 1997a). Rarely, however, do young children attribute the somatic symptoms to going crazy; rather, they are more likely to think that something is wrong with them physically and that they might die. Children as young as 8 years of age report high levels of anxiety sensitivity and elevated internal attributions in response to negative outcomes; these cognitive processes, in turn, appear to serve as important risk factors for future development of PD (Ginsburg & Drake, 2002; Mattis & Ollendick, 1997a; Ollendick, 1998).

Risk Factors Associated With the Development of PAs and PD

PANIC ATTACKS   Female sex, puberty, negative affectivity (NA: an increased sensitivity to negative stimuli with resulting distress and fearfulness), anxiety sensitivity (AS: an increased tendency to respond fearfully to anxiety symptoms), internal attributions of responsibility in response to negative events, and the presence of MDD have been associated with the onset of full-blown PAs (Hayward et al., 1992, 2000; Mattis & Ollendick, 1997a). Other studies have shown a significant association between AS and panic in both Caucasian and African-American adolescent populations (Ginsburg & Drake, 2002; Kearney et al., 1997; Lau et al., 1996). Although the findings are less conclusive, family conflict and stress have also been shown to be predictive of attacks in some adolescents (King, Ollendick, Mattis, et al., 1997; Macaulay & Kleinknecht, 1989).

PANIC DISORDER   Female sex, MDD, high AS, and family history of MDD and PD have been associated with higher prevalence of PD (e.g., Biederman et al., 2001; Horesh, Amir, Kedem, Goldberger, & Kotler, 1997; Kearney et al., 1997). The association with female sex, however, may be accounted for by the higher prevalence of MDD in females (Hayward et al., 2000). Earlier studies suggested that childhood separation anxiety disorder might herald the development of PD during late adolescence and adulthood (see review by Silove, Manicavasagar, Curtis, & Blaszcynski, 1996). However, more recent studies have been negative in this regard (Craske, Poulton, Tsao, & Plotkin, 2001; Essau et al., 1999; Hayward et al., 2000).

Diagnosis

COMORBIDITY   Up to 90% of patients with PD have comorbidity with other anxiety disorders (e.g., separation anxiety disorder, social phobia, general anxiety disorder) and mood disorders (Alessi & Magen, 1988; Alessi et al., 1987; Biederman et al., 1997; Birmaher et al., 2002; Essau et al., 2000). For example, Birmaher and colleagues (2002) found 42 patients with PD in a large sample ($n = 2,025$) of outpatient children and adolescents assessed with the Schedule for Affective Disorders and Schizophrenia for School-Age Children–Present Episode (K-SADS; Chambers et al., 1985). In comparison with youth with non-PD psychiatric disorders ($n = 1,983$), patients with PD were significantly older (15.3 vs. 14.3 years, $p < .01$), had significantly more comorbid MDD (50% vs. 30.4%, $p < .01$), bipolar disorder (19.0% vs. 6.8%, $p < .007$), and had significantly more anxiety disorders—in particular, general anxiety and separation anxiety disorders (for all anxiety disorders, rates of 8% to 50% vs. 0.5% to 10%, $p < 0.04$). When only compared with patients with other anxiety disorders without PD ($n = 407$), patients with PD were significantly older and had more bipolar disorder (19% vs. 5.4%, $p < .004$), but no other diagnostic differences were found. Biederman et al. (1997) also reported high incidence of bipolar disorder (52% vs. 15% vs. 0%) in a sample of 26 outpatients with PD in comparison with psychiatric ($n = 372$) and normal controls ($n = 144$). It is interesting that approximately 20% of adults with PD have bipolar disorder (Bowen, South, & Hawkes, 1994), and adults with BPD have high incidence of PD when compared with nonbipolar psychiatric and depressed controls (21% vs. 8% vs. 0%, $p < .05$; Chen & Dilsaver, 1995). Also, in a community study, Lewinsohn, Klein, and Seeley (1995) reported significantly more BPD in adolescents with PD (11%) than in normal controls (0.9%, $p < .001$).

PD is also comorbid with other psychiatric disorders, including attention-deficit/hyperactivity disorder (6% to 50%) and oppositional defiant disorder (6% to 50%), reflecting the clinical settings where the samples were ascertained (Biederman et al., 1997; Last & Strauss, 1989).

In patients with recurrent PAs, 10% to 90% may develop avoidance of places or situations (i.e., agoraphobia) where escape or help may be unavailable if they experience a PA (Biederman et al., 1997; Kearney et al., 1997). These patients usually avoid separation from caretakers, crowded places (school, movies, etc.), buses, bridges, tunnels, and being far from home, unless they are accompanied by others and feel safe. Ollendick (1995) reported a wide variety of agoraphobic situations endorsed by adolescents with PD: churches, malls, parties, grocery stores, restaurants, theaters, auditoriums, and schools. Avoidance of such situations precludes the adolescent from engaging in a host of normative experiences and socializing events.

It has been reported that PD patients are at high risk for suicide, but it is not clear whether this is due to the high comorbidity with mood disorders (APA, 1998). PD has also been associated with medical and neurological conditions such as migraine and, more controversially, with mitral valve prolapse (APA, 1998).

DIFFERENTIAL DIAGNOSIS   Inasmuch as PAs can occur in the contexts of other psychiatric disorders, medical illness, use of substances or medications, or when the person is confronted with fearful or threatening situations, the need to consider the presence of other disorders in a person with PAs is evident. Patients with other psychiatric disorders—including mood disorders, schizophrenia, and other anxiety disorders (e.g., social phobia, separation anxiety, posttraumatic stress disorder)—can and frequently do experience PAs (APA, 1994, 1998). In this case, the diagnosis of PD is only made if the PA is not explained solely by the other psychiatric disorder. For example, if separation-anxious youths experience PAs only when they are separated from their parent(s), or social-anxious youths have PAs only when exposed to potentially embarrassing situations or situations in which they might be socially evaluated, no diagnosis of PD would be made.

Patients with certain medical conditions (e.g., hyperthyroidism, hyper-parathyroidism, pheocromocytoma) may experience general anxiety symptoms that resemble PAs, and thus they may be misdiagnosed with PD. On the contrary, given that PD is accompanied by high incidence of somatic symptoms, patients with PD can be and frequently are misdiagnosed with pulmonary (e.g., asthma), cardiovascular (e.g., angina, arrhythmias, myocardial infarction), neurological (e.g., seizures, vestibular dysfunctions, syncope), and gastrointestinal (e.g., irritable bowel syndrome) illnesses (APA, 1998). Therefore, clinicians need to be aware of these conditions and to show good clinical judgment when these medical illnesses need to be ruled out.

Nocturnal episodes of PAs are manifested similarly to PAs that occur only during the day, but because they happen suddenly during the night, they need to be differentiated from nocturnal seizures (Herskowitz, 1986; Kushner, Clayton, Crow, & Knopman, 2000) and night terrors. Night terrors occur during the deep sleep stage of sleep (usually after midnight). During night terror episodes, children are agitated, confused, and usually their eyes are open. They have no response to external stimuli and no recall of the event the next morning. Patients with nocturnal seizures are unconscious and do not remember what happened during the night; when they awake, their sheets may be in disarray and may be stained with blood (if an injury was sustained, or if the tongue or lips were bitten), and there will be urine or feces if the patient lost control of his or her sphincter.

Substances, including street drugs (e.g., cocaine, caffeine) and over-the-counter medications, and acute withdrawal from these substances (e.g., benzodiazepines, alcohol) can also induce PAs. In these instances, PD is only diagnosed if the PAs have occurred before or lasted long enough after the substance has been discontinued (APA, 1994).

Finally, a child can be experiencing anxiety symptoms and PAs due to exposure to real current or past threatening situations, such as sexual or physical abuse and exposure to violence. Such possibilities should be routinely explored in the clinical interview

LONGITUDINAL COURSE

No longitudinal studies of children and adolescents with PD have been published. In adults, this disorder has been reported to wax and wane, with periods of frequent PAs and periods where the PAs ameliorate or seemingly disappear altogether. In longitudinal studies of cases presented to tertiary institutions, approximately one third of the adult patients show improvement, one third remain with subsyndromal symptoms, and one third continue to fulfill criteria for PD (APA, 1994, 1998). Even if the patients improve, they may continue to have some episodes with some symptoms of PAs but not the full criteria for a PA (e.g., limited-symptom attacks of less than four symptoms).

ASSESSMENT

This section describes the psychiatric interviews, clinician-based questionnaires, and self-reports that are useful for the assessment of PD. In addition, some scales to measure cognitive distortions associated with PD and other scales that can be used to measure overall improvement are highlighted.

Psychiatric Interviews

These interviews include, among others the Schedule for Affective Disorders and Schizophrenia for School-Age Children, Present Episode and Lifetime versions (K-SADS-PL; Kaufman et al., 1997), the Anxiety Disorders Interview Schedule for Children and Parents (ADIS-C/P; Silverman & Albano, 1996), and the National Institute of Mental Health (NIMH) Diagnostic Interview Schedule for Children, Version 2.3 (DISC 2.3; Shaffer et al., 1996). All include sections to evaluate symptoms of PD, and their psychometric characteristics have been found to be acceptable (see King, Ollendick, Murphy, & Tonge, 1997, for a review). Clinician preference determines which of these interviews will be chosen for use. We recommend the K-SADS or the ADIS-C/P. The ADIS-C/P, for example, is designed specifically for the diagnosis of childhood anxiety and phobic disorders, including PD. The child interview makes use of visual analogue scales and pictorial material to facilitate accurate child ratings of interference and agoraphobic avoidance. There is also a parent version of the interview schedule that is typically administered after the child interview. Children are provided the following probe (their parents receive a paraphrased version): "Okay, we just talked about how sometimes people get scared because they are afraid of a specific thing, like being scared of a dog or being scared of the dark. But sometimes people feel really scared for no reason at all! They are not in a scary place and there is nothing scary around. But, all of a sudden, out of the blue, they feel really scared and they don't know why. Has that ever happened to you?" Assuming a positive response to this probe, additional questions about PA symptoms, frequency of PAs, and worry about additional PAs are pursued. Finally, the child is asked, "Okay, I want to know how much you feel this problem has messed things up in your life. That is, how much has it messed things up for you with friends, in school, or at home? How much does it stop you from doing things you would like to do?" The child is then asked to show the clinician the extent of interference, on a nine-point "Interference Thermometer." Guidelines are provided to assist the clinician in the formulation of composite diagnoses based on both child and parent interview data.

We have found the parent interview to be particularly useful with children but less so with adolescents. Younger children (i.e., those less than 11 years of age) appear to be less reliable and accurate in their reports of anxiety disorders and phobias on such interviews. Adolescents, however, have been shown to provide reliable and valid information on structured diagnostic interviews and other reports of internalizing symptoms (see Edelbrock & Costello, 1985). Although structured interviews such as these appear useful, further studies, including research with larger samples of youth with PD, are sorely needed. To date, these interviews have been used sparingly with children and adolescents with PD; still, their psychometric properties with other anxiety and affective disorders are good, and they show considerable promise.

Clinician-Based Rating Scales

The only specific clinician rating scale for the assessment of PD is the Multiple Collaborative Panic Disorder Severity Scale (MCPAS; Shear et al., 1997), but this scale has been mainly used in older adolescent and adult studies. The Hamilton Anxiety Rating Scale (HARS; Clark & Donovan, 1994) has been validated for the assessment of general anxiety symptoms in adolescents. It includes some somatic symptoms applicable to PD, but it is not specific for this disorder. Recently, the Pediatric Anxiety Rating Scale (PARS) was developed by the NIMH Research Units for Pediatric Psychopharmacology (RUPP, 2002) for the assessment of multiple anxiety disorders. This scale includes symptoms relevant to PD, but it has not been used in samples of children and adolescents with this disorder.

Self-Reports

The only self-report instrument designed specifically to evaluate PAs is the Panic Attack Questionnaire (PAQ; Norton, Dorward, & Cox, 1986). The PAQ consists of a series of questions about PAs, including their occurrence, frequency, intensity, and duration. PAs are defined as follows: "Panic attacks involve very intense feelings of fear or anxiety that come on very suddenly and unexpectedly, and usually reach a peak very quickly. During a PA you feel that something terrible is about to happen to you such as losing control or even dying. Many people experience changes in their breathing. Other physical changes such as the shakes might occur." Other questions explore antecedents to the PAs, the situations in which they occur, and their level of interference in daily life. This questionnaire has been used exclusively with adolescents 13 years of age and older (see King et al., 1997) and young adults. If it is used as the sole source of information about PAs, however, it is likely to result in a number of false positives (i.e., responses not indicative of true PAs; see Hayward et al., 1989). Still, this instrument is very useful in guiding the clinician in obtaining information about the various facets of the PAs and their probable relation to PD versus other anxiety or medical disorders.

In addition to the PAQ, the Panic Attributional Checklist (Mattis & Ollendick, 1997a, 2002) has recently been developed and used to assess cognitive responses to the somatic and physical symptoms of PAs. The checklist is unique, in that it asks the child or adolescent to read a scenario and to imagine or pretend that he or she is actually experiencing the feelings described. The scenario is as follows: "Imagine that you are sitting in your bedroom at home. Try to picture your bedroom in your mind as best you can. Imagine that you are sitting on your bed and reading a book. All of a sudden, out of the blue, you start to breathe very fast. You are also having difficulty catching your breath and you feel short of breath, as if you have just been running. At the same time, you feel dizzy and unsteady, as if you might faint. Your heart is beating very fast and you can feel some pain in your chest. There's a feeling of tightness in your throat and, at the same time, you feel sick in your stomach. Your hands are tingling and you feel hot. You notice that you are shaking and sweating. It's a strange feeling." The child or adolescent is then asked to imagine these feelings while reviewing a list of 16 thoughts someone might have when experiencing these feelings. The thoughts tap four different classes of attributions: *external noncatastrophic* (e.g., "I'd think I was feeling this way because of the temperature or the weather"), *external catastrophic* (e.g., "I'd think something or someone was trying to kill me"), *internal noncatastrophic* (e.g., "I'd think I was worried about something"), and *internal catastrophic* (e.g., "I'd think I must be dying").

Most children between 8 and 14 years of age tended to make internal noncatastrophic attributions when imaging the physical feelings associated with panic. However, a subset of children and adolescents did make internal catastrophic attributions, regardless of age. Youngsters who made such attributions tended to score high on the Anxiety Sensitivity Index (discussed later in this chapter) and also described themselves as generally fearful and anxious. Although the Panic Attribution Checklist is in its psychometric infancy, we have found it useful in our clinical practice. It has been most useful in helping us pinpoint the nature of the youngster's response to the physical symptoms of panic and in helping us identify meaningful targets with our cognitive-behavioral interventions.

A third self-report instrument we have found to be useful in the assessment of PD and its comorbid disorders is the Childhood Anxiety Sensitivity Index (CASI; Silverman, Fleisig, Rabian, & Peterson, 1991; Silverman, Ginsburg, & Goedhart, 1999). Anxiety sensitivity is defined as the belief that anxiety or fear will cause negative events such as illness, incompetence, or embarrassment. In its simplest form, it refers to "fear of fear" (Reiss & McNally, 1985). Individuals with high anxiety sensitivity may be more likely to develop PD, because they tend to make more negative attributions about the symptoms of anxiety (see Hayward et al., 2000; Mattis & Ollendick,

1997a). As noted by Silverman and colleagues (1991), "Anxiety would be a more dreadful thing for those who believe that it can lead to severe consequences (e.g., a heart attack) than for those who do not" (p. 162). The CASI is a brief 18–item questionnaire; respondents are requested to indicate whether the item at hand disturbs them none, some, or a lot (e.g., "It scares me when I have trouble catching my breath," "It scares me when my heart beats fast"). Acceptable psychometric properties have been reported for children and adolescents ranging in age from 7 to 16 years (see King, Ollendick, & Murphy, 1997, for a review).

Many other self-report instruments evaluate numerous anxiety symptoms, including PD symptomatology. For example, the Fear Survey Schedule for Children–Revised (FSSC-R; Ollendick, 1983; Ollendick, King, & Frary, 1989; Weems, Silverman, Saavedra, Pina, & Lumpkin, 1999), the Revised Children's Manifest Anxiety Scale (RCMAS; Reynolds & Richmond, 1985), and the Beck Anxiety Inventory (BAI; Beck, Epstein, Brown, & Steer, 1988) all possess adequate psychometric properties and have been used productively with children and adolescents. Newer self-report instruments that show considerable promise include the Multidimensional Anxiety Scale for Children (MASC; March, Parker, Sullivan, Stallings, & Conners, 1997; March & Sullivan, 1999) and the Screen for Childhood Anxiety Related Disorders (SCARED; Birmaher et al., 1997, 1999; Khetarpal-Monga et al., 2000; Muris, Merckelbach, Gadet, Moulaert, & Tierney, 1999). Although both of these recently developed instruments have been found to be useful with children and adolescents, an added advantage of the SCARED is that it contains a parent version as well. Overall, the older self-report instruments, such as the FSSC-R, RCMAS, and BAI, evaluate general symptoms of fear and anxiety and are less specific for the assessment of anxiety symptoms that characterize specific disorders such as PD. Moreover, although these various self-reports have shown good psychometric properties, they have not been validated in large samples of children and adolescents with PD. Considerable more research is required to evaluate their clinical utility.

Self-Monitoring Forms

In addition to self-report instruments, we have found self-monitoring forms indispensable in our assessment and treatment of youngsters with PD. Self-monitoring requires the individual to first self-observe and then to systematically self-record occurrences of PAs and related PD phenomena. Use of such recording forms can help the clinician determine antecedent and consequent conditions associated with PAs, as well as their frequency, intensity, and duration. They can also be used to record youngsters' cognitions about the PAs and how they deal with the PAs on a regular basis. When self-monitoring procedures are used with children and adolescents, it is imperative that the behaviors to be recorded are well defined and that the recording procedures are not complicated or time-consuming. Recently, Ollendick (1995) successfully used such forms in the cognitive-behavioral treatment of adolescents with PD and agoraphobia (PDAG). In this study, each adolescent was provided with a Panic Attack Record (PAR) form (a simple index card) similar to that used by Rapee, Craske, and Barlow (1990) in their treatment of adults with PDAG. The adolescents were instructed to monitor the date, time, duration, location, circumstance, and symptoms experienced (the 13 *DSM-IV* symptoms of PAs) during their PAs. They were asked to record this information daily during the coming week. The PAR was reviewed at the beginning of each subsequent session, difficulties in monitoring were addressed, and the adolescent was requested to monitor attacks for the next week. These records, along with reports of self-efficacy for coping with panic in the various agoraphobic situations and reports of avoidance of the agoraphobic situations, were used to evaluate treatment outcome. In addition, these monitoring forms were used to adjust and monitor the treatment program itself. In this manner, treatment was self-correcting, allowing for maximal behavioral and cognitive change (see Mattis & Ollendick, 2002, and Ollendick, 1998, for additional detail on use of monitoring forms in clinical practice).

In brief, these interviews, questionnaires, and forms can be used to evaluate progress in treatment as well as treatment response following cessation of treatment. For example, presence of PD symptoms on the K-SADS or ADIS-C/P and a significant reduction in PD symptoms from self-report and self-monitoring forms (e.g., 50% reduction) can be determined. Other instruments that are used to evaluate the overall clinical and functional response, such as the Clinical Global Impression Scale (CGIS; Guy, 1976), have also been widely used. However, we are less confident of the reliability, validity, and clinical utility of these more global measures of change. Moreover, even if the symptoms have improved, it is imperative to assess the child's psychosocial and school functioning. General scales such as the Children's Global Assessment Scale (C-GAS; Shaffer et al., 1983) and Quality of Life Scales (see review by Mendlowicz & Stein, 2000) may prove productive and useful in this regard. It is important to evaluate the presence of other nonanxious psychiatric disorders that require different interventions, such as depressive, bipolar, and disruptive disorders. Finally, it is recommended to assess anticipated side effects before starting any pharmacological treatment, because parents and patients may attribute side effects to the medications, when in fact these somatic symptoms may be manifestations of the PD or other anxiety and mood disorders. We have found the Side Effects Form for Children and Adolescents (SEFCA; Klein et al., 1994) to be useful in this regard. Obviously, we believe that careful and ongoing assessment is a prerequisite to effective and evidence-based practice. We now turn our attention to the treatment of PD in youths.

TREATMENT

This section describes the psychosocial and pharmacological treatments for PD. Most of the studies in adults and all of the studies in youth so far published address the acute treatment of PD. Studies evaluating the effects of continuation (to avoid relapses) and maintenance (to avoid recurrences— new episodes) are scarce in the adult literature and nonexistent in the youth literature. Given the paucity of studies in youth, most of the recommendations described in this section are extrapolated from the adult literature. However, these recommendations need to be taken cautiously, because adult treatments do not always take into account developmental factors, and children may respond differently to psychological and psychopharmacological treatments than their adult counterparts do (Ollendick & Vasey, 1999).

Psychoeducation

For any treatment modality, education about the disorder is indicated. Patients and parents should be educated about the clinical characteristics, pathophysiology, longitudinal course, assessment, and treatment of PD. Psychoeducation can increase parents' and patients' compliance with treatment, reduction of anxiety, and improvement in the children's self-esteem (e.g., the children can understand that having PAs is not a sign of weakness) and family relationships (e.g., parents understand that their children are not pretending; parents may diminish the self-blame). Although no studies have been published on the effects of psychoeducation for parents and children with PD, for other disorders (depression, bipolar, schizophrenia), psychoeducation alone and in combination with active treatments has been found to be helpful (e.g., Brent, Poling, McKain, & Baugher, 1993).

Acute Treatment: Psychosocial Interventions

Effective psychosocial treatment models for the treatment of PD have been based largely on cognitive and cognitive-behavioral theories. The primary proponents of the cognitive model have been David Clark, Paul Salkovskis, and Aaron Beck (Beck & Emery, 1985; Clark, Salkovskis, & Chalkley, 1985; Salkovskis, Jones, & Clark, 1986). In its simplest form, this model suggests that the insidious spiral into panic is due to catastrophic misinterpretations of otherwise normal bodily sensations. Implicit in this theorizing is the notion that nothing particularly unique is occurring in the individual from a neurobiological perspective; rather, it is primarily a psychological account of the development and maintenance of panic. Mild chest pain experienced after exercise, for example, might be interpreted in an at-risk or psychologically vulnerable individual as an impending heart attack and as an indicator that the person might actually die. Individual differences in the tendency to misinterpret somatic events would differentiate the person who develops PAs from the person who does not. Persons high in anxiety sensitivity might more likely be vulnerable to the onset of PAs and eventual PD. Treatment, according to this model, consists largely of a mixture of cognitive techniques and behavioral experiments designed to modify the faulty misinterpretations of bodily sensations and the processes that maintain them. Considerable support for this cognitive model has been garnered in recent years for the treatment of PAs and PD, at least with adults (cf. Clark, 1996; Clark et al., 1999). To our knowledge, this approach has not been used or evaluated with children and adolescents.

The primary proponent of the cognitive-behavioral model has been David Barlow, and the treatment evolving from this perspective has come to be called *panic control treatment*. According to Barlow (1988), several risk factors are required in order for PAs and PD to develop. First, a person must have the tendency to be neurobiologically overreactive to stress. In particular, some individuals seem to react to the stress of negative life events with considerable apprehension, believing that some drastic or terrible thing will happen to them. Such apprehension leads to a fight-or-flight response that is, in all probability, triggered prematurely and unnecessarily (i.e., the response exceeds the stimulus event). Barlow refers to this premature, unnecessary, and extreme response as a false alarm. Over time, through a process of conditioning, false alarms become associated with bodily sensations (e.g., rapid heartbeat, difficulty breathing), and PAs may follow. Following repeated conditioning trials, the person becomes extremely sensitive to the physical sensations, so that even slight bodily changes associated with, for example, exercise or fatigue may trigger an alarm reaction and a resultant PA. Subsequently, the individual develops anxious apprehension over the possibility that future alarms or PAs will occur. This tendency to develop anxious apprehension is viewed as a psychological vulnerability that arises from developmental experiences with predictability and control. Finally, avoidance behavior may develop, depending on the person's coping skills and perceptions of safety. Treatment from this model is threefold: relaxation training and breathing retraining to address neurobiological sensitivities to stress, interoceptive exposure to address heightened somatic symptoms, and cognitive restructuring to address faulty misinterpretations associated with the somatic symptoms. In effect, this model consists of cognitive therapy (similar to that espoused by Beck, Clark, and Salkovskis) as well as behavioral therapy (breathing retraining, interoceptive exposure). Considerable support for this cognitive-behavioral model has been accumulated in recent years in the treatment of PAs and PD, especially with adults (Barlow, Gorman, Shear, & Woods, 2000; Barlow & Lehman, 1996).

Recently, Mattis and Ollendick (1997b) adapted Barlow's model of panic to children and suggested a pathway through which stressful separation experiences, combined with individual differences in temperament characteristics and attachment styles, might result in development of panic. In effect, they proposed that children respond to stressful separation experiences differently depending on their temperaments (in particular, behavioral inhibition) and the nature of their attachment relationships with significant adults (in particular, insecure-ambivalent/resistant relationships). Children who are characterized by this constellation of events are at high risk for the development of PAs and eventual PD. Inasmuch as these children have difficulty being soothed and comforted by their caregivers in times of stress (e.g., separations), they experience intense alarm reactions and have little sense of predictability or control over these stressors. These at-risk children learn to associate distress in such situations with physical or somatic symptoms (e.g., pounding heart, shaky hands), resulting in a cascade of false alarms. Next, as suggested by Mattis and Ollendick, the child begins to display anxious apprehension over the possibility of future alarms or PAs. Anxious apprehension is viewed as a psychological vulnerability, encapsulated in the notion of anxiety sensitivity (i.e., the development of fear of anxiety symptoms). PA symptoms are likely to occur when these at-risk children have little control over what will happen to them and little ability to predict what will happen to them. Agoraphobic avoidance develops when the children begin to withdraw from unfamiliar people and situations as a way of coping with and reducing their distress (Mattis & Ollendick, 2002).

Treatment studies based on Barlow's model and Mattis and Ollendick's adaptation of it have been sparse; however, two single-case studies lend initial support to its use, and one large-scale treatment outcome study appears promising. In the first study, Barlow and Seidner (1983) treated three adolescent agoraphobics with an early precursor of panic control treatment. The adolescents were treated in a 10-session group-therapy format and were accompanied by their mothers, who were enlisted to facilitate behavior change. Treatment consisted of panic management procedures, cognitive restructuring, and instructions to engage in structured homework sessions, which involved graduated exposure to feared situations. Parents were instructed on the nature of agoraphobia and procedures for dealing with anxiety that were neither reinforcing of anxiety-related behaviors nor punishing to the adolescent. Parents encouraged and supported their teens to practice between sessions and practiced with them at least once a week. Following treatment, two of the three adolescents showed marked improvement in their symptoms; however, the other adolescent did not show significant change. In fact, for this latter adolescent, treatment resulted in a slight increment in phobic avoidance. Barlow and Seidner argued that treatment outcome was related to level of parent-adolescent conflict; that is, for the two families in which a reasonably good parent-adolescent relationship was evident, treatment was successful, but for the remaining family, the presence of pronounced parent-adolescent conflict appeared to interfere with treatment outcome. Although this single-case study was uncontrolled and only two of the three adolescents responded positively, the treatment appeared promising.

In the second study, Ollendick (1995) used a controlled multiple baseline design across four adolescents with PDAG to illustrate the controlling effects of a version of panic control treatment. The adolescents ranged in age from 13 to 17 years of age; however, their PAs reportedly began when they were between 9 and 13 years of age—nearly 4 years, on average, prior to the beginning of treatment. Adolescents were treated individually but, as in Barlow and Seidner's (1983) study, their mothers were enlisted to facilitate behavior change. Treatment consisted of information about panic, relaxation training and breathing retraining, cognitive restructuring, interoceptive exposure, participant modeling (e.g., therapist and then parent demonstrating approach behavior in agoraphobic situations), in-vivo exposure, and praise and social reinforcement. Treatment varied in duration but lasted between 10 and 12 sessions. Treatment was effective for all four adolescents in eliminating PAs, reducing agoraphobic avoidance, decreasing accompanying negative mood states, and increasing self-efficacy for coping with previously avoided situations and PAs, should they occur in the future. Follow-up over a 6-month interval affirmed the lasting effects of the treatment. As noted by Ollendick, this single-case study design did not allow the mechanisms of change to be detected. Multiple cognitive-behavioral treatment components were used, and parents were recruited to facilitate and encourage change in their adolescents. Any one of these components, either alone or in concert with other components, might have been responsible for the changes observed. Future research will need to identify the effective ingredients in randomized clinical control trials with children and adolescents.

Presently, Mattis and her colleagues are undertaking a randomized controlled trial of a developmental adaptation of panic control treatment and a wait-list condition in the treatment of PD in adolescents. Three aspects of PD are addressed in this intervention: (1) the cognitive aspect of PD or the tendency to misinterpret physical sensations as catastrophic; (2) the tendency to hyperventilate or overbreathe, thus creating or intensifying physical sensations of panic; and (3) conditioned fear reactions to the physical sensations. Key components of treatment include correcting misinformation about panic, breathing retraining, cognitive restructuring, and interoceptive and in-vivo exposure. In the interoceptive exposure component of treatment, the adolescents are taught to face their primary fear, namely, the physical sensations of panic.

Exercises such as shaking one's head from side to side for 30 seconds, running in place for 1 minute, holding one's breath for 30 seconds, spinning in a chair for 1 minute, hyperventilating for 1 minute, and breathing through a thin straw for 2 minutes are used to facilitate exposure to the interoceptive physical sensations. Adolescents are informed that they will be learning different tools to address their panic and resultant anxiety. Specifically, "changing my breathing" is described as a tool for reducing the frequency and intensity of unwanted or undesired physical sensations; "being a detective" is introduced as the process of evaluating and changing anxious, worrisome, and nonproductive thoughts; and "facing my fears" is the strategy for reducing avoidance through interoceptive and graduated in-vivo exposure exercises. The adolescent is further informed that the goal of using these tools is to break the cycle of panic by reducing physical panic sensations, anxious thoughts, and avoidance, while also altering the relations among the components. For example, reducing physical sensations through breathing retraining will also change anxious thoughts associated with the sensations and, in turn, reduce the likelihood that avoidance of the situation will be necessary or desired. Twelve sessions, all manualized, are enacted. Although the randomized trial is still underway, initial findings clearly support the efficacy of this innovative adaptation of panic control treatment (Mattis, personal communication, March 2003).

At this time, it is obvious that psychosocial treatments have been used only sparingly with adolescents and not at all with children. The reasons for this state of affairs is not at all clear, especially since very similar procedures have been used effectively with children and adolescents with other forms of phobic and anxiety disorders (see Ollendick & King, 1998, 2000, for reviews). Many of these cognitive-behavioral treatments enjoy empirically validated status. It is perhaps even more alarming that no other psychosocial treatments (i.e., interpersonal psychotherapy, psychodynamic therapy, family therapy) have been evaluated with children and adolescents who present with PAs or PD. Clearly, the development and evaluation of psychosocial treatments for PAs and PD in children and adolescents are in an embryonic period and sorely in need of careful and systematic inquiry.

Acute Treatment: Pharmacological Interventions

There are no randomized controlled trials (RCTs) for the treatment of childhood-onset PD (Kutcher & Mackenzie, 1988). In adults, RCTs comparing the following classes of medications with placebo have been found efficacious for the treatment of PD: the selective serotonin reuptake inhibitors, or SSRIs (60% to 80% vs. 36% to 60%); the tricyclic antidepressants, or TCAs (45% to 70% vs. 15% to 50%); and the high-potency benzodiazepines (55% to 75% vs. 15% to 50%). The SSRIs have been the first choice, due to their easier administration and side effects profile, and they are much less dangerous in case of overdose. Although the monoamine oxidase inhibitors (MAOIs) are also efficacious for the treatment of PD in adults (APA, 1998), they are used mainly for patients who have not responded to any other treatments because of the risk of hypertensive crisis and dietary restrictions.

In children and adolescents, anecdotal case reports have shown that benzodiazepines (e.g., Biederman, 1987; Kutcher & Mackenzie, 1988; Lepola, Leinonen, & Koponen, 1996; Simeon & Ferguson, 1987; Simeon et al., 1992) and SSRIs (e.g., Fairbanks et al., 1997; Renaud, Birmaher, Wassick, & Bridge, 1999) may be effective in the treatment of children and adolescents with PD. For example, in a prospective open study, Renaud and colleagues (1999) treated 12 children and adolescents with PD with SSRIs for a period of 6 to 8 weeks. If necessary, a high-potency benzodiazepine was used temporarily. Patients were followed for 6 months and evaluated periodically with clinician-based and self-report rating scales for anxiety and depression, functioning, and side effects. Using the Clinical Global Improvement Scale (CGIS) as the outcome measure, 75% of patients showed much to very much improvement with SSRIs without experiencing significant side effects. After controlling for changes in depressive symptoms, self-report and clinician-based anxiety scales yielded similar results. At the end of the trial, eight patients (67%) no longer fulfilled criteria for PD, and four patients (33%) remained with significant residual symptoms.

On the basis of the adult literature, clinical experience, results of several open studies, and the fact that SSRIs have been found efficacious for the treatment of children and adolescents with other anxiety disorders (RUPP, 2001; Birmaher et al., 2003) and major depressive disorder (e.g., Emslie et al., 1997), it appears that SSRIs are a safe and promising treatment for children and adolescents with PD. However, RCTs evaluating the effects of SSRIs in youth are needed. Given the low prevalence of this disorder in children and adolescents, the participation of multiple centers would be required to have meaningful results.

Until these studies are carried out, based on our clinical experience and the adult literature, the first pharmacological treatment choice to treat PD in youngsters is SSRIs. These medications should be initiated with low doses (e.g., fluoxetine 5 mg/day, fluvoxamine 12.5 mg/day, paroxetine 10 mg/day, sertraline 25 mg/day) to avoid the potential exacerbation of panic symptoms that sometimes have been observed in adult patients with PD (e.g., APA, 1998). Starting with low doses also diminishes the risk of producing side effects, especially in patients who already are highly sensitive to experiencing somatic symptoms and whose parents usually also have anxiety disorders and may be overanxious about the appearance of any minor side effect.

It appears that for an appropriate acute trial, SSRIs should be administered for at least 12 weeks (APA, 1998). Patients who have not shown improvement within 6 to 8 weeks should be reevaluated with regard to diagnosis, compliance with treatment, and the presence of comorbid disorders or medical/neurological and psychosocial problems. These patients may require changes in medications, combination treatment with psychotherapy, or both (e.g., cognitive-behavioral therapy, as noted previously).

For patients who do not tolerate or respond to at least two trials with SSRIs, other types of medications that have been found useful for the treatment of adults with PD can be tried, such as venlafaxine, nefazodone, or the TCAs (APA, 1998). If TCAs are used, close monitoring of the patient's blood pressure, pulse, electrocardiogram, as well the development of other TCA side effects (e.g., anticholinergic effects), is needed.

As indicated previously, the high-potency benzodiazepines (e.g., alprazolam) are efficacious for the treatment of adults with PD (APA, 1998). However, due to the risk of developing tolerance and dependence after long-term benzodiazepine use, it is better to consider the temporal use of these medications for situations in which rapid control of symptoms is necessary (for example, a patient with frequent severe PAs who requires frequent visits to the medical or psychiatric emergency room, a child refusing to go to school because he or she is afraid to have a PA at school, or a patient with recurrent fainting episodes). When these circumstances occur, there is indication to combine the benzodiazepines with SSRIs, and after several weeks, to taper down the benzodiazepines for several weeks (e.g., 12 weeks) at rates no higher than 10% of the dose per week (APA, 1998). The benzodiazepines are generally contraindicated in patients with substance abuse. Because some SSRIs (e.g., fluvoxamine) may interfere with the benzodiazepines' metabolism and increase the patient's blood levels (Leonard, March, Rickler, & Allen, 1997), caution is recommended. In this case, lower doses of benzodiazepines may be sufficient.

PD usually is accompanied by other psychiatric disorders. Treatment of these comorbid conditions is essential to improve the patient's functioning. Fortunately, two of the common comorbid disorders, depression and other anxiety disorders, may also respond to SSRIs, CBT, or both (Birmaher et al., 1994; Birmaher et al., 2003; Brent et al., 1997; Emslie et al. 1997; Kendall et al., 1997; RUPP, 2001).

Finally, given that children and adolescents are dependent on their parents, that PD as well as other anxiety disorders and depression run in families (e.g., Biederman et al., 2001), and that parental psychiatric disorders may affect the treatment response and course of several psychiatric illnesses, it is important to offer treatment to parents as well.

Acute Treatment: Combined Interventions

To date, no controlled clinical trials have examined the joint efficacy of psychosocial and pharmacologic treatments. Given the independent promise of both treatments, however, there is reason to believe that synergistic effects will occur as has been evidenced in the treatment of other anxiety disorders with children and adolescents, as well as with adults. Still, research into their combined effects, such as the studies pursued with adult populations, is needed (e.g., Barlow et al., 2000) before firm conclusions can be offered.

Continuation and Maintenance Treatments

As with other psychiatric and medical illnesses, after achieving response to treatment for PD, it is important to continue the same treatment (CBT, medications, or both) to prevent relapses. During these phases, patients probably need to be seen less frequently, depending on their clinical status. Unfortunately, very little research in adults (APA, 1998) and none in youth have been conducted with regard to the continuation and maintenance treatment phases for PD. In adults, it has been recommended to continue the medications for at least 12 to 18 months. Thereafter, if the patient is judged to be stable, it has been recommended that medications be reduced very slowly to avoid withdrawal side effects that may mimic the relapse of PAs, and to avoid relapses or recurrences (APA, 1998). Some patients may require treatment for years.

Prevention

It has been proposed that children at risk of developing PD may have one or more of the following predisposing factors: (a) a temperamental vulnerability to developing anxiety disorders, (b) a tendency to worry too much or focus on somatic symptoms, (c) a predisposition to catastrophize (to make things seem worse than they are), and (d) a tendency to use avoidance behaviors to cope with stress(see Ollendick, 1998). If these conditions prove to be risk factors for the development of PD, certain interventions may be helpful to prevent PD relapses, recurrences, and new onsets. For example, group CBT interventions have been found efficacious for the prevention of new onset of major depression in school-age youth with subsyndromal symptoms of depression (Clarke, Rohde, Lewinsohn, Hops, & Seeley, 1999) and in the onset and development of subsyndromal symptoms of anxiety disorders (Dadds, Spence, Holland, Barrett, & Laurens, 1997). Similar interventions might well prove useful in the development and onset of PD in particular.

There are several groups of children and adolescents who appear be at risk of developing anxiety disorders, including PD, and for whom primary preventive interventions may be indicated. These children include the so-called behavioral-inhibited children (Kagan, Reznick, & Snidman, 1988); the offspring of parents who are anxious, depressed, or both—in particular, those of parents with early-onset PD (≤ 20 years old; Goldstein, Wickramaratne, Horwath, & Weissman, 1997); and, more controversially, children with separation anxiety disorder (Craske et al., 2001; Silove et al., 1996).

Behavioral inhibition occurs in 10% to 15% of Caucasian children and is manifested by the tendency to withdraw, to seek a parent, and to inhibit play and vocalization following encounters with unfamiliar events or people (Kagan et al., 1988). As toddlers, these children are introverted and quiet, with increased vigilance and reduced exploratory behavior. In comparison with uninhibited children, these children have low thresholds for arousal in the amygdala and hypothalamic circuits, resulting in increased sympathetic arousal (Hirshfeld et al., 1992). Parents of children with behavioral inhibition usually have anxiety disorders, including PD (Biederman et al., 1990). Conversely, offspring of parents with PD and agoraphobia have high rates of behavioral inhibition. Children with *persistent* behavioral inhibition have higher rates of anxiety disorders than children who are not inhibited and children who do not show persistent inhibition (Biederman et al., 1990; Hirshfeld et al., 1992).

Children who have high stress reactivity, poor self-regulatory ability, and failure to regulate distress through caregiver contact are at high risk of experiencing high stress reactivity in situations where escape is blocked or difficult. After repeated experiences of separation, these children may conceptualize separation and associated alarms as frightening experiences and develop anxious apprehension over the possibility that they will recur with time, leading to increased anxiety sensitivity and anxious attributions of internal responsibility for the negative outcomes associated with these experiences (Mattis & Ollendick, 1997a; Ollendick, 1998). Finally, avoidance (agoraphobia, separation anxiety) may occur in the absence of safety signals (a secure base), effective coping skills, and self-efficacy for the mastery of such stressful situations (Ollendick, 1995).

CONCLUSIONS

The study of PAs and PD in children and adolescence is truly in its own stage of early development. Although it was initially thought that children could not develop PAs and PD due to cognitive limitations, it now seems clear that children (and adolescents) can and do develop these disorders. Moreover, as with adults, these disorders are frequently comorbid with other anxiety and affective disorders and, albeit less frequently, comorbid with externalizing disorders such as substance abuse and conduct disturbance. The effects of these disorders on the developing child are considerable; many of these children experience academic, behavioral, emotional, and social difficulties. Still, the developmental course of PD is poorly understood at this time and is need of careful examination and inquiry. Presently, promising assessment devices including psychiatric diagnostic interviews, behavior rating scales, self-report instruments, and self-monitoring and behavioral observation forms exist for the study of these children and adolescents. Treatment, especially treatment guided by a stages-of-treatment model, is not well established at this time. As in the assessment arena, promising psychosocial and pharmacological interventions exist. However, RCTs with children and adolescents are lacking, and little has been done in terms of the combination of psychosocial and pharmacological treatments. Hence, although we know much about PAs and PD in children and adolescents, much remains to be learned.

REFERENCES

Alessi, N. E., & Magen, J. (1988). Panic disorders in psychiatrically hospitalized children. *American Journal of Psychiatry, 145,* 1450–1452.

Alessi, N. E., Robbins, D. R., & Dilsaver, S. C. (1987). Panic and depressive disorders among psychiatrically hospitalized adolescents. *Psychiatry Research, 20,* 275–283.

American Psychiatric Association. (1994). *Diagnostic and statistical manual of mental disorders: DSM-IV* (4th ed.). Washington, DC: Author.

American Psychiatric Association. (1998). Practice guidelines for the treatment of patients with panic disorder. *American Journal of Psychiatry, 155,* 1–34.

Barlow, D. H. (1988). *Anxiety and its disorders: The nature and treatment of anxiety and panic.* New York: Guilford Press.

Barlow, D. H., Gorman, J. M., Shear, M. K., & Woods, S. W. (2000). Cognitive-behavioral therapy, imipramine, or their combination for panic disorder: A randomized controlled trial. *Journal of the American Medical Association, 283*(19), 2529–2536.

Barlow, D. H., & Lehman, C. L. (1996). Advances in the psychosocial treatment of anxiety disorders: Implications for national health care. *Archives of General Psychiatry, 53,* 727–735.

Barlow, D. H., & Seidner, A. L. (1983). Treatment of adolescent agoraphobics: Effects on parent-adolescent relations. *Behaviour Research and Therapy, 21,* 519–526.

Battaglia, M., Bertella, S., Bajo, S., Binaghi, F., & Bellodi, L. (1998). Anticipation of age at onset in panic disorder. *American Journal of Psychiatry, 155,* 590–595.

Beck, A. T., & Emery, G. (1985). *Anxiety disorders and phobias: A cognitive perspective.* Philadelphia: Center for Cognitive Therapy.

Beck, A. T., Epstein, N., Brown, G., & Steer, R. A. (1988). An inventory for measuring clinical anxiety: Psychometric properties. *Journal of Consulting and Clinical Psychology, 56,* 893–897.

Biederman, J. (1987). Clonazepam in the treatment of prepubertal children with panic-like symptoms. *Journal of Clinical Psychiatry, 48*(Suppl.), 38–41.

Biederman, J., Faraone, S. V., Hirshfeld-Becker, D. R., Friedman, D., Robin, J. A., & Rosenbaum, J. F. (2001). Patterns of psychopathology and dysfunction in high-risk children of parents with panic disorder and major depression. *American Journal of Psychiatry, 158*(1), 49–57.

Biederman, J., Faraone, S. V., Marrs, A., Moore, P., Garcia, J., Ablon, S., Mick, E., et al. (1997). Panic disorder and agoraphobia in consecutively referred children and adolescents. *Journal of the American Academy of Child and Adolescent Psychiatry, 36,* 214–223.

Biederman, J., Rosenbaum, J. F., Hirshfeld, D. R., Faraone, S. V., Bolduc, E. A., Gersten, M., Meminger, S. R., et al. (1990). Psychiatric correlates of behavioral inhibition in young children of parents with and without psychiatric disorders. *Archives of General Psychiatry, 47,* 21–26.

Birmaher, B., Axelson, D. A., Monk, K., Kalas, C., Clark, D. B., Ehmann, M., Bridge, J., Heo, J., & Brent, D. A. (2003). Fluoxetine for childhood anxiety disorders. *Journal of the American Academy of Child and Adolescent Psychiatry, 42*(4), 415–423.

Birmaher, B., Brent, D. A., Chiappetta, L., Bridge, J., Monga, S., & Baugher, M. (1999). Psychometric properties of the Screen for Child Anxiety Related Emotional Disorders (SCARED): A replication study. *Journal of the American Academy of Child and Adolescent Psychiatry, 38,* 1230–1236.

Birmaher, B., Kennah, A., Brent, D., Ehmann, M., Bridge, J., & Axelson, D. (2002). Is bipolar disorder specifically associated with panic disorder in youths? *Journal of Clinical Psychiatry, 63*(5), 414–419.

Birmaher, B., Khetarpal, S., Brent, D. A., Cully, M., Balach, L., Kaufman, J., McKenzie-Neer, S. (1997). The Screen for Child Anxiety Related Emotional Disorders (SCARED): Scale construction and psychometric characteristics. *Journal of the American Academy of Child and Adolescent Psychiatry, 36*(4), 545–553.

Birmaher, B., Waterman, G. S., Ryan, N. D., Cully, M., Balach, L., Ingram, J., & Brodsky, M. (1994). Fluoxetine for childhood anxiety disorders. *Journal of the American Academy of Child and Adolescent Psychiatry, 33,* 993–999.

Bowen, R., South, M., & Hawkes, J. (1994). Mood swings in patients with panic disorder. *Canadian Journal of Psychiatry, 39*, 91–94.

Brent, D. A., Holder, D., Kolko, D., Birmaher, B., Baugher, M., Roth, C., Iyengar, S., et al. (1997). A clinical psychotherapy trial for adolescent depression comparing cognitive, family, and supportive therapy. *Archives of General Psychiatry, 54*, 877–885.

Brent, D. A., Poling, K., McKain, B., & Baugher, M. (1993). A psychoeducational program for families of affectively ill children and adolescents. *Journal of the American Academy of Child & Adolescent Psychiatry, 32*, 770–774.

Chambers, W. J., Puig-Antich, J., Hirsch, M., Paez, P., Ambrosini, P. J., Tabrizi, M. A., & Davies, M. (1985). The assessment of affective disorders in children and adolescents by semistructured interview: Test-retest reliability of the Schedule for Affective Disorders and Schizophrenia for School-age Children, Present Episode Version. *Archives of General Psychiatry, 42*, 696–702.

Chen, Y.-W., & Dilsaver, S. C. (1995). Comorbidity of panic disorder in bipolar illness: Evidence from the Epidemiologic Catchment Area Survey. *American Journal of Psychiatry, 152*, 280–282.

Clark, D. B., & Donovan, J. E. (1994). Reliability and validity of the Hamilton Anxiety Rating Scale in an adolescent sample. *Journal of the American Academy of Child and Adolescent Psychiatry, 33*, 354–360.

Clark, D. M. (1996). Panic disorder: From theory to therapy. In P. M. Salkovskis (Ed.), *Frontiers of cognitive therapy* (pp. 318–344). New York: Guilford Press.

Clark, D. M., Salkovskis, P. M., & Chalkley, A. J. (1985). Respiratory control as a treatment for panic attacks. *Journal of Behavior Therapy and Experimental Psychiatry, 16*, 23–30.

Clark, D. M., Salkovskis, P. M., Hackmann, A., Wells, A., Ludgate, J., & Gelder, M. (1999). Brief cognitive therapy for panic disorder: A randomized controlled trial. *Journal of Consulting and Clinical Psychology, 67*, 583–589.

Clarke, G. N., Rohde, P., Lewinsohn, P. M., Hops, H., & Seeley, J. R. (1999). Cognitive-behavioral treatment of adolescent depression: Efficacy of acute group treatment and booster sessions. *Journal of the American Academy of Child and Adolescent Psychiatry, 38*, 272–279.

Craske, M. G., Poulton, R., Tsao, J. C. I., & Plogkin, D. (2001). Paths to panic disorder/agoraphobia: An exploratory analysis from age 3 to 21 in an unselected birth cohort. *Journal of the American Academy of Child and Adolescent Psychiatry, 40*, 556–563.

Dadds, M. R., Spence, S. H., Holland, D. E., Barrett, P. M., & Laurens, K. R. (1997). Prevention and early intervention for anxiety disorders: A controlled trial. *Journal of Consulting and Clinical Psychology, 65*, 627–635.

Edelbrock, C. S., & Costello, A. J. (1985). Validity of the NIMH Diagnostic Interview Schedule for Children: A comparison between psychiatric and pediatric referrals. *Journal of Abnormal Child Psychology, 13*(4), 579–595.

Emslie, G. J., Rush, A. J., Weinberg, W. A., Kowatch, R. A., Hughes, C. W., Carmody, T., & Rintelmann, J. (1997). A double-blind, randomized, placebo-controlled trial of fluoxetine in children and adolescents with depression. *Archives of General Psychiatry, 54*, 1031–1037.

Essau, C. A., Conradt, J., & Petermann, F. (1999). Frequency of panic attacks and panic disorder in adolescents. *Depression and Anxiety, 9*, 19–26.

Essau, C. A., Conradt, J., & Petermann, F. (2000). Frequency, comorbidity, and psychosocial impairment of anxiety disorders in German adolescents. *Journal of Anxiety Disorders, 14,* 263–279.

Fairbanks, J. M., Pine, D. S., Tancer, N. K., Dummit, E. S., III, Kentgen, L. M., Asche, B. K., & Klein, R. G. (1997). Open fluoxetine treatment of mixed anxiety disorders in children and adolescents. *Journal of the American Academy of Child and Adolescent Psychiatry, 7,* 17–29.

Ginsburg, G. S., & Drake, K. L. (2002). Anxiety sensitivity and panic attack symptomatology among low-income African-American adolescents. *Journal of Anxiety Disorders, 16*(1), 83–96.

Goldstein, R. B., Wickramaratne, P. J., Horwath, E., & Weissman, M. M. (1997). Familial aggregation and phenomenology of "early"-onset (at or before age 20 years) panic disorder. *Archives of General Psychiatry, 54,* 271–278.

Guy, W. (1976). *ECDEU Assessment Manual of Psychopharmacology.* DHEW Publication ADM 76–338. Rockville, MD: National Institute of Mental Health, Psychopharmacology Research Branch.

Hayward, C., Killen, J. D., Hammer, L. D., Litt, I. F., Wilson, D. M., Simmonds, B., & Taylor, C. B. (1992). Pubertal stage and panic attack history in sixth- and seventh-grade girls. *American Journal of Psychiatry, 149,* 1239–1243.

Hayward, C., Killen, J. D., Kraemer, H. C., & Barr Taylor, C. (2000). Predictors of panic attacks in adolescents. *Journal of the American Academy of Child and Adolescent Psychiatry, 39,* 207–214.

Hayward, C., Killen, J. D., Kraemer, H. C., Blair-Greiner, A., Strachowski, D., Cunning, D., & Barr Taylor, C. (1997). Assessment and phenomenology of nonclinical panic attacks in adolescent girls. *Journal of Anxiety Disorders, 11,* 17–32.

Hayward, C., Killen, J. D., & Taylor, C. B. (1989). Panic attacks in young adolescents. *American Journal of Psychiatry, 146,* 1061–1062.

Herskowitz, J. (1986). Neurologic presentations of panic disorder in childhood and adolescence. *Developmental Medicine and Child Neurology, 28,* 617–623.

Hirshfeld, D. R., Rosenbaum, J. F., Biederman, J., Bolduc, E. A., Faraone, S. V., Snidman, N., Reznick, J. S., & Kagan, J. (1992). Stable behavioral inhibition and its association with anxiety disorder. *Journal of the American Academy of Child and Adolescent Psychiatry, 31,* 103–111.

Horesh, N., Amir, M., Kedem, P., Goldberger, Y., & Kotler, M. (1997). Life events in childhood, adolescence and adulthood and the relationship to panic disorder. *Acta Psychiatrica Scandinavica, 96,* 373–378.

Kagan, J., Reznick, J. S., & Snidman, N. (1988). Biological bases of childhood shyness. *Science, 240,* 167–171.

Kaufman, J., Birmaher, B., Brent, D. A., Rao, U., Flynn, C., Moreci, P., Williamson, D., et al. (1997). Schedule for Affective Disorders and Schizophrenia for School-Age Children–Present and Lifetime Version (K-SADS-PL): Initial reliability and validity data. *Journal of the American Academy of Child and Adolescent Psychiatry, 36,* 980–988.

Kearney, C. A., Albano, A. M., Eisen, A. R., Allan, W. D., & Barlow, D. H. (1997). The phenomenology of panic disorder in youngsters: An empirical study of a clinical sample. *Journal of Anxiety Disorders, 11,* 49–62.

Kendall, P. C., Flannery-Schroeder, E., Panichelli-Mindel, S., Southam-Gerow, M., Henin, A., & Warman, M. (1997). Therapy for youth with anxiety disorders: A second randomized clinical trial. *Journal of Consulting and Clinical Psychology, 65,* 366–380.

Khetarpal-Monga, S., Birmaher, B., Chiappetta, L., Brent, D., Kaufman, J., Bridge, J., & Cully, M. (2000). The screen for child anxiety related emotional disorders (SCARED): Convergent and divergent validity, *Depression and Anxiety, 12,* 85–91.

King, N. J., Gullone, E., Tonge, B. J., & Ollendick, T. H. (1993). Self-reports of panic attacks and manifest anxiety in adolescents. *Behaviour Research and Therapy, 31,* 111–116.

King, N. J., Ollendick, T. H., Mattis, S. G., Yang, B., & Tonge, B. (1997). Nonclinical panic attacks in adolescents: Prevalence, symptomatology and associated features. *Behaviour Change, 13,* 171–183.

King, N. J., Ollendick, T. H., & Murphy, G. C. (1997). Assessment of childhood phobias. *Clinical Psychology Review, 17,* 667–687.

King, N. J., Ollendick, T. H., Murphy, G. C., & Tonge, B. (1997). Behavioural assessment of childhood phobias: A multimethod approach. *Scandinavian Journal of Behaviour Therapy, 26,* 3–10.

Klein, R. G., Abikoff, H., Barkley, R. A., Campbell, M., Leckman, J. F., Ryan, N. D., Solanto, M. V., et al. (1994). Clinical trials in children and adolescents. In R. F. Prien & D. S. Robinson (Eds.), *Clinical evaluation of psychotropic drugs: Principles and guidelines* (pp. 501–546). New York: Raven Press.

Kushner, M. G., Clayton, P. J., Crow, S., & Knopman, D. (2000). Seizure disorder is in the differential diagnosis of panic disorder. *Psychosomatics, 41,* 436–438.

Kutcher, S., & Mackenzie, S. (1988). Successful clonazepam treatment of adolescents with panic disorder. *Journal of Clinical Psychopharmacology, 8,* 299–301.

Last, C. G., & Strauss, C. C. (1989). Panic disorder in children and adolescents. *Journal of Anxiety Disorders, 3,* 87–95.

Lau, J. J., Calamari, J. E., & Waraczynski, M. (1996). Panic attack symptomatology and anxiety sensitivity in adolescents. *Journal of Anxiety Disorders, 10,* 355–364.

Leonard, H. L., March, J., Rickler, K. C., & Allen, A. J. (1997). Pharmacology of the selective serotonin reuptake inhibitors in children and adolescents. *Journal of the American Academy of Child and Adolescent Psychiatry, 36,* 725–736.

Lepola, U., Leinonen, E., & Koponen, H. (1996). Citalopram in the treatment of early-onset panic disorder and school phobia. *Pharmacopsychiatry, 29,* 30–32.

Lewinsohn, P. M., Klein, D. N., & Seeley, J. R. (1995). Bipolar disorders in a community sample of older adolescents: Prevalence, phenomenology, comorbidity, and course. *Journal of the American Academy of Child and Adolescent Psychiatry, 34,* 454–463.

Macaulay, J. L., & Kleinknecht, R. A. (1989). Panic and panic attacks in adolescents. *Journal of Anxiety Disorders, 3,* 221–241.

March, J. S., Parker, J., Sullivan, K., Stallings, P., & Conners, C. K. (1997). The Multidimensional Anxiety Scale for Children (MASC): Factor structure, reliability, and validity. *Journal of the American Academy of Child and Adolescent Psychiatry, 36,* 554–565.

March, J. S., & Sullivan, K. (1999). Test-retest reliability of the Multidimensional Anxiety Scale for Children. *Journal of Anxiety Disorders, 13,* 349–358.

Mattis, S. G., & Ollendick, T. H. (1997a). Children's cognitive responses to the somatic symptoms of panic. *Journal of Abnormal Child Psychology, 25,* 47–57.

Mattis, S. G., & Ollendick, T. H. (1997b). Panic in children and adolescents: A developmental analysis. In T. H. Ollendick & R. J. Prinz (Eds.), *Advances in clinical child psychology* (Vol. 19, pp. 27–74). New York: Plenum Press.

Mattis, S. G., & Ollendick, T. H. (2002). *Panic disorder and anxiety in adolescents.* London: British Psychological Society.

Mendlowicz, M. V., & Stein, M. B. (2000). Quality of life in individuals with anxiety disorders. *American Journal of Psychiatry, 157,* 669–682.

Moreau, D. L., & Follet, C. (1993). Panic disorder in children and adolescents. *Child and Adolescent Psychiatric Clinics of North America, 2,* 581–602.

Moreau, D. L., & Weissman, M. M. (1992). Panic disorder in children and adolescents: A review. *American Journal of Psychiatry, 149,* 1306–1314.

Muris, P., Merckelbach, H., Gadet, B., Moulaert, V., & Tierney, S. (1999). Sensitivity of the Screen for Child Anxiety Related Emotional Disorders. *Journal of Psychopathology and Behavioral Assessment, 21,* 323–335.

Nelles, W. B., & Barlow, D. H. (1988). Do children panic? *Clinical Psychology Review, 8,* 359–372.

Norton, G. R., Dorward, J., & Cox, B. J. (1986). Factors associated with panic attacks in nonclinical subjects. *Behavior Therapy, 17,* 239–252.

Ollendick, T. H. (1983). Reliability and validity of the Revised Fear Survey Schedule for Children (FSSC-R). *Behaviour Research and Therapy, 21,* 685–692.

Ollendick, T. H. (1995). Cognitive-behavioral treatment of panic disorder with agoraphobia in adolescents: A multiple baseline design analysis. *Behavior Therapy, 26,* 517–531.

Ollendick, T. H. (1998). Panic disorder in children and adolescents: New developments, new directions. *Journal of Clinical Child Psychology, 27,* 234–245.

Ollendick, T. H., & King, N. J. (1994). Assessment and treatment of internalizing problems: The role of longitudinal data. *Journal of Consulting and Clinical Psychology, 62,* 918–927.

Ollendick, T. H., & King, N. J. (1998). Empirically supported treatments for children with phobic and anxiety disorders: Current status. *Journal of Clinical Child Psychology, 27,* 156–167.

Ollendick, T. H., & King, N. J. (2000). Empirically supported treatments for children and adolescents. In P. C. Kendall (Ed.), *Child and adolescent therapy: Cognitive-behavioral procedures* (2nd ed., pp. 386–425). New York: Guilford Press.

Ollendick, T. H., King, N. J., & Frary, R. (1989). Fears in children and adolescents: Reliability and generalizability across gender, age, and nationality. *Behaviour Research and Therapy, 27,* 19–26.

Ollendick, T. H., Mattis, S. G., & King, N. J. (1994). Panic in children and adolescents: a review. *Journal of Child Psychology and Psychiatry, 35,* 113–134.

Ollendick, T. H., & Vasey, M. W. (1999). Developmental theory and the practice of clinical child psychology. *Journal of Clinical Child Psychology, 28,* 457–466.

Pine, D. S., Cohen, P., Gurley, D., Brook, J., & Ma, Y. (1998). The risk for early-adulthood anxiety and depressive disorders in adolescents with anxiety and depressive disorders. *Archives of General Psychiatry, 55,* 56–64.

Pollack, M. H., Otto, M. W., Sabatino, S., Majcher, D., Worthington, J. J., McArdle, E. T., & Rosenbaum, J. F. (1996). The relationship of childhood anxiety to adult panic disorder: Correlates and influence on course. *American Journal of Psychiatry, 153,* 376–381.

Rapee, R. M., Craske, M. G., & Barlow, D. H. (1990). Subject-described features of panic attacks using self-monitoring. *Journal of Anxiety Disorders, 4,* 171–181.

Reiss, S., & McNally, R. J. (1985). The expectancy model of fear. In S. Reiss & R. R. Bootzin (Eds.), *Theoretical issues in behavior therapy*. New York: Academic Press.

Renaud, J., Birmaher, B., Wassick, S. C., & Bridge, J. (1999). Use of selective serotonin reuptake inhibitors for the treatment of childhood panic disorder: A pilot study. *Journal of Child and Adolescent Psychopharmacology, 9,* 73–83.

Reynolds, C. R., & Richmond, B. O. (1985). *Revised Children's Manifest Anxiety Scale (RCMAS) Manual*. Los Angeles: Western Psychological Services.

RUPP [Research Units on Pediatric Psychopharmacology Anxiety Study Group] (2001). Fluvoxamine for the treatment of anxiety disorders in children and adolescents. *New England Journal of Medicine, 344*(17), 1279–1285.

RUPP [Research Units on Pediatric Psychopharmacology Anxiety Study Group] (2002). The Pediatric Anxiety Rating Scale (PARS): Development and psychometric properties. *Journal of the American Academy of Child and Adolescent Psychiatry, 41,* 1061–1069.

Salkovskis, P. M., Jones, D. R. O., & Clark, D. M. (1986). Respiratory control in the treatment of panic attacks: Replication and extension with concurrent measurement of behaviour and CO_2. *British Journal of Psychiatry, 148,* 526–532.

Shaffer, D., Fisher, P., Dulcan, M. K., Davies, M., Piacentini, J., Schwab-Stone, M. E., Lahey, B. B., et al. (1996). The NIMH Diagnostic Interview Schedule for Children Version 2.3 (DISC-2.3): Description, acceptability, prevalence rates, and performance in the MECA study. *Journal of the American Academy of Child and Adolescent Psychiatry, 35,* 865–877.

Shaffer, D., Gould, M. S., Brasic, J., Ambrosini, P., Fisher, P., Bird, H., & Aluwahlia, S. (1983). A children's global assessment scale (C-GAS). *Archives of General Psychiatry, 40,* 1228–1231.

Shear, K. M., Brown, T. A., Barlow, D. H., Money, R., Sholomskas, D. E., Woods, S. W., Gorman, J. M., et al. (1997). Multicenter Collaborative Panic Disorder Severity Scale. *American Journal of Psychiatry, 154,* 1571–1575.

Silove, D., Manicavasagar, V., Curtis, J., & Blaszczynski, A. (1996). Is early separation anxiety a risk factor for adult panic disorder? A critical review. *Comprehensive Psychiatry, 37,* 167–179.

Silverman, W. K., & Albano, A. M. (1996). *Anxiety Disorders Interview Schedule for DSM-IV*. San Antonio, TX: Graywind Publications/Psychological Corporation.

Silverman, W. K., Fleisig, W., Rabian, B., & Peterson, R. A. (1991). Childhood Anxiety Sensitivity Index. *Journal of Clinical Child Psychology, 20,* 162–168.

Silverman, W. K., Ginsburg, G. S., & Goedhart, A. W. (1999). Factor structure of the Childhood Anxiety Sensitivity Index. *Behaviour Research and Therapy, 37,* 903–917.

Simeon, J., & Ferguson, B. (1987). Alprazolam effects in children with anxiety disorders. *Canadian Journal of Psychiatry, 32,* 570–574.

Simeon, J., Ferguson, B., Knott, V., Roberts, N., Gauthier, B., Dubois, C., & Wiggins, D. (1992). Clinical, cognitive and neurophysiological effects of alprazolam in children with overanxious and avoidant disorders. *Journal of the American Academy of Child and Adolescent Psychiatry, 31,* 29–33.

Strauss, J., Birmaher, B., Bridge, J., Axelson, D., Chiappetta, L., Brent, D., & Ryan, N. (2000). Anxiety disorders in suicidal youth. *Canadian Journal of Psychiatry, 45*(8), 739–745.

Thyer, B. A., Parrish, R. T., Curtis, G. C., Nesse, R. M., & Cameron, O. G. (1985). Ages of onset of *DSM-III* anxiety disorders. *Comprehensive Psychiatry, 26,* 113–122.

Von Korff, M., Eaton, W., & Keyl, P. (1985). The epidemiology of panic attacks and panic disorder: Results of three community surveys. *American Journal of Epidemiology, 122,* 970–981.

Weems, C. F., Silverman, W. K., Saavedra, L. M., Pina, A. A., & Lumpkin, P. W. (1999). The discrimination of children's phobias using the Revised Fear Survey Schedule for Children. *Journal of Child Psychology & Psychiatry & Allied Disciplines, 40,* 941–952.

Weissman, M. M., Bland, R. C., Canino, G. J., Faravelli, C., Greenwald, S., Hwu, H., Joyce, P. R., et al. (1997). The cross-national epidemiology of panic disorder. *Archives of General Psychiatry, 54,* 305–309.

World Health Organization. (1992–1994). ICD-10: International statistical classification of diseases and related health problems (10th rev.). Geneva, Switzerland: Author.

12

GENERALIZED ANXIETY DISORDER

Philip C. Kendall, Sandra Pimentel,
Moira A. Rynn, Aleta Angelosante,
& Alicia Webb

Sarah, an 11-year-old in fifth grade, was known for noticing the little things. She also anticipated unfavorable outcomes and, until her friends called her weird, she would often speculate that there was risk around the next corner. Sarah worried about saving receipts from purchases, the unfairness of the U.S. voting system, and the one time that she stepped on and killed a bug. She frequently experienced stomachaches and headaches and frequently had trouble falling asleep. Because Sarah would get wrapped up in her thoughts and conversations about these and other experiences, she found that she was afraid to try new things, intolerant of uncertainty, and that she was becoming the kid who was less likely to be called by friends.

Generalized anxiety disorder (GAD) is the manifestation of excessive worry in one or more areas of one's life. Others often see children with GAD as "little adults" because their worries may focus on keeping schedules, family finances, relationships, and perfectionism—themes that are more typically concerns for adults. Such children may not be disruptive or acting-out in their behavior, so their difficulties may go unnoticed by parents, family, and teachers. However, some of these children may show their distress through temper tantrums, especially when faced with unexpected changes in plans. Their internal distress interferes with their overall adjustment. This chapter describes the phenomenon of GAD in children and discusses useful assessment tools and therapies (both pharmacotherapy and psychotherapy) for the identification and treatment of this disorder.

CLINICAL FEATURES

Children with GAD often express worries about topics considered more typical of adult concern. Such worries can include punctuality, the health and safety of self and family members, and catastrophic events such as hurricanes or war. These children may also exhibit perfectionistic behavior, for example, meticulously doing and even redoing minor assignments (e.g., making a list, homework) until they feel that these are perfect. Unfortunately, as many of these worries and behaviors may be valued by parents, teachers, and other adults (who view such a child as simply more mature or diligent than most), these patterns may be encouraged by adults' inadvertently reinforcing them. Although they can be adaptive for some, when these patterns interfere with other aspects of maturation and adjustment, they become a clinical concern.

Other characteristic concerns of children with GAD include excessive worry about more typical kid stuff. These concerns often involve their competencies in academic, social, or athletic domains, even if they are not being evaluated. These children may be extremely self-conscious, often seeking excessive reassurance. Reassurance-seeking behavior can inhibit performance, because children may not be able to move forward during a task without constant feedback that they are doing well.

Whether the child is displaying adult concerns or more age-appropriate ones, the child with GAD may be very compliant and conforming; though unlikely to display disruptive behavior, he or she can become oppositional when stressed. Moreover, many of the features of GAD (e.g., perfectionism, timeliness, academic or social concerns) are socially desirable in modest quantities. These attributes can make the detection of GAD in children somewhat difficult. Most often, children are not brought in for treatment by their parents until they begin to display excessive distress or their academic or social functioning begins to falter.

Somatic complaints are another element of GAD in children. These children may experience excessive headaches, muscle aches, sleep disturbance, restlessness, or gastrointestinal distress for which no medical explanation can be found (Eisen & Engler, 1995; Kendall & Pimentel, 2003). Anxiety is often associated with physiological symptoms, usually related to the autonomic nervous system. These symptoms are similar to those mentioned above but can also include enuresis, sweating, and jitteriness (Barrios & Hartmann, 1988; Kendall et al., 1991).

DIAGNOSIS AND CLASSIFICATION

In the *Diagnostic and Statistical Manual of Mental Disorders: DSM-IV* (American Psychiatric Association [APA], 1994), the prior category of overanxious disorder (OAD) has been reclassified as GAD. Further, the broad categorization of "anxiety disorders of childhood or adolescence" no longer exists. Despite these organizational changes, there is evidence for diagnostic consistency between OAD and GAD (Kendall & Warman, 1996).

The hallmark symptom of GAD is unrealistic or excessive worry for a minimum of 6 months. This anxious distress must be present on more days than not and must encompass a variety of domains, including (among others) academic or athletic performance, social interaction, and health concerns. The child must find this worry difficult to control—for example, being unable to be soothed either by parental reassurance or distraction with pleasurable activities. Whereas adults must exhibit at least three somatic symptoms, children must exhibit only one physical symptom, such as sleep disturbance, muscle tension, irritability, concentration difficulties, fatigue, or restlessness. Recent data (Kendall & Pimentel, 2003) document that GAD youth report many of these somatic symptoms. Also of interest, both diagnostically and clinically, are the findings that (a) children diagnosed with GAD and their parents do not necessarily agree on the presence or absence of specific somatic symptoms experienced by the child, and (b) parents endorse significantly more somatic symptoms than their GAD children. Because the physical symptom criteria were developed with adults in mind, headaches and stomachaches (common somatic complaints among GAD children) are, unfortunately, not listed as relevant criteria. Further examination of the GAD criteria as applied to children (or as defined by children—the developmental expression of the GAD) is suggested for future editions of the *DSM*—an important step, given that the specific criteria needed for the diagnosis are the same for children as for adults, with the exception of somatic symptoms.

ASSOCIATED FEATURES

In addition to clinical features and diagnostic criteria, children with GAD also have some behavioral and cognitive similarities they share in common. In the behavioral realm, these children engage in a great deal of avoidance. For instance, children who attended our clinic (the Child and Adolescent Anxiety Disorders Clinic [CAADC] at Temple University) endorsed many of the following: avoidance of schoolwork for fear of making mistakes, avoidance of school for fear of social or academic evaluation, and avoidance of sports or group activities due to excessive doubts about their abilities (Kendall, Krain, & Treadwell, 1999). In addition, these children reported frequenting the school nurse's office with somatic complaints, attempting to use somatic complaints to avoid tests or other evaluative activities, and asking an unreasonable number of questions about upcoming events.

In the cognitive realm, children with GAD evidence thought processes that may be described as distorted. For example, they may catastrophize or exaggerate the importance of even minor events. A middle school–aged child may become extremely distressed about a "bad" (average) grade on a test. Rather than experiencing mere disappointment, to the GAD child, the grade becomes evidence of incompetence that can snowball into worries and expectations of present and future failure (e.g., not getting into the college of his or her choice). Perfectionism appears related to these distorted cognitive processes, wherein even the smallest error can be equated with widespread failure. To prevent disaster, therefore, the child thinks he or she must make perfect all homework and extensively prepare for every test. Excessive reassurance-seeking seems also to run parallel, as such children need frequent reassurance that they are doing well in order to accomplish tasks. Without such reassurance, they may be unable to advance through the required steps to completion.

Some degree of self-focused attention and fluctuating self-concept is a part of normal development, but in children with GAD, a high degree of self-consciousness is seen, which can be linked to cognitive distortions about self. Studies have found that children with GAD (and some other anxiety disorders) endorsed significantly more negative and uncertain statements about themselves than did nonanxious youth (Ronan & Kendall, 1997). Whereas anxious children endorsed more negative self-statements than normal controls, they endorsed the same number of positive self-statements. Therapeutically, then, it is not crucial to attempt to increase positive self-talk to reduce anxiety and increase psychological well-being; instead, it is more beneficial to focus on decreasing the level of negative self-talk (Kendall, 1984; Treadwell & Kendall, 1996).

The negative and uncertain self-concepts of GAD youth can be associated with fears of peer evaluation and embarrassment through poor performance. Because these children entertain a high frequency of negative self-talk, it is not surprising that they believe their peers are going to evaluate them negatively and that they will somehow embarrass themselves. Accordingly, these beliefs can lead the GAD child to avoid age-appropriate behavior and activities, such as parties, school events, and sports. They may not even join clubs because they are too worried about anticipated social evaluation for the activities to be enjoyable—they may mistakenly look upon the activities as chores. When anxious children do engage in activities, they are less likely to be involved and enthusiastic, perhaps because they are viewing the activities as chores rather than as fun. The outcome perpetuates the beliefs, as peers are more likely to reject or avoid them because of their indifference or peripheral involvement in the activity. For example, Strauss, Last, Hersen, and Kazdin (1988) found that GAD children were liked significantly less by peers and were often neglected in social situations. Evidence also suggests that anxious children anticipate more negative outcomes when faced with a social situation than do nonanxious children (Chansky & Kendall, 1997). Parents and teachers rate these children as significantly less socially adept, to the point of being maladjusted. Not surprisingly then, these children also have less social self-confidence and high levels of social anxiety.

USING THE DECISION TREE FOR DIFFERENTIAL DIAGNOSIS

If the symptom pattern described for GAD youth were specific to GAD and not seen in youth with other anxiety disorders, differential diagnosis would be much simpler than in fact is the case. The social problems that children with GAD experience are similar to those of other disorders (e.g., social anxiety disorder, aka social phobia) and therefore call into question the meaningfulness of the difference between GAD and social anxiety disorder. In fact, GAD shares many features of several other anxiety disorders. To arrive at a diagnosis of GAD, it is recommended that the diagnostic evaluator rule out a number of alternate explanations when presented with a case of excessive or unrealistic anxiety.

Consistent with the notion of a diagnostic decision tree (see the *DSM-IV*; APA, 1994), the diagnostic evaluator first determines whether symptoms of anxiety, fear, avoidance, or increased arousal are better accounted for by other diagnoses. To that end, GAD should be distinguished from anxiety that is focused solely on social interactions or performances, as in social phobia. If, however, social concerns are only one area of concern, and the child also has excessive amounts of worry in other areas (e.g., the health of his or her parents), then GAD may be the more appropriate diagnosis.

GAD should also be separated from anxiety that is centered on recurrent, unexpected panic attacks (panic disorder) and from agoraphobia, in which the fear concerns being in places from which escape might be difficult or embarrassing. GAD should be further differentiated from fear that is limited to specific objects or situations, as in specific phobia, or worry in the form of obsessions or compulsions, as in obsessive-compulsive disorder (OCD). In GAD, the anxiety is not focused solely on situations involving separation from attachment figures, as in separation anxiety disorder. Also, although jittery behavior, restlessness, or trouble concentrating can be seen in youth with both attention-deficit/hyperactivity disorder (ADHD) and GAD, the former does not have the added component of worry or undue concern about the future and the latter does not have the degree of attention problems seen in ADHD children. That is, children with GAD may be jittery and restless, but such behavior occurs primarily as part of the worrying process.

When the excessive worry (on more days than not) has lasted for less than 6 months, GAD is not diagnosed, and one may consider a diagnosis of adjustment disorder with anxious features. If the anxiety were the result of a psychosis or mood disorder or use of a substance (e.g., medication, drug of abuse, or toxin), GAD would not be diagnosed. Finally, given the presence of somatic complaints in GAD, it is important to examine organic causes for these symptoms to determine if a medical condition exists (Walker & Greene, 1989).

ISSUES OF COMORBIDITY

Is it possible to for a child to be diagnosed with GAD as well as another Axis I disorder? The answer is decidedly yes. For example, both anorexia nervosa and GAD may be diagnosed when the focus of the worry for GAD extends beyond weight gain. Similarly, if restlessness or jitteriness exists even when the child is not actively worrying, and other symptoms of ADHD are present, both ADHD and GAD may be diagnosed.

Although *DSM-IV* shifted from OAD to GAD in an effort to help increase specificity and decrease symptom overlap with other disorders, it remains unclear whether this goal has been fully achieved. Specifically, there continue to be several overlapping features between GAD and separation anxiety disorder (SAD) and social anxiety disorder, perhaps contributing to the high comorbidity rates between these disorders (Kendall & Brady, 1995).

Researchers have found that children with OAD (*DSM-III-R*; APA, 1987) quite often meet criteria for a secondary anxiety diagnosis. For instance, in clinic samples, 57% of children with a primary diagnosis of OAD received a secondary diagnosis of an anxiety disorder (Last, Hersen, Kazdin, Finkelstein, & Strauss, 1987). Another report indicated that 36% of OAD children had at least one additional anxiety diagnosis, and 18% had two or more additional anxiety diagnoses (Last, Strauss, & Francis, 1987). Moreover, those children diagnosed with SAD were most likely to receive a secondary diagnosis of OAD.

Seeming to differ with age, low to moderate comorbidity rates also exist for GAD and nonanxiety-related diagnoses. Younger children more often received a concurrent SAD or ADHD diagnosis, whereas older children more often had concurrent simple phobia or major depression (Brady & Kendall, 1992; Last, Hersen, et al., 1987). Several studies examined the comorbidity rates of depression and OAD, with rates ranging from 9 to 33% (Bowen, Offord, & Boyle, 1990; Last, Strauss, et al., 1987; for a review, see Brady & Kendall, 1992). Kendall and colleagues (1997) reported a comorbidity rate of 6% for anxiety disorders and depression in children in a randomized child clinical trial. Also commonly comorbid with primary OAD diagnoses are oppositional disorders (Last, Strauss, et al., 1987). It seems clear that, using the language of today's youth, "comorbidity rules": It is more common for a child identified as having GAD to have other, comorbid diagnoses than it is for the child to receive the single diagnosis.

DEVELOPMENTAL DIFFERENCES

Preliminary data has provided evidence for developmental differences in symptom report between older versus younger children with OAD/GAD (Strauss, Lease, Last, & Francis, 1988). In particular, significant differences were reported in the overall number of symptoms endorsed by older versus younger children. Reporting more than five of seven GAD symptoms, the children over age 12 endorsed more symptoms than did the children under the age of 12. In fact, 28% of the older group, versus only 4% of the younger group, met all seven GAD criteria. The researchers also found that older children scored significantly higher than younger ones on three instruments: the trait and state subscales of the State-Trait Anxiety Inventory–Children (STAIC; Spielberger, 1973); the worry/oversensitivity factor of the Revised

Children's Manifest Anxiety Scale (RCMAS; Reynolds & Richmond, 1978); and the Children's Depression Inventory (CDI; Saylor, Finch, Spirito, & Bennett, 1984). When their scores were compared with the instruments' normative data, members of the older group were found to exhibit elevated anxiety and depression, whereas the younger group was in the normal (nondeviant) range.

Given these findings, it seems that, with age, children's manifestation of GAD changes in both content and in symptom number (see also Kendall & Pimentel, 2003). Older children, over the age of 12, present with a higher number of overall symptoms, as well as more anxiety about past events. This increase in symptom report may be somewhat GAD-specific, rather than a mere function of increased age, as findings in youth with SAD often reveal that younger children report more symptoms than do older children (Francis, Last, & Strauss, 1987).

EPIDEMIOLOGY

Prior to *DSM-IV*, children experiencing excessive worry would have been classified as having OAD. Given evidence finding no significant differences between the anxiety disorders for children in *DSM-III-R* and those in *DSM-IV* (Kendall & Warman, 1996), it is possible to extend research findings on OAD to research on GAD.

Epidemiological studies of OAD reported it present in 3% of adolescents (Bell-Dolan & Brazeal, 1993). Higher rates of OAD/GAD have been found in other studies of youth aged 12 to 18—as high as 10.8% (Costello, Stouthamer-Loeber, & DeRosier, 1993). It is important to note that most pediatric epidemiological data are based on symptomatology, and not actual anxiety disorder diagnoses (Orvaschel & Weissman, 1986). Using anxiety symptoms, the review by Orvaschel and Weissman included children aged 3 to 12 and concluded that girls were more likely than boys to display anxiety, albeit with wide variations across ages.

In a study reported by Silverman and Nelles (1988) focusing on children referred to general psychological clinics, prevalence rates were found to be approximately 14%. When studying children specifically referred to anxiety clinics, however, the rates were found to be anywhere from 15% (Last, Strauss, et al., 1987) to 58% (Kendall et al., 1997). Children who received the diagnosis of GAD also appeared to be significantly older than those diagnosed with either SAD or specific phobia (Albano, Chorpita, DiBartolo, & Barlow, 1995).

Gender differences have not been found for the diagnosis of GAD in children aged 9 to 13 (Last, Strauss, et al., 1987; Kendall et al., 1997). However, after early adolescence, GAD is found to be more prevalent in women than in men. This difference appears to be a result of fewer anxious men, rather than an increase with age in the number of anxious women (Velez, Johnson, & Cohen, 1989).

ETIOLOGY

Research on the etiology of GAD has largely been ignored. Early adult twin research did not implicate genetic factors in the development of anxiety disorders (Torgersen, 1983), although more recent studies have suggested a possible genetic contribution to GAD in adults (Brown, 1999). Studies of this nature have not yet focused on childhood GAD. In addition to genetic factors, research on temperament, parenting styles, and early stressors is warranted.

Cognitive paradigms have received some attention in the study of etiology of anxiety disorders in adults (Barlow, 1988) and youth. Some of the hypothesized cognitive factors include self-questioning and negative self-talk, expectations of peril, and personal schemata focused on threat. Combinations of these cognitive concepts may contribute to the development of dysfunctional anxiety symptoms and disorders, in both children and adults (Kendall, 1991). The context of cognitive processing is important, as it is the way in which one perceives behavior in context that gives it meaning. Over time, the child experiences similar behaviors and interprets them in a similar manner. Eventually the child begins to anticipate the behavior and becomes anxious in advance (i.e., expectancies of peril, anticipatory distress). Additional research is needed to understand the role of cognitive-processing factors in childhood anxiety disorders such as GAD.

Very little longitudinal research has been done to study the course of GAD, particularly among children. What little information we have comes from retrospective reports from the adult literature. Several studies have found that most adults with GAD report an onset dating back to childhood, or they cannot report a clear age of onset because they relate that they have been worriers all of their lives (Noyes, Clancy, Crowe, Hoenk, & Slymen, 1992).

Can etiology vary depending on the age of the appearance of GAD? Is early-onset GAD more biologically driven, with adult-onset GAD more linked to specific environmental stressors (Brown, 1999)? There are mixed reports about the possibility of significant differences between adults whose GAD began in childhood versus those with adult onset. Hoehn-Saric, Hazlett, and McLeod (1993) reported that individuals with early-onset GAD had more extensive psychiatric histories, including childhood inhibitions and phobias. This group also scored higher on levels of trait anxiety, worry, neuroticism, and depression. However, Brown (1999) used the same cutoff point for determining late-onset and found no significant between-group differences. Future research should include prospective studies, to allow a more accurate portrayal of the course of GAD.

ASSESSMENT

The assessment and diagnosis of childhood anxiety disorders requires that the researcher or clinician be cognizant of several issues. First, one must be aware of normative behavior and normative developmental changes in children's fears: Some fear and anxiety is normal, and normal fear and anxiety in children have been well documented (Gullone & King, 1993). In addition, there must be sensitivity to cultural and gender issues in assessment (e.g., Dong, Yang, & Ollendick, 1994; Fonseca, Yule, & Erol, 1994; King, Gullone, & Ollendick, 1992). Developmental cognitive differences must be considered, because children, particularly those under the age of 11, have difficulty answering complex (emotion-related) questions (Schniering, Hudson, & Rapee, 2000). Clearly, the accuracy of their reports depends on the acquisition of specific cognitive and language skills, as well as an understanding of self, emotions, and the perceptions of others (Schniering et al., 2000). Most often referred for mental health services by a parent or teacher, the child with GAD may not understand why he or she is in treatment. Another important consideration is social desirability as a threat to report accuracy, because anxious children may be especially likely to respond in socially desirable ways due to the very concerns about performance and negative evaluation that are a part of their presenting pattern.

Assessment of anxiety and its disorders has generally followed a tripartite model, consistent with Lang's (1968) model. The examination of three domains of anxiety is warranted: cognitive, behavioral, and physiological. Clinical interviews, self-report measures, clinician ratings, ratings by others (parents, teachers), behavioral observations, and—to a lesser extent—physiological recordings are strategies that can be employed to elicit expressions of anxiety across these three response channels. To date, research on task performance measures (e.g., the Stroop test) has not yet produced any specific instrument to assess child anxiety. The selection of assessment strategies can be guided by consideration of several goals: (a) to provide reliable and valid measurement of symptoms in or across the multiple domains (e.g., cognitive, behavioral, psychological), (b) to discriminate between disorders (selection/classification), (c) to evaluate current severity, (d) to reconcile multiple sources of information (e.g., parent and child ratings), and (e) to enable the evaluation of therapeutic change (Kendall & Flannery-Schroeder, 1998; Stallings & March, 1995). Although no one single instrument or procedure can meet all of these goals, several acceptable assessment tools do exist. In this section, we provide an overview of an illustrative though not exhaustive selection of the instruments currently available for measuring anxiety in children and adolescents.

Clinical Interviews

The clinical interview, historically speaking, has been the most common method of assessing children (Greenspan, 1981). The recent emergence of highly structured interviews offers the clinician or researcher the advantage of gathering interview data in a manner that will be consistent with diagnostic categories such as those provided in *DSM*. It is worth noting that structured interviews may be more appropriate than unstructured ones for anxious children, who have been shown to respond better to specific, rather than open-ended, questions (Ollendick & Francis, 1988). Examples of structured and diagnostically oriented interviews include the Child Assessment Schedule (CAS; Hodges, Kline, Fitch, McKnew, & Cytryn, 1981); the Anxiety Disorders Interview Schedule for Children/Parents (ADIS-C/P; Silverman & Albano, 1997); the Schedule for the Assessment of Conduct, Hyperactivity, Anxiety, Mood, and Psychoactive Substances (CHAMPS; Mannusa & Klein, 1987); the National Institute of Mental Health (NIMH) Diagnostic Interview Schedule for Children and Adolescents (DISC 2.3; Shaffer et al., 1996); the Diagnostic Interview for Children and Adolescents (DICA; Herjanic & Reich, 1982); and the Schedule for Affective Disorders and Schizophrenia for School-Aged Children (K-SADS; Puig-Antich & Chambers, 1978). With few exceptions, these interviews generally have low informant reliability for diagnosing anxiety disorders, underscoring the difficulty of diagnosing anxiety disorders in youth (Silverman & Nelles, 1988). Perhaps due to the complications associated with child assessment and the difficulty in deciding a gold standard to which diagnosis can be compared, studies of criterion validity have shown mixed results (Silverman, 1994).

To date, there is no universally accepted approach to the comprehensive assessment of all childhood anxiety disorders. Notwithstanding, the ADIS-C/P (Silverman & Albano, 1997) appears the most appropriate and comprehensive tool, because it was developed specifically to assess for *DSM-IV* anxiety diagnoses (assessing symptomatology, course, etiology, and severity) and to screen for other common childhood disorders (Silverman, 1991). Comprised of both child and parent interview components, the ADIS-C/P is a semistructured interview that enlists an interviewer-observer format, such that information is drawn through both the interviews and through clinical observation. Final, or composite, diagnoses are based on the level of severity endorsed in each interview (child and parent) and the agreement in identification of pathology between parent and child interviews. Among its strengths are favorable psychometric properties (March & Albano, 1998; Silverman & Eisen, 1992; Silverman & Nelles, 1988), clinically sensitive sections for the diagnosis of distinct anxiety disorders, and sections to screen for other disorders (comorbid conditions).

Clinician Rating Scales

The Anxiety Rating for Children-Revised (ARC-R; Bernstein, Crosby, Perwien, & Borchardt, 1996) is a clinician rating scale for anxiety symptomatology. It is comprised of two subscales: the anxiety subscale and the physiological subscale, measuring somatic symptoms (e.g., muscular, sensory, cardiovascular, respiratory, gastrointestinal, and autonomic). Cronbach's alphas (.69 to .79) and test-retest reliability were high for the two subscales, and the anxiety subscale discriminated well between children with and without an anxiety disorder (Bernstein, Crosby, et al., 1996).

   The Pediatric Anxiety Rating Scale (PARS; Research Unit on Pediatric
Psychopharmacology [RUPP] Anxiety Study Group, 1997) is a clinician-
rated anxiety severity rating scale for children and adolescents. The PARS
consists of a 50-item anxiety symptom checklist and seven anxiety severity
ratings specifically addressing the combined severity of symptoms of SAD,
social phobia, and GAD. Recent reliability data was excellent (calculated
Interclass correlation [ICC] > .97) and consistent across a broad range of
anxiety severity (RUPP Anxiety Study Group, 1998).

Self-Reports

Self-report inventories are widely used measures for assessing child anxiety
in both research and clinical settings. Self-report measures allow the presence and content of fears and anxieties to be assessed, but such measures
alone may not be sufficient for assigning specific diagnoses. Several scales
are useful in assessing children with GAD:

1. Revised Children's Manifest Anxiety Scale (RCMAS; Reynolds
   & Richmond, 1978)
2. State-Trait Anxiety Inventory for Children (STAIC; Spielberger,
   1973)
3. Youth Self-Report (Achenbach, 1987)
4. Multidimensional Anxiety Scale for Children (MASC; March,
   Parker, Sullivan, Stallings, & Conners, 1997)
5. Spence Children's Anxiety Scale (SCAS; Spence, 1997)
6. Screen for Child Anxiety Related Emotional Disorders
   (SCARED; Birmaher et al., 1997; Muris, Merckelbach, Gadet,
   Moulaert, & Tierney, 1999)
7. Positive and Negative Affect Scale for Children (PANAS-C;
   Laurent, Potter, & Catanzaro, 1994)

   The RCMAS is a 37-item scale with dichotomous (*yes/no*) answers that
yield an overall anxiety score and several scaled subscores tapping physiological manifestations of anxiety, worry and oversensitivity, and fear/con-
centration (Reynolds & Richmond, 1978). A lie subscale reflects a child's
tendency to respond in a socially desirable manner. Recent research (Chu,
Marrs-Garcia, Mennin, & Kendall, 2000) supports the utility of the RCMAS
in determining clinically significant diagnoses of GAD. High reliability and
test-retest reliability (.68 to .98; Reynolds & Paget, 1981, 1983; Reynolds
& Richmond, 1985; Witt, Heffer, & Pfeiffer, 1990) as well as concurrent
validity for the measure have been reported (Spielberger, 1973).
   The STAIC (Spielberger, 1973) is comprised of two 20-item inventories: the State scale, designed to assess present state and situationally linked
anxiety, and the Trait scale, to assess stable anxiety across situations. Scores
are standardized and normative data are available (Spielberger, 1973). Test-
retest reliability has been reported at .63 to .72 for the State scale (Finch,

Kendall, Montgomery, & Morris, 1975) and .44 to .65 for the Trait scale (Finch, Montgomery, & Deardorff, 1974). Data have been reported that support the state-trait distinction in children (Finch, Kendall, & Montgomery, 1976; Finch et al., 1975), but the STAIC may best serve as a general screening instrument (see Barrios & Hartmann, 1988) given a lack of correspondence between STAIC A-State and A-Trait scores and actual *DSM* anxiety disorder categories.

The Youth Self-Report (YSR, Achenbach, 1987) is comprised of 17 items measuring social competencies and 103 items measuring behavioral problems. Symptoms are organized through factor-analytic techniques that divide them into two broadband factors: internalizing and externalizing disorders. Good test-retest reliability for the YSR has been reported. An advantage to this child self-report measure is that it can be compared with corresponding parent and teacher reports of child functioning, the Child Behavior Checklist (CBCL; Achenbach, 1991b) and the Teacher Report Form (TRF; Achenbach, 1991a; see the "Other Informants: Parent and Teacher Reports" section of this chapter).

Recently, the MASC (March et al., 1997) was developed to address the issue of a multidimensional conceptualization of anxiety. To that end, this self-report scale addresses the major domains of anxiety in children and adolescents. It is a 39-item self-report inventory containing 4 major factors: physical symptoms (e.g., tension), social anxiety (e.g., rejection), harm avoidance (e.g., perfectionism), and separation anxiety. This factor structure has been shown to hold across gender and age, and test-retest reliability (.79 to .93) has been shown to be excellent over 3 weeks and 3 months (March & Albano, 1998).

Other recent developments are the SCAS (Spence, 1997) and the SCARED (Birmaher et al., 1997; Muris et al., 1999). The SCAS is 44-item self-report measuring anxiety on a four-point scale via the following six subscales: (1) separation anxiety, (2) social phobia, (3) OCD, (4) panic-agoraphobia, (5) GAD, and (6) fears of physical injury. It has been shown to have adequate test-retest reliability (.51) across a 6-month interval and acceptable concurrent and convergent validity. The SCARED is a 66-item self-report measuring anxious symptomatology through nine *DSM-IV*-linked subscales: (1) panic disorder, (2) GAD, (3) social phobia, (4) SAD, (5) OCD, (6) PTSD, (7) specific phobia—animal type, (8) specific phobia—blood/injection/injury type, and (9) specific phobia—situational/environmental type (Muris et al., 1999). With these nine subscales corresponding to specific anxiety diagnoses, the SCARED has this advantage over scales comprised of items relevant to overall anxious symptomatology (Schniering et al., 2000). In addition to good discriminant validity, the SCARED evidences high test-retest reliability (.86) and acceptable concurrent or convergent validity (Birmaher et al., 1997). A parent report form is available for the SCARED.

A more global measure of anxiety, the PANAS-C (Laurent et al., 1994) is a child version of the Positive and Negative Affect Schedule (PANAS;

Watson, Clarke, & Tellegen, 1988) that was developed in light of Clark and Watson's (1991) tripartite model of depression and anxiety. This model holds that (a) depression is specifically characterized by anhedonia or low positive affect (PA), (b) anxiety is specifically characterized by physiological hyperarousal (PH), and (c) general negative affect (NA) is a nonspecific factor that relates to both depression and anxiety. Similar in content, format, and instructions to the original scale, the PANAS-C is comprised of 12 positive items (e.g., *happy, proud, joyful*) and 15 negative items (e.g., *sad, upset, scared*). Overall, the PANAS-C can be used to differentiate anxiety from depression in youngsters and has evidenced sufficient reliability and validity—coefficient alphas are .91 to .92 for PA and .88 to .95 for NA (Joiner & Lonigan, 2000; Laurent et al., 1994, Laurent et al., 1999).

The topic of anxiety sensitivity has recently begun to receive attention among child anxiety researchers and clinicians (Laurent, Schmidt, Catanzaro, Joiner, & Kelley, 1998). Anxiety sensitivity is the propensity to react to autonomic arousal with fear, or more basically, it is the extent to which an individual is afraid of becoming anxious. When children with high anxiety sensitivity become anxious in response to a stressor, they are prone to worrying about the negative repercussions of the anxiety, producing additional anxiety and, ultimately, possibly developing panic and other anxiety disorders (Laurent et al., 1998). Consistent with cognitive theories of anxiety, the notion of anxiety sensitivity holds that cognitive misinterpretation is critical to the generation of anxiety; however, diverging here from cognitive theories, it is a stable traitlike characteristic (Laurent et al., 1998; Reiss, 1991; Reiss & McNally, 1985). Few published studies have examined the anxiety-sensitivity construct in children. Two modifications of the widely used adult Anxiety Sensitivity Index (ASI; Reiss, Peterson, Gursky, & McNally, 1986) exist for use with children: the Child Anxiety Sensitivity Index (CASI; Silverman, Fleisig, Rabian, & Peterson, 1991; see reviews by Chorpita, Albano, & Barlow, 1996; Lau, Calamari, & Waraczynski, 1996; Ollendick, 1995; Rabian, Peterson, Richters, & Jensen, 1993) and the Anxiety Sensitivity Index for Children (ASIC; Laurent & Stark, 1993; Laurent et al., 1998). Generally, research conducted using the child versions of the ASI has provided promising initial psychometric data (Laurent et al., 1998; Laurent & Stark, 1993; Mattis & Ollendick, 1997; Silverman et al., 1991).

Although not specific to GAD, supplemental tools measuring other anxiety disorders (e.g., specific phobias, social anxiety disorder) are essential to the assessment process due to the aforementioned high comorbidity rates in the anxiety disorders. For example, the Fear Survey Schedule for Children-Revised (FSSC-R; Ollendick, 1983) is an 80-item tool using a three-point scale to measure specific fears in several areas (e.g., school, home, social, physical, animal, travel). Another tool, the Social Phobia and Anxiety Inventory for Children (SPAI-C; Beidel, Turner, & Morris, 1995) is a 26-item inventory with a three-point scale measuring social concerns (e.g., assertiveness, social interactions, public performance). The Social Anxiety

Scale for Children–Revised (SASC-R; La Greca & Stone, 1993) is a 22-item self-report enlisting a five-point scale and three factors to assess social anxiety: fear of negative evaluation, social avoidance and distress in new situations, and general social avoidance. Acceptable psychometric properties have been reported for the FSSC-R, the SPAI-C, and the SASC-R (Beidel et al., 1995; Ginsburg, La Greca, & Silverman, 1998; La Greca & Stone, 1993; Ollendick, 1983).

Cognitive Measures

A promising area of self-report in childhood anxiety is the assessment of cognitive-processing factors that may be associated with the disorder. An individual's cognitive processing of environmental (e.g., social, contextual) information may be inaccurate (distorted) in a manner that is consistent with the purported psychopathology. Cognitive processing has been divided into cognitive contents, cognitive processes, cognitive products, and cognitive schema, and several of these processing factors have been implicated in the etiology and maintenance of anxiety in adults (e.g., Ingram & Kendall, 1987; Kendall & Ingram, 1987, 1989). Unfortunately, less empirical attention has been paid to cognitive-processing factors in child populations (Kendall & Ronan, 1990). There are several adult measures of anxious cognition, but there are few child measures. Indeed, many of the existing child measures are essentially downward extensions of an adult scale with minor semantic alterations (Schniering et al., 2000). For example, both Ambrose and Rholes (1993) and Laurent and Stark (Thought Checklist [TCC]; Laurent & Stark, 1993) modified the adult Cognition Checklist (CCL; Beck, Brown, Steer, Eidelson, & Riskind, 1987) for use with children. It is unclear, however, whether these adult-derived scales are optimal measures of children's thoughts (Schniering et al., 2000).

Two measures have been designed specifically to assess cognitive processing (e.g., self-talk) in children: the Negative Affectivity Self-Statement Questionnaire (NASSQ; Ronan, Kendall, & Rowe, 1994) and the Coping Questionnaire for Children (Kendall, 1994; Kendall et al., 1997). The NASSQ is a 55-statement inventory developed to assess the cognitive contents of anxious/dysphoric children, measuring the more global construct of negative affectivity as well as the specific cognition of anxiety and of depression. A factor analysis of the NASSQ revealed four factors: depressive self-statements, anxiety/somatic self-statements, negative affect self-statements, and positive affect self-statements (Lerner et al., 1999). Analyses indicate favorable reliability, concurrent validity, and construct validity, as well as discriminant validity, supporting its ability to differentiate both psychometrically defined and clinic cases of anxious and nonanxious children. in addition to discriminating between anxious and depressive self-talk (Lerner et al., 1999; Ronan et al., 1994; Treadwell & Kendall, 1996; see also Ronan & Kendall, 1997).

The NASSQ has been used further in the CAADC as a weekly assessment tool, along with the A-State, in order to gauge session-by-session change. The NASSQ was shortened to two different versions, one for ages 7 to 10 and another for ages 11 to 15. Each version is comprised of only 10 questions, in order to make weekly assessment tolerable to the child. The items were chosen to be indicative of common self-statements that children with anxiety make, and were chosen to be age appropriate. The A-State is also used to measure state anxiety across sessions.

The Coping Questionnaire–Child (or Parent) version (CQ-C, CQ-P; Kendall, 1994; Kendall et al., 1997) is an instrument for assessing the child's self-perceived ability to cope with anxious distress in challenging situations. The CQ-C requires the child to identify his or her three most anxiety-provoking situations and rate his or her ability to cope with the situation on a seven-point scale. Among the advantages of the CQ, the parent can also rate the child's ability to cope with these situations using the complementary parent version of the tool measure (Kendall, 1994; see also the next section of this chapter). Analyses indicate adequate internal consistency and strong test-retest reliability and document its usefulness as a clinically sensitive measure of improvement (Kendall & Marrs-Garcia, 1999).

Other Informants: Parent and Teacher Reports

The child's self-report and the clinician's interview data are crucial, yet parent and teacher reports can offer additional and important perspectives. Nevertheless, there are potential limitations to using other informants for assessing internalizing disorders in children. In addition to concerns about the retrospective nature of parent/teacher accounts and the possibility of rater bias, parents and teachers may not be aware of the nature or extent of the child's inner pressures and distress (Kendall & Flannery-Schroeder, 1998). There is also a body of literature documenting a low concordance between child and parent reports of anxiety (see R. G. Klein, 1991). And, although findings are mixed (see Krain & Kendall, 2000), some studies (e.g., Frick, Silverthorn, & Evans, 1994) found that mothers tend to overreport their children's anxiety symptoms, particularly in cases of high maternal anxiety. This finding highlights the importance of clinician awareness of parental anxiety level (Bernstein, Borchardt, & Perwien, 1996) when seeking parent input for the purpose of making a child diagnosis.

From the many available measures, we have chosen three for examination here, reports that tap other informants' data that may be useful in assessing anxiety in youth. These are the CBCL (Achenbach & Edelbrock, 1983) and the TRF (Achenbach, 1991a; Achenbach and Edelbrock, 1986), which can be used in combination with the YSR (Achenbach, 1987; see also the "Self-Reports" section of this chapter), as well as the CQ-P (Kendall, 1994).

The CBCL (Achenbach, 1991b), a widely used parent rating scale, has acceptable reliability, validity, and normative data. The 118-item CBCL assesses behavioral problems and social competencies, providing data about the child's level of disturbance on specific factors. Although the tool provides adequate discrimination between externalizing disorders and internalizing disorders, it neither identifies nor differentiates between *DSM-IV* subtypes of anxiety. The CBCL also provides data on the child's participation in social activities and interactions with age peers for evaluation of change. A subset of 16 CBCL items, the CBCL–Anxiety Scale (CBCL-A; Kendall, Henin, MacDonald, & Treadwell, 1999) was found to have test-retest reliability and internal consistency and to reliably distinguish between anxiety-disordered and nondisordered youth. Additional research is warranted to determine the usefulness of the CBCL-A in the prediction and identification of anxiety disorders in youth.

The teacher version of the CBCL, the TRF (Achenbach, 1991a; Achenbach & Edelbrock, 1986), allows the child's primary teacher to rate the child's classroom functioning. In combination with the parent-rated CBCL, the TRF allows a consideration and comparison of the child's anxious behavior at home and in the school setting and may be especially relevant for children whose generalized anxiety involves social and evaluative situations. As suggested earlier, the classroom behavior of anxious youth, particularly GAD children, may not be viewed by teachers as problematic (e.g., perfectionism, or cautiousness, may preferred by someone in charge of a class of youths). Also, teachers may not be aware of a child's internal distress. Therefore, TRF scores may not reflect the level of anxiety experienced by the child.

For the CQ-P, the parents rate their perception of their child's ability to face and cope with the three most anxiety-provoking situations identified by the child in his or her interview. The CQ-P shows moderate interrater agreement and has been shown to be sensitive to treatment effects (Kendall & Marrs-Garcia, 1999).

Behavioral Observations

Ideally, there would be a single behavioral code that could be observed, counted, and used to make valid diagnostic statements. Unfortunately, such is not the case for GAD (and GAD is certainly not alone in this situation).

The behavioral assessment of childhood anxiety can include many structured and unstructured observations. Unstructured observations take place throughout the assessment process, especially during the clinical interview, when diagnosticians can spend time with the child and note any behaviors suggestive of anxiety (possibly fidgeting, fingernail biting, avoiding eye contact, and speaking softly). The parent and teacher rating scales are also based on unstructured observations of the child's behavior in naturalistic settings. These observations are important but can be limited by observer bias and, particularly in the case of parent and teacher ratings, may lack appropriate observer training.

Structured observation strategies such as behavioral avoidance tasks (BATs) involve direct observation by trained raters in naturalistic settings such as the schoolroom or playground. As an example, consider a BAT for the assessment of anxious distress related to eating in public. A situation could be arranged to mimic a cafeteria, with food and trays available and a variety of seating options—alone, with one other person, or with multiple people. In this BAT, the child participant would be rated by trained observers as to the degree of approach/avoidance to the distressing situation. In other words, how far along the continuum from not eating at all to eating among people did the participant progress? Although the BAT method has advantages because trained raters assess a child's behavior against a list of operationalized behaviors, it is limited by the absence of standardized procedures, occasionally preventing cross-study comparisons. However, as recommended by Glennon and Weisz (1978), Kendall and colleagues (1997) implemented a coding system to apply to observations of a videotaped task performance. Of six observational codes (gratuitous verbalizations, gratuitous body movements, task avoidance, fingers in mouth, absence of eye contact, trembling voice), no one code was independently pathognomic; however the total of behaviors was indicative of diagnostic status.

Neither unstructured nor structured behavioral observations are by themselves entirely sufficient for a diagnosis, as no single coded behavioral frequency appears to be pathognomic to childhood anxiety. The lack of diagnostic specificity linked to specific behaviors may be due to an overlap of symptomatology of the internalizing disorders (see also Brady & Kendall, 1992; Cole, Truglio, & Peeke, 1997; Finch, Lipovsky, & Casat, 1989; Joiner, Catanzaro, & Laurent, 1996; Jolly & Dykman, 1994; Kendall & Watson, 1989; King, Ollendick, & Gullone, 1991; Lonigan, Carey, & Finch, 1994) as well as the wide variability in behavioral manifestations of anxiety in children.

Physiological Recordings

The physiological assessment of anxiety has received wide attention in the adult literature (e.g., Himadi, Boice, & Barlow, 1985), yet relatively little empirical data on these indicators exist in the child and adolescent population (Barrios & Hartmann, 1988; Beidel, 1988). Reported physiological indicators include increased heart rate (Beidel, 1988), changes in perspiration (Tal & Miklich, 1976), increased palmar sweating (Lore, 1966), increased adrenergic activity (Rogeness, Cepeda, Macedo, Fischer, & Harris, 1990), and increased baseline zygomatic muscle tension (Turner, Beidel, & Epstein, 1991). Opponents of the use of physiological assessment methods have cited the large imbalance between the extensive cost (in time and money) of gathering such information, and its relatively modest yield (Barlow & Wolfe, 1981; Schniering et al., 2000). Furthermore, the most commonly used physiological techniques, such as cardiovascular and electrodermal measures, lack adequate child normative data. During physiological assessment, children also tend to show idiosyncratic response patterns, and measures can be influenced by expectancy effects, emotions other than anxiety, and incidental motoric and perceptual activity (Schniering et al., 2000; Wells & Virtulano, 1984; Werry, 1986).

Despite these limitations and reported setbacks, continued investigation of the physiological assessment of childhood anxiety may be warranted. Further empirical investigation of autonomic responsivity in anxious children would increase our understanding of the psychophysiological expression of anxiety and help to develop normative data in this area. These efforts would be important in informing a comprehensive picture of the expression of anxiety through biological, cognitive, and behavioral assessments.

Family Assessment

Family assessment, albeit an important and theoretically rich arena for inquiry, is a relatively underexplored method for assessing childhood anxiety. Most models of anxiety in childhood (e.g., cognitive-behavioral model; Kendall, 1985, 1991) acknowledge the influence of the family and other social contexts on the presentation and maintenance of the anxiety disorder. In recent years, efforts in the treatment of childhood anxiety disorders have begun to combine interventions directed at both the anxious child and his or her family. Family involvement in child anxiety treatment has been implicated, because some etiological evidence points to a familial role in the development or maintenance of child anxiety (Cobham, 1998), and some treatment outcome evidence suggests the benefits of interventions with a combined child and parent focus (e.g., Barrett, Dadds, & Rapee, 1996; Cobham, Dadds, & Spence, 1999; Howard & Kendall, 1996). Unfortunately, however, there is a paucity of established techniques to assess family functioning, particularly with regard to the GAD child. One tool, the Family Assessment Device (FAD; Epstein, Baldwin, & Bishop, 1983), based on the McMaster model of family functioning, measures six dimensions of family functioning (e.g., communication, affective involvement, behavior control) and has been reported to possess adequate test-retest reliability and to differentiate between clinician-rated healthy and unhealthy families (Miller, Epstein, Bishop, & Keitner, 1985; Miller, Kabacoff, Keitner, Epstein, & Bishop, 1986). However, the FAD was not found to differentiate anxious and nonanxious youth in a study with our clinic sample (Hedtke, 2002).

Another tool, the Family Environment Questionnaire (FEQ; Caster, Inderbitzen, & Hope, 1999), is a 27-item self-report modification of the Parent Attitudes Toward Child-Rearing Scale (PATCS; Bruch, Heimberg, Berger, & Collins, 1989), which assesses adults' retrospective reports of their childhood family environment. The PATCS was modified in four ways: (1) item wording was changed from past to present to reflect youths' current perceptions, (2) the language was simplified, (3) youth are asked to indicate how true an item is for their mothers and fathers separately, and (4) eight new items assessing youths' self-perceptions of sociability were added. The FEQ enlists a five-point scale and consists of four subscales as per the PATCS (isolation, others' opinion, shame, family sociability) as well as a fifth subscale, self-sociability (Caster et al., 1999). It has a parallel 19-item parent self-report form inquiring about the individual parent's attitudes and behaviors across the four core subscales. Psychometric properties of the FEQ student and parent versions are acceptable (Caster et al., 1999).

A third instrument, the Family Adaptability and Cohesion Evaluation Scale II (FACES-II; Olson, Bell, & Portner, 1982), is comprised of 30 items rated on a five-point scale to measure the cohesion (enmeshed to disengaged) and adaptability (flexible to rigid) dimensions in the family. Subjects rate both their current and ideal families. Test-retest reliability (.80 to .83) and Cronbach's alphas (.78 to .80) are high, and standardized norms are available (Olson et al., 1983). Continued research is needed to determine the reliability and validity of specific family functioning measures for anxious children.

Another tool, the Children's Report of Parent's Behavior Inventory (CRPBI; Schaefer, 1965; Schludermann & Schludermann, 1970) contains 108 child-rated items descriptive of maternal child-rearing behaviors. The parent version (Schwarz, Barton-Henry, & Pruzinsky, 1985) assesses mothers' ratings of their own parenting behavior and can also aggregate parenting scores across multiple raters (e.g., both mother and father). The CRPBI contains 18 subscales representing three dimensions: (1) acceptance/rejection—the extent to which the parent expresses care and affection for the child (e.g., *Tells me how much she loves me*); (2) autonomy/psychological control—the extent to which parents control their children through indirect psychological methods such as inducing guilt or anxiety and withdrawing love (e.g., *Feels hurt when I don't follow her advice*); and, 3) firm or lax control—the extent to which parents consistently enforce compliance by making rules or threatening punishment (e.g., *Sees to it that I know exactly what I may or may not do*). In both parent and child forms, the degree of similarity between the described behavior and the mother's behavior is rated via a three-point scale (0 = *like*, 1 = *somewhat like*, 2 = *not like*). Internal consistency for the three dimensions is high for both children's (.77 to .95) and mothers' (.77 to .87) reports (Schwarz et al., 1985).

Assessment Summary

The assessment of GAD in children requires a multimethod approach, drawing information from a semistructured clinical interview, child self-report, parent and teacher ratings, behavioral observations, task performance, and perhaps even physiological indices. There is merit in the consideration of and inclusion of family history and patterns of interaction. Assessors and diagnosticians need to be aware of each method's advantages and disadvantages, particularly if forced to rely on a single assessment method. It is best when multiple strategies are used to assess and diagnose GAD, to inform treatment planning, and to sensitively evaluate treatment process and outcome.

TREATMENT

Although a wide range of treatments has been used over the years, including various medications as well as various psychological approaches (e.g., behavioral, psychodynamic), only a very small number of treatments have warranted the esteemed label of *empirically supported*. In the following sections, our descriptions of the treatment of GAD in youth emphasizes the treatments that have received empirical support. We describe cognitive-behavioral therapy in some detail and review the information that is available on medications.

Selecting the Initial Treatment

In selecting the initial treatment for children with generalized anxiety, it is important to consider the weight of empirical research. According to the criteria set by the APA Task Force on Promotion and Dissemination of Psychological Procedures (1995) and Chambless and Hollon (1998) for determining and defining empirically supported therapies, cognitive-behavioral therapy (CBT) has been found to be efficacious in treating anxiety in children (see also Kazdin & Weisz, 1998, and Ollendick & King, 2000). The results of several randomized clinical trials using cognitive-behavioral treatment conducted by two different research groups support the application of this approach (Barrett et al., 1996; Kendall, 1994; Kendall et al., 1997). In the first randomized clinical trial investigating the efficacy of CBT for 9- to 13-year-old children with a primary diagnosis of OAD/GAD, SAD, or social phobia, Kendall (1994) compared a manual-based CBT to wait-list control. At posttreatment assessment, 64% of treated children no longer received their principal anxiety disorder diagnosis, with treatment gains maintained at 1-year follow-up. Longer-term follow-up assessments revealed that children continued to maintain these gains 2 to 5 years (mean of 3.35 years) after treatment (Kendall & Southam-Gerow, 1996). These positive outcomes and the efficacy of CBT were replicated in a second randomized clinical trial of 9- to 13-year-olds with a primary anxiety disorder (Kendall et al., 1997).

Barrett and colleagues (1996) added a family management component to individual child CBT and produced promising results. In this clinical trial, 79 children aged 7 to 14 who met a primary diagnosis of OAD/GAD, SAD, or social phobia were randomly assigned to a CBT group, a CBT-plus-family-management group (CBT+FAM), or a wait-list control group. Sixty percent of children in both treatment conditions received a nondiagnosis status, compared to less than 30% of the wait-list children. At 1-year follow-up, 70% of the CBT and 95% of the CBT+FAM children did not have their anxiety diagnosis. In the following sections, we first describe CBT and then discuss medications for the treatment of GAD.

Cognitive-Behavioral Therapy

The cognitive-behavioral approach (e.g., Kendall, 1994; Kendall et al., 1997) that has been evaluated in the studies discussed above is a manual-based approach (Kendall, Kane, Howard, & Siqueland, 1990) that integrates elements of cognitive information processing associated with anxiety with behavioral techniques (e.g., relaxation, imaginal and in-vivo exposure, role playing) known to be useful in the reduction of anxiety. The overall goal of treatment is to help children learn to recognize their signs of anxious arousal and to use these signs as cues for the employment of acquired anxiety-management strategies.

In CBT, children with anxiety participate in a structured 16- to 20-week treatment program that is divided into two segments: education and practice. The first half of treatment (the first eight sessions or so) is a period of training, education, and skill building, during which the therapist works with the child to recognize signs of anxiety, to acquire relaxation skills, and to identify anxious cognitive processing. Through self-monitoring homework assignments and in-session role playing, the child learns about anxiety and, more important, the cognitive, somatic, emotional, and behavioral aspects of his or her own personal anxious experience. These sessions also allow the child to think about various ways to overcome anxiety. The therapist and child work together to create a personalized FEAR plan that is used by the child to cope when anxiety-provoking situations arise. The steps of the FEAR plan include:

*F*eeling frightened?

*E*xpecting bad things to happen?

*A*ttitudes and actions

*R*esults and rewards

Each step is part of the learning that takes place during the first half of treatment. In learning these four steps symbolized by the acronym *FEAR*, the child is armed with a coping plan that he or she can then practice during the second half of treatment.

Education and Skill-Building

During initial sessions, the anxious child learns to distinguish between various bodily reactions to emotions as well as the somatic reactions that are specific to his or her anxiety. If the child is *feeling frightened*, he or she learns that this is the important first signal for managing unwanted anxiety. Coupled with this awareness, the child is taught relaxation exercises that may help in development of greater awareness of and control over physiological and muscular reactions to anxiety (see King, Hamilton, & Ollendick, 1988). These exercises are audiotaped for the child to listen to and practice at home. Given the somatic complaints associated with GAD in children (APA, 1994; see also Kendall & Pimentel, 2003), this segment of the plan may be especially beneficial for children whose worry is accompanied by more severe somatic symptoms (see also Eisen & Silverman, 1998). In this way, children with

GAD may develop an awareness of their physiological responses to anxiety and use this as an early warning signal to initiate relaxation procedures.

Next, GAD children are taught how to identify and modify anxious cognition (their internal dialogue). In this second step of the FEAR plan, children learn to ask, "Am I *expecting bad things to happen?*" Therapist and child then discuss such thoughts and the child is encouraged to ask himself or herself what the various possibilities are that may occur in a given situation. Given the theorized link between cognition, emotion, and behavior (Ingram, Kendall, & Chen, 1991), it is believed that helping a child to challenge his or her distorted or unrealistic cognition will promote more constructive ways of thinking and less dysfunctional emotional and behavioral responses. For example, the perfectionistic nature of many children with generalized anxiety can be challenged as these children become better able to examine, test, and reduce their negative self-talk; modify unrealistic expectations; generate more realistic and positive self-statements; and create a plan to cope with their concerns. To achieve this, therapists use strategies such as cognitive modeling, rehearsal, social reinforcement, and role playing. It should be noted that, as described earlier, the idea here is not necessarily to fill the child with positive self-talk. Rather, the ameliorative power rests in the reduction of negative self-talk, or the "power of non-negative thinking" (Kendall, 1984, p. 177). This phenomenon is supported by recent evidence indicating that changing children's anxiety-ridden and negative self-talk—but not positive self-talk—mediates the changes in anxiety that are associated with treatment-produced gains (Treadwell & Kendall, 1996).

Tied closely to the previous step in the FEAR plan, children learn problem-solving skills that help them to devise a behavioral plan to cope with their anxiety. With *attitudes and actions* that help, children learn to recognize the problem, brainstorm and generate alternatives to managing their anxiety, weigh the consequences of each possible alternative, and then choose and follow through with the plan (see D'Zurilla & Goldfried, 1971; D'Zurilla & Nezu, 1999). The therapist serves as a model during each phase of problem solving by reminding the child that problems and challenges are part of life, for example, or by brainstorming ideas without judgment. With the acquisition of problem-solving skills, children develop confidence in their ability to handle anxiety-provoking situations as well as everyday challenges that arise.

The fourth and final step in the FEAR plan, *results and rewards,* allows children to judge the effectiveness of their efforts and reward themselves for these efforts. Children learn to identify those things they liked about how they handled a situation and those things that they want to do differently. Here, children are encouraged to reward both complete and partial successes. Children with generalized anxiety may place exceedingly high standards for achievement on themselves and can be unforgiving and critical of themselves if they fail to meet these standards. Therefore, it is important for the therapist to emphasize and encourage self-reward for effort and partial success, despite seeming imperfections. With this step comes the culmination of the child's learning and integrating the four-step coping plan symbolized by the FEAR acronym. What to do with it next?

Practice, Practice, Practice

The second half of treatment focuses on practicing the newly acquired skills. In these sessions, the child is prepared for and exposed to various situations that are likely to induce anxiety. The child is first exposed to imaginary and low-anxiety situations and gradually is exposed to moderate-anxiety and then high-anxiety situations. Through imaginal and in-vivo exposures, the therapist assists the child in preparing for the exposure by, for example, discussing aspects of the situation that are likely to be troubling, working through the steps of the plan, and rehearsing. The in-vivo exposures are extremely important, as these situations provide the child real opportunities to practice using the steps of the FEAR plan. Thus, they should be tailored to address the specific worries of the GAD child. For example, in-vivo exposures for 11-year-old Sarah could revolve around her fear of trying new things or her intolerance of uncertainty by placing her in such situations and allowing her to practice the FEAR plan.

The therapist also facilitates children's postexperience processing of the exposures, helping them to evaluate their performances and think of a reward. In so doing, the therapist helps to frame the current exposure experience in terms of a pattern for future coping. When designing the graduated hierarchy of exposures, it is beneficial for the therapist and child to collaborate to create in-vivo exposures that are meaningful and memorable for the child.

Homework assignments are an important feature of this program. Throughout the treatment, children complete STIC, or *show-that-I-can* tasks in a personal notebook, which allow them to practice their steps and to use their skills outside of session. Rewards (e.g., stickers) are provided upon completion of STIC assignments to encourage children to work on these tasks throughout the week. Children earn bigger rewards (e.g., baseball cards, music CDs) after they complete four assignments.

"Going Hollywood"

Starting with 3 or 4 weeks left, the therapist and child begin to discuss how the child will create and produce a "commercial" about his or her experiences in the program, to be presented during the last session of the treatment. Children are encouraged to use their imagination and create a videotape, audiotape, or booklet describing their experiences with the FEAR plan to help in telling other children about strategies for coping with anxiety. This effort is designed not only to help children organize their experiences, but also to afford them the opportunity to go public with their newly acquired skills and to recognize their accomplishments. The commercial also serves as a tangible reward that children can take home with them once the treatment is completed, and although it may not be described as such, it is an in-vivo exposure task with emotional, social, creative, and organizational features.

Therapist Roles

Throughout the various parts of the treatment, the therapist assumes several roles. He or she is a coach, a collaborator, a teacher, and a trainer. Modeling, as derived from the social-learning paradigm (see Bandura, 1969, 1986), is a strategy employed by the therapist, in which nonfearful behavior is demonstrated in the fear-producing situation to illustrate appropriate responses for the child. It is important to note that the therapist functions as a coping model, demonstrating coping skills in each new situation. The child is then invited to participate with the therapist in role playing (e.g., tag along; Ollendick & Cerny, 1981). To make role plays less threatening, the therapist may role-play a situation first as the child follows along. The therapist described to the child what he or she is feeling and asks if the child is experiencing similar or different feelings. Gradually, the child increases his or her involvement in the role plays and in describing the anxious experience, while the therapist's input decreases. Ultimately, children are encouraged to role-play scenes alone as they acquire their new skills. To reinforce the therapist's role as a coping model and to normalize the experience of anxiety for the child, therapist self-disclosure may be appropriate. The therapist can reveal past experiences that are relevant to the child's anxious experience, describing aloud his or her own feelings or thoughts in these situations. Such self-disclosure also helps to create a comfortable atmosphere, with sessions becoming a forum for openly discussing feelings.

Developmental Considerations

The treatment manual described (Kendall et al., 1990) was designed for children between the ages of 8 and 13 years. Also designed for this age range, the *Coping Cat Workbook* (Kendall, 1992) contains exercises that parallel treatment sessions in an effort to facilitate the child's involvement in the program and the acquisition of skills (the therapist's manual and workbook for teenagers is called the *C.A.T. Project*). Although some manual-based treatments have acquired the reputation of being somewhat rigid, the therapist working with this program is allowed flexibility, as life can be breathed into the treatment program to better fit the needs and functioning of the child (Kendall, Chu, Gifford, Hayes, & Nauta, 1998). Although adaptations can be made when working with older children, younger children may not have yet developed the cognitive skills necessary to participate fully in or benefit maximally from this intervention, and children with IQs below 80 may not have the prerequisite skills. Additionally, with developmental considerations, it is important to be cognizant of possible age-related increases in physiological functioning, emotional vulnerability, social and peer pressures, and comorbid conditions, as well as any other changes that these children may be experiencing.

Relapse Prevention

The ultimate goal of treatment is to equip the child with skills that will help him or her manage anxious distress. The goal of treatment is not to "cure" anxiety (see Kendall, 1989). Because some form of anxious arousal is likely to persist, modifying dysfunctional expectations and distorted processing styles can help to make possible more adaptive functioning. The use of in-vivo exposure tasks in treatment provides performance-based experiences of coping that bolster confidence for future situations. Therapeutic intervention is the first step—a step that helps to realign the maladaptive developmental trajectories of these children so that they are better able to address the inevitable challenges emerging in their lives. Upon completion of the treatment program, the guiding principle is for the child to continue to practice the skills learned.

There are several strategies that help to guide children toward consolidation of treatment-produced gains. First, the therapist should shape and encourage effort attributions regarding the management of anxiety. Children are encouraged always to reward their hard work and coping efforts, even if the successes are only partial.

A second principle for continued posttreatment functioning includes introducing children to the concept of lapses in efforts, rather than relapses (see Brownell, Marlatt, Lichtenstein, & Wilson, 1986; Marlatt & Gordon, 1985). Mistakes and partial successes are not viewed as incompetence or inability; rather, they can be constructively framed as vital to and inextricably linked to the learning process. Within this framework, children can label and accept inevitable setbacks as temporary and then proceed to work through problem solving. Mistakes are viewed as an acceptable part of the learning process and not as excuses for giving up or confirming anxious cognitions.

Working with Families

In assessing and addressing anxiety in children, parental involvement is paramount. Although the treatment program discussed is focused on helping the child think and behave differently, parents are encouraged to participate in a supportive role. During the assessment period, parental responses to inventories and input in a structured interview are required for the child to receive a GAD diagnosis. Once treatment has begun, the therapist meets with the parents after the third session to collaborate with them on treatment plans. Parents are given the opportunity to discuss any concerns, and they are encouraged to provide information that may be useful for treatment. When appropriate, they are encouraged to help their children practice relaxation skills and participate in in-vivo exposures, and they can be integral to the reward process.

When working with children, it is critical to be mindful of specific problems that families of anxious children may be experiencing, especially given the role that parents may play in their child's treatment (see Kazdin & Weisz, 1998). Problems may include increased rates of anxiety disorders (for a review see Carey & Gottesman, 1981) or other pathologies such as depression or alcoholism (e.g., Noyes, Clancy, Crowe, Hoenk, & Slyman, 1978; Solyom, Beck, Solyom, & Hugel, 1974). Additional consideration should be given to issues that are stemmed in parenting, such as parental over-protectiveness and guilt regarding the problems their children are experiencing (see Chorpita & Barlow, 1998).

Given the increased clinical and empirical attention highlighting the potential contributing role of the family in the genesis and maintenance of childhood anxiety (see Fauber & Long, 1991; Ginsburg, Silverman, & Kurtines, 1995; Sanders, 1996) and the positive outcomes of initial research that has introduced more family focused CBT (Barrett et al., 1996; Howard & Kendall, 1996), a family intervention has been developed. The same principles and strategies discussed above are used, but parents attend and are directly involved in sessions. A manual describing this program is available (Howard, Chu, Krain, Marrs-Garcia, & Kendall, 2000). Although we support and encourage the collaborative input of parents during child-focused treatment as well as the continued development of family-focused programs, we recognize the need for continued research and empirical evaluation of when it is most therapeutically beneficial to include, or not include, parents in the treatment of their child's anxiety disorder.

Brief Case Illustration: Sarah

Sarah, whom we introduced at the beginning of this chapter, illustrates how a child with GAD can learn to successfully manage her anxiety. The diffuse and sometimes adult nature of her worry became a problem because it began to interfere with her ability to enjoy a normal childhood. For Sarah, feeling frightened was signaled by the onset of her stomach-aches and headaches. Thus, she was able to learn to use these as cues for implementing coping skills and the FEAR plan. Given her somatic complaints, relaxation training was an especially useful tool for her. In earlier treatment sessions, she learned to combat her negative self-talk and expecting bad things to happen by learning to generate possible favorable outcomes or alternatives to situations in addition to the unfavorable scenarios she was accustomed to envisioning. Because Sarah was afraid to try new things, for example, finding attitudes and actions that could help and deciding on a coping plan to try in a new situation (i.e., during in-vivos) prepared her for managing her anxiety. Sarah needed to learn to reward herself for her efforts, whatever the outcome. The importance of this in Sarah's case was manifold: First, she was rewarded for *trying* something new, whether or not she was successful. Second, she learned to re-ward herself for any partial successes, encouraging her to overlook the little things or imperfections she tended to worry about. And finally, she learned that outcomes may not always be so unfavorable. Given her tendency to predict unfavorable outcomes, in-vivo exposures provided her the opportunities to test and evaluate these predictions and to reward herself for the process of trying, which was important. Additionally, therapy, as a new experience for Sarah, served as a very real and ongoing in-vivo exposure; in many ways, she was already trying and was reminded of and rewarded for that.

Pharmacotherapy

There is limited data on pharmacotherapy of anxiety disorders, with the exception of OCD (March et al., 1998), despite the continuous increase in the use of psychotropic medications in both adult and children populations (Pincus et al., 1998; Zito et al., 2000). Few adequately designed studies are available that establish the safety and efficacy of any class of medication for childhood GAD (Allen, Leonard, & Swedo, 1995; Bernstein et al., 1996). Medication options for the treatment of GAD in children and ado-lescents includes the benzodiazepines, the nonbenzodiazepine anxiolytic buspirone, the selective serotonin reuptake inhibitors (SSRIs), and tricy-clic antidepressants (TCAs). All have demonstrated efficacy in adult anxi-ety disorders such as panic disorder (den Boer & Westerberg, 1998), GAD (Rickels, Downing, Schweizer, & Hassman, 1993), and social phobia (Jefferson, 1995; Katzelnick et al., 1995). Recently, venlafaxine was shown to be effective in the treatment of adult GAD (Derivan, Entsuah, Haskins, Rudolph, & Aguiar, 1997; Haskins, Rudolph, Pallay, & Derivan, 1997; Rickels, Pollack, Sheehan, & Haskins, 2000) and may also be a candidate for use with childhood GAD.

Whether or Not to Use Medication Can Be a Dilemma

Deciding when to use a medication for the treatment of childhood GAD can be a challenge, as in Sarah's case, especially when no comparative effi-cacy data exists for CBT versus medication. Often, initiation of medication treatment is determined by a practitioner's clinical judgment or bias. For example, Sarah constantly worried about everyday activities, such as events that might occur the next day at school, safety issues for herself and family, and catching illnesses from other children. What if such a child also com-plains of nightly difficulty with falling asleep, midnight awakenings due to nightmares, several daily visits to the nurse's office with multiple somatic complaints that lead to school refusal? What if her grades had begun to drop, and she was too fatigued to participate in after-school activities with class-mates? In Sarah's case, she also described decreased enjoyment of most activities and that she even avoided birthday parties, but she denied feeling sad. According to parent and teacher reports, she was displaying more irritability and tearfulness. Clearly, one first option was to recommend a trial of CBT as outlined earlier in this chapter. However, the level of symptoms such a child presents with may warrant consideration of the addition of medication, even at the onset of treatment.

Before starting a medication, a detailed medical and family history should be obtained, as well as laboratory measures as indicated. For example, if a child complains of feeling heat intolerance with warm, moist skin, weight loss, and rapid heart rate, it would be reasonable to do baseline thyroid studies. The prescribing clinician, with the consent of parent and child, should consult with the child's primary care physician to be aware of any additional medical issues, and to be sure that the child has had a recent physical exam. This will also build collaboration with the primary care physician that will support the treatment being recommended to the family. Both the parent and child need to be informed about the risks and benefits to medication treatment and informed consent must be obtained prior to initiating treatment. It is important to be clear with the child and parent concerning what target symptoms will be monitored to determine the medication effectiveness. The remainder of this section reviews the primary medication classes used for the treatment of childhood GAD (for an in-depth review, see Velosa & Riddle, 2000).

Benzodiazepines

The benzodiazepines bind to the gamma-aminobutyric acid receptor (GABA) membrane chloride channel complexes, which lead to enhanced CNS inhibition through the neurotransmitter GABA. Besides its anxiolytic affect, benzodiazepines are also used for their anticonvulsant, hypnotic, and muscle-relaxant properties (Brawman-Mintzer & Lydiard, 1997). Although there exists an extensive literature on the effectiveness of benzodiazepines in adult anxiety disorders (Rickels et al., 1983; Rickels, Schweizer, Case, & Greenblatt, 1990), there have been only a few studies, with small sample sizes, to examine the use of benzodiazepines in childhood anxiety disorders (Graae, Milner, Rizzotto, & Klein, 1994; Simeon et al., 1992). Most of the studies involved children and adolescents with additional comorbidities such as major depression, panic disorder, and school refusal (Bernstein, Garfinkel, & Borchardt, 1990; Kutcher & Mackenzie, 1988). Biederman (1987) treated three prepubertal children who presented with panic symptoms, plus each had one additional anxiety disorder (SAD, avoidant disorder, or OAD). The children were treated with clonazepam, two with 0.5 mg per day and one with 3 mg per day, with positive results and no side effects. Simeon et al. (1992) enrolled 30 patients, 8 to 16 years of age, with the primary diagnosis of OAD or avoidant disorder in a double-blind placebo controlled study for 4 weeks treated with alprazolam. There was some improvement in the patients on alprazolam (88%) as compared to placebo (62%); however, this difference was not statistically significant.

The most common side effects from benzodiazepines are drowsiness, headache, nausea, and fatigue. The side effects are dose related and can lead to tremor, slurred speech, and ataxia (Rickels, 1990b; Rickels, Case, & Schweitzer, 1991). There have been reports of paradoxical reactions in which the child experiences overexcitement, irritability, and perceptual disorganization. Another concern is the potential risk of dependence and withdrawal associated with the benzodiazepines, which rules them out as a front-line treatment. If children and adolescents are treated with benzodiazepines, it is recommended that treatment continue for a limited amount of time and at the lowest possible dose and, as clinically indicated, that the dose be increased every 3 to 4 days. Once treatment is completed, the benzodiazepine should be gradually tapered to avoid any risk of withdrawal symptoms, such as insomnia, gastrointestinal complaints, rebound anxiety, and concentration difficulties (Coffey, 1993; Kutcher, Reiter, Gardener, & Klein, 1992; Velosa & Riddle, 2000).

Although not recommended as a first choice of treatment, benzodiazepines may be effective for the child experiencing severe physical symptoms (that interfere with the child's everyday functioning) and serve as a useful adjunct for the first 2 weeks of the CBT.

Buspirone

Buspirone, a partial agonist at the serotonin 5–HT1A receptor, is a non-benzodiazepine anxiolytic. Although it has been shown to have both anxiolytic and antidepressants affects in adults (Rickels, 1990a; Rickels, Amsterdam, et al., 1991), buspirone does not appear to be a highly effective or broad-spectrum anxiolytic in adults (Pohl, Balon, Yergani, & Gershon, 1989; Sheehan, Raj, Sheehan, & Soto, 1990); so it would not appear to be a first choice for study with children. There is some evidence of improvement in open-label trials with children diagnosed with anxiety and depressive disorders (Kutcher et al., 1992; Simeon et al., 1994). Common side effects are headache, nausea, and dizziness (Riddle et al., 1999). The recommended dosage for children is 0.2 to 0.6 mg per kilogram of body weight three times a day; for adolescents, it is 5 to 10 mg three times a day, with 5 to 10 mg increases every 4 days to the maximum dose of 60 mg per day (Werry & Aman, 1999). There is no evidence of withdrawal with this medication, and its effects should be seen within 6 weeks.

Tricyclic Antidepressants

Dysregulation of both the noradrenergic and serotonin system of the central nervous system is believed to be part of the explanation for the development of GAD. In general, the TCAs' therapeutic effectiveness is through the metabolism and reuptake of the monoamine neurotransmitters (or both) for the treatment for GAD (Brawman-Mintzer & Lydiard, 1997). The significant and often hard-to-tolerate side effects are due to the TCAs' blockade at the muscarinic/cholinergic, histamine (H1), and alpha-adrenergic receptors. The most common side effects are constipation, nausea, orthostatic hypotension, sedation, and weight gain (Werry & Aman, 1993). The majority of clinical trials performed using TCAs did not have children and adolescents with GAD only, but rather the much more complicated comorbid group of school-refusing children.

Several placebo-controlled studies of TCAs for anxiety-based school-refusal children provide conflicting results. Gittelman-Klein and Klein (1973) studied a group of these children (N = 16; ages 6 to 14). This double-blind study comparing placebo to imipramine (25 to 200 mg per day) for 6 weeks with the addition of a behavioral plan showed that the imipramine group improved a mean of 80% on two dependent variables for anxiety, with 81.25 % returning to school. In another double-blind study comparing placebo to clomipramine (40 to 75 mg per day) for the treatment of anxiety-based school-refusal children (N = 51; ages 9 to 15), there was a mean improvement of 63.10% across three dependent measures of anxiety (Berney et al., 1981). Bernstein and colleagues (1990) completed two studies with children suffering from anxiety-based school refusal. Both studies compared imipramine and alprazolam—one in an open-label fashion and the other in a double-blind method. In the double-blind study, the mean improvement for both treatment conditions on two dependent measures of anxiety was 50%.

D. F. Klein, Mannuzza, Chapman, and Fyer (1992) studied 20 children diagnosed with SAD who received either placebo or imipramine (dose range of 75 to 225 mg per day) for 6 weeks. At the end of the study, there were no significant differences between the two treatment groups. Bernstein and colleagues (2000) recently reported that the combination of imipramine and CBT was significantly more effective than CBT alone in the treatment of school refusal of adolescents with comorbid depression and anxiety. The group treated with imipramine showed a faster treatment response in symptoms of depression and rate of return to school, when compared with a placebo group. With all of these studies, there are issues with the study design, subject population, and the addition of various forms of psychotherapy. None of the studies were designed to examine children with the primary diagnosis of GAD; however, these studies did provide the basic foundation for research that would follow to examine a clearer diagnostic group of anxiety disorders in children.

Another issue of concern with TCA use in children is associated with a growing recognition of cardiac risk. There have been reports of children who suddenly died while being treated with appropriate dosages of desipramine (Popper & Ziminitzky, 1995; Riddle, Geller, & Ryan, 1993; Riddle, Nelson, et al., 1991; Varley & McClellan, 1997). Given the uncertain clinical efficacy of TCAs for anxiety-disordered children (including those with GAD) and the significant side effects, particularly the cardiac risk, this class of medication is not a first choice. When these medications are used, the child or adolescent needs to have baseline vital signs, including sitting and standing blood pressure with pulse, as well as a baseline electrocardiogram (EKG). Once the therapeutic dose is reached, the EKG should be repeated and a serum level should be checked. This should be repeated with each significant dose adjustment.

Serotonin Reuptake Inhibitors

At this time, evidence-based medicine suggests the SSRIs as potential candidates for the treatment of childhood GAD and SAD. The safety of the SSRIs recommends them as a choice, as does their notable effectiveness in treating depression, which may be comorbid with childhood GAD and SAD. The SSRIs have shown preliminary efficacy in the treatment of adult anxiety disorders including GAD, panic disorder, and social phobia (Pohl, Wolkow, & Clary, 1998). Given the clinical similarity between these disorders and childhood anxiety disorders such as SAD and GAD, the favorable response to SSRIs provides an initial rationale for considering these medications in younger populations.

Another rationale for choosing an SSRI is the widespread use of SSRIs by pediatricians and child psychiatrists to treat both childhood depression and anxiety disorders. With the exception of one recently published study of fluoxetine in depression (Emslie et al., 1997), only very limited open-label studies exist to provide empirical support for the use of SSRI compounds in depression. However, one open-label study of adolescents with major depression provides some preliminary data on the efficacy of sertraline with depression (McConville et al., 1996).

There is some evidence currently available for the use of SSRIs to treat childhood GAD. Given the clinical similarity between GAD and SAD and the favorable response of adult patients with GAD to such SSRIs as paroxetine (Rickels et al., submitted) and venlafaxine, there is some rationale for using these medications in younger populations. Again, the majority of the studies include patients with GAD, SAD, social phobia, selective mutism, and anxiety disorder not otherwise specified. Fluoxetine has shown some preliminary benefit in a retrospective review of 21 patients who were treated openly for OAD, SAD, and social phobia, and in other case series (Birmaher et al., 1994: Manassis & Bradley, 1994). In another study, children and adolescents were diagnosed with one to several anxiety disorders. Those who failed an adequate trial of psychotherapy were treated openly with fluoxetine for approximately 9 weeks and showed significant improvement in symptoms (Fairbanks et al., 1997). The dose range was 20 to 40 mg per day. Rynn, Siqueland, and Rickels (2001) randomized ($N = 22$) children meeting the diagnosis of GAD to receive either placebo or 50 mg (maximum dose) of sertraline for 9 weeks. The Hamilton Anxiety Scale total (Hamilton, 1959), its psychic and somatic factors, and two clinical global scales—the severity (CGS-S) and improvement (CGS-I < 3)—showed significant treatment differences in favor of sertraline over placebo from Week 4 on. Self-report measures reflected these results of treatment. The main side effects of the sertraline-treated children as compared with those of the placebo-treated children were dry mouth (55% vs. 27%), drowsiness (73% vs. 45%), leg spasms (36% vs. 9%), and restlessness (55% vs. 27%).

The Research Unit on Pediatric Psychopharmacology Anxiety Study Group (2000) completed a randomized, controlled clinical trial of 8 weeks of fluvoxamine (maximum dose of 300 mg) versus placebo for 128 children and adolescents with GAD (51%), SAD (63%), social phobia (62%), and allowed for comorbid ADHD/ADD and oppositional-defiant disorder. In the fluvoxamine-treated group, 76% had a CGI less than 4, as compared with 29% in the placebo group. After being treated openly with supportive psychoeducational psychotherapy for 3 weeks, those children who did not improve were randomly assigned to either fluvoxamine or placebo treatment for 8 weeks. The two side effects seen more commonly in the children treated with fluvoxamine were increased motor activity and abdominal discomfort. There have been previous reports of activation or agitation with the SSRIs, and it appears to be dose related (Apter et al., 1994; Riddle, Hardin, & King, 1990; Riddle, King, & Hardin, 1991). With these recent positive studies, it appears that SSRIs are emerging as the first-line medication treatment for childhood anxiety disorders.

There are no specific laboratory tests required for the prescribing of SSRIs. One particular concern for the prescribing clinician is the risk for drug-drug interactions. The SSRIs inhibit specific isoenzymes in the P450 cytochrome system (2D6, 1A2, 2C, and 3A4), and this effect is different for each medication (for a review, see Leonard, March, Rickler, & Allen, 1997). It is important for the clinician to obtain a detailed medication history, including over-the-counter medications.

In prescribing SSRIs, it is recommended to initiate the medication at a low dose—for example, with sertraline, 25 mg per day for the first 7 days and then an increase to 50 mg per day, increasing slowly as clinical response dictates. As can be seen from the information presented, there still remains a lack of information about the amount of these medications required by this particular anxiety disorder. Once a therapeutic dose is reached, this dose should be maintained for 6 to 8 weeks to assess its efficacy.

Withdrawal symptoms have been reported with the discontinuation of SSRIs, including nausea, headache, dizziness, and agitation (Labellarte, Walkup, & Riddle, 1998). Therefore, these medications should not be abruptly discontinued. From the available evidence on the effects of medications, it appears that perhaps the SSRIs would be a first-line psychopharmacological treatment for childhood GAD, if the clinical course warranted their use, given their safety and tolerability.

Stages of Treatment

When considering stages of treatment, four dimensions can be identified: initial treatment, management of partial response, addressing treatment-refractory clients, and maintenance issues. As noted previously, the selection of a preferred treatment is best guided by the data, especially data gathered in a randomized clinical trial. Much of the evidence to date informs us about the choice of an initial treatment to be undertaken for a GAD youth. There is a noted absence of studies about what to do at the various other stages of treatment.

Studies have evaluated the efficacy and relative efficacies of treatments for children identified with the disorder, and these data guide our treatment choices. However, it is likely that some of the cases treated in these studies had prior experience with one or another treatment and may or may not have been partially refractory to those earlier treatments. More detailed analyses of initial treatment response may reveal useful information about the moderating role of prior treatment experiences in the efficacy of the treatment being evaluated. The field has, nevertheless, made meaningful progress in identifying at least a few initial treatments for GAD in youth that are quite promising.

We know little about what to do when the youthful patient is among those whose response to treatment is not favorable. Even when approximately two thirds of cases respond favorable to CBT, for example, there are still one third of the cases who did not respond well and may need something additional. The needs of both the partial responder and the refractory patient have not yet been addressed in systematic research. On might speculate that, in the CBT approach, a combination of more practice, increased exposure tasks, and help with the use of the FEAR plan in new, challenging situations would be worthwhile. One might also speculate that a combination of approaches may be valuable. The matter of the nonresponsive client is complicated by the fact that a nonresponder to one treatment approach (e.g., psychosocial, or medication) may then seek the other as a way to rectify the less-than-optimal previous outcomes. Again, more information is needed about prior treatment history and its effect on the evaluation of a current intervention, and there is a dramatic need for studies of the preferred treatment for cases in which the response to treatment was less than satisfactory.

With regard to maintenance, follow-up data for CBT have been reported. Several of the initial outcome studies reported follow-ups of 1 year, and separate follow-ups of 3.5 years and 6 years have also appeared in the literature. The good news supported by the evidence is that, for those whose treatment response was favorable, the effects seem to be maintained at a comparable rate. In contrast, there has yet to be a study of the effects of additional (booster sessions) or alternate treatment procedures on the maintenance of treatment effects.

The use of the combination of medications and CBT for the treatment of GAD has several potential merits and a few potential enigmas. First, the GAD youth who is nonresponsive to one of the approaches may be responsive to the other or their combination. The differences in the two treatments are apparent, and the GAD child may find the combination to be more effective than either monotherapy. However, the child who is refractory to one approach may carry other features (third variables, so to speak) that also contribute to the child's being refractory to the second approach or to the combined approach. Second, on the optimistic side, it may be that the combined treatment effect is additive—medications reduce initial distress and prepare the client for a more active and involved participation in CBT. However, a less optimistic view of the combined treatment is that a medication may detract from the efficacy of CBT. That is, if it is exposure to the situation and the facing of the unwanted emotional distress in that situation that contribute to the efficacy of CBT, then it is possible that the medication-produced nonanxious condition will prevent the CBT participant from experiencing anxiety in the exposure in-vivo tasks. That is, the effectiveness of the medications could undermine one of the thought-to-be-active aspects of CBT (habituation to anxiety in the situation).

Treatment Summary

The treatment of GAD requires consideration of psychological and pharmacological approaches and should be guided by the empirical data. The data suggest that the problems associated with GAD are treatable with moderate degrees of success, and that there is merit to consideration of the inclusion of parents in the treatment of the child's disorder. What is needed, clearly, are additional studies of the effects of medications and the relative effectiveness of CBT, both alone and in combination with medications.

REFERENCES

Achenbach, T. M. (1987). *Manual for the Youth Self-Report and Profile.* Burlington: University of Vermont Department of Psychiatry.

Achenbach, T. M. (1991a). *Integrative guide for the 1991 CBCL/4–18, YSR, and TRF Profiles.* Burlington: University of Vermont Department of Psychiatry.

Achenbach, T. M. (1991b). *Manual for the Child Behavior Checklist/4–18 and 1991 Profile.* Burlington: University of Vermont Department of Psychiatry.

Achenbach, T. M., & Edelbrock, C. S. (1983). *Manual for the Child Behavior Checklist and Revised Child Behavior Profile.* Burlington, VT: University Associates in Psychiatry.

Achenbach, T. M., & Edelbrock, C. S. (1986). *Manual for the Teacher's Report Form and Teacher Version of the Child Behavior Profile.* Burlington: University of Vermont Department of Psychiatry.

Albano, A. M., Chorpita, B. F., DiBartolo, P. M., & Barlow, D. H. (1995). *Comorbidity of DSM-III-R anxiety disorders in children and adolescents.* Unpublished manuscript, State University of New York at Albany.

Allen, A., Leonard H., & Swedo, S. E. (1995). Current knowledge of medications for the treatment of childhood anxiety disorders. *Journal of the American Academy of Child and Adolescent Psychiatry, 34,* 976–986.

Ambrose, B., & Rholes, W. S. (1993). Automatic cognitions and symptoms of depression and anxiety in children and adolescents: An examination of the content specificity hypothesis. *Cognitive Therapy and Research, 17,* 289–308.

American Psychiatric Association. (1987). *Diagnostic and statistical manual of mental disorders: DSM-III-R* (3rd ed., rev.). Washington, DC: Author.

American Psychiatric Association. (1994). *Diagnostic and statistical manual of mental disorders: DSM-IV* (4th ed.). Washington, DC: Author.

American Psychological Association Task Force on Promotion and Dissemination of Psychological Procedures. (1995). Training in and dissemination of empirically-validated psychological treatments: Report and recommendations. *Clinical Psychologist, 48,* 3–24.

Apter, A., Ratzoni, G., King, R., Weizman, A., Doncy, I., Ginder, M., & Riddle, M. (1994). Fluvoxamine open-label treatment of adolescent inpatients with obsessive-compulsive disorder or depression. *Journal of the American Academy of Child and Adolescent Psychiatry, 33,* 342–348.

Bandura, A. (1969). *Principles of behavior modification.* New York: Holt, Rinehart & Winston.

Bandura, A. (1986). *Social learning theory.* Englewood Cliffs, NJ: Prentice-Hall.

Barlow, D. (1988). *Anxiety and its disorders: The nature and treatment of anxiety and panic.* New York: Guilford Press.

Barlow, D., & Wolfe, B. E. (1981). Behavioral approaches to anxiety disorders: A report on the NIMH-SUNY, Albany, Research Conference. *Journal of Consulting and Clinical Psychology, 49,* 448–454.

Barrett, P. M., Dadds, M. R., & Rapee, R. M. (1996). Family treatment of childhood anxiety: A controlled trial. *Journal of Consulting and Clinical Psychology, 64,* 333–342.

Barrios, B. A., & Hartmann, D. B. (1988). Fears and anxieties. In E. J. Mash & L. G. Terdal (Eds.) *Behavioral assessment of childhood disorders* (2nd ed., pp. 196–264). New York: Guilford Press.

Beck, A. T., Brown, G., Steer, R. A., Eidelson, T. J., & Riskind, J. H. (1987). Differentiating anxiety and depression: A test of the cognitive content-specific hypothesis. *Journal of Abnormal Psychology, 96,* 179–183.

Beidel, D. C. (1988). Psychophysiological assessment of anxious emotional states in children. *Journal of Abnormal Psychology, 97,* 80–82.

Beidel, D. C., Turner, S. M., & Morris, T. L. (1995). A new inventory to assess childhood social anxiety and phobia: The social phobia and anxiety inventory for children. *Psychological Assessment, 7,* 73–79.

Bell-Dolan, D. J., & Brazeal, T. J. (1993). Separation anxiety disorder, overanxious disorder, and school refusal. *Child and Adolescent Psychiatric Clinics of North America, 2,* 563–580.

Berney, T., Kolvin, I., Bhate, S. R., Garside, R. F., Jeans, J., Kay, B., & Scarth, L. (1981). School phobia: A therapeutic trial with clomipramine and short-term outcome. *British Journal of Psychiatry, 138,* 110–118.

Bernstein, G. A., Borchardt, C. M., & Perwien, A. R. (1996). Anxiety disorders in children and adolescents: A review of the past 10 years. *Journal of the American Academy of Child & Adolescent Psychiatry, 35,* 1110–1119.

Bernstein, G. A., Brochardt, C. M., Perwien, A. R., et al. (2000). Imipramine plus cognitive-behavioral therapy in the treatment of school refusal. *Journal of the American Academy of Child and Adolescent Psychiatry, 3,* 276–283.

Bernstein, G. A., Crosby, R. D., Perwien, A. R., & Borchardt, C. M. (1996). Anxiety rating scale for children-revised: Reliability and validity. *Journal of Anxiety Disorders, 10,* 97–114.

Bernstein, G. A., Garfinkel, B. D., & Borchardt, C. M. (1990). Comparative studies of pharmacotherapy for school refusal. *Journal of the American Academy of Child and Adolescent Psychiatry, 29,* 773–781.

Biederman, J. (1987). Clonazepam in the treatment of prepubertal children with panic-like symptoms. *Journal of Clinical Psychiatry, 48*(Suppl.), 38–41.

Birmaher, B., Khetarpal, S., Brent, D., Cully, M., Balach, L., Kaufman, J., & McKenzie Neer, S. (1997). The Screen for Child Anxiety Related Emotional Disorders (SCARED): Scale construction and psychometric characteristics. *Journal of the American Academy of Child and Adolescent Psychiatry, 36,* 545–553.

Birmaher, B., Waterman, G. S., Ryan, N., Cully, M., Balach, L., Ingram, J., & Brodsky, M. (1994). Fluoxetine for childhood anxiety disorders. *Journal of the American Academy of Child and Adolescent Psychiatry, 33,* 993–999.

Bowen, R. C., Offord, D. R., & Boyle, M. H. (1990). The prevalence of generalized anxiety disorder and separation anxiety disorder: Results from the Ontario Child Health Study. *Journal of the American Academy of Child and Adolescent Psychiatry, 29,* 753–758.

Brady, E., & Kendall, P. (1992). Comorbidity of anxiety and depression in children and adolescents. *Psychological Bulletin, 111,* 244–255.

Brawman-Mintzer, O., & Lydiard, R. B. (1997). Biological basis of generalized anxiety disorder. *Journal of Clinical Psychiatry, 58*(Suppl. 3), 16–25.

Brown, T. A. (1999). Generalized anxiety disorder and obsessive-compulsive disorder. In T. Millon, P. H. Blaney, & R. D. Davis (Eds.), *Oxford textbook of psychopathology* (114–125). New York: Oxford University Press.

Brownell, K. D., Marlatt, G. A., Lichtenstein, E., & Wilson, G. T. (1986). Understanding and preventing relapse. *American Psychologist, 41,* 765–782.

Bruch, M. A., Heimberg, R. G., Berger, P., & Collins, T. M. (1989). Social phobia and perceptions of early parental and personal characteristics. *Anxiety Research, 2,* 57–63.

Cantwell, D. P., & Baker, L. (1989). Anxiety disorders. In L. K. G. Hsu & M. Hersen (Eds.), *Recent developments in adolescent psychiatry* (pp. 161–199). New York: Wiley.

Carey, G., & Gottesman, I. (1981). Twin and family studies of anxiety, phobic, and obsessive disorders. In D. F. Klein & J. Rabkin (Eds.), *Anxiety: New research and changing concepts* (pp. 117–133). New York: Raven Press.

Caster, J. B., Inderbitzen, H. M., & Hope, D. (1999). Relationship between youth and parent perceptions of family environment and social anxiety. *Journal of Anxiety Disorders, 13,* 237–251.

Chambless, D., & Hollon, S. (1998). Defining empirically supported treatments. *Journal of Consulting and Clinical Psychology, 66,* 5–17.

Chansky, T. E., & Kendall, P. C. (1997). Social expectations and self-perceptions of children with anxiety disorders. *Journal of Anxiety Disorders, 11,* 297–315.

Chorpita, B., Albano, A. M., & Barlow, D. (1996). Child anxiety sensitivity index: Considerations for children with anxiety disorders. *Journal of Clinical Child Psychology, 25,* 77–82.

Chorpita, B., & Barlow, D. (1998). The development of anxiety: The role of control in the early environment. *Psychology Bulletin, 124,* 3–21.

Chu, B. C., Marrs-Garcia, A. L., Mennin, D. S., & Kendall, P. C. (2000, November). *Determining clinically significant diagnoses of generalized anxiety in youth: A receiver operating characteristic (ROC) analysis approach.* Poster session presented at the 34th meeting of the Association for the Advancement of Behavior Therapy, New Orleans, LA.

Clark, L. A., & Watson, D. (1991). Tripartite model of anxiety and depression: Psychometric evidence and taxonomic implications. *Journal of Abnormal Psychology, 100,* 316–336.

Cobham, V. E. (1998). The case for involving the family in the treatment of childhood anxiety. *Behaviour Change, 15,* 203–212.

Cobham, V. E., Dadds, M. R., & Spence, S. H. (1999). Anxious children and their parents. *Journal of Clinical Child Psychology, 28,* 220–231.

Coffey, B. J. (1993). Review and update: Benzodiazepines in childhood and adolescence. *Psychiatric Annals, 23,* 332–339.

Cole, D. A., Truglio, R., & Peeke, L. (1997). Relation between symptoms of anxiety and depression in children: A multitrait-multimethod-multigroup assessment. *Journal of Consulting and Clinical Psychology, 65,* 110–119.

Costello, E. J., Costello, A. J., Edelbrock, C., Burns, B., Dulcan, M. K., Brent, D., & Janiszewski, S. (1988). Psychiatric disorders in pediatric primary care: Prevalence and risk factors. *Archives of General Psychiatry, 45,* 1107–1116.

Costello, E. J., Stouthamer-Loeber, M., & DeRosier, M. (1993). *Continuity and change in psychopathology from childhood to adolescence.* Paper presented at the Annual Meeting of the Society for Research in Child and Adolescent Psychopathology, Santa Fe, NM.

den Boer, J., & Westerberg, G. M. (1988). Effect of serotonin and noradrenaline uptake inhibitor in panic disorder: A double-blind comparative study with fluvoxamine and maprotiline. *Informational Clinical Psychopharmacology, 3,* 59–74.

Derivan, A. T., Entsuah, R., Haskins, T., Rudolph, R., & Aguiar, L. (1997, December). *Double-blind, placebo-controlled study of once-daily venlafaxine XR and buspirone in outpatients with generalized anxiety disorder (GAD).* Paper presented at the annual meeting of the American College of Neuropsychopharmacology, Honolulu, HI.

Dong, Q., Yang, B., & Ollendick, T. H (1994). Fears in Chinese children and adolescents and their relations to anxiety and depression. *Journal of Child Psychology and Psychiatry and Allied Disciplines, 35,* 351–363.

D'Zurilla, T. J., & Goldfried, M. R. (1971). Problem-solving and behavior modification. *Journal of Abnormal Psychology, 78,* 107–126.

D'Zurilla, T. J., & Nezu, A. M. (1999). *Problem-solving therapy: A social competence approach to clinical intervention* (2nd ed.). New York: Springer.

Eisen, A. R., & Engler, L. B. (1995). Chronic anxiety. In A. R. Eisen, C. A. Kearney, & C. E. Schaefer (Eds.), *Clinical handbook of anxiety disorders in children and adolescents* (pp. 223–250). Northvale, NJ: Jason Aronson.

Eisen, A. R., & Silverman, W. K. (1998). Prescriptive treatment for generalized anxiety disorder in children. *Behavior Therapy, 29,* 105–121.

Emslie, G. J., Rush, A. J., Weinberg, W. A., Kowatch, R. A., Hughes, C. W., Carmody, T., & Rintelmann, J. (1997). A double-blind, randomized, placebo-controlled trial of fluoxetine in children and adolescents with depression. *Archives of General Psychiatry, 54,* 1031–1037.

Epstein, N., Baldwin, L., & Bishop, D. (1983). The McMaster Family Assessment Device. *Journal of Marital and Family Therapy, 9,* 171–180.

Fairbanks, J. M., Pine, D. S., Tancer, N. K., Dummit, E. S., Kentgen, L. M., Martin

J., Asche, B. K., et al. (1997). Open fluoxetine treatment of mixed anxiety disorders in children and adolescents. *Journal of the American Academy of Child and Adolescent Psychiatry, 7,* 17–29.

Fauber, R. L., & Long, N. (1991). Children in context: The role of the family in child psychotherapy. *Journal of Consulting and Clinical Psychology, 59,* 813–820.

Finch, A. J., Kendall, P. C., & Montgomery, L. E. (1976). Qualitative differences in the experience of state-trait anxiety in emotionally disturbed and normal children. *Journal of Personality Assessment, 40,* 522–530.

Finch, A. J., Kendall, P. C., Montgomery, L. E., & Morris, T. (1975). Effect of two types of failure on anxiety. *Journal of Abnormal Psychology, 84,* 583–585.

Finch, A. J., Montgomery, L. E., & Deardorff, P. A. (1974). Children's manifest anxiety scale: Reliability with emotionally disturbed children. *Psychological Reports, 34,* 658.

Finch, A. J., Jr., Lipovsky, J. A., & Casat, C. D. (1989). Anxiety and depression in children and adolescents: Negative affectivity or separate constructs. In P. C. Kendall & D. Watson (Eds.), *Anxiety and depression: Distinctive and overlapping features* (pp. 171–202). San Diego, CA: Academic Press.

Fonseca, A. C., Yule, W., & Erol, N. (1994). Cross-cultural issues. In T. H. Ollendick, N. J. King, & W. Yule (Eds.), *International handbook of phobic and anxiety disorders in children and adolescents* (pp. 67–84). New York: Plenum Press.

Francis, G., Last, C. G., & Strauss, C. C. (1987). Expression of separation anxiety disorder: The roles of age and gender. *Child Psychiatry and Human Development, 18,* 82–89.

Frick, P. J., Silverthorn, P., Evans, C. (1994). Assessment of childhood anxiety using structured interviews: Patterns of agreement among informants and association with maternal anxiety. *Psychological Assessment, 6,* 372–379.

Ginsburg, G. S., La Greca, A. M., & Silverman, W. K. (1998). Social anxiety in children with anxiety disorders: Relation with social and emotional functioning. *Journal of Abnormal Child Psychology, 26,* 175–185.

Ginsburg, G. S., Silverman, W. K., Kurtines, W. K. (1995). Family involvement in treating children with phobic and anxiety disorders: A look ahead. *Clinical Psychology Review, 15,* 457–473.

Gittelman-Klein, R., & Klein, D. F. (1973). School phobia: diagnostic considerations in the light of imipramine effects. *Journal of Nervous and Mental Disorders, 156,* 199–215.

Glennon, B. & Weisz, J. R. (1978). An observational approach to the assessment of anxiety in young children. *Journal of Consulting and Clinical Psychology, 46,* 1246–1257.

Graae, F., Milner, J., Rizzotto, L., & Klein, R. G. (1994). Clonazepam in childhood anxiety disorders. *Journal of the American Academy of Child and Adolescent Psychiatry, 33,* 372–376.

Greenspan, S. I. (1981). *The clinical interview of the child.* New York: McGraw-Hill.

Gullone, E., & King, N. J. (1993). The fear of youth in the 1990s: Contemporary normative data. *Journal of Genetic Psychology, 154,* 137–153.

Hamilton, M. A. (1959). The assessment of anxiety status by rating. *British Journal of Medical Psychology, 32,* 50–55.

Haskins, T., Rudolph, R., Pallay, A., & Derivan, A. (1997, December). *Double-*

blind, placebo-controlled study of once-daily venlafaxine XR in outpatients with generalized anxiety disorder (GAD). Paper presented at the annual meeting of the American College of Neuropsychopharmacology, Honolulu, HI.

Herjanic, B., & Reich, W. (1982). Development of a structured psychiatric interview for children: Agreement between child and parent on individual symptoms. *Journal of Abnormal Child Psychology, 10,* 307–324.

Himadi, W. G., Boice, R., & Barlow, D. H. (1985). Assessment of agoraphobia: Triple response measurement. *Behavior Research and Therapy, 23,* 311–323.

Hodges, K., Kline, J., Fitch, P., McKnew, D., & Cytryn, L. (1981). The Child Assessment Schedule: A diagnostic interview for research and clinical use. *Catalog of Selected Documents in Psychology, 11,* 56.

Hoehn-Saric, R., Hazlett, R. L., & McLeod, D. R. (1993). Generalized anxiety disorder with early and late onset of anxiety symptoms. *Comprehensive Psychiatry, 34,* 291–298.

Howard, B. L., Chu, B., Krain, A., Marrs-Garcia, A., & Kendall, P. C. (1999). *Cognitive-behavioral family therapy for anxious children: Therapist manual* (2nd ed.). Ardmore, PA: Workbook Publishing (WorkbookPub@aol.com).

Howard, B. L., & Kendall, P. C. (1996). Cognitive-behavioral family therapy for anxiety disordered children: A multiple baseline evaluation. *Cognitive Therapy and Research, 20,* 423–443.

Ingram, R. E., & Kendall, P. C. (1987). The cognitive side of anxiety. *Cognitive Therapy and Research, 11,* 523–537.

Ingram, R. E., Kendall, P. C., & Chen, A. H. (1991). Cognitive-behavioral interventions. In C. R. Snyder & D. R. Forsyth (Eds.), *Handbook of social and clinical psychology: The health perspective* (pp. 509–522). New York: Pergamon Press.

Jefferson, J. (1995). Social phobia, a pharmacological treatment overview. *Journal of Clinical Psychiatry, 56,* 18–24.

Joiner, T. E., Jr., Catanzaro, S., & Laurent, J. (1996). The tripartite structure of positive and negative affect, depression, and anxiety in child and adolescent psychiatric inpatients. *Journal of Abnormal Psychology, 105,* 401–409.

Joiner, T. E., Jr., & Lonigan, C. J. (2000). Tripartite model of depression and anxiety in youth psychiatric inpatients: Relations with diagnostic status and future symptoms. *Journal of Clinical Child Psychology, 29,* 372–382.

Jolly, J. B., & Dykman, R. A. (1994). Using self-report data to differentiate anxious and depressive symptoms in adolescents: Cognitive content specificity and global distress? *Cognitive Therapy and Research, 18,* 25–38.

Katzelnick, D., Kobak, K. A., Greist, J. H., Jefferson, J. W., Mantle, J. M., & Serlin, R. C. (1995). Sertraline for social phobia: A double-blind, placebo-controlled cross-over study. *American Journal of Psychiatry, 152,* 1368–1371.

Kazdin, A., & Weisz, J. (1998). Identifying and developing empirically supported child and adolescent treatments. *Journal of Consulting and Clinical Psychology, 66,* 100–110.

Kendall, P. C. (1984). Behavioral assessment and methodology. In G. T. Wilson, C. M. Franks, K. D. Brownell, & P. C. Kendall (Eds.), *Annual review of behavior therapy: Theory and practice* (Vol. 9). New York: Guilford Press.

Kendall, P. C. (1985). Toward a cognitive-behavioral model of child psychopathology and a critique of related interventions. *Journal of Abnormal Child Psychology, 13,* 357–372.

Kendall, P. C. (1989). The generalization and maintenance of behavior change:

Comments, considerations and the "no-cure" criticism. *Behavior Therapy, 20,* 357–364.

Kendall, P. C. (1991). Guiding theory for treating children and adolescents. In P. C. Kendall (Ed.), *Child and adolescent therapy: Cognitive behavioral procedures* (pp. 3–24). New York: Guilford Press.

Kendall, P. C. (1992). *Coping cat workbook.* Ardmore, PA: Workbook Publishing (WorkbookPub@aol.com).

Kendall, P. C. (1994). Treating anxiety disorders in children: Results of a randomized clinical trial. *Journal of Consulting and Clinical Psychology, 62,* 100–110.

Kendall, P. C., & Brady, E. U. (1995). Comorbidity in the anxiety disorders of childhood. In K. D. Craig & K. S. Dobson (Eds.), *Anxiety and depression in adults and children.* Newbury Park, CA: Sage.

Kendall, P. C., Chansky, T. E., Friedman, M., Kim, R., Kortlander, E., Sessa F. M., & Siqueland, L. (1991). In P. C. Kendall (Ed.), *Child and adolescent therapy: Cognitive-behavioral procedures* (pp. 131–164). New York: Guilford Press.

Kendall, P. C., Chu, B., Gifford, A., Hayes, C., Nauta, M. (1998). Breathing life into a manual: Flexibility and creativity with manual-based treatments. *Cognitive and Behavioral Practice, 5,* 177–198.

Kendall, P. C., & Flannery-Schroeder, E. (1998). Methodological issues in treatment research for anxiety disorders in youth. *Journal of Abnormal Child Psychology, 26,* 27–38.

Kendall, P. C., Flannery-Schroeder, E., Panichelli-Mindel, S., Southam-Gerow, M. Henin, A., & Warman, M. (1997). Therapy for youth with anxiety disorders: A second randomized clinical trial. *Journal of Consulting & Clinical Psychology, 65,* 366–380.

Kendall, P. C., Henin, A., MacDonald, J. P., & Treadwell, K. R. H. (1999). *Parent ratings of anxiety in children: Development and validation of the CBCL-A.* Manuscript submitted for publication.

Kendall, P. C., & Ingram, R. (1987). The future of cognitive assessment of anxiety: Let's get specific. In L. Michelson & M. Ascher (Eds.), *Anxiety and stress disorders: Cognitive-behavioral assessment and treatment.* New York: Guilford Press.

Kendall, P. C., & Ingram, R. (1989). Cognitive-behavioral perspectives: Theory and research on depression and anxiety. In P. C. Kendall & D. Watson (Eds.), *Anxiety and depression: Distinctive and overlapping features.* New York: Academic Press.

Kendall, P. C., Kane, M., Howard, B., & Siqueland, L. (1990). *Cognitive-behavioral therapy for anxious children: Treatment manual.* Ardmore, PA: Workbook Publishing.

Kendall, P. C., Krain, A. L., & Treadwell, K. R. H. (1999). Generalized anxiety disorder. In R. Ammerman, C. Last, & M. Hersen (Eds.), *Handbook of prescriptive treatments for children and adolescents* (2nd ed.). Needham, MA: Allyn & Bacon.

Kendall, P. C., & Marrs-Garcia, A. (1999). *Psychometric analyses of a therapy-sensitive measure: The Coping Questionnaire (CQ).* Manuscript submitted for publication.

Kendall, P. C., & Pimentel, S. (2003). On the physiological symptom constellation in youth with generalized anxiety disorder (GAD). *Journal of Anxiety Disorders, 17*(2), 211–221.

Kendall, P. C., & Ronan, K. R. (1990). Assessment of childhood anxieties, fears, and phobias: Cognitive-behavioral models and methods. In C. R. Reynolds & R. W. Kamphaus (Eds.), *Handbook of psychological and educational assessment of children: Personality, behavior, and context* (pp. 223–244). New York: Guilford Press.

Kendall, P. C., & Southam-Gerow, M. (1996). Long-term follow-up of treatment for anxiety disordered youth. *Journal of Consulting and Clinical Psychology, 65,* 883–888.

Kendall, P. C., & Warman, M. (1996). Anxiety disorders in youth: Diagnostic consistency across *DSM-III-R* and *DSM-IV. Journal of Anxiety Disorders, 10,* 452–463.

Kendall, P. C., & Watson, D. (Eds.). (1989). *Anxiety and depression: Distinctive and overlapping features.* New York: Academic Press.

King, N. J., Gullone, E., & Ollendick, T. H. (1992). Manifest anxiety and fearfulness in children and adolescents. *Journal of Genetic Psychology, 153,* 63–73.

King, N. J., Hamilton, D. I., & Ollendick, T. H. (1988). *Children's phobias: A behavioral perspective.* London: Wiley.

King, N. J., Ollendick, T. H., & Gullone, E. (1991). Negative affectivity in children and adolescents: Relations between anxiety and depression. *Clinical Psychology Review, 11,* 441–459.

Klein, D. F., Mannuzza, S., Chapman, T., & Fyer, A. J. (1992). Child panic revisited. *Journal of the American Academy of Child and Adolescent Psychiatry, 31,* 112–116.

Klein, R. G. (1991). Parent-child agreement in clinical assessment of anxiety and other psychopathology: A review. *Journal of Anxiety Disorders, 5,* 187–198.

Krain, A. L., & Kendall, P. C. (2000). The role of parental emotional distress in parent report of child anxiety. *Journal of Clinical Child Psychology, 29,* 328–335.

Kutcher, S., & Mackenzie, S. (1988). Successful clonazepam treatment of adolescents with panic disorder. *Journal of Clinical Psychopharmacology, 8,* 299–301.

Kutcher, S. P., Reiter, S., Gardener, D. M., & Klein, R. G. (1992). The pharmacotherapy of anxiety disorders in children and adolescents. *Psychiatric Clinics of North America, 15,* 41–66.

Labellarte, M. J., Walkup, J. T., & Riddle, M. A. (1998). The new antidepressants: Selective serotonin reuptake inhibitors. *Pediatric Clinics of North America, 45,* 1137–1155.

La Greca, A. M., & Stone, W. L. (1993). The Social Anxiety Scale for Children–Revised: Factor structure and concurrent validity. *Journal of Clinical Child Psychology, 22,* 17–27.

Lang, P. J. (1968). Fear reduction and fear behavior: Problems in treating a construct. In J. M. Schleen (Ed.), *Research in psychotherapy.* Washington, DC: American Psychological Association.

Last, C. G., Hersen, M., Kazdin, A. E., Finkelstein, R., & Strauss, C. C. (1987). Comparison of *DSM-III* separation anxiety and generalized anxiety disorders: Demographic characteristics and patterns of comorbidity. *Journal of the American Academy of Child and Adolescent Psychiatry, 26,* 527–531.

Last, C. G., Strauss, C. C. & Francis, G. (1987). Comorbidity among childhood anxiety disorders. *Journal of Nervous and Mental Disease, 175,* 726–730.

Lau, J., Calamari, J., & Waraczynski, M. (1996). Panic attack symptomatology and anxiety sensitivity in adolescents. *Journal of Anxiety Disorders, 10,* 355–364.

Laurent, J., Catanzaro, S. J., Joiner, T. E., Rudolph, K. D., Potter K. I., Lambert, S., Osborne, L., et al. (1999). A measure of positive and negative affect for children: Scale development and preliminary validation. *Psychological Assessment, 11,* 326–338.

Laurent, J., Potter, K., & Catanzaro, S. J. (1994). *Assessing positive and negative affect in children: The development of the PANAS-C.* Paper presented at the 26th annual convention of the National Association of School Psychologists, Seattle, WA.

Laurent, J., Schmidt, N. B., Catanzaro, S. J., Joiner, T. E., Jr., & Kelley, A. M. (1998). Factor structure of a measure of anxiety sensitivity in children. *Journal of Anxiety Disorders, 12,* 307–331.

Laurent, J., & Stark, K. D. (1993). Testing the cognitive content specificity hypothesis with anxious and depressed youngsters. *Journal of Abnormal Psychology, 102,* 226–237.

Leonard, H. L., March, J., Rickler, K. C., & Allen, A. J. (1997). Pharmacology of the selective serotonin reuptake inhibitors in children and adolescents. *Journal of the American Academy of Child and Adolescent Psychiatry, 36,* 725–736.

Lerner, J., Safren, S. A., Henin, A., Warman, M., Heimberg, R. G., & Kendall, P. C. (1999). Differentiating anxious and depressive self-statements in youth: Factor structure of the Negative Affect Self-Statement Questionnaire among youth referred to an anxiety disorders clinic. *Journal of Clinical Child Psychology, 28,* 82–93.

Lonigan, C. J., Carey, M. P., & Finch, A. J., Jr. (1994). Anxiety and depression in children and adolescents: Negative affectivity and the utility of self-reports. *Journal of Consulting and Clinical Psychology, 62,* 1000–1008.

Lore, R. (1966). Palmar sweating and transitory anxieties in children. *Child Development, 37,* 115–123.

Manassis, K., & Bradley, S. (1994). Fluoxetine in anxiety disorders [Letter to the editor]. *Journal of the American Academy of Child and Adolescent Psychiatry, 33,* 761.

Mannusa, S., & Klein, R. (1987). *Schedule for the Assessment of Conduct, Hyperactivity, Anxiety, Mood, and Psychoactive Substances (CHAMPS).* New York: Authors.

March, J. S., & Albano, A. M. (1998). New developments in assessing pediatric anxiety disorders. In T. Ollendick and R. Prinz (Eds.), *Advances in clinical child psychology* (Vol. 20). New York: Plenum Press.

March, J. S., Biederman, J., Wolkow, R., Safferman, A., Mardekian, J., Cook, E. H., Cutler, N. R., et al. (1998). Sertraline in children and adolescents with obsessive-compulsive disorder: A multicenter randomized controlled trial. *Journal of the American Medical Association, 280,* 1752–1756.

March, J. S., Parker, J., Sullivan, K., Stallings, P., & Conners, C. (1997). The Multidimensional Anxiety Scale for Children (MASC): Factor structure, reliability and validity. *Journal of the American Academy of Child and Adolescent Psychiatry, 36,* 554–565.

Marlatt, G. A., & Gordon, J. J. (1985). *Relapse prevention.* New York: Guilford Press.

Mattis, S. G., & Ollendick, T. H. (1997). Panic in children and adolescents: A developmental analysis. *Advances in Clinical Child Psychology, 19,* 27–74.

McConville, B. J., Minnery, K. L., Sorter, M. T., West, S. A., Friedman, L. M., & Christian, K. (1996). An open study of the effects of sertraline on adolescent major depression. *Journal of Child and Adolescent Psychopharmacology, 6,* 41–51.

Miller, I., Epstein, N., Bishop, D., & Keitner, G. (1985). The McMaster Family Assessment Device: Reliability and validity. *Journal of Marital and Family Therapy, 11,* 345–356.

Miller, I., Kabacoff, R., Keitner, G., Epstein, N., & Bishop, D. (1986). Family functioning in the families of psychiatric patients. *Comprehensive Psychiatry, 27,* 302–312.

Muris, P., Merckelbach, H., Gadet, B., Moulaert, V., & Tierney, S. (1999). Sensitivity for treatment effects of the screen for child anxiety related emotional disorders. *Journal of Psychopathology and Behavioral Assessment, 21,* 323–335.

Noyes, R., Clancy, J., Crowe, R., Hoenk, P. R., & Slymen, D. J. (1978). The familial prevalence of anxiety neurosis. *Archives of General Psychiatry, 35,* 1057–1059.

Noyes, R., Woodman, C., Garvey, M. J., Cook, B. L., Suelzer, M., Chancy, J., & Anderson, D. J. (1992). Generalized anxiety disorder vs. panic disorder: Distinguishing characteristics and patterns of comorbidity. *Journal of Nervous and Mental Disease, 180,* 369–379.

Ollendick, T. H. (1983). Reliability and validity of the Revised Fear Survey Schedule for Children (FSSC-R). *Behavior Research and Therapy, 21,* 685–692.

Ollendick, T. H. (1995). Cognitive behavioral treatment of panic disorder with agoraphobia in adolescents: A multiple baseline design analysis. *Behavior Therapy, 26,* 517–531.

Ollendick, T. H., & Cerny, J. A. (1981). *Clinical behavior therapy with children.* New York: Plenum Press.

Ollendick, T. H., & Francis, G. (1988). Behavioral assessment and treatment of childhood phobias. *Behavior Modification, 12,* 165–204.

Ollendick, T. H., & King, N. J. (2000). Empirically supported treatments for children and adolescents. In P. C. Kendall (Ed.), *Child and Adolescent Therapy* (pp. 386–425). New York: Guilford Press.

Olson, D. H., Bell, R., & Portner, J. (1982). *Family Adaptability and Cohesion Evaluation Scales II.* (Available from Life Innovations, Family Inventories Project, PO Box 190, Minneapolis, MN 55440–0190)

Olson, D. H., McCubbin, H. I., Barnes, H., Larsen, A., Muxen, M., & Wilson, M. (1983). *Families: What makes them work?* Beverly Hills, CA: Sage.

Orvaschel, H., & Weissman, M. M. (1986). Epidemiology of anxiety disorders in children: A review. In R. Gittelman (Ed.), *Anxiety disorders of childhood* (pp. 58–72). New York: Guilford Press.

Pincus, H. A., Tanielian, T. L., Marcus, S. C., Olfson, M., Zarin, D. A., Thompson, J., & Magno, Z. J. (1998). Prescribing trends in psychotropic medications: Primary care, psychiatry, and other medical specialties. *Journal of the American Medical Association, 279,* 526–531.

Pohl, R., Balon, R., Yergani, V. K., & Gershon, S. (1989). Serotonergic anxiolytics in the treatment of panic disorder: A controlled study with buspirone. *Psychopathology, 22,* 60–67.

Pohl, R. B., Wolkow, R. M., & Clary, C. M. (1998). Sertraline in the treatment of panic disorder: a double-blind multicenter trial. *American Journal of Psychiatry, 155,* 1189–1195.

Popper, C. W., & Ziminitzky, B. (1995). Sudden death putatively related to desipramine treatment in youth: A fifth case and a review of speculative mechanisms. *Journal of Child and Adolescent Psychopharmacology, 5,* 283–300.

Puig-Antich, J., & Chambers, W. (1978). *The Schedule for Affective Disorders and Schizophrenia for School-Age Children (Kiddie-SADS).* New York: New York State Psychiatric Institute.

Rabian, B., Peterson, R., Richters, J., & Jensen, P. (1993). Anxiety sensitivity among anxious children. *Journal of Clinical Child Psychology, 22,* 441–446.

Reiss, S. (1991). Expectancy model of fear, anxiety, and panic. *Clinical Psychology Review, 11,* 141–153.

Reiss, S., & McNally, R. J. (1985). The expectancy model of fear. In S. Reiss & R. R. Bootzin (Eds.), *Theoretical issues in behavior therapy* (pp. 107–121). New York: Academic Press.

Reiss, S., Peterson, R., Gursky, D., & McNally, R. (1986). Anxiety sensitivity, anxiety frequency, and the prediction of fearfulness. *Behaviour Research and Therapy, 24,* 1–8.

Research Units of Pediatric Psychopharmacology Anxiety Study Group. (2000, May 30–June 2). A multi-site double-blind placebo-controlled trial of fluvoxamine for children and adolescents with anxiety disorders. Presented at the 40th New Clinical Drug Evaluation Unit Annual Meeting, Boca Raton, Florida.

Reynolds, C. R., & Paget, K. D. (1981). Factor analysis of the Revised Children's Manifest Anxiety Scale for blacks, whites, males, and females with a national normative sample. *Journal of Consulting and Clinical Psychology, 49,* 352–359.

Reynolds, C. R., & Paget, K. D. (1983). National normative and reliability data for the Revised Children's Manifest Anxiety Scale. *School Psychology Review, 12,* 324–336.

Reynolds, C. R., & Richmond, B. O. (1978). What I Think and Feel: A revised measure of children's manifest anxiety. *Journal of Abnormal Psychology, 6,* 271–280.

Reynolds, C. R., & Richmond, B. O. (1985). *Revised Children's Manifest Anxiety Scale.* Los Angeles: Western Psychological Service.

Rickels, K. (1990a). Buspirone in clinical practice. *Journal of Clinical Psychiatry, 9*(Suppl.), 51–54.

Rickels, K. (1990b). Discontinuation studies with alprazolam. *Journal of Psychiatry Research, 24,* 57–58.

Rickels, K., Amsterdam, J., Clary, C., Puzzuoli, G., & Schweizer, E. (1991). Buspirone in major depression: A controlled study. *Journal of Clinical Psychiatry, 52,* 34–38.

Rickels, K., Case, W. G., & Schweizer, E. (1991, June). Management of benzodiazepine discontinuation. Biological Psychiatry I. *Proceedings of 5th World Congress of Biological Psychiatry, Florence, Italy,* 778–779.

Rickels, K., Csanalosi, I., Greisman, P., Cohen, D., Werblowsky, J., Ross, H. A., Harris, H. (1983). A controlled clinical trial of alprazolam for the treatment of anxiety. *American Journal of Psychiatry, 140,* 82–85.

Rickels, K., Downing, R., Schweizer, E., & Hassman, H. (1993). Antidepressants for the treatment of generalized anxiety disorder: A placebo-controlled comparison of imipramine, trazodone and diazepam. *Archives of General Psychiatry, 50,* 884–895.

Rickels, K., Pollack, M. H., Sheehan, D. V., & Haskins, J. T. (2000). Efficacy of extended-release venlafaxine in nondepressed patients with generalized anxiety disorder. *American Journal of Psychiatry, 157,* 968–974.

Rickels, K., Schweizer, E., Case, W. G., & Greenblatt, D. J. (1990). Long-term therapeutic use of benzodiazepines: I. Effects of abrupt discontinuation. *Archives of General Psychiatry, 47,* 899–907.

Riddle, M. A., Bernstein, G. A., Cook, E. H., Leonard, H., L., March, J. S., & Swanson, J. M. (1999). Anxiolytics, adrenergic agents and naltrexone. *Journal of the American Academy of Child and Adolescent Psychiatry, 38,* 546–556.

Riddle, M. A., Geller, B., & Ryan, N. (1993). Case study: Another sudden death with a child treated with desipramine. *Journal of the American Academy of Child and Adolescent Psychiatry, 32,* 792–797.

Riddle, M. A., Hardin, M. T., & King, R. A. (1990). Fluoxetine treatment of children and adolescents with Tourette's and obsessive-compulsive disorders: Preliminary clinical experience. *Journal of the American Academy of Child and Adolescent Psychiatry, 29,* 45–48.

Riddle, M. A., King, R. A., Hardin, M. T., Scahill, L., Ort, S. I., & Leckman, J. F. (1991). Behavioral side effects of fluoxetine in children and adolescents. *Journal of Child and Adolescent Psychopharmacology, 1,* 193–198.

Riddle, M. A., Nelson, J. C., Kleinman, C. S., Rasmusson, A., Leckman, J. F., King, R. A., & Cohen, D. J. (1991). Case study: Sudden death in children receiving Norpramin: A review of three reported cases and commentary. *Journal of the American Academy of Child and Adolescent Psychiatry, 30,* 104–108.

Rogeness, G. A., Cepeda, C., Macedo, C. A., Fischer, C., & Harris, W. R. (1990). Differences in heart rate and blood pressure in children with conduct disorder, major depression, and separation anxiety. *Psychiatry Research, 33,* 199–206.

Ronan, K. R., & Kendall, P. C. (1997). Self-talk in distressed youth: States-of-mind and content specificity. *Journal of Clinical Child Psychology, 26,* 330–337.

Ronan, K., Kendall, P. C, & Rowe, M. (1994). Negative affectivity in children: Development and validation of a self-statement questionnaire. *Cognitive Therapy and Research, 18,* 509–528.

RUPP [Research Units on Pediatric Psychopharmacology Anxiety Study Group] (2001). Fluvoxamine for the treatment of anxiety disorders in children and adolescents. *New England Journal of Medicine, 344*(17), 1279–1285.

Rynn, M., Siqueland, L., Rickels, K., & Garcia-Espana, F. (2000, December). Treatment outcome of children with anxiety disorders. In *Scientific Abstract of the 39th Annual Meeting of the American College of Neuropsychopharmacology,* San Juan, Puerto Rico.

Sanders, M. (1996). New directions in behavioral family intervention with children. In T. Ollendick & R. Prinz (Eds.), *Advances in clinical child psychology* (Vol. 18). New York: Plenum.

Saylor, C. F., Finch, A. J., Spirito, A., & Bennett, B. (1984). The Children's Depression Inventory: A systematic evaluation of psychometric properties. *Journal of Consulting and Clinical Psychology, 52,* 955–967.

Schaefer, E. S. (1965). A configural analysis of children's reports of parent behavior. *Journal of Consulting Psychology, 27,* 552–557.

Schludermann, E., & Schludermann, S. (1970). Replicability of factors in children's report of parent behavior (CRPBI). *Journal of Psychology, 76,* 239–249.

Schniering, C. A., Hudson, J. L., & Rapee, R. M. (2000). Issues in the diagnosis and assessment of anxiety disorders in children and adolescents. *Clinical Psychology Review, 20,* 453–478.

Schwarz, J. C., Barton-Henry, M. L., & Pruzinsky, T. (1985). Assessing child-rearing behaviors: A comparison of ratings made by mother, father, child, and sibling on the CRPBI. *Child Development, 56,* 462–479.

Shaffer, D., Fisher, P., Dulcan, M. K., Davis, D., Piacentini, J., Schwab-Stone, M., Lahey, B., et al. (1996). The NIMH Diagnostic Interview Schedule for Children, Version 2.3. (DISC-2.3): Description, acceptability, prevalence rates, and performance in the MECA study. *Journal of the American Academy of Child and Adolescent Psychiatry, 49,* 865–877.

Sheehan, D. V., Raj, A. B., Sheehan, K. H., & Soto, S. (1990). Is buspirone effective for panic disorder? *Journal of Clinical Psychopharmacology, 10,* 3–11.

Silverman, W. K. (1991). *Guide to the use of the Anxiety Disorders Interview Schedule for Children–Revised (child and parent versions).* Albany, NY: Graywind Publications.

Silverman, W. K. (1994). Structured diagnostic interviews. In T. H. Ollendick, N. J. King, & W. Yule (Eds.), *International handbook of phobic and anxiety disorders in children and adolescents* (pp. 293–316). New York: Plenum Press.

Silverman, W. K., & Albano, A. M. (1997). *The Anxiety Disorders Interview Schedule for Children (DSM-IV),* San Antonio, TX: Graywind Publications/Psychological Corporation.

Silverman, W. K., & Eisen, A. R. (1992). Age differences in the reliability of parent and child reports of child anxious symptomatology using a structured interview. *Journal of the American Academy of Child and Adolescent Psychiatry, 31,* 117–124.

Silverman, W. K., Fleisig, W., Rabian, B., & Peterson, R. (1991). The Childhood Anxiety Sensitivity Index. *Journal of Clinical Child Psychology, 20,* 162–168.

Silverman, W. K., & Nelles, W. B. (1988). The anxiety disorders interview schedule for children. *Journal of the American Academy of Child and Adolescent Psychiatry, 27,* 772–778.

Simeon, J. G., Ferguson, H. B., Knott, V., Roberts, N., Gauthier, B., Dubois, C., & Wiggins, D. (1992). Clinical, cognitive, and neurophysiological effects of alprazolam in children and adolescents with overanxious and avoidant disorders. *Journal of the American Academy of Child and Adolescent Psychiatry, 31,* 29–33.

Simeon, J. G., Knott, V. J., Dubois, C., Wiggins, D., Geraets, I., Thatte, S., & Miller, W. (1994). Buspirone therapy of mixed anxiety disorders in childhood and adolescence: A pilot study. *Journal of Child and Adolescent Psychopharmacology, 4,* 159–170.

Solyom, M. D., Beck, P., Solyom, C., & Hugel, R. (1974). Some etiological factors in phobic neurosis. *Canadian Psychiatric Association Journal, 19,* 69–78.

Spence, S. H. (1997) Structure of anxiety symptoms among children: A confirmatory factor-analytic study. *Journal of Abnormal Psychology, 106,* 280–297.

Spielberger, C. (1973). *Preliminary manual for the State-Trait Anxiety Inventory for Children ("How I Feel Questionnaire").* Palo Alto, CA: Consulting Psychologists Press.

Stallings, P., & March, J. S. (1995). Assessment. In J. S. March (Ed.), *Anxiety disorders in children and adolescents* (pp. 125–147). New York: Guilford Press.

Strauss, C. C., Last, C. G., Hersen, M., & Kazdin, A. E. (1988). Association be-tween anxiety and depression in children and adolescents with anxiety disor-ders. *Journal of Abnormal Child Psychology, 16,* 57–68.

Strauss, C. C., Lease, C., Last, C. G., & Francis, G. (1988). Overanxious disor-der: An examination of developmental differences. *Journal of Abnormal Child Psychology, 16,* 433–443.

Tal, A., & Miklich, D. R. (1976). Emotionally induced decreases in pulmonary heart flow rates in asthmatic children. *Psychosomatic Medicine, 38,* 190–200.

Torgersen, S. (1983). Genetic factors in anxiety disorders. *Archives of General Psychiatry, 40,* 1085–1089.

Treadwell, K. H., & Kendall, P. C. (1996). Self-talk in anxiety-disordered youth: States-of-mind, content specificity, and treatment outcome. *Journal of Con-sulting and Clinical Psychology, 64,* 941–950.

Turner, S. M., Beidel, D. C., & Epstein, L. H. (1991). Vulnerability and risk for the anxiety disorders. *Journal of Anxiety Disorders, 5,* 151–166.

Varley, C. K., & McClellan, J. (1997). Case study: Two additional sudden deaths with tricyclic antidepressants. *American Journal of Child and Adolescent Psy-chiatry, 36,* 390–394.

Velez, C. N., Johnson, J., & Cohen, P. (1989). A longitudinal analysis of selected risk factors for childhood psychopathology. *Journal of the American Acad-emy of Child and Adolescent Psychiatry, 28,* 861–864.

Velosa, J. F., & Riddle, M. A. (2000). Pharmacologic treatment of anxiety disor-ders. In M. Lewis, A. Martin, & L. Scahill (Eds.), *Child and Adolescent Psy-chiatric Clinics of North America: Psychopharmacology* (Vol. 9, pp. 119–133). Philadelphia: W. B. Saunders.

Walker, L. S., & Greene, J. W. (1989). Children with recurrent abdominal pain and their parents: More somatic complaints, anxiety, and depression than other patient families? *Journal of Pediatric Psychology, 14,* 231–243.

Watson, D., Clark, L. A., & Tellegen, A. (1988). Development and validation of brief measures of positive and negative affect: The PANAS scales. *Journal of Personality and Social Psychology, 54,* 1063–1070.

Wells, K. C., & Virtulano, L. A., (1984). Anxiety disorders in childhood. In S. E. Turner (Ed.), *Behavioral theories and treatment of anxiety.* New York: Ple-num Press.

Werry, J. S. (1986). Diagnosis and assessment. In R. Gittelman (Ed.), *Anxiety disorders of childhood* (pp. 73–100). New York: Guilford Press.

Werry, J. S., & Aman, M. G. (1993). Anxiolytics, sedatives, and miscellaneous drugs. In J. S. Werry & M. G. Aman (Eds.), *Practitioner's guide to psychoac-tive drugs for children and adolescents* (2nd ed., pp. 391–415). New York: Plenum Medical Book Company.

Witt, J. C., Heffer, R. W., & Pfeiffer, J. (1990). Structured rating scales: A review of self-report and informant rating processes, procedures, and issues, In C. R. Reynolds & R. W. Kamphaus (Eds.). *Handbook of psychological and edu-cational assessment of children: Personality, behavior, and context* (pp. 364–394). New York: Guilford Press.

Zito, M. J. M., Safer, D. J., dosReis, S., Gardner, J. F., Boles, M., & Lynch, F. (2000). Trends in the prescribing of psychotropic medications to preschoolers. *Journal of the American Medical Association, 283,* 1025–1030.

13

PEDIATRIC OBSESSIVE-COMPULSIVE DISORDER

MARTIN E. FRANKLIN, MOIRA A. RYNN,
EDNA B. FOA, & JOHN S. MARCH

Approximately one in 200 young people suffers from obsessive-compulsive disorder (OCD) (Flament et al., 1988), which can result in significant functional impairment (Laidlaw, Falloon, Barnfather, & Coverdale, 1999; Leonard et al., 1993). Despite this, pediatric OCD often goes undiagnosed or is inadequately treated, leading to considerable morbidity and comorbidity extending into adulthood. As we describe in this chapter, considerable progress has been made in the last decade in developing and evaluating treatments for this condition in children and adolescents. It is hoped that broad dissemination of information about pediatric OCD in venues such as this book will lead to increased identification of children suffering from this condition, followed by proper referral and clinical care.

In this chapter, we review the extant literature pertaining to the clinical manifestation, diagnosis, assessment, and treatment of OCD in children and adolescents. In general, the literature on pharmacotherapy for pediatric OCD is better developed than is the cognitive-behavioral therapy (CBT) literature, and here we describe several ongoing studies that shed additional light on the relative efficacy of initial treatment strategies. Like many treatment providers, we also recognize that not all patients respond fully to the currently available initial treatments, so we discuss clinical considerations when this is the case. Information from the OCD Expert Consensus Guidelines (March, Frances, Kahn, & Carpenter, 1997) is used to structure that discussion, and areas where the guidelines have received empirical support are emphasized.

CLINICAL MANIFESTATION AND DIAGNOSIS

Children and adolescents with OCD suffer from anxiety-evoking thoughts and images (obsessions) that prompt overt behaviors or mental acts (compulsions) intended to reduce obsessional distress and the likelihood of a feared disastrous consequence (e.g., illness resulting from contamination). These OCD symptoms can result in significant distress and functional impairment, leaving some youngsters unable to complete schoolwork, pursue their hobbies, or socialize with peers. Passive avoidance is also a common feature of OCD in children and adolescents, such as refusal to enter situations that provoke their obsessional anxiety (e.g., writing and reading, for fear of having to repeat). From the adult literature, it is clear that there is a range of insight into the senselessness of OCD concerns, with approximately 30% of OCD patients reporting very little or no insight (Foa et al., 1995). Although not studied empirically, clinical experience suggests that poor insight into the senselessness of symptoms may be quite common in pediatric OCD, and thus the *DSM-IV* does not require past or present insight for diagnosis of OCD in children and adolescents (APA, 1994). Poor insight is a negative predictor of response to CBT in adults (Foa, Abramowitz, Franklin, & Kozak, 1999), quite possibly because these fixed beliefs compromise homework compliance. Although no comparable empirical data are available for children, degree of insight should be examined carefully prior to beginning treatment with a child suffering from OCD. Furthermore, family beliefs about the senselessness of symptoms should also be explored, because parents who believe the feared consequences will occur may also discourage compliance with CBT assignments.

Pediatric OCD is formally similar to OCD in adults, yet the content of obsessions and compulsions is likely to be influenced by developmental factors. For example, younger children are generally more magical in their thinking and thus may have more superstitious OCD symptoms (e.g., "If I don't retrace my steps, something really bad will happen to my little sister"). Furthermore, advances in language development may make it easier for adults with contamination fears to articulate the feared consequence of becoming contaminated (e.g., contracting AIDS) than a younger person might be. Because introspection is generally challenging for children, those youngsters with OCD may have greater difficulty articulating obsessions and may instead refer to their physical reactions ("If I don't do my washing, then my tummy will feel really bad"). Additionally, some children who are well aware of their obsessional content may be embarrassed about verbalizing it or fearful that saying their disastrous consequences aloud will magically cause them to occur.

As with adults, some pediatric OCD patients are able to identify feared consequences of not ritualizing (e.g., books will be stolen if the locker is not checked), whereas others experience anxiety and distress in the absence of articulated consequences. Presence or absence of feared consequences has implications for CBT that are discussed in detail later in the chapter.

Furthermore, although the logic of some patients' feared consequences is shared by many in their culture (e.g., contracting disease via direct contact with a public toilet seat), other patients' fears are extremely unusual (e.g., losing their essence by discarding trash that has touched them). It is important to recognize that bizarre content does not preclude a diagnosis of OCD and that patients with such unusual fears may also be responsive to CBT (Franklin, Tolin, March, & Foa, 2001).

Modern classification schemes for OCD have focused on ritualistic activity (i.e., compulsions) rather than on the obsessive content. Although many patients have more than one form of ritual, the predominant one typically determines how the individual's OCD symptoms are usually classified. Thus, patients are described as washers, checkers, orderers, and so on.

Ritualistic washing is the most common compulsion in children and adolescents and is typically performed to decrease discomfort associated with contamination obsessions. For example, individuals who fear contact with AIDS "germs" clean themselves and their environment excessively to prevent either contracting AIDS themselves or spreading it to others. Most washers can identify a specific disaster that will occur if they refrain from compulsive washing, although developmental factors affect this ability. For some washers, the state of being contaminated itself generates tremendous discomfort. To decrease this distress, they feel compelled to engage in washing rituals.

Another common compulsion is repetitive checking, which is typically performed to prevent an anticipated catastrophe. Developmental factors influence content here as well, because children and adolescents with checking rituals may worry more about losing items out of their book bags than they would about the car being stolen. Youngsters with such fears will repeatedly check in order to make sure that the feared consequence has not happened, yet the repetition itself may increase rather than decrease anxiety in the long run. Some repeaters are similar to checkers in that they, too, are typically driven by the wish to prevent disasters; however, they often differ from checkers in that their rituals are unrelated logically to their feared consequences. For example, it is logical (if excessive) to check the front door lock many times if one fears a burglary, but illogical to walk up and down the stairs repeatedly to prevent a loved one's death in a motor vehicle accident. As we described above, some OCD subtypes may exhibit more ticlike behavior, in that there is not a feared consequence to be avoided but simply negative affect to be alleviated. This may be especially true in younger OCD sufferers, although this hypothesis awaits empirical confirmation.

Other common pediatric compulsions include ordering, counting, and hoarding. Hoarding is atypical in that many hoarders engage in little compulsive activity and are perhaps better characterized as avoidant. Instead of going to great lengths to collect materials to save, many hoarders simply avoid discarding items they encounter in everyday life (e.g., newspapers, string) for fear of not having them available in the future. Over long periods of time, consistent avoidance of discarding can result in overwhelming accumulations, even in the absence of active gathering rituals. Clearly, the accumulation of massive amounts of hoarded material is less common in children, because they have had less time to do so than have adults, but hoarding behaviors and fears of discarding items should be evaluated nevertheless. Hoarded material can also vary from items of some monetary value (e.g., complete sets of Pokemon cards) to those that are worthless (e.g., chicken bones, empty milk containers); diagnosis is more complicated when the hoarded material can be viewed as "collectibles." The difference between hoarding and collecting in children may be best illustrated by example: A child who collected action figures would routinely discuss his collections with his friends at school, who had similar collections in their own homes. However, the child being treated for hoarding also felt that he had to keep the ripped cardboard boxes that the figures came in, the wrapping paper that covered the boxes if they were given as presents, and he had four of each figure "in case something happened to the main ones."

With respect to comorbidity, of 70 children and adolescents in the large-scale NIMH sample (which excluded children with mental retardation, eating disorders, and Tourette's syndrome), only 26% of the study patients had OCD as the sole disorder at baseline (Swedo, Rapoport, Leonard, Lenane, & Cheslow, 1989). Clinically, comorbidity, especially with the oppositional and tic disorders, appears to predict non- or partial response to both pharmacotherapy and CBT, but the hypothesis remains untested in pediatric patients. Thus, although these comorbid conditions do not currently present a contraindication to CBT or to pharmacotherapy, careful assessment of them and consideration of their implications appears to be necessary in clinical settings.

In summary, children and adolescents with OCD typically present with both obsessions and compulsions, although the youngest sufferers may have difficulty identifying specific obsessions. As is the case with adults, the cardinal feature of OCD in youth is neutralizing: When the patient describes anxiety-inducing thoughts or images and attempts to relieve this anxiety or reduce the chances that feared consequences will occur by performing some overt or covert neutralizing behavior, the OCD diagnosis should be considered. Functional impairment is required for diagnosis as well, because subclinical obsessions and compulsions are probably ubiquitous. Insight into the senselessness of obsessional concerns, on the other hand, is not required for diagnosis in children and adolescents. Obsessional content can range from exaggerated concerns shared by most in the culture (e.g., fear of burglary resulting from leaving the front door unlocked) to highly unusual and illogical fears (e.g., loss of one's soul due to failure to neutralize a feared mental image). Comorbidity with anxiety disorders, tic disorders, ADHD, and mood disorders is also apparently common (e.g., Last & Strauss, 1989; Swedo et al., 1989), and therefore careful evaluation is needed to gather a sufficiently detailed clinical picture that can be used to guide discussion of treatment alternatives.

ASSESSMENT

An adequate assessment of pediatric OCD should include a comprehensive evaluation of current and past OCD symptoms, current OCD symptom severity and associated functional impairment, and a survey of comorbid psychopathology. In addition, the strengths of the child and family should be evaluated, as well as their knowledge of OCD and its treatment. There are many self-report and clinician-administered instruments that can be used to guide this type of assessment. We typically mail several relevant self-report questionnaires (e.g., Multidimensional Anxiety Scale for Children [MASC] and MASC OC Screener; March, 1998) for the family to complete prior to the intake visit, then review these materials before meeting with the child. If it is apparent from these materials that comorbid depression or other anxiety problems besides OCD are prominent, we focus on these symptoms as well in the intake. The Anxiety Disorders Interview Schedule for Children (ADIS-C; Albano & Silverman, 1996) is a semistructured interview that can be used to examine comorbid problems in greater detail; we use the ADIS in our current collaborative study examining the relative efficacy of CBT, sertraline, combined treatment, and pill placebo (Franklin, Foa, & March, in press).

For surveying history of OCD symptoms and current symptom severity, we use the Children's Yale Brown Obsessive-Compulsive Scale (CY-BOCS) checklist and severity scale (Scahill et al., 1997). Before administering this scale, it is important to determine whether the child should be interviewed with or without the parent present. In our randomized controlled trial, we conduct a conjoint interview, directing questions to the child but soliciting parental feedback as well. In nonresearch settings, there is more flexibility, and the decision to interview the child alone or with a parent present can be made by discussing these choices with the parent in advance, observing the child and family's behavior in the waiting area and even during the interview, if necessary. For example, if it becomes clear that a patient is reluctant to discuss certain symptoms with a parent present (e.g., sexual obsessions), the therapist can skip that item on the CY-BOCS checklist and save some time at the end of the interview to revisit these potentially sensitive issues alone with the patient. Our mantra in the clinic is "get the information," meaning that if parental presence increases the validity of the assessment then do that; if not, then interview the child alone.

Prior to administering the CY-BOCS, the therapist should explain the concepts of obsessions and compulsions, using examples if the child or parent has difficulty grasping the concepts. We also take this opportunity to tell children and adolescents about the prevalence, nature, and treatment of OCD, which may increase their willingness to disclose their specific symptoms. Children may be particularly vulnerable to feeling as if they are the only ones on earth with obsessive fears of hurting a loved one, so we preface the examples with "I once met a kid who . . . " to dispel this myth and minimize the accompanying sense of isolation. During the intake, it is also important to observe the child's behavior and inquire if certain behaviors (e.g., unusual movements, vocalizations) are compulsions designed to neutralize obsessions or to reduce distress. Tic disorders are commonly comorbid with OCD, and it is important to try to make a differential diagnosis, because compulsions and tics would be targeted by different treatment procedures. Furthermore, as mentioned previously, some children who are aware of their obsessional content may be fearful of saying the fears aloud. Surveying common obsessions with a checklist instead of asking the child to disclose the fears tends to help with this problem, as does encouragement on the part of the therapist (e.g., "Lots of the kids I see have a hard time talking about these kinds of fears"). We have found that flexibility in manner of disclosing the obsession is warranted. Thus, for example, we allow the child to write down the fears or nod as the therapist describes examples of similar fears to help the child share OCD problems. In this way, we can convey to the child and family that we recognize the difficulty associated with disclosure. We also use examples from children we have evaluated in the past (e.g., "I remember a few months ago when a kid about your age told me she would be scared to touch her dog for fear she might lose control and hurt him"), although we let the children and families know that we are careful not to violate confidentiality when citing such examples. Below are brief descriptions of our core assessments.

CHILDREN'S YALE-BROWN OBSESSIVE-COMPULSIVE SCALE   The primary instrument for assessing OCD is the Y-BOCS, which assesses obsessions and compulsions separately on time consumed, distress, interference, degree of resistance, and control (Goodman, Price, Rasmussen, Mazure, Delgado, et al., 1989; Goodman, Price, Rasmussen, Mazure, Fleischmann, et al., 1989). We use the pediatric version (Scahill, Riddle, McSwiggin-Hardin, et al., 1997) to inventory past and present OCD symptoms, initial severity, total OCD severity, relative preponderance of obsessions and compulsions, and degree of insight. The CY-BOCS is a clinician-rated instrument merging data from clinical observation and parent and child report.

ANXIETY DISORDERS INTERVIEW FOR CHILDREN   The child and adolescent ADIS is a semistructured interview for assessing *DSM-IV* anxiety disorders in youth that shows excellent psychometric properties for internalizing conditions relative to other available instruments, such as the DISC (Silverman, 1991). The ADIS uses an interviewer-observer format, thereby allowing the clinician to draw information from the interview and from clinical observations. Scores are derived regarding *specific diagnoses* and *level of diagnosis-related interference*. Adequate psychometric properties have been demonstrated (Silverman & Nelles, 1998; Silverman & Rabian, 1995).

CHILDREN'S OCD IMPACT SCALE (COIS)   We also obtain child and parent versions of the OCD Impact Scale, which shows preliminary evidence favoring psychometric adequacy and sensitivity to change (Piacentini, Jaffer, Liebowitz, & Gitow, 1992), for use in analyses of functional impairment from OCD. This instrument enables us to estimate whether the CY-BOCS improvements result in normalization as assessed by functional impairment. A new and shorter version of this scale has been developed recently, and the psychometric properties of this scale appear to be favorable (Piacentini, Jaffer, Bergman, McCracken, & Keller, 2001).

MULTIDIMENSIONAL ANXIETY SCALE FOR CHILDREN   The MASC has four factors and six subfactors—physical anxiety (tense/restless, somatic/autonomic), harm avoidance (perfectionism, anxious coping), social anxiety (humiliation/rejection, performance anxiety), and separation anxiety—and is in use in a variety of NIMH-funded treatment outcome studies. The MASC shows test-retest reliability in clinical (intraclass correlation coefficient [ICC] > .92) and school samples (ICC >.85); convergent/divergent validity is similarly superior (March, 1998; March & Sullivan, 1999).

CHILDREN'S DEPRESSION INVENTORY (CDI)   The CDI (Kovacs, 1985) is a 27-item self-report scale that measures cognitive, affective, behavioral, and interpersonal symptoms of depression. Each item consists of three statements, of which the child is asked to select the one statement that best describes his or her current functioning. Items are scored from 0 to 2; therefore, scores on the CDI can range from 0 to 54. The CDI shows adequate reliability and validity (Kovacs, 1985). This scale is useful in assessing for symptoms of depression, which assists in tailoring the treatment plan.

MEDICAL HISTORY   Pediatric OCD patients' medical histories should also be surveyed, with particular attention to the presence of recurrent strep infection. Although children with streptococcal-precipitated OCD (pediatric autoimmune neuropsychiatric disorders associated with streptococcal infection, or PANDAS) may require somewhat different treatment(s), experts agree that the base rate of PANDAS given to OCD is currently unknown and that the diagnosis cannot be assigned retrospectively at this juncture (Leonard et al., 1999; Swedo et al., 1998). Current research diagnostic criteria for PANDAS require at least two prospectively documented episodes of exacerbations in OCD and tic symptoms associated with streptococcal infection. Unfortunately, an unambiguous retrospective diagnosis of PANDAS is next to impossible in a clinically referred population of youth with OCD (Giulino et al., 2002). Clinically, children who have unambiguous cases of PANDAS should be referred for appropriate treatment of their Group A beta-hemolytic streptococcal (GABHS) infection. Once the child has been treated for strep, the clinician should then also consider the CBT and selective serotonin reuptake inhibitor (SSRI) pharmacotherapy described later in this chapter.

In brief, the aforementioned scales, interviews, and questionnaires may be useful in generating relevant clinical information at pretreatment and in helping us to evaluate treatment gains once treatment has ended. In our research-oriented settings, this is part of routine clinic practice, and perhaps the development of an efficient packet for evaluating outcome may stimulate more interest in effectiveness research in real-world clinical settings. Until our measurements have been streamlined and boiled down to their essential components, however, financial, time, and personnel constraints may limit the more general usefulness of our battery.

TREATMENT OVERVIEW

Evidence-based clinical practice guidelines that employ a stages-of-treatment model are assuming increasing importance in pediatric psychiatry. Most discussions of practice guidelines focus only on selection of initial treatment or management of treatment-refractory patients. However, maximum clinical utility requires a stages-of-treatment model that addresses selection of initial treatment, management of partial response, maintenance treatment, treatment resistance, and comorbidity. We were instrumental in developing the only two practice guidelines that so far have been published for the treatment of OCD in youth: The Expert Consensus Guidelines (March et al., 1997) and the American Academy of Child and Adolescent Psychiatry (AACAP) Practice Parameters for OCD (King, 1995). Both recommend starting with CBT or CBT plus an SSRI, depending on severity and pattern of comorbidity; both recommend that patients started on SSRI monotherapy who are partial responders be augmented with CBT. As shown in Table 13.1, a variety of options are recommended by OCD experts in the face of partial response and treatment resistance. For example, experts generally consider CBT a first-line augmentation strategy and medication augmentation a second-line option.

With or without concomitant medication, exposure and response (ritual) prevention is the cornerstone of treatment for children and adolescents with OCD. As applied to OCD, the exposure principle relies upon the fact that anxiety usually attenuates after sufficient duration of contact with a feared stimulus (Foa & Kozak, 1986). Thus, a child with fear of germs should be encouraged to confront relevant feared situations until his or her anxiety decreases. Repeated exposure is associated with decreased anxiety across exposure trials, with anxiety reduction largely specific to the domain of exposure, until the child no longer fears contact with specifically targeted phobic stimuli (March & Mulle, 1995). Adequate exposure depends on blocking the negative reinforcement effect of rituals or avoidance behavior, a process termed *response prevention*. For example, a child with germ worries must not only touch "germy things," but must also refrain from ritualized washing until his or her anxiety diminishes substantially. Exposure/response prevention (EX/RP) is typically implemented in a gradual fashion (sometimes termed graded exposure), with exposure targets under the patient's or, less desirably, the therapist's control (March & Mulle, 1996). Intensive prescriptive approaches work equally well for children who

Table 13.1. Executive Summary from OCD Expert Consensus Guidelines (March, Frances, Kahn, & Carpenter, 1997)

Obsessive-Compulsive Disorder Executive Summary
A. Consensus Recommendations for First-Line Treatments by Clinical Situation

(**Bold italics** indicate treatments of choice)

SELECTING THE INITIAL TREATMENT STRATEGY AND THE SEQUENCE OF TREATMENTS

Age-specific considerations
- Prepubescent children: CBT first for milder or more severe OCD
- Adolescents: CBT first for milder OCD; CBT + SRI for more severe OCD
- Adults: CBT first for milder OCD; CBT + SRI or SRI alone first for more severe OCD

Considerations based on overall efficacy, speed, and durability of treatment
- Milder OCD: CBT alone, or CBT + SRI
- More severe OCD: CBT + SRI

Considerations based on tolerability and patient acceptability
- Milder OCD: CBT alone, or CBT + SRI
- More severe OCD: CBT + SRI, or SRI alone

Selecting CBT strategy

Obsessions and compulsions	EX/RP (exposure/response prevention) EX/RP + CT (cognitive therapy)

Tailoring treatment for specific symptoms

Contamination fears, symmetry rituals, counting/repeating, hoarding, aggressive urges	EX/RP
Scrupulosity and moral guilt, pathological doubt	CT

Intensity of CBT
- Gradual (i.e., weekly): Recommended for most patients (usually 13–20 sessions)
- Intensive (i.e., daily): Recommended when speed is of the essence, or for patients who have not responded to gradual CBT or who have extremely severe symptoms

Selecting a specific medication: Use a serotonin reuptake inhibitor (SRI)

- Fluvoxamine - Fluoxetine - Clomipramine - Sertraline - Paroxetine	Recommendations for timing - Inadequate response to average SRI dose: Push to maximum dose in 4–9 weeks from start of treatment - Inadequate response after 4–6 additional weeks at maximum dose: Switch to another SRI

Treatment resistance

If no response or partial response to CBT alone	Add an SSRI; add more CBT with changes in approach
If no response or partial response to SSRI alone	Add CBT or switch to another SSRI
If no response to combined CBT and SSRI	Switch to another SSRI
If partial response to combined CBT and SSRI	Switch to another SSRI Add more CBT with changes in approach Augment with another medication
After failing trials of 2–3 SSRIs + CBT	Try clomipramine
If no response or partial response to combined CBT and 3 SRI trials (one of which was clomipramine)	Augment with another medication (select agent based on associated features) Add more CBT with changes in approach

Table 13.1. (continued)

Obsessive-Compulsive Disorder Executive Summary
A. Consensus Recommendations for First-Line Treatments by Clinical Situation

Maintenance treatment

When to use long-term medication	After 3–4 mild/moderate relapses or 2–4 severe relapses despite adequate CBT
How to stop medication	Gradually taper meds after 1–2 years while continuing monthly CBT (decrease meds by 25% and wait 2 months before next decrease)
Frequency of office visits	
Full recovery with CBT alone	Monthly for the next 3–6 months
Partial recovery with CBT alone	Weekly to monthly for the next 3–6 months
Full or partial recovery with medications	Monthly for the next 3–6 months

B. Consensus Recommendations for First-Line Psychosocial Treatments

Cognitive-behavioral therapy For OCD, CBT involves exposure plus response prevention (EX/RP) combined with cognitive therapy (CT)	• When available, use CBT for every patient with OCD except those who have very severe symptoms or who are unwilling to participate in CBT • Add when patient has been a nonresponder or partial responder to SRI alone • Use alone if patient is intolerant to side effects of medication or is pregnant or has a medical condition that contraindicates medication • Comorbidity with other psychiatric disorders for which CBT may be helpful, especially if modified for the comorbid disorder
Exposure plus response prevention (EX/RP)	• Especially helpful for contamination or other fears, symmetry rituals, counting/repeating, hoarding, aggressive urges
Cognitive therapy	• Especially helpful for scrupulosity, moral guilt, and pathological doubt
Treatment format and intensity	
Format:	• Especially helpful for contamination or other fears Individual weekly therapy sessions combined with homework or therapist-assisted out-of-office (in vivo) techniques; consider adding family therapy when appropriate
Frequency:	• Especially helpful for contamination or other fears 13–20 sessions typically required to treat an uncomplicated OCD patient
Intensity:	• Especially helpful for contamination or other fears Gradual, i.e., weekly: Recommended for most patients Intensive, i.e., daily: Recommended when speed is of the essence or patients have not responded to gradual CBT or have very severe symptoms
Maintenance Schedule:	• Especially helpful for contamination or other fears Schedule: Monthly booster sessions for 3–6 months

(continued)

Table 13.1. (continued)

C. Consensus Recommendations for First-Line Somatic Treatments

Selective serotonin reuptake inhibitors (SSRIs) (Fluvoxamine, Fluoxetine, Sertraline, Paroxetine)	• Combine with CBT or use alone in adults with moderate to severe symptoms • Add when no response or partial response to CBT alone • Rather than clomipramine when anticholinergic, cardiovascular, sexual, sedative, or weight-gain side effects are a concern • Comorbidity with other psychiatric disorders for which an SSRI may be helpful
Clomipramine	• Use after 2–3 failed SSRI trials • Augment SSRI in partially responsive or nonresponsive patient • Less likely than SSRIs to cause insomnia, akathisia, nausea, or diarrhea • Comorbidity with other psychiatric disorders for which a TCA may be helpful

D. Consensus Recommendations for OCD Complicated by Comorbid Illness

Comorbidity	
Pregnancy	CBT alone
Heart disease	CBT alone, or CBT + SSRI
Renal disease	CBT alone, or CBT + SSRI
Tourette's syndrome	CBT + conventional antipsychotic + SRI
Attention-deficit/hyperactivity disorder	CBT + SSRI + psychostimulant
Panic disorder or social phobia	CBT + SSRI
Major depressive disorder	CBT + SRI (start SRI first for severe symptoms)
Bipolar disorder (I or II)	CBT + mood stabilizer alone, or CBT + mood stabilizer + SRI
Opposition/conduct/antisocial disorder	CBT + family therapy +SRI
Schizophrenia	SRI + neuroleptic

Note. CBT = cognitive behavioral therapy. SRI (serotonin reuptake inhibitor) refers to the five compounds clomipramine, fluoxetine, fluvoxamine, paroxetine, and sertraline; SSRI (selective SRI) refers to all but clomipramine.

subscribe in advance to this approach (Franklin et al., 1998). Intensive approaches may be especially useful for treatment-resistant OCD or in cases in which a very rapid response is needed.

As shown in Table 13.2, the protocol used by March and Foa in their NIMH study (discussed in a later section), which is fairly typical of gradual exposure (March & Mulle, 1998), consists of 14 visits over 12 weeks, spread across five phases: (1) psychoeducation, (2), cognitive training, (3) mapping OCD, (4), exposure and response prevention, and (5) relapse prevention and generalization training. Except for Weeks 1 and 2, where patients come twice weekly, all visits are administered on a once-per-week basis, last 1 hour, and include one between-visit 10-minute telephone contact, sched-

Table 13.2.   Cognitive-Behavioral Therapy Treatment
Protocol

Treatment Week	Goals
Weeks 1 and 2	Psychoeducation
	Cognitive training
Week 2	Mapping obsessive-compulsive disorder
	Cognitive training
Weeks 3 to 12	Exposure and response prevention
Weeks 11 to 12	Relapse prevention
Visits 1, 7, and 11	Parent sessions

uled during Weeks 3 to 12. Each session includes a statement of goals, review of the preceding week, provision of new information, therapist-assisted practice, homework for the coming week, and monitoring procedures. Although family psychopathology is neither necessary nor sufficient for the onset of OCD, families affect and are affected by the disorder (Lenane, 1989). Clinical observations suggest that a combination of individual and family sessions is best for most patients (March & Mulle, 1998). Similarly, OCD commonly but not universally exerts an adverse effect on school performance, either directly through schoolwork-related rituals or indirectly by competing with time available for completing schoolwork. School interventions based on a behavioral consultation model that takes into account relevant comorbidities, including the nonverbal learning disorders (which are important), are often critical to the success of the overall treatment program (Adams, Waas, March, & Smith, 1994; March & Mulle, 1998).

Until the mid-1980s, psychopharmacological interventions in OCD were thought to be largely ineffective. Positive effects were attributed to relief of depressive symptoms or to a reduction in overall anxiety. However, it is now clear that drug treatment can benefit most pediatric patients with OCD (Leonard, March, Rickler, & Allen, 1997). Clomipramine (Anafranil, manufactured by CIBA-Geigy) was the first medication to be studied in treating OCD in children and adolescents. Clomipramine differs from imipramine in structure only by the addition of a chloro-substituent to the fused-ring system. This change markedly increases the potency of serotonin reuptake inhibition. Following completion of multicenter placebo-controlled double-blind trials, the FDA approved clomipramine for the treatment of OCD in patients age 8 and older in 1989. Clomipramine is a nonselective tricyclic compound (a serotonin reuptake inhibitor, or SRI). The selective serotonin reuptake inhibitors (SSRIs) fluvoxamine (Luvox, manufactured by Solvay), sertraline (Zoloft, manufactured by Pfizer), paroxetine (Paxil, manufactured by GlaxoSmithKline), fluoxetine (Prozac, manufactured by Lilly) and citalopram (Celexa, manufactured by Forrest) also are likely effective treatments for OCD in youth. Controlled studies now support the efficacy of all but citalopram in the treatment of pediatric OCD. On the basis of large multicenter trials, fluvoxamine (ages 8 to 18) and sertraline (ages 6 to 18) recently received FDA approval for use in treatment of pediatric OCD.

Clinically relevant lessons originating from the multicenter trials include the following:

1. Patients with OCD show little or no placebo effect, in contrast to depressed patients treated with medications.
2. Clinical effects begin at 3 weeks and plateau at 10 weeks.
3. SRIs produce about a 30% reduction in OCD symptoms, corresponding to a rating of *moderately improved* to *markedly improved* on a measure of patient satisfaction.
4. The SRIs are not a panacea for all patients, given that subjects (on average) remained in the mildly to moderately ill range at the conclusion of the trial.

Side effects and magnitude of improvement in pediatric trials are comparable to those seen in adult trials. The absence of typical tricyclic side effects, including cardiac toxicity, give the SSRIs significant advantages over clomipramine, which is usually given only after two or three failed SSRI trials. Although many patients will respond early to one of the serotonin reuptake inhibitors, a substantial minority will not respond until after 8 or even 12 weeks of treatment at therapeutic doses. Thus, it is important to wait until at least 8 weeks have passed, with the patient at a therapeutic dose, before changing agents or undertaking augmentation regimes.

EMPIRICAL STUDIES OF TREATMENT OUTCOME

CBT Involving EX/RP

Despite widespread acceptance of CBT as the treatment of choice for OCD (Franklin et al., 1998; March & Mulle, 1996), the empirical literature still awaits a robust randomized controlled trial of CBT against control and active comparison treatments. Two trials of relevance are currently underway: our own randomized controlled study of CBT, sertraline, combined treatment, and PBO (Franklin et al., in press), and a study being conducted at UCLA in which CBT is being compared to relaxation, a cognitive-behavioral treatment that does not include exposure and ritual-prevention components (Piacentini, 1999). These studies collectively will answer several important questions about the relative efficacy of initial treatments, the maintenance of treatment gains over time, and whether EX/RP is better than a cognitive-behavioral treatment that does not target obsessions and compulsions directly. In the meantime, however, we review here the initial pilot studies that set the stage for both of these NIMH-funded outcome trials and fueled enthusiasm for the potential benefits of CBT for pediatric OCD.

ACUTE STUDIES   Using a treatment manual developed in response to deficiencies identified in a systematic literature review and extensive clinical experience, March, Mulle, and Herbel (1994) conducted an open trial of manualized CBT for moderately to severely ill children and adolescents with OCD. The treatment manual, which was explicitly designed to facilitate patient and parental compliance, exportability, and empirical evaluation, was used to treat 15 consecutive child and adolescent patients with OCD, all but one of whom had previously been stabilized on pharmacotherapy with an SRI. Statistical analyses showed a significant benefit for treatment immediately posttreatment and maintenance of gains at follow-up. Nine patients experienced at least a 50% reduction in symptoms as measured by the CY-BOCS at posttreatment; six were asymptomatic according to the National Institute of Mental Health (NIMH) Global Obsessive-Compulsive Scale. No patients relapsed at follow-up intervals as long as 18 months. Booster behavioral treatment allowed medication discontinuation in six patients. No patient refused treatment; two discontinued prematurely. The overall conclusion from this preliminary study was that CBT, in combination with SRI pharmacotherapy, showed promise as a safe, acceptable, and effective treatment for OCD in children and adolescents (March et al., 1994).

In a subsequent single case study, March and Mulle used a within-subject multiple baseline design plus global ratings across treatment weeks, to treat an 8-year-old girl with OCD by using CBT alone (March & Mulle, 1995). Eleven weeks of treatment produced complete resolution in OCD symptoms; treatment gains were maintained at 6-month follow-up. Figure 13.1 illustrates the progress of treatment at each week for each symptom baseline. Each box represents a treatment week. The y (vertical) axis represents SUDS (fear thermometer) scores for each symptom present at baseline on the symptom hierarchy, which are depicted as bars on the x (horizontal) axis. Symptom reduction in each baseline was specific to the exposure or response prevention targets for that baseline, or both. As is often the case, once their patient got the idea, generalization across baselines appeared, with some slowing down again as she reached the most difficult symptoms at the top of the symptom hierarchy.

Using similar protocols, others have also shown reductions in OCD with cognitive-behavioral approaches (Albano, Knox, & Barlow, 1995; Piacentini, Gitow, Jaffer, & Graae, 1994; Wever & Rey, 1997). Furthermore, Franklin et al. (1998) examined the efficacy of cognitive-behavioral treatment involving exposure and ritual prevention in 14 children and adolescents. Seven received intensive treatment (mean = 18 sessions over 1 month), and seven received weekly treatment (mean = 16 sessions over 4 months). Eight of these patients received concurrent treatment with SRIs, and six received CBT alone. Twelve of the 14 patients were at least 50% improved over pretreatment CY-BOCS severity, and the vast majority remained improved at follow-up; mean reduction in CY-BOCS was 67% at posttreatment and 62% at follow-up (mean time to follow-up = 9 months). No differences were apparent between those who received

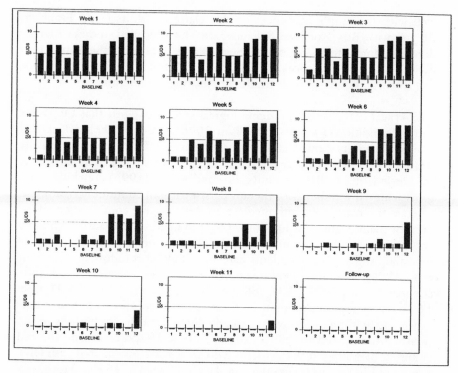

Figure 13.1. Multiple baselines over time (adapted from March & Mulle, 1995). Symptom key: 1 = touching mouth; 2 = snacking after touching plants; 3 = not washing for meals; 4 = wearing turtlenecks again; 5 = touching something sticky; 6 = touching dish liquid; 7 = using towel again; 8 = touching cat; 9 = using Ajax; 10 = using Windex; 11 = using toxic paint; 12 = touching sick people

gradual versus intensive exposure or in those who received or did not receive medication. In the only published study in pediatric OCD that directly compared CBT and SRI monotherapies, de Haan, Hoogduin, Buitelaar, and Keijsers (1998) randomly assigned pediatric patients to treatment with CBT or clomipramine, finding that CBT was superior to clomipramine in reducing OCD symptoms as measured by the CY-BOCS. Moreover, the percentages of symptom reduction for both conditions were quite similar to what has been found already in CBT and pharmacotherapy studies conducted to date.

Taken together, results from different groups using similar approaches thus suggest that CBT is a safe, acceptable, and effective short-term treatment for pediatric OCD. With a few exceptions, the pilot studies have examined CBT's effects in patients who were already receiving SRI pharmacotherapy, so the separate effects of CBT cannot be disentangled in such designs. However, the only direct comparison study yet published supported the efficacy of CBT alone, so the limited evidence available so far suggests that CBT may also be an effective stand-alone therapy, which converges well with the ample evidence for this claim in adults (e.g., Franklin, Abramowitz, Bux, Zoellner, & Feeny, 2002). Controlled studies with random assignment to conditions are needed now to evaluate the relative efficacy of cognitive-behavioral, pharmacological, and combined treatments, and fortunately several such studies are nearing completion.

LONG-TERM OUTCOMES   Epidemiological studies suggest that OCD is a chronic condition (Rasmussen & Eisen, 1990). On the other hand, clinical research in adults shows that long-term outcomes for patients successfully treated with CBT alone or CBT plus medication are generally favorable. In a review of EX/RP for adults, Foa and Kozak (1996) concluded that gains achieved with behavior therapy persist without continuing treatment, whereas those achieved with medication alone require continuing medication for maintenance. As in adults, OCD in children and adolescents is a chronic mental illness in many patients. For example, in the first NIMH follow-up study, 68% of patients had clinical OCD at follow-up (Flament et al., 1990). In a subsequent more systematic 2- to 7-year follow-up study (Leonard et al., 1993), 43% still met diagnostic criteria for OCD; only 11% were totally asymptomatic. Seventy percent continued to take medication at the time of follow-up, clearly illustrating the limitations of the treatments received by these patients. Clinical experience and limited empirical data suggest that patients who are successfully treated with CBT alone tend to stay well (Franklin et al., 1998; March, 1995). Moreover, since relapse commonly follows medication discontinuation, the finding of March et al. (1994) that improvement persisted in six of nine responders following the withdrawal of medication provides limited support for the hypothesis that behavior therapy inhibits relapse when medications are discontinued.

SRI Pharmacotherapy

Numerous adult studies have established the efficacy of SRI pharmacotherapy for adult OCD (for a review, see Greist, Jefferson, Kobak, Katzelnick, & Serlin, 1995). In the last decade, encouraging findings from these trials and the formal similarity between adult and pediatric OCD spawned considerable interest in examining the same compounds as treatments for children and adolescents suffering from OCD. In a later section of the chapter, we describe the outcome of randomized controlled trials in pediatric OCD, which collectively inform us that SRI pharmacotherapy is efficacious for pediatric OCD as well. At the same time, it appears from these data that partial response is the norm, and that most patients who participated in these RCTs probably met the minimum OCD severity criteria at posttreatment. These findings suggest that more efficacious treatments are needed, and perhaps the combination of SRI pharmacotherapy with CBT is among the most promising possibilities to increase the percentage of pediatric OCD sufferers whose symptoms remit following a course of treatment(s).

ACUTE STUDIES   The clomipramine multicenter registration trial (DeVeaugh-Geiss et al., 1992) led to the first FDA approval of an SRI in pediatric OCD. Since then, fluvoxamine (for ages 8 to 18) and sertraline (for ages 6 to 18) have also obtained FDA labeling. Using a double-blind, placebo-controlled crossover design, Riddle et al. (1992), in an underpowered study, found that 20 mg of fluoxetine was marginally superior to PBO. Fluoxetine also seemed to improve OCD symptoms in patients with tic disorders with little effects on tics per se (Scahill, Riddle, King, et al., 1997). Open trials of fluvoxamine (Apter et al., 1994) and sertraline (Cook, Charak, Trapani, & Zelko, 1994) eventually gave way to industry-funded multicenter registration trials supporting the short-term efficacy of both fluvoxamine (Riddle et al., 2001) and sertraline (March et al., 1998). Open studies currently support the use of citalopram and paroxetine (Rosenberg, Stewart, Fitzgerald, Tawile, & Carroll, 1999; Thomsen, 1997); an unpublished placebo substitution trial provides limited support for the efficacy of paroxetine (D. Cartwright, GlaxoSmithKline, personal communication, December 2001). To date no study has compared the relative efficacy of one SRI versus another using a pediatric OCD sample, although the individual trials themselves do not indicate the superiority of any particular SRI over another.

The short-term efficacy of SRIs relative to placebo having been established, several caveats about pharmacotherapy for pediatric OCD need to be emphasized. First, the mean CY-BOCS reductions from the controlled studies described above suggest that most patients remain at least somewhat symptomatic following treatment. Second, approximately one third of pediatric OCD patients fail to respond at all to a particular SRI (DeVeaugh-Geiss et al., 1992). Third, side effects prevent a certain percentage of OCD patients from taking SRIs or tolerating therapeutic dosages. Fourth, although the short-term safety and tolerability of SRIs appears to be acceptable (e.g., March et al., 1998), little is known about the long-term effects of continued treatment in children and adolescents. In the absence of this information, some parents remain reluctant even to begin a trial of pharmacotherapy with an SRI. Finally, as is the case with adults, some pediatric OCD patients who are contamination fearful are unwilling to consider taking medication of any kind for fear that they will be harmed by foreign substances or by germs they believe could have been introduced during the packaging process. Thus, the development of alternative and/or augmentative treatment strategies is clearly needed.

LONG-TERM OUTCOMES   Paralleling the adult findings (e.g., Pato, Zohar-Kadouch, Zohar, & Murphy, 1988), relapse following clomipramine withdrawal was almost universal in a small pediatric OCD sample, indicating that, for maintenance, treatment is necessary (Leonard et al., 1991). The rate of relapse on SRI discontinuation has yet to be established in children, although it is currently under investigation. Analysis of long-term open-label extension studies of clomipramine (DeVeaugh-Geiss et al., 1992), fluvoxamine (Walkup, personal communication, December 2001) and sertraline (Cook et al., 2001), which are confounded with intercurrent CBT and high dropout rates, suggest modest incremental improvement but not normalization over 52 weeks of SRI treatment.

Combined Interventions

No published controlled trials have examined the efficacy of CBT and SRI pharmacotherapy, which seems logically to be the most potentially useful combination available. As discussed above, empirical data clearly support the efficacy of SRI pharmacotherapy, some limited data are quite encouraging with respect to CBT's potential benefits, and the one randomized comparison of monotherapies showed an advantage of CBT over clomipramine. Franklin et al.'s (in press) randomized controlled trial will be completed shortly and will provide a wealth of information about relative efficacy and durability of these monotherapies versus combined treatment. Combined treatment was applied simultaneously rather than sequentially, which means that questions about treatment sequencing cannot be answered by that study. Future studies of combined treatments that employ different experimental designs, such as initial treatment with SSRI pharmacotherapy followed by CBT or visa versa, will therefore be needed.

Continuation and Maintenance Treatments

Little research has been done in pediatric OCD to examine the maintenance of gains over time associated with CBT or pharmacotherapy. The few open studies of CBT augmentation of SRI pharmacotherapy that have included follow-up suggest maintenance of gains over time (e.g., Franklin et al., 1998; Wever & Rey, 1997); medication discontinuation at follow-up was also noted in six of nine patients who received CBT augmentation of SRI pharmacotherapy (March et al., 1994). As we discussed above, it appears that SRI pharmacotherapy may need to be continued indefinitely to preserve benefits and that continued treatment over the course of a year is not associated with further symptom reduction. In the context of our soon-to-be-completed RCT, we will examine maintenance of gains for patients who received CBT alone, sertraline alone, or combined treatment, which will allow us to test the hypothesis that CBT protects SRI patients from relapse following pharmacotherapy discontinuation.

PREVENTION

Perhaps because OCD's cause is multidetermined, and because attention has only recently been given to even syndromal OCD in children and adolescents, little research has been conducted pertaining to the prevention of pediatric OCD. Treatment of subsyndromal OCD symptoms in children and adolescents would appear to be a potentially fruitful avenue to pursue, yet it is difficult to know—without data from large-scale longitudinal studies—what percentage of children and adolescents with subclinical symptoms would go on to develop full-blown OCD without any intervention. Thus, a carefully selected matched control group that received no intervention would be essential in determining the efficacy of a prevention program targeted at the subclinical cases. Another possibility for prevention research is to develop and examine programs in children and adolescents who are at increased risk for the development of OCD, namely the offspring of adults with OCD. Here again, insufficient information is available to inform the development of such programs, that is, which of these potentially vulnerable children are in need of intervention and which will not go on to develop OCD. Children with elevations on putative cognitive risk factors such as thought suppression and thought-action fusion (Salkovskis, 1985) may also be potentially at risk for the development of OCD, and therefore a potentially useful group for longitudinal study and perhaps prevention interventions down the road. Furthermore, examining prevention programs in children who present with more than one of these risk factors may also be useful, although the utility of such approaches rests on thin empirical ice as it is.

CONCLUSIONS

Despite obvious limitations in the research literature, CBT has become the psychotherapeutic treatment of choice for OCD in children and adolescents. Whereas pharmacotherapy with an SSRI is clearly the first-line medication strategy in community practice as recommended in the Expert Consensus Guidelines, the public health would be best served if most young persons with OCD first received CBT that has been optimized for treating childhood-onset OCD. Then, if the patients were not rapidly responsive, either more intensive CBT or concurrent pharmacotherapy with an SSRI would be used (March et al., 1997; Franklin et al., 1998). Because CBT may improve both short- and long-term outcomes in drug-treated patients, we further suggest that all patients who receive medication also should receive concomitant CBT. In this regard, arguments advanced against CBT for OCD—such as symptom substitution, danger of interrupting rituals, uniformity of learned symptoms, and incompatibility with pharmacotherapy—have all proven unfounded.

Perhaps the most insidious myth is that CBT is a simplistic treatment that ignores real problems. We believe that the opposite is true. Helping patients make rapid and difficult behavior changes over short time intervals takes both clinical savvy and focused treatment. Currently, state-of-the art treatments for pediatric OCD are best delivered by a multidisciplinary team, usually but not always located in a subspecialty clinic setting (March, Mulle, Stallings, Erhardt, & Conners, 1995). Unfortunately, the Expert Consensus Guidelines' recommendation to start with CBT presupposes the ready availability of this treatment, and unfortunately this is rarely the case. Thus, translation of specialty practice to community settings or, alternatively, triage of OCD patients into subspecialty OCD referral clinics is essential if demonstrably effective treatments, such as CBT for OCD, are to be made available to the children and adolescents suffering from this disorder (March et al., 1995; Kendall & Southam-Gerow, 1995).

REFERENCES

Adams, G. B., Waas, G. A., March, J. S., & Smith, M. C. (1994). Obsessive-compulsive disorder in children and adolescents: The role of the school psychologist in identification, assessment, and treatment. *School Psychology Quarterly, 9,* 274–294.

Albano, A. M., Knox, L. S., & Barlow, D. H. (1995). Obsessive-compulsive disorder. In A. Eisen & C. Kearney & C. Schafer (Eds.), *Clinical handbook of anxiety disorders in children and adolescents.* (pp. 282–316). Northvale, NJ: Jason Aaronson.

Albano, A. M., & Silverman, W. K. (1996). *Anxiety Disorders Interview Schedule for DSM-IV: Child Version.* San Antonio, TX: Psychological Corporation.

American Psychiatric Association. (1994). *Diagnostic and statistical manual of mental disorders: DSM-IV* (4th ed.). Washington, DC: Author.

Apter, A., Ratzoni, G., King, R. A., Weizman, A., *Iancu, I., Binder, M., & Riddle, M. A.* (1994). Fluvoxamine open-label treatment of adolescent inpatients with obsessive-compulsive disorder or depression. *Journal of the American Academy of Child and Adolescent Psychiatry, 33,* 342–348.

Cook, E., Charak, D., Trapani, C., & Zelko, F. (1994). Sertraline treatment of obsessive-compulsive disorder in children and adolescents: Preliminary findings. *Scientific Proceeding of the AACAP Annual Meeting, New York, 57–58.*

Cook, E. H., Wagner, K. D., March, J. S., Biederman, J., Landau, P., Wolkow, R., & Messig, M. (2001). Long-term sertraline treatment of children and adolescents with obsessive-compulsive disorder. *Journal of the American Academy of Child and Adolescent Psychiatry, 40,* 1175–1181.

de Haan, E., Hoogduin, K. A. L., Buitelaar, J. K., & Keijsers, G. P. J. (1998). Behavior therapy versus clomipramine for the treatment of obsessive-compulsive disorder in children and adolescents. *Journal of the American Academy of Child and Adolescent Psychiatry, 37,* 1022–1029.

DeVeaugh-Geiss, J., Moroz, G., Biederman, J., Cantwell, D., Fontaine, R., Greist, J. H., Reichler, R., et al. (1992). Clomipramine hydrochloride in childhood and adolescent obsessive-compulsive disorder: A multicenter trial. *Journal of the American Academy of Child and Adolescent Psychiatry, 31,* 45–49.

Flament, M. F., Koby, E., Rapoport, J. L., Berg, C. J., Zahn, T., Cox, C., Denckla, M., & Lenane, M. (1990). Childhood obsessive-compulsive disorder: a prospective follow-up study. *Journal of Child Psychology & Psychiatry & Allied Disciplines, 31,* 363–380.

Flament, M. F., Whitaker, A., Rapoport, J. L., Davies, M., Berg, C. Z., Kalikow, K., Sceery, W., et al. (1988). Obsessive-compulsive disorder in adolescence: an epidemiological study. *Journal of the American Academy of Child and Adolescent Psychiatry, 27,* 764–771.

Foa, E. B., Abramowitz, J. S., Franklin, M. E., & Kozak, M. J. (1999). Feared consequences, fixity of belief, and treatment outcome in OCD. *Behavior Therapy, 30,* 717–724.

Foa, E. B., & Kozak, M. J. (1986). Emotional processing of fear: Exposure to corrective information. *Psychological Bulletin, 99,* 20–35.

Foa, E. B., & Kozak, M. J. (1996). Psychological treatment for obsessive-compulsive disorder. In M. R. Mavissakalian & R. F. Prien (Eds.), *Long-term treatments of anxiety disorders* (pp. 285–309). Washington, DC: American Psychiatric Press.

Foa, E. B., Kozak, M. J., Goodman, W. K., Hollander, E., Jenike, M., & Rasmussen, S. (1995). *DSM-IV* field trial: Obsessive-compulsive disorder. *American Journal of Psychiatry, 152,* 90–94.

Franklin, M., Foa, E., & March, J. S. (in press). The pediatric OCD treatment study (POTS): Rationale, design, and methods. *Journal of Child and Adolescent Psychopharmacology.*

Franklin, M. E., Abramowitz, J. S., Bux, D. A., Zoellner, L. A., & Feeny, N. C. (2002). Cognitive-behavioral therapy with and without medication in the treatment of obsessive-compulsive disorder. *Professional Psychology: Research and Practice, 33,* 162–168.

Franklin, M. E., Kozak, M. J., Cashman, L. A., Coles, M. E., Rheingold, A. A., & Foa, E. B. (1998). Cognitive-behavioral treatment of pediatric obsessive-compulsive disorder: An open clinical trial. *Journal of the American Academy of Child and Adolescent Psychiatry, 37,* 412–419.

Franklin, M. E., Tolin, D. F., March, J. S., & Foa, E. B. (2001). Intensive cognitive-behavior therapy for pediatric OCD: A case example. *Cognitive and Behavioral Practice, 8,* 297–304.

Giulino, L., Gammon, P., Sullivan, K., Franklin, M., Foa, E., Maid, R., & March, J. (2002). Is parental report of upper respiratory infection at the onset of OCD suggestive of pediatric autoimmune neuropsychiatric disorder associated with streptococcal infection? *Journal of Child and Adolescent Psychopharmacology, 12,* 157–164.

Goodman, W. K., Price, L. H., Rasmussen, S. A., Mazure, C., Delgado, P., Heninger, G. R., & Charney, D. S. (1989). The Yale-Brown Obsessive-Compulsive Scale: II. Validity. *Archives of General Psychiatry, 46,* 1012–1016.

Goodman, W. K., Price, L. H., Rasmussen, S. A., Mazure, C., Fleischmann, R. L., Hill, C. L., Heninger, G. R., et al. (1989). The Yale-Brown Obsessive-Compulsive Scale: I. Development, use, and reliability. *Archives of General Psychiatry, 46,* 1006–1011.

Greist, J. H., Jefferson, J. W., Kobak, K. A., Katzelnick, D. J., & Serlin, R. C. (1995). Efficacy and tolerability of serotonin transport inhibitors in obsessive-compulsive disorder: A meta-analysis. *Archives of General Psychiatry, 52,* 53–60.

Kendall, P. C., & Southam-Gerow, M. A. (1995). Issues in the transportability of treatment: the case of anxiety disorders in youths. *Journal of Consulting and Clinical Psychology, 63,* 702–708.

King, R. A. (1995). Practice parameters for the psychiatric assessment of children and adolescents: American Academy of Child and Adolescent Psychiatry. *Journal of the American Academy of Child and Adolescent Psychiatry, 34,* 1386–1402.

Kovacs, M. (1985). The Children's Depression Inventory (CDI). *Psychopharmacology Bulletin, 21,* 995–998.

Laidlaw, T. M., Falloon, I. R., Barnfather, D., & Coverdale, J. H. (1999). The stress of caring for people with obsessive-compulsive disorders. *Community Mental Health Journal, 35,* 443–450.

Last, C. G., & Strauss, C. C. (1989). Obsessive-compulsive disorder in childhood. *Journal of Anxiety Disorders, 3,* 295–302.

Lenane, M. (1989). Families in obsessive-compulsive disorder. In J. Rapoport (Ed.), *Obsessive-compulsive disorder in children and adolescents* (pp. 237–249). Washington, DC: American Psychiatric Press.

Leonard, H. L., March, J., Rickler, K. C., & Allen, A. J. (1997). Pharmacology of the selective serotonin reuptake inhibitors in children and adolescents. *Journal of the American Academy of Child and Adolescent Psychiatry, 36,* 725–736.

Leonard, H. L., Swedo, S. E., Garvey, M., Beer, D., Perlmutter, S., Lougee, L., Karitani, M., et al. (1999). Post-infectious and other forms of obsessive-compulsive disorder. *Child and Adolescent Psychiatry Clinics of North America, 8,* 497–511.

Leonard, H. L., Swedo, S. E., Lenane, M. C., Rettew, D. C., Cheslow, D. L., Hamburger, S. D., & Rapoport, J. L. (1991). A double-blind desipramine substitution during long-term clomipramine treatment in children and adolescents with obsessive-compulsive disorder. *Archives of General Psychiatry, 48,* 922–927.

Leonard, H. L., Swedo, S. E., Lenane, M. C., Rettew, D. C., Hamburger, S. D., Bartko, J. J., & Rapoport, J. L. (1993). A 2– to 7–year follow-up study of 54 obsessive-compulsive children and adolescents. *Archives of General Psychiatry, 50,* 429–439.

March, J. (1995). Cognitive-behavioral psychotherapy for children and adolescents with OCD: A review and recommendations for treatment. *Journal of the American Academy of Child and Adolescent Psychiatry, 34,* 7–18.

March, J. (1998). *Manual for the Multidimensional Anxiety Scale for Children (MASC).* Toronto, Canada: Multi-Health Systems.

March, J., Biederman, J., Wolkow, R., Safferman, A., Mardekian, J., Cook, E. H., Cutler, N. R., et al. (1998). Sertraline in children and adolescents with obsessive-compulsive disorder: A multicenter randomized controlled trial [see comments]. *Journal of the American Medical Association, 280,* 1752–1756.

March, J., Frances, A., Kahn, D., & Carpenter, D. (1997). Expert consensus guidelines: Treatment of obsessive-compulsive disorder. *Journal of Clinical Psychiatry, 58*(Suppl. 4), 1–72.

March, J., & Mulle, K. (1995). Manualized cognitive-behavioral psychotherapy for obsessive-compulsive disorder in childhood: A preliminary single case study. *Journal of Anxiety Disorders, 9,* 175–184.

March, J., & Mulle, K. (1996). Banishing obsessive-compulsive disorder. In E. Hibbs & P. Jensen (Eds.), *Psychosocial treatments for child and adolescent disorders* (pp. 82–103). Washington, DC: American Psychological Press.

March, J., & Mulle, K. (1998). *OCD in children and adolescents: A cognitive-behavioral treatment manual.* New York: Guilford Press.

March, J., Mulle, K., & Herbel, B. (1994). Behavioral psychotherapy for children and adolescents with obsessive-compulsive disorder: An open trial of a new protocol driven treatment package. *Journal of the American Academy of Child and Adolescent Psychiatry, 33,* 333–341.

March, J., Mulle, K., Stallings, P., Erhardt, D., & Conners, C. (1995). Organizing an anxiety disorders clinic. In J. March (Ed.), *Anxiety disorders in children and adolescents* (pp. 420–435). New York: Guilford Press.

March, J. S., & Sullivan, K. (1999). Test-retest reliability of the Multidimensional Anxiety Scale for Children. *Journal of Anxiety Disorders, 13,* 349–358.

Pato, M. T., Zohar-Kadouch, R., Zohar, J., & Murphy, D. L. (1988). Return of symptoms after discontinuation of clomipramine in patients with obsessive-compulsive disorder. *American Journal of Psychiatry, 145,* 1521–1525.

Piacentini, J. (1999). Cognitive behavioral therapy of childhood OCD. *Child and Adolescent Psychiatric Clinics of North America, 8,* 599–617.

Piacentini, J., Gitow, A., Jaffer, M., & Graae, F. (1994). Outpatient behavioral treatment of child and adolescent obsessive-compulsive disorder. *Journal of Anxiety Disorders, 8,* 277–289.

Piacentini, J., Jaffer, M., Bergman, R. L., McCracken, J., & Keller, M. (2001). *Measuring impairment in childhood OCD: Psychometric properties of the COIS.* Paper presented at the annual meeting of the American Academy of Child and Adolescent Psychiatry, Honolulu, HI.

Piacentini, J., Jaffer, M., Liebowitz, M., & Gitow, A. (1992). Systematic assessment of impairment in youngsters with obsessive-compulsive disorder: The OCD impact scale. *AABT Proceedings.* New York: AABT.

Rasmussen, S. A., & Eisen, J. L. (1990). Epidemiology of obsessive-compulsive disorder. *Journal of Clinical Psychiatry, 51*(Suppl. 2), 10–13.

Riddle, M., Reeve, E., Yaryura-Tobias, J., Yang, H., Claghorn, J., Gaffney, G., Greist, J., et al. (2001). Fluvoxamine for children and adolescents with obsessive-compulsive disorder: A randomized, controlled, multicenter trial. *Journal of the American Academy of Child and Adolescent Psychiatry, 40,* 222–229.

Riddle, M. A., Scahill, L., King, R. A., Hardin, M. T., Anderson, G. M., Ort, S. I., Smith, J. C., et al. (1992). Double-blind, crossover trial of fluoxetine and placebo in children and adolescents with obsessive-compulsive disorder. *Journal of the American Academy of Child and Adolescent Psychiatry, 31,* 1062–1069.403403

Rosenberg, D. R., Stewart, C. M., Fitzgerald, K. D., Tawile, V., & Carroll, E. (1999). Paroxetine open-label treatment of pediatric outpatients with obsessive-compulsive disorder. *Journal of the American Academy of Child and Adolescent Psychiatry, 38,* 1180–1185.

Salkovskis, P. M. (1985). Obsessional compulsive problems: A cognitive behavioral analysis. *Behaviour Research and Therapy, 23,* 571–583.

Scahill, L., Riddle, M. A., King, R. A., Hardin, M. T., Rasmusson, A., Makuch, R. W., & Leckman, J. F. (1997). Fluoxetine has no marked effect on tic symptoms in patients with Tourette's syndrome: A double-blind placebo-controlled study [In Process Citation]. *Journal of Child and Adolescent Psychopharmacology, 7,* 75–85.

Scahill, L., Riddle, M. A., McSwiggin-Hardin, M., Ort, S. I., King, R. A., Goodman, W. K., Cicchetti, D., & Leckman, J. F. (1997). Children's Yale-Brown Obsessive-Compulsive Scale: Reliability and validity. *Journal of the American Academy of Child and Adolescent Psychiatry, 36,* 844–852.

Silverman, W. K. (1991). Diagnostic reliability of anxiety disorders in children using structured interviews [Special issue: Assessment of childhood anxiety disorders]. *Journal of Anxiety Disorders, 5,* 105–124.

Silverman, W. K., & Nelles, W. B. (1988). The anxiety disorders interview schedule for children. *Journal of the American Academy of Child and Adolescent Psychiatry, 27,* 772–778.

Silverman, W. K., & Rabian, B. (1995). Test-retest reliability of the *DSM-III-R* childhood anxiety disorders symptoms using the Anxiety Disorders Interview Schedule for Children. *Journal of Anxiety Disorders, 9,* 139–150.

Swedo, S. E., Leonard, H. L., Garvey, M., Mittleman, B., Allen, A. J., Perlmutter, S., Dow, S., et al. (1998). Pediatric autoimmune neuropsychiatric disorders associated with streptococcal infections: Clinical description of the first 50 cases. *American Journal of Psychiatry, 155,* 264–271.

Swedo, S. E., Rapoport, J. L., Leonard, H., Lenane, M., & Cheslow, D. (1989). Obsessive-compulsive disorder in children and adolescents: Clinical phenomenology of 70 consecutive cases. *Archives of General Psychiatry, 46,* 335–341.

Thomsen, P. H. (1997). Child and adolescent obsessive-compulsive disorder treated with citalopram: Findings from an open trial of 23 cases. *Journal of Child and Adolescent Psychopharmacology, 7,* 157–166.

Wever, C., & Rey, J. M. (1997). Juvenile obsessive-compulsive disorder. *Australian and New Zealand Journal of Psychiatry, 31,* 105–113.

14

POSTTRAUMATIC STRESS DISORDER

Judith A. Cohen & Anthony P. Mannarino

CLINICAL MANIFESTATION

Posttraumatic stress disorder (PTSD) is unique among *DSM-IV* disorders in that its diagnosis depends on exposure to an extremely traumatic event. This traumatic event must be of potentially life- or health-threatening magnitude to the child or another individual. The child must have either personally experienced the event, witnessed someone being exposed to the event, or learned about its being experienced by someone close to the child. Examples of such events to which children may be exposed are sexual abuse; kidnapping; physical assaults at school, home, or in the community; serious motor vehicle accidents; natural or man-made disasters; and life-threatening illnesses such as cancer or severe burn injuries.

Children with PTSD respond to such events with intense fear, horror or helplessness, as well as some degree of disorganized or agitated behavior. They also develop characteristic symptoms that fall into the categories of reexperiencing, avoidance/numbing, and hyperarousal. There are developmental variations in how these symptoms may be manifested, with symptoms in younger children sometimes having less clear direct reference to the traumatic event.

Reexperiencing symptoms typically include frightening, intrusive trauma-related memories or thoughts, or recurring dreams or nightmares about the event. In younger children these may take a more generic form (for example, fears or dreams of frightening animals or monsters) that may be difficult to distinguish from normal childhood fears and nightmares. Less frequently, children may have episodes in which they report or appear to be reliving the event, behaving as if it were happening in the present moment. In younger children, this may take the form of repetitive play (posttraumatic play). Reminders of the event often trigger intense psychological distress, physiological arousal, or both. These triggers may be particularly idiosyncratic in children and may not have an obvious connection to the traumatic event.

Children with PTSD typically try to avoid encountering traumatic reminders or triggers (for example, a child involved in a serious automobile accident may refuse to ride in cars) and also try to avoid thoughts or discussions about the trauma. Adolescents may use drugs or alcohol to decrease reexperiencing symptoms or to avoid thinking about the traumatic event. Children may become amnestic for an important aspect of the traumatic experience but may remember other aspects with extreme clarity. Children may also say that they forget specifics of the trauma to avoid having to discuss it. Emotional numbing and having a sense of a foreshortened future (for example, not believing that one is going to live until adulthood) are common symptoms of PTSD, but children may have difficulty reporting affective constriction or their concept of the future due to age-appropriate limitations in language or cognitive development. Adolescents may engage in reckless or self-mutilating behavior in an attempt to lessen emotional numbing.

Hyperarousal symptoms may include angry outbursts, irritability, sleep disturbance, difficulty concentrating, shortened attention span, feeling jittery or displaying motor hyperactivity, somatic complaints such as stomachaches or headaches, increased startle response, and hypervigilance. Younger children typically do not make a cognitive connection between the traumatic event and these symptoms; parent and teacher reports are often necessary to determine whether such symptoms were preexisting or developed after the traumatic experience.

DIAGNOSIS AND CLASSIFICATION

The diagnosis of PTSD depends on the presence of a traumatic stressor as just described, one or more reexperiencing symptoms, at least three avoidance/numbing symptoms, and two or more symptoms of hyperarousal. The duration of symptoms must exceed 1 month and must cause clinically significant distress or impairment in an important area of functioning. Types of PTSD include *acute* (duration of less than 3 months), *chronic* (duration of 3 months or more), and *with delayed onset* (if onset of symptoms is at least 6 months after the most recent PTSD stressor).

Several authors have questioned whether the *DSM-IV* diagnostic criteria for PTSD are valid for younger children. Scheeringa, Zeanah, Drell, and Larrieu (1995) pointed out that 8 of these 18 criteria require the child to verbally describe internal states and experiences in a way that most developmentally normal preschool children would not be capable of, and that alternative criteria for this age group may be more appropriate. Because the criteria for PTSD were not field tested in children, it is difficult to determine whether they are adequate for identifying this disorder in younger children or those with delayed development.

Childhood PTSD has substantial comorbidity with other psychiatric conditions. Several studies have documented that major depressive disorder (MDD) and dysthymic disorder (depressive disorder not otherwise specified, in *DSM-IV*) are frequently present in children with PTSD (Brent et al., 1995; Goenjian et al., 1995; Hubbard, Realmuto, Northwood, & Masten, 1995; Kinzie, Sack, Angell, Manson, & Rath, 1986; Kiser, Heston, Milsap, & Pruitt, 1991; McCloskey & Walker, 2000; Singer, Anglin, Song, & Lunghofer, 1995; Stoddard, Norman, & Murphy, 1989; Weine et al., 1995; Yule & Udwin, 1991). In many cases, PTSD precedes the development of depressive disorders. Several authors have hypothesized that PTSD predisposes children to MDD (Goenjian et al., 1995; Reinhertz et al., 1993; Yehuda & McFarlane, 1995). Children who develop PTSD in response to maltreatment may be even more likely than other traumatized children to develop depressive symptoms; the 1-year prevalence of MDD in representative preadolescent child protective service caseloads has been found to be approximately 20% (Kaufman, 1991; Pelcovitz et al., 1994).

Several researchers have also documented the high rate of generalized anxiety disorder (GAD), separation anxiety disorder, agoraphobia, and other anxiety disorders in children with PTSD (Brent et al., 1995; Clark et al., 1995; Goenjian et al., 1995; Kiser et al., 1991; Lonigan, Shannon, Taylor, Finch, & Sallec, 1994; McCloskey & Walker, 2000; Singer et al., 1995; Yule & Udwin, 1991). The results of one study that examined the relationship of predisaster functioning and the development of PTSD in children following Hurricane Andrew indicate that children's predisaster anxiety level predicted the presence of PTSD symptoms at both 3 and 7 months after the hurricane (La Greca, Silverman, & Wasserstein, 1998). This study suggests that other anxiety disorders predispose children to developing PTSD rather than the reverse (as is more typically the case with MDD).

An interesting preliminary finding indicated that preexisting bipolar disorder (manic type) in children strongly predicted subsequent traumatic exposure during a 4-year follow-up period (Wozniak et al., 1999). This study only included children with comorbid attention-deficit/hyperactivity disorder (ADHD) diagnoses, so it may be the coexistence of these two disorders that puts children at increased risk for experiencing trauma. It is worth noting that ADHD alone was not found to increase the risk of such exposure, which suggests that impulsivity and poor judgment alone (which occur independently in both disorders) do not account for this increased risk. These authors noted that, because bipolar disorder is so strongly familial, children with this diagnosis are more likely to be exposed to family members with severe psychiatric disturbances, who may either perpetrate violence or place the child at greater risk for traumatic exposure (Wozniak et al., 1999). They also discussed the possibility that the irritability and mood lability that often occurs following traumatic exposure may be due to undetected preexisting bipolar disorder rather than to the traumatic experience per se.

ADHD is frequently diagnosed in children exposed to traumatic life events, whether or not these children meet diagnostic criteria for PTSD (Cuffe, McCullough, & Pumariega, 1994; Glod & Teicher, 1996). Some researchers have found that traumatized children present with ADHD more frequently than with PTSD (DeBellis et al., 1994; Looff, Grimley, Kuiler, Martin, & Shunfield, 1995; McLeer, Callaghan, Henry, & Wallen, 1994). This may be because ADHD is a relatively common childhood disorder that often precipitates clinical referral (Costello et al., 1996) or because PTSD is mistaken for ADHD in younger children; it is also possible that children with preexisting ADHD are more vulnerable to traumatic experiences or to developing PTSD in reaction to such exposure, or both. Two studies that addressed this issue found that, in outpatient child psychiatry clinic cohorts, a diagnosis of ADHD did not increase the risk of traumatic exposure (Ford et al., 1999; Wozniak et al., 1999). Another study demonstrated that the presence of PTSD hyperarousal symptoms in children with ADHD was largely due to overlapping diagnostic criteria (i.e., the particular hyperarousal symptoms these children had were irritability, angry outbursts, and decreased concentration rather than hypervigilance and increased startle reaction). These studies suggest that many of these traumatized children have true ADHD, and that such symptoms are not simply developmental manifestations of PTSD (Wozniak et al., 1999).

In addition to ADHD, other externalizing disorders such as oppositional defiant disorder (ODD) and conduct disorder (CD) have been noted in children with PTSD (Arroyo & Eth, 1985; Ford et al., 2000; McCloskey & Walker, 2000; Steiner et al., 1997). Ford et al. (2000) presented evidence supporting the idea that PTSD may exacerbate ODD symptoms, and that traumatic exposure in childhood may contribute to the hypothesized progression from ADHD to ODD to conduct disorder (Biederman et al., 1996). It is possible that children who develop PTSD in response to exposure to interpersonal violence are more likely to display significant anger and behavioral problems than children exposed to other types of traumatic experiences (Singer et al., 1995). Several authors have offered theoretical explanations for this, including victim identification with the aggressor or modeling of inappropriate behaviors (Berliner & Wheeler, 1987). Clinical interventions that inadvertently encourage the child to externalize responsibility for his or her own negative behavior (Ryan, 1989) and PTSD-related loss of impulse control can also lead to increased anger and aggression (Steiner et al., 1997).

There is also significant comorbidity between PTSD and substance abuse disorders in adolescents (Arroyo & Eth, 1985; Brent et al., 1995; Clark et al., 1995; Looff et al., 1995; Sullivan & Evans, 1994), perhaps in part because drugs and alcohol may be used to self-medicate disturbing reexperiencing or hyperarousal symptoms of PTSD. It is interesting that a study of young adults found that traumatic exposure in the absence of PTSD did not lead to substance abuse, nor did preexisting substance abuse predispose this cohort to either traumatic experiences or the development of PTSD (Chilcoat & Breslau, 1998). These authors concluded that drug abuse in young children with PTSD most likely occurs as an attempt to self-medicate the PTSD symptoms.

Finally, there is preliminary evidence of comorbidity between PTSD and dissociative disorders, in children who have been physically or sexually abused (Famularo, Fenton, Augustyn, & Zuckerman, 1996; Spiegel, 1984). One recent study found very high correlations between history of traumatic exposure and dissociative symptoms, particularly depersonalization, among delinquent adolescents (Carrion & Steiner, 2000). Borderline personality disorder (BPD) has been found to have high comorbidity with PTSD in sexually abused females; in some studies, more than half of females with BPD diagnoses reported a history of childhood sexual abuse (Herman, Perry, & van der Kolk, 1989; Stone, 1990). Some authors have speculated that BPD may in fact be a particularly severe form of PTSD rather than a separate diagnostic category (Goodwin, 1985; Herman & van der Kolk, 1987). This has yet to be empirically examined.

The differential diagnosis of childhood PTSD includes adjustment disorders, other anxiety disorders, mood disorders, and (rarely) psychotic disorders. There is some room for clinician judgment in determining whether the identified stressor qualifies as being extreme. If the child symptomatically meets PTSD criteria but the clinician does not judge the stressor to be sufficiently severe, an adjustment disorder diagnosis may be given. Conversely, if in response to an extreme stressor the child develops only mild symptoms or has some PTSD symptoms but not enough to reach diagnostic criteria, an adjustment disorder diagnosis is appropriate.

In the presence of a known extreme stressor, it is important to distinguish PTSD from other psychiatric conditions that either predated or developed subsequent to the traumatic event. Stress is known to exacerbate anxiety and depressive disorders in particular; it is possible that a child's symptoms from such a disorder were unrecognized until the traumatic event either worsened the symptoms or focused parental attention on them to the point of seeking professional help. Obtaining a careful history from the child and parents (and possibly from other informants such as teachers or other caretakers) may clarify this issue. It is also possible for any psychiatric disorder to newly appear after a traumatic event, either in response to stress or coincidentally; clinical assessment should not be limited to PTSD symptoms just because the child experienced a PTSD-type trauma.

Because a diagnosis of PTSD requires that the symptoms develop after exposure to a specific stressor, the child who had PTSD symptoms prior to the identified stressor poses a diagnostic dilemma. It is possible that such a child experienced previous undisclosed traumatic events that account for the symptoms; this scenario emphasizes the importance of routinely screening for past child abuse, exposure to domestic violence, and other common forms of childhood trauma. However, it is also possible that such a child has another psychiatric condition that accounts for the symptoms, because both depressive and anxiety disorders have considerable symptomatic overlap with PTSD (Brent et al., 1995). For example, children with obsessive-compulsive disorder (OCD) typically have recurrent intrusive thoughts and hypervigilance and may also display avoidant behaviors. However, in children with OCD, the symptoms are not related to a traumatic event as they would be with PTSD.

Flashbacks and other intense reexperiencing phenomena may mimic hallucinations, illusions, or other psychotic symptoms. Dissociative symptoms such as flat affect, disorganized behavior, and social withdrawal may present in a manner similar to psychotic disorders, which are typically unrelated to traumatic exposure. It has been suggested that children with severe PTSD resulting from physical or sexual abuse may be particularly likely to display transient frank psychotic symptoms when placed in a frightening situation, such as being physically restrained on an inpatient psychiatric unit. If the evaluating clinician is unaware of the traumatic history, it may be extremely difficult to distinguish this presentation from a true psychotic disorder. Additionally, PTSD may present with symptoms very similar to a psychotic depressive disorder, or these two conditions may coexist (Lindley, Carlson, & Sheikh, 2000). Determining the correct diagnosis in such a case would also be a difficult and challenging task.

DEVELOPMENTAL COURSE

The developmental course of childhood PTSD has not been adequately studied. Longitudinal studies have failed to control for the impact of intervening treatment, exposure to additional traumatic stressors, comorbid psychiatric conditions, and a variety of other factors that would be expected to have an impact on recovery. Studies have demonstrated both that childhood PTSD has a substantial spontaneous remission rate (Boyle et al., 1995; Green et al., 1994; Milgram, Toubiana, Klingman, Raviv, & Goldstein, 1988; Laor et al., 1997) and that PTSD persists for months to years in many children (Hubbard et al., 1995; La Greca, Vernberg, Silverman, & Prinstein, 1996; Macksoud & Aber, 1996; McFarland, 1987; Nader, Pynoos, Fairbanks, & Frederick, 1990; Shaw et al., 1995; Stoddard et al., 1989). Although there is some information with regard to risk factors in developing and maintaining PTSD symptoms for selected subgroups of children (Pine & Cohen, 2002), not enough is known in this regard.

As discussed above, there are also variations in the presentation of PTSD depending on the child's developmental level. Typically, children are more likely to exhibit the full range of PTSD symptoms as they mature. Thus, adolescents often meet full adult criteria for *DSM-IV* PTSD, although those with chronic PTSD who have experienced severe or repeated stressors may have a predominance of dissociative symptoms such as depersonalization, derealization, intermittent angry or aggressive outbursts, self-mutilation, and substance abuse (Goodwin, 1988; Hornstein, 1996). As noted in *DSM-IV*, elementary school-aged children may develop omen formation (Terr, 1983), in which they believe that there were specific warning signs that the traumatic event was about to occur and that vigilance against specific signs may prevent or warn of a future traumatic event. Children in this developmental stage may be particularly prone to sleep disturbances or a skewed sense of time during the traumatic event. Their reexperiencing symptoms may take the form of traumatic reenactment (recreating aspects of the event in play or drawings) or intrusive thoughts and nightmares, or both. Because they are typically present oriented and have a limited future perspective, they may have difficulty comprehending questions about a foreshortened future. Very young children may be able to report only a few PTSD symptoms, for the reasons noted previously. Therefore, preschool children, toddlers, and infants may present with symptoms of general anxiety such as separation difficulties; fears of strangers, monsters, or the dark; preoccupation with or avoidance of words or symbols that have no apparent link to the traumatic event; and sleep disturbance (Drell, Siegel, & Gaensbauer, 1993). Scheeringa et al. (1995) have proposed alternative PTSD criteria for children in early developmental stages, but only preliminary validity of their criteria has been demonstrated to date (Scheeringa et al., 2003). There is thus ongoing discussion but little agreement regarding the appropriate criteria to use for identifying PTSD in very young children.

It is important to recognize that PTSD may have profoundly deleterious effects on normal cognitive functioning and neurodevelopment (DeBellis et al., 1999), and therefore early identification and treatment is critical to optimal development.

ASSESSMENT

The assessment of PTSD in children requires careful and direct clinical interviewing of both the child and parents or primary caretaker of the child. Typically, the child and parents are interviewed separately, as their perspective on the child's symptoms may be different. It should be noted that if one or both parents are the alleged perpetrators of the identified traumatic event (for example, domestic violence or child abuse), the other parent or another caretaking adult should be interviewed. The child and parent should be questioned about the child's exposure to a variety of traumatic events, in addition to discussing the identified traumatic experience, because many children will have been exposed to multiple traumas (Ismail, Cohen, Mannarino, Goessler, & Guthrie, 2000). The child may perceive the trauma that led to the clinical assessment as less stressful than a previous traumatic event. It is also possible for a recent trauma to trigger PTSD symptoms related to a previous experience (for example, physical assault by a boyfriend may trigger PTSD symptoms related to an adolescent girl's past sexual abuse). In addition to the direct questioning, interviews and self-report instruments such as the Traumatic Events Screening Inventory for Children

(TESI-C; Ford et al., 1999) ask children and adolescents about exposure and severity of response to a variety of stressful life events.

One of the current controversies about assessing PTSD symptoms in children is whether children's self-reports of traumatic exposure are of adequate reliability. Concerns about children's suggestibility (either in therapy or in nonclinical situations) and the imperfection of childhood memory have resulted in debate as to whether it is necessary to obtain independent validation that the alleged traumatic exposure really occurred, prior to diagnosing PTSD. It is of interest that this question has only arisen with regard to child abuse and not with other forms of childhood traumatization. In abuse cases, parental report with regard to traumatic exposure or symptomatology may be unreliable, either because the parent is unaware that abuse has occurred or because the parent is the perpetrator and therefore has strong motivation to deny that the abuse occurred. In response to these concerns, many clinical programs now require an independent forensic examination in cases of alleged child abuse before treatment can be initiated. Whether this has improved or detracted from optimal care for these children is an unanswered question. Clinicians should be aware that there are substantial differences between forensic and clinical evaluations, which have been discussed elsewhere (Appelbaum, 1997; Strasburger, Guthiel, & Brodsky, 1997). There is agreement that, optimally, these roles should be performed by different professionals (Greenberg & Shuman, 1997). It is important to note that clinicians in either forensic or clinical roles are required to comply with state reporting laws when child abuse or neglect is suspected.

Assuming adequate information that the child has been exposed to the reported traumatic event, the next step in assessing for PTSD involves direct questioning about each of the symptom clusters included in this diagnosis. The use of developmentally appropriate language is critical in this regard, as is insight into the developmental variations in symptom presentation that are discussed above. In addition to careful clinical interviewing, a number of structured and semistructured interviews are available to assess the presence of PTSD symptoms in children and adolescents. Most of these are quite time-consuming to administer and must be given by an interviewer who is experienced both in evaluating children of different developmental levels and in asking about PTSD symptoms. For these reasons, it is unlikely that these instruments will have much utility in typical clinical practice, much less for screening in routine settings such as pediatric clinics or schools. The structured interviews that are currently available to assess childhood PTSD are summarized in Table 14.1. As noted there, the instruments differ not only in their demonstrated psychometric properties, but also in terms of which *DSM* version they were designed for. They are similar in that all use consensus ratings for each symptom; that is, the child and parent are interviewed separately, and the interviewer makes a clinical judgment about the presence and severity of each symptom based on the answers given. This involves assessing the relative reliability of each reporter when the two reports are not in agreement—a very common occurrence

Table 14.1. Semistructured Interviews Used to Assess PTSD in Children and Adolescents

Measure (Source)	Reliability and Validity Data
Schedule for Affective Disorders and Schizophrenia for School-Age Children-Present and Lifetime Version, PTSD Scale (Kaufman et al., 1997)[1]	High interrater reliability, good test-retest reliability
Diagnostic Interview for Children and Adolescents, PTSD Section (Famularo et al., 1996)[2]	None
Diagnostic Interview Schedule for Children, PTSD Section (Garrison et al., 1995)[2]	None
KID-Structured Clinical Interview for *DSM-IV*, PTSD Section (Hubbard, Realmuto, Northwood, & Masten, 1995; Matzer, Silva, Silvan, Chawdury, & Natasi, 1997)[1]	Good test-retest reliability
Clinician-Administered PTSD Scale for Children and Adolescents, *DSM-IV* Version (Nader et al., 1996; personal communication, 2000)[1]	High concurrent validity and interrater reliability
Childhood PTSD Interview-Child Form (Fletcher, 1997)[1]	High interrater reliability, strong construct and convergent validity

Note. PTSD = posttraumatic disorder.
[1] Based on *DSM-IV* diagnostic criteria.
[2] Based on *DSM-III* diagnostic criteria.

when comparing child and parent reports for many psychiatric conditions (Kazdin, 1995). Typically, in this situation the parent report is considered more reliable when asking about behavioral symptoms (which children tend to underreport), whereas the child is considered more accurate in reporting internalized symptoms of which the parent may not be aware. Preliminary data suggest that parent report is especially critical when assessing PTSD in very young children (Scheeringa, Peebles, Cook, & Zeanah, 2001). However, clinical judgment may indicate exceptions to these assumptions. Because of the time and expertise required to administer these interviews, they are generally used only in research settings.

At this time, the most frequently used assessment interviews for PTSD are the PTSD section of the Kiddie Schedule for Affective Disorders and Schizophrenia (K-SADS-PL) section and the Clinician Administered PTSD Schedule for Children and Adolescents (CAPS-CA), both of which were written to assess *DSM-IV* PTSD diagnostic criteria. Although the CAPS is considered the gold standard for assessing adult PTSD in noncombat populations (Foa & Tolin, 2000), the child and adolescent version (CAPS-CA) does not yet appear to have attained such widespread acceptance.

In addition to structured interviews, many shorter self- and parent-report instruments have strong psychometric properties. At least one recent study has indicated that the PTSD Symptom Scale–Interview Version (PSS-I), a 24-item questionnaire, was as accurate at diagnosing adult PTSD as the more lengthy CAPS structured interview (Foa & Tolin, 2000). This is good news for most practitioners, who need a time- and cost-efficient method of identifying this disorder. Because both of these instruments have validated child versions, it is hoped that similar data may soon be available for child and adolescent cohorts.

Other brief instruments have been shown to possess good validity and reliability and to be useful in routine settings such as schools (March, Amaya-Jackson, Murray, & Schulte, 1998) and pediatric clinics (Ismail et al., 2000). Self- and parent-report instruments that evaluate the presence of PTSD symptoms in children are described in Table 14.2. Again, they vary according to how extensively their psychometric properties have been evaluated and whether each generates an actual PTSD diagnosis or a score that correlates with PTSD symptom severity. Only two parent-report instruments have been designed and tested for use in very young children, one of which is specifically for use in sexually abused children. Efforts are continuing to develop better instrumentation for the assessment of this disorder in children.

There are ongoing controversies about how to optimally diagnose childhood PTSD. This disorder may be overdiagnosed by clinicians who are not adequately familiar with *DSM-IV* diagnostic requirements and assume that traumatic exposure and related emotional distress are sufficient to meet criteria. This has led to recent attempts to better educate clinicians about this disorder (American Academy of Child and Adolescent Psychiatry, 1998). On the other hand, underdiagnosis is clearly a problem, because much if not most child traumatization is not identified (Ismail et al., 2000; Singer et al., 1995), and without recognition of exposure, symptoms are unlikely to be noticed unless they reach a very high level of severity (such as suicidality or violence toward others). Often a PTSD diagnosis is missed because clinicians fail to ask about traumatic exposure. Frequently, children do not make the connection between current symptoms and past traumatic experiences unless directly asked about the traumatic event (Almqvist & Brandell-Forsberg, 1997; Pynoos & Eth, 1986; Wolfe, Sas, & Wekerle, 1994). Yet, despite this, many clinicians are hesitant to ask about traumatic exposure due to the child's, parent's, or clinician's avoidance of discussing potentially painful events, or the clinician's concern with tainting the child's description of the traumatic event if subsequent legal proceedings occur (Benedek, 1985). The available empirical evidence suggests that it is essential to ask children directly about possible traumatic exposure and about PTSD symptoms as they relate to that experience, to accurately diagnose this disorder (Almqvist & Brandell-Forsberg, 1997; Wolfe et al., 1994).

There is also ongoing controversy about how many symptoms in each of the three PTSD clusters children must have for a diagnosis of PTSD (Saigh, 1988). For example, it has been noted that reexperiencing and avoidant symptoms are in some ways opposite manifestations of trauma-related emotional distress, and as such they may not occur at the same time but may alternate, with one cluster being more prominent at one point,

Table 14.2. Instruments That Measure PTSD Symptoms in Children and Adolescents

Measure	Format	Reliability and Validity Data	Age	Comments
PTSD Reaction Index (Frederick, 1985; Goenijian et al., 1995; Pynoos et al., 1987; Pynoos, Rodriguez, Steinberg, Stuber, & Frederick, 1998)	20-item self-report (may also be used as semistructured interview)	High correlation with clinical diagnosis; no psychometric data available for *DSM-IV* version	Not specified	*DSM-IV* version has child, adolescent, and parent forms. Most commonly used instrument in published research studies; composite score indicates severity of PTSD symptoms, does not measure PTSD severity.
Child PTSD Symptom Scale (Foa, Johnson, Feeny, & Treadwell, 2001)	24-item child self-report	High internal consistency, test-retest reliability, and convergent validity with reaction index and discriminant validity	Not specified	Designed for research as well as clinical use; includes a 7-item scale assessing adaptive functioning.
Children's PTSD Inventory (March, 1999; Saigh, 1989, 1998)	Self-report with five subscales (exposure, reexperiencing, avoidance, hyperarousal, degree of distress)	High interrater reliability; sensitivity and specificity of diagnosis, high correlation with clinical diagnosis	Not specified	Only instrument that provides discrete diagnosis of no PTSD or acute, chronic, or delayed-onset PTSD.
Checklist for PTSD Symptoms in Infants and Young Children (Scheeringa, Zeanan, Drell, & Larrieu, 1995; Scheeringa, Peebles, Cook, & Zeanah, 2001)	Clinician-rated symptom inventory using a standard observation/interactional procedure with children and semistructured interviews with children and parents	High preliminary interrater reliability for most symptoms; high discriminant validity and procedural validity	0–3 years	Alternative assessment method for diagnosing PTSD in infants and toddlers.
Posttraumatic Symptom Inventory for Children (Eisen, 1997)	30-item interview	High internal consistency, preliminary convergent validity	4–8 years	Specifically designed for use in younger children.
When Bad Things Happen Scale (Fletcher, 1997)	95-item self-report	High internal consistency and convergent validity	≥ third grade	Includes a parent report version (Parent Report of Child's Reaction to Stress).

(*continued*)

Table 14.2. (*continued*)

Measure	Format	Reliability and Validity Data	Age	Comments
PTSD Checklist/Parent Report (Ford et al., 1996, 1999)	17-item parent report	High internal consistency, good interrater reliability, strong convergent and construct validity	Not specified	Standardized on pediatric medical trauma population.
Checklist of Child Distress Symptoms (Martinez & Richters, 1993)	25-item self-report	High interrater and concurrent validity	6–17 years	Specifically designed for use in children; has a parallel parent-report version.
CCDS–Parent Report (Richters & Martinez, 1990)	28-item parent report	High interrater and concurrent validity	6–17 years	Parallels child version.
Levonn (Richters, Martinez, & Valla, 1990)	40-item self-report pictorial/visual thermometer rating scale in response to questions read to child	None	< 6 years	Only self-report instrument for preschool children.
Child Stress Reaction Checklist (Saxe et al., 1997)	35-item parent, teacher, or medical staff report	High preliminary interrater reliability and construct validity	Not specified	Standardized on acutely burned children; also measures acute stress disorder.
Child and Adolescent PTSD Checklist (Amaya-Jackson, 1995; Amaya-Jackson et al., 2000)	28-item self-report	High internal consistency, criterion validity with CAPS-CA, high test-retest reliability	Not specified	Psychometrics established in diverse populations (outpatient, inpatient, incarcerated, exposed to a wide variety of acute and chronic stressors).
Child and Adolescent Trauma Survey (March, Amaya-Jackson, Murray, & Schulte, 1998; March, Amaya-Jackson, Terry, & Costanzo, 1997)	12-item self-report	High internal and test-retest reliability	Not specified	
Screen for Child Anxiety Related Emotional Disorders–Revised (SCARED-R) Traumatic Stress Disorder Scale (Birmaher et al., 1997; Muris, Merckelbach, Korver, & Meesters, 2000)	4 items embedded in a 70-item self-report measure	Preliminary convergent validity	Not specified	

and the other being more prominent at another time (M. Horowitz, 1976; Miller & Veltkamp, 1988; Schwarz & Kowalski, 1991). Others have suggested that if children have very effective avoidant and numbing responses, they will appear to be largely unaffected by traumatic events, when in fact these symptoms are masking other PTSD symptoms (Arroyo & Eth, 1995; Stuber, Nader, Yasuda, Pynoos, & Cohen, 1991). Avoidant (denial) symptoms, and the child's ability to link such symptoms to a traumatic event, are by definition difficult if not impossible to assess (Green et al., 1991). For this reason alone, requiring three avoidant symptoms in children may be too stringent a criteria to accurately identify many children with PTSD. As noted previously, alternative criteria have been suggested for younger children (Scheeringa et al., 2001; Scheeringa et al., 1995), although these have only received preliminary psychometric evaluation (Scheeringa et al., 2003). Because the *DSM-IV* PTSD criteria have not been validated in children or adolescents, this debate will likely continue, with many suggesting the need for developmental-stage-specific diagnostic criteria for this disorder (Benedek, 1985; Drell et al., 1993; Green et al., 1991; F. D. Horowitz, 1996).

Perhaps it is more important to consider whether there is a clinically relevant distinction between children who meet full versus partial PTSD criteria, or whether meeting full criteria is a somewhat arbitrary cutoff point without true clinical implications. At this time, there is no clear evidence to document that children meeting full versus partial PTSD criteria need different types of treatment. At least one study has documented that sub-syndromal levels of PTSD lead to similar functional impairment in children as full-blown PTSD (Carrion et al., 2002). Thus, it makes sense to offer treatment to children with PTSD symptoms that are causing some significant functional impairment, regardless of whether or not the child meets full diagnostic criteria for this disorder.

The assessment tree in Figure 14.1 illustrates the decision-making process in determining a correct diagnosis, to assist in treatment planning and evaluation of treatment outcome.

TREATMENT

Compared with treatments for other childhood anxiety disorders, the treatment of PTSD has received relatively little empirical evaluation. Only a few treatments have been subjected to randomized clinical trials (RCTs) for this population. Thus, it is possible that treatments other than those discussed in the following section may be efficacious in treating this disorder.

Trauma-focused cognitive-behavioral therapies (CBTs) have received most empirical support to date. Other treatment modalities that have been studied include eye movement desensitization and reprocessing (EMDR), nondirective supportive therapy, psychological debriefing, and pharmacotherapy. Anecdotal reports using psychoanalytic techniques have been published (e.g., Gaensbauer, 1994), but due to the absence of empirical data, these are not discussed here.

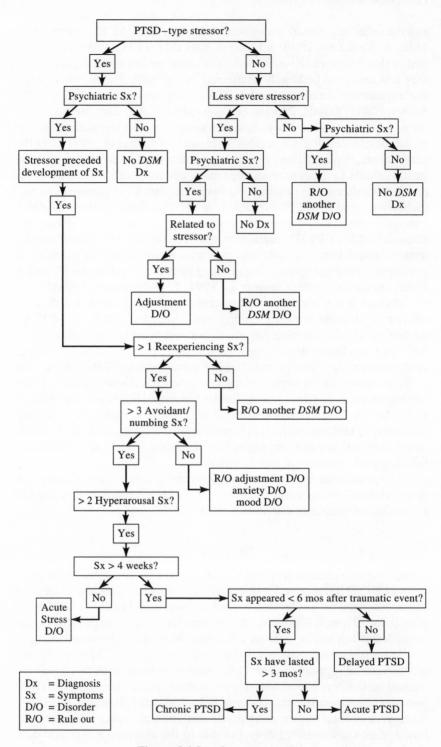

Figure 14.1. Assessment tree

Selected Treatment: Trauma-Focused
Cognitive-Behavioral Therapy

The only treatment modality that has demonstrated efficacy in comparative RCTs is trauma-focused CBT. Although the studies cited have used
different CBT treatment manuals, these interventions shared several basic
CBT components, including gradual exposure techniques (creating a narrative of the child's traumatic experience), cognitive processing of the traumatic event, psychoeducation, and training in stress-reduction techniques
such as relaxation and positive self-talk (Cohen, Berliner, & Mannarino,
2000; Deblinger & Heflin, 1996). Most included a parental treatment component. Three studies comparing the efficacy of CBT to either standard
community care (SCC) or nondirective supportive therapy (NST) demonstrated that CBT was superior in decreasing PTSD symptoms as well as other
symptoms in cohorts of sexually abused children. Deblinger, Lippmann,
and Steer (1996) compared CBT delivered only to the child, only to the
parent, or to child and parent, to SCC and found that providing CBT to
the child (whether or not the parent received CBT) resulted in significantly
greater improvement in PTSD symptoms. This study also found that providing CBT to the nonoffending parent resulted in significantly greater
improvement in the child's self-reported depressive symptoms and in
parenting practices. Cohen and Mannarino (1996, 1997) demonstrated that
CBT was superior to NST in improving PTSD symptoms in sexually abused
preschoolers (3 to 7 years old), including sexually inappropriate behaviors.
CBT also resulted in greater improvement in general behavioral problems
for this cohort. In a parallel study, these researchers demonstrated that at
posttreatment, treatment completers receiving TF-CBT experienced significantly greater improvement in depression and social competence than
those receiving NST (Cohen & Mannarino, 1998), while at the 1-year
follow-up, the TF-CBT completers had significantly greater improvement
in PTSD and dissociative symptoms than the NST completers (Cohen,
Mannarino, & Knudsen, 2003). This study also demonstrated the superiority of TF-CBT in an intent-to-treat analysis, with regard to depressive,
anxiety, and sexual problems. The only multisite treatment study for child
PTSD to date (Cohen, Deblinger, Mannarino, & Steer, 2003) demonstrated
the superiority of TF-CBT over Rogerian-based supportive child-centered
therapy in improving PTSD, depressive, anxiety, and behavioral symptoms.
Other studies comparing CBT with another active treatment have not found
significant group times time effects (Berliner & Saunders, 1996; Celano,
Hazzard, Webb, & McCall, 1996).

Two studies compared trauma-focused CBT to no-treatment controls
and found CBT to be efficacious in decreasing PTSD symptoms in children. Chemtob, Hamada, and Nakashima (1996) randomly assigned children exposed to a hurricane to either CBT or a wait-list control condition
and found significantly more improvement in PTSD symptoms in the children receiving CBT. Goenjian et al. (1997) compared trauma-focused psy-

chotherapy with no treatment for children exposed to an earthquake and found that, although the treatment group experienced improvement in PTSD symptoms, PTSD symptoms actually worsened in the no-treatment group; the latter group also experienced worsening of depressive symptoms over time. Although the therapy provided in this study was not labeled CBT by the authors, the description of the interventions was consistent with other CBT modalities, in that it was comprised of exposure, cognitive reframing, and psychoeducational components.

Two treatment studies of trauma-focused CBT have used a delayed or staggered start design to control for the effect of the passage of time. March et al. (1998) utilized a staggered start design, providing group CBT in school settings to children exposed to single-episode traumatic stressors. This study demonstrated that PTSD symptoms improved only after CBT was initiated and continued to improve as treatment progressed. Deblinger, McLeer, and Henry (1990) used a delayed start design to demonstrate that PTSD symptoms in sexually abused children remained high until individual CBT was provided, and that CBT resulted in significant improvement in these symptoms.

Thus, a variety of empirical treatment studies have demonstrated that trauma-focused CBT is efficacious in decreasing PTSD symptoms in children exposed to a variety of stressors. In addition, a series of single case studies have supported the efficacy of exposure techniques in reducing PTSD symptoms in children and adolescents (Saigh, 1986, 1989; Saigh, Yule, & Inamdar, 1996). Because CBT has stronger empirical support than any other tested treatment modality for this population, at present, it may be considered the first-line treatment for this population.

Experimental Treatments: Eye Movement Desensitization and Reprocessing

Eye movement desensitization and reprocessing (EMDR) is a newer treatment that has received a great deal of recent attention in both academic journals and the popular press. Although several studies have supported its efficacy in decreasing PTSD symptoms in adults, other researchers have demonstrated that the eye movements used in this intervention are not the essential ingredient of this treatment approach (Pitman et al., 1996). In the absence of eye movements, EMDR consists of exposure and cognitive-reprocessing techniques, typically provided in relatively few treatment sessions. For this reason, many have conceptualized EMDR as a variety of CBT (Cohen, Berliner, & Mannarino, 2000). Two studies have examined the efficacy of this treatment for children with PTSD. Chemtob, Nakashima, and Carlson (2002) demonstrated that, following exposure to a hurricane, children receiving four sessions of EMDR experienced significantly greater improvement in PTSD and anxiety symptoms than children assigned to a wait-list control condition. Jaberghaderi et al. (2002) compared TF-CBT to EMDR for Iranian sexually abused girls and found these two interventions to be comparable in efficacy. If future studies replicate these findings, EMDR may become an important treatment approach for these children. However, support for this intervention must be considered preliminary at this time.

Supportive Therapies

As noted above, one study demonstrated that nondirective supportive therapy (NST) for sexually abused preschool children and their nonoffending parents was not as efficacious as CBT in decreasing PTSD symptoms and sexually inappropriate behaviors (Cohen & Mannarino, 1996, 1997). This protocol used nondirective play therapy for the child subjects and nondirective supportive counseling for the parents. A parallel study of older children (8- to 14-year-olds) failed to find significant group by time differences between these two treatments at posttreatment with regard to PTSD; at 12 months posttreatment, however, treatment completers in the TF-CBT group showed significantly greater improvement in PTSD than those in the NST group (Cohen, Mannarino, & Knudsen, 2003). Although child-centered supportive therapy (CCT) resulted in significant improvement in PTSD and other symptoms in a subsequent multisite study, it was less effective than TF-CBT in this regard (Cohen, Deblinger, Mannarino, & Steer, 2003). Unless future studies support the efficacy of supportive therapy for treating childhood PTSD, this treatment approach should probably not be considered a first-line treatment for this population.

Psychoanalytic Therapy

One study compared sexually abused children randomly assigned to receive up to 18 sessions of group psychoeducation or up to 30 sessions of individual psychoanalytic therapy (Trowell et al., 2002). Although the psychoanalytic treatment group demonstrated significantly greater improvement in PTSD symptoms, it is not clear whether this was due to differences in the type of treatment (psychoanalytic versus psychoeducation), the modality of treatment (individual versus group), or the dosage of treatment (30 versus 18 sessions). An earlier study that compared psychodynamic therapy to behavioral therapy for sexually abused children (Downing et al., 1988) found behavioral therapy to be superior in improving sexualized behaviors, but other aspects of PTSD were not measured in this study. Further research on the efficacy of psychoanalytic and psychodynamic treatments for childhood PTSD is warranted.

Psychological Debriefing

One study of psychological debriefing was conducted with a small number of children following a school bus accident (Stallard & Law, 1993). This three-session intervention consisted of psychoeducation and encouragement to verbalize feelings about the stressful event. No control or comparison condition was included. Symptoms of PTSD, anxiety, and depression decreased from pre- to posttreatment in this study. This study has not been replicated, and a recent adult study has indicated that psychological debriefing may in fact be detrimental rather than beneficial (Hobbs, Mayou, Harrison, & Warlock, 1996). In the absence of empirically rigorous evidence that supports this intervention, it should therefore not be viewed as a first-line treatment approach for childhood PTSD.

Pharmacological Interventions

Although no placebo-controlled RCTs of pharmacologic interventions have been conducted in children with PTSD, a number of open (noncontrolled) medication trials have been published. Most of these have evaluated the use of catecholamine drugs. The most rigorous was an *A-B-A* design (comparing no medication to medication) evaluating the efficacy of propranalol in 11 sexually or physically abused children (Famularo, Kinscherff, & Fenton, 1988). This study demonstrated significant decreases in PTSD symptoms in children who were given propranolol, and worsening of symptoms when the medication was discontinued. Clonidine was found to reduce PTSD in two small uncontrolled studies, one using twice-a-day dosing (Perry, 1994) and the other using clonidine patches (Harmon & Riggs, 1996). The only published study examining the efficacy of a dopamine-blocking agent in treating childhood PTSD was conducted by Horrigan (1998). Risperidone was given to 18 children with severe PTSD and various comorbid psychiatric disorders. Thirteen of the subjects experienced remission of PTSD symptoms following this treatment. The anticonvulsant carbamazepine was evaluated in one study and was found to produce PTSD symptom remission in 22 of 28 children (Looff et al., 1995). Finally, an open study of the serotonergic medication citalopram indicated that this medication was as effective and efficient in decreasing PTSD in children and adolescents with PTSD as it was in as adults with PTSD (Seedat et al., 2002). Serotonin reuptake inhibitors such as citalopram have favorable side-effect profiles compared with those of other medications used to treat PTSD. Because no placebo-controlled trials of any medication have been conducted in children with this disorder, pharmacologic interventions do not currently have the necessary empirical support to be considered first-line treatments. However, for children with comorbid conditions known to respond to pharmacologic treatments (such as MDD or panic disorder), pharmacologic treatment should be considered, particularly if TF-CBT interventions are unsuccessful in producing symptom remission.

Summary of Stages of Treatment

Clearly, compared with research on treatment for other childhood anxiety disorders, the treatment research for PTSD is at a very early stage. More empirical research is needed to better inform practitioners of best treatment practices for this population. At present, TF-CBT is the only intervention with adequate empirical support to be considered a first-line treatment approach for this disorder. Given the current state of knowledge, it is recommended that trauma-focused CBT be used first when treating children with significant PTSD symptoms. Because it is not clear what components of TF-CBT are essential for symptom resolution, it is not possible to prescribe which of these should be used first, or to state whether integrating CBT components into other treatment modalities will have comparable efficacy in resolving PTSD symptoms.

A national expert consensus survey (Foa, Davidson, & Francis, 1999) indicated that CBT, either alone or in combination with a selective serotonin reuptake inhibitor (SSRI), is recommended as the first-line treatment for children and adolescents with PTSD. This survey also recommended that children with treatment-resistant PTSD be treated with a medication that works on multiple neurotransmitter systems (for example, venlafaxine or bupropion).

For children who have comorbid psychiatric conditions such as MDD or OCD, for which CBT and pharmacotherapy are known to be efficacious, CBT should be provided either alone or in combination with the appropriate medication for the child's comorbid disorder. If CBT alone is ineffective in resolving the child's symptoms, the appropriate medication should be added.

At the present time, there is no clear evidence to direct treatment selection for children who do not respond to TF-CBT. More research is needed to address this important question. It is likely that other treatment modalities will be found that effectively reduce PTSD symptoms in traumatized children. We also currently have no empirical information from randomized clinical trials on the optimal management of partial treatment responders, treatment resistance, and maintenance or discontinuation of treatment for childhood PTSD. It is to be hoped that new research will be available in the near future to guide such decisions.

SUMMARY

Exposure to traumatic life events in childhood can lead to the development of PTSD. Childhood PTSD is associated with serious deleterious effects, including interruption of normal neurodevelopment, smaller brain size, and lower IQ. Assessment of this disorder in children can be challenging, and it is not clear whether current diagnostic criteria are adequate to identify children with this disorder. Since children with substantial PTSD symptoms who do not meet full *DSM-IV* PTSD criteria have similar functional impairment to those with the diagnosis, those with significant PTSD symptoms should receive similar treatments regardless of diagnostic status. Trauma-focused CBT currently has the strongest empirical support and currently should be considered a first-line treatment for childhood PTSD.

More research is needed to identify other effective treatments. Dissemination and implementation of effective treatments among community providers will greatly enhance the optimal treatment of childhood PTSD.

REFERENCES

Almqvist, K., & Brandell-Forsberg, M. (1997). Refugee children in Sweden: Posttraumatic stress disorder in Iranian preschool children exposed to organized violence. *Child Abuse and Neglect, 21*(4), 351–366.

Amaya-Jackson, L. (1997). *The Child PTSD Checklist.* Unpublished manuscript, Duke University School of Medicine.

Amaya-Jackson, L., Newman, E., Lipschitz, D., Rosenbalm, K. D., Billingslea, E., & Ymanis, N. (2000). *The Child and Adolescent PTSD Checklist in three clinical populations.* Paper presented at the Annual Meeting of the American Academy of Child and Adolescent Psychiatry, New York.

American Academy of Child and Adolescent Psychiatry. (1998). Practice parameters for the assessment and treatment of children and adolescents with posttraumatic stress disorder. *Journal of the American Academy of Child and Adolescent Psychiatry, 10*(Supplement), S4–S26.

Appelbaum, P. S. (1997). Ethics in evolution: The incompatibility of clinical and forensic functions. *American Journal of Psychiatry, 154*(4), 445–446.

Arroyo, W., & Eth, S. (1995). Assessment following violence: Witnessing trauma. In E. Peled, P. G. Jaffe, & J. L. Edleson (Eds.), *Ending the cycle of violence: Community responses in children of battered women.* Thousand Oaks, CA: Sage.

Benedek, E. I. (1985). Children and psychic trauma: A brief review of contemporary thinking. In S. Eth & R. S. Pynoos (Eds.), *Posttraumatic stress disorder in children.* Washington, DC: American Psychiatric Press.

Berliner, L., & Saunders, B. E. (1996). Treating fear and anxiety in sexually abused children: Results of a controlled 2-year follow-up study. *Child Maltreatment, 1,* 294–309.

Berliner, L., & Wheeler, J. R. (1998). Treating the effects of sexual abuse on children. *Journal of Interpersonal Violence, 2*(4), 415–434.

Biederman, J., Faraone, S. V., Milberger, S., Jetton, J. G., Chen, L., Mick, E., Greene, R. W., et al. (1996). Is childhood oppositional defiant disorder a precursor to adolescent conduct disorder? *Journal of the American Academy of Child and Adolescent Psychiatry, 35,* 1193–1204.

Birmaher, B., Brent, D. A., Chiappetta, L., Bridge, J., Monga, S., & Baugher, M. (1999). Psychometric properties of the Screen for Child Anxiety Related Emotional Disorders (SCARED): A replication study. *Journal of the American Academy of Child and Adolescent Psychiatry, 38*(10), 1230–1236.

Boyle, S., Bolton, D., Nurrish, J., O'Ryan, D., Udwin, O., & Yule, W. (1995). *The Jupiter sinking follow-up: Predicting psychopathology in adolescence following trauma.* Paper presented at the 11th Annual Meeting of the International Society for Traumatic Stress Studies, Boston.

Brent, D. A., Perper, J. A., Moritz, G., Liotus, L., Richardson, D., Canobbio, R., Schweers, J., et al. (1995). Posttraumatic stress disorder in peers of adolescent suicide victims. *Journal of the American Academy of Child and Adolescent Psychiatry, 34*(2), 209–215.

Carrion, V. G., & Steiner, H. (2000). Trauma and dissociation in delinquent adolescents. *Journal of the American Academy of Child and Adolescent Psychiatry, 39*(3), 353–359.

Carrion, V. G., Weems, C. F., Ray, R., & Reiss, A. L. (2002). Toward an empirical definition of pediatric PTSD: The phenomenology of PTSD symptoms in youth. *Journal of the American Academy of Child and Adolescent Psychiatry, 41*, 166–173.

Celano, M., Hazzard, A., Webb, C., & McCall, C. (1996). Treatment of traumagenic beliefs among sexually abused girls and their mothers: An evaluation study. *Journal of Abnormal Child Psychology, 24*, 1–16.

Chemtob, C., Hamada, R., & Nakashima, J. (1996). *Psychosocial intervention for post-disaster trauma symptoms in elementary school children: A controlled field study.* Unpublished manuscript, University of Hawaii.

Chemtob, C., Nakashima, J., & Carlson, J. (2002). Brief treatment for elementary school children with disaster-related posttraumatic stress disorder: A field study. *Journal of Clinical Psychology, 58*, 99–112.

Chilcoat, H. D., & Breslau, N. (1998). Posttraumatic stress disorder and drug disorders: Testing causal pathways. *Archives of General Psychiatry, 55*, 913–917.

Clark, D. B., Bukstein, O. G., Smith, M. G., Kaczynski, N. A., Mezzich, A. C., & Donovan, J. E. (1995). Identifying anxiety disorders in adolescents hospitalized for alcohol abuse or dependence. *Psychiatric Services, 46*, 618–620.

Cohen, J. A., Berliner, L., & Mannarino, A. P. (2000). Treatment of traumatized children: A review and synthesis. *Journal of Trauma, Violence and Abuse, 1*(1), 29–46.

Cohen, J. A., Deblinger, E., Mannarino, A. P., & Steer, R. (2003). A multisite randomized controlled treatment study for sexually abused children. Paper presented at the annual meeting of the American Professional Society on the Abuse of Children, Chicago, July.

Cohen, J. A., & Mannarino, A. P. (1993). A treatment model for sexually abused preschoolers. *Journal of Interpersonal Violence, 8*(1), 115–131.

Cohen, J. A., & Mannarino, A. P. (1996). A treatment outcome study for sexually abused preschool children: Initial findings. *Journal of the American Academy of Child and Adolescent Psychiatry, 35*, 42–50.

Cohen, J. A., & Mannarino, A. P. (1997). A treatment study of sexually abused preschool children: Outcome during a one year follow-up. *Journal of the American Academy of Child and Adolescent Psychiatry, 36*(9), 1229–1235.

Cohen, J. A., & Mannarino, A. P. (1998). Interventions for sexually abused children: Initial treatment outcome findings. *Child Maltreatment, 3*, 17–26.

Costello, E. J., Angold, A., Burns, B. J., Stangl, D. K., Tweed, D. L., Erkanli, A., & Worthman, C. M. (1996). The Great Smoky Mountains Study of Youth: Goals, designs, methods, and the prevalence of *DSM-III-R* disorders. *Archives of General Psychiatry, 53*, 1129–1136.

Cuffe, S. P., McCullough, E. L., & Pumariega, A. J. (1994). Comorbidity of attention-deficit/hyperactivity disorder and posttraumatic stress disorder. *Journal of Child and Family Studies, 3*(3), 327–336.

DeBellis, M. D., Chrousos, G. P., Dorn, L, D., Burke, L., Helmers, K., Kling, M. A., Trickett, P. K., et al. (1994). H-P-A axis dysregulation in sexually abused girls. *Journal of Clinical Endocrinology and Metabolism, 78*, 249–255.

DeBellis, M. D., Keshavan, M. S., Clark, D. B., Casey, B. J., Giedd, J. N., Boring,

A. M., Frustacik, & Ryan N. D. (1999). Developmental traumatology, Part II: Brain development. *Biological Psychiatry, 45,* 1271–1284.

Deblinger, E., & Heflin, A. H. (1996). *Cognitive behavioral interventions for treating sexually abused children.* Thousand Oaks, CA: Sage Publications.

Deblinger, E., Lippmann, J., & Steer, R. (1996). Sexually abused children suffering posttraumatic stress symptoms: Initial treatment outcome findings. *Child Maltreatment, 1*(40), 310–321.

Deblinger, E., McLeer, S. V., & Henry, D. (1990). Cognitive behavioral treatment for sexually abused children suffering posttraumatic stress: Preliminary findings. *Journal of the American Academy of Child and Adolescent Psychiatry, 29,* 747–752.

Downing, J., Jenkins, S. J., & Fisher, G. L. (1988). A comparison of psychodynamic and reinforcement treatment with sexually abused children. *Elementary School Guidance Counseling, 22,* 291–298.

Drell, M. J., Siegel, C. H., & Gaensbauer, T. J. (1993). Posttraumatic stress disorder. In C. H. Zeanah (Ed.), *Handbook of infant mental health.* New York: Guilford Press.

Eisen, M. (1997). Posttraumatic Symptom Survey for Children. In E. Carlson (Ed.), *Trauma assessments: A clinician's guide.* New York: Guilford Press.

Famularo, R., Fenton, T., Augustyn, M., & Zuckerman, B. (1996). Persistence of pediatric posttraumatic stress after two years. *Child Abuse and Neglect, 20*(12), 1245–1248.

Famularo, R., Kinscherff, R., & Fenton, T. (1988). Propranolol treatment for childhood posttraumatic stress disorder, acute type: A pilot study. *American Journal of Diseases of Children, 142,* 1244–1247.

Fletcher, K. (1997). When Bad Things Happen Scale. In E. Carlson (Ed.), *Trauma assessment: A clinician's guide* (pp. 257–258). New York: Guilford Press.

Foa, E. B., Davidson, R. T., & Francis, A. (Eds.). (1999). Expert consensus guideline series: Treatment of posttraumatic stress disorder. *Journal of Clinical Psychiatry, 60*(Suppl. 16), 17.

Foa, E. B., Johnson, K. M., Feeny, N. C., & Treadwell, K. R. H. (2001). The Child PTSD Symptom Scale: A preliminary examination of its psychometric properties. *Journal of Clinical Child Psychology, 30*(3), 376–384.

Foa, E. B., & Tolin, D. F. (2000). Comparison of the PTSD Symptom Scale Interview Version and the Clinician Administered PTSD Scale. *Journal of Traumatic Stress, 13,* 181–192.

Ford, J. D., Racusin, R., Daviss, W. B., Ellis, C. G., Thomas, J., Rogers, K., Reiser, J., et al. (1999). Trauma exposure among children with ODD and ADHD. *Journal of Consulting and Clinical Psychology, 67,* 786–789.

Ford, J. D., Racusin, R., Ellis, C. G., Daviss, W. B., Reiser, J., Fleisher, A., & Thomas, J. (2000). Child maltreatment, other trauma exposure, and posttraumatic symptomatology among children with oppositional defiant and attention deficit hyperactivity disorders. *Child Maltreatment, 5*(3), 205–217.

Ford, J. D., Thomas, J. E., Rogers, K. C., Racusin, R. J., Ellis, C. G., Schiffman, J. G., Daviss, W. B., et al. (1996, November). *Assessment of children's PTSD following abuse or accidental trauma.* Paper presented at the Annual Meeting of the International Society for Traumatic Stress Studies, San Francisco.

Frederick, C. J. (1985). Children traumatized by catastrophic situations. In S. Eth & R. S. Pynoos (Eds.), *Posttraumatic stress disorder in children.* Washington, DC: American Psychiatric Press.

Gaensbauer, T. J. (1994). Therapeutic work with a traumatized toddler. *Psychoanalytic Study of the Child, 49,* 412–433.

Garrison, C. Z., Bryant, E. S., Addy, C. L., Spurrier, P. G., Freedy, J. R., & Kilpatrick, D. G. (1995). Posttraumatic stress disorder in adolescents after Hurricane Andrew. *Journal of the American Academy of Child and Adolescent Psychiatry, 34*(9), 1193–1201.

Glod, C. A., & Teicher, M. H. (1996). Relationship between early abuse, PTSD, and activity levels in prepubertal children. *Journal of the American Academy of Child and Adolescent Psychiatry, 35*(10), 1384–1393.

Goenjian, A. K., Karayan, I., Pynoos, R. S., Minassian, D., Najarian, L. M., Steinberg, A. M., & Fairbanks, L. A. (1997). Outcome of psychotherapy among early adolescents after trauma. *American Journal of Psychiatry, 154*(4), 536–542.

Goenjian, A. K., Pynoos, R. S., Steinberg, A. M., Najarian, L. M., Asarnow, J. R., Karayan, J., Ghurabi, M., et al. (1995). Psychiatric comorbidity in children after the 1988 earthquake in Armenia. *Journal of the American Academy of Child and Adolescent Psychiatry, 34*(9), 1174–1184.

Goodwin, J. (1985). Posttraumatic symptoms in incest victims. In S. Eth & R. S. Pynoos (Eds.), *Posttraumatic stress disorder in children.* Washington, DC: American Psychiatric Press.

Goodwin, J. (1988). Posttraumatic stress symptoms in abused children. *Journal of Traumatic Stress, 1*(4), 475–488.

Green, B. L., Grace, M. C., Vary, M. G., Kramer, T. L., Gleser, G. C., & Leonard, A. C. (1994). Children of disaster in the second decade: A 17-year follow-up of the Buffalo Creek survivors. *Journal of the American Academy of Child and Adolescent Psychiatry, 33,* 71–79.

Green, B. L., Korol, M., Grace, M. C., Vary, M. G., Leonard, A. C., Gleser, G. C., & Smitson-Cohen, S. (1991). Children and disaster: Age, gender and parental effects on posttraumatic stress disorder symptoms. *Journal of the American Academy of Child and Adolescent Psychiatry, 30*(6), 945–951.

Greenberg, S. A., & Shuman, D. W. (1997). Irreconcilable conflict between the therapeutic and forensic roles. *Professional Psychology: Research and Practice, 28,* 50–57.

Harmon, R. J., & Riggs, P. D. (1996). Clinical perspectives: Clonidine for posttraumatic stress disorder in preschool children. *Journal of the American Academy of Child and Adolescent Psychiatry, 35*(9), 1247–1249.

Herman, J. L., Perry, J. C., & van der Kolk, B. A. (1989). Childhood trauma in borderline personality disorder. *American Journal of Psychiatry, 146,* 490–495.

Herman, J. L., & van der Kolk, B. A. (1987). Traumatic antecedents of borderline personality disorder. In B. A. van der Kolk (Ed.), *Psychological trauma.* Washington, DC: American Psychiatric Press.

Hobbs, M., Mayou, R., Harrison, B., & Warlock, P. (1996). A randomized trial of psychological debriefing for victims of road traffic accidents. *British Medical Journal, 31*(3), 1438–1439.

Hornstein, N. L. (1996). Complexities of psychiatric differential diagnosis in children with dissociative symptoms and disorders. In J. Silberg (Ed.), *The dissociative child.* Lutherville, MD: Sidran Press.

Horowitz, F. D. (1996). Developmental perspectives on child and adolescent posttraumatic stress disorder. *Journal of School Psychology, 34*(2), 189–191.

Horowitz, M. (1976). *Stress response syndromes.* New York: Jason Aronson.

Horrigan, J. (1998, December 18). Risperidone appears effective for children and adolescents with severe PTSD. *Psychiatric News*, p. 8.

Hubbard, J., Realmuto, G. M., Northwood, A. K., & Masten, A. S. (1995). Comorbidity of psychiatric diagnoses with posttraumatic stress disorder in survivors of childhood trauma. *Journal of the American Academy of Child and Adolescent Psychiatry, 34*(9), 1167–1173.

Ismail, A., Cohen, J. A., Mannarino, A. P., Goessler, M., & Guthrie, R. (2000, February). *Incidence of PTSD in a pediatric primary care population.* Peter B. Henderson Outstanding Paper Award presented at the American Association of Directors of Psychiatry Residency Training Annual Meeting, San Juan, Puerto Rico.

Jaberghaderi, N., Greenwald, R., Rubin, A., Dolatubadim, S., & Zand, S. O. (2002). A comparison of CBT and EMDR for sexually abused Iranian girls. Unpublished ms., Allame Tabatabee University, Teheran, Iran.

Kaufman, J. (1991). Depressive disorders in maltreated children. *Journal of the American Academy of Child and Adolescent Psychiatry, 30*, 257–265.

Kaufman, J., Birmaher, B., Brent, D., Rao, U., Flynn, C., Moreci, P., Williamson, D., et al. (1997). Schedule for Affective Disorders and Schizophrenia for School-Age Children–Present and Lifetime Version (K-SADS-PL): Initial reliability and validity data. *Journal of the American Academy of Child and Adolescent Psychiatry, 36*(7), 980–988.

Kazdin, A. (1995). Scope of child and adolescent psychotherapy research: Limited sampling of dysfunctions, treatment, and client characteristics. *Journal of Clinical and Consulting Psychology, 24*(2), 125–140.

Kinzie, J. D., Sack, W. H., Angell, R. H., Manson, S., & Rath, B. (1986). The psychiatric effects of massive trauma on Cambodian children: I. The children. *Journal of the American Academy of Child and Adolescent Psychiatry, 25*(3), 370–376.

Kiser, L. J., Heston, J., Milsap, P. A., & Pruitt, D. B. (1991). Physical and sexual abuse in childhood: Relationships with posttraumatic stress disorder. *Journal of the American Academy of Child and Adolescent Psychiatry, 30*, 776–783.

La Greca, A. M., Silverman, W. K., & Wasserstein, S. B. (1998). Children's pre-disaster functioning as a predictor of posttraumatic stress following Hurricane Andrew. *Journal of Consulting and Clinical Psychology, 66*(6), 883–892.

La Greca, A. M., Vernberg, E. M., Silverman, W. K., & Prinstein, M. J. (1996). Symptoms of posttraumatic stress in children after Hurricane Andrew: A prospective study. *Journal of Consulting and Clinical Psychology, 64*(4), 712–723.

Laor, N., Wolmer, L., Mayes, L. C., Gershon, A., Weizman, R., & Cohen, D. T. (1997). Israeli preschool children under Scuds: A 30-month follow-up. *Journal of the American Academy of Child and Adolescent Psychiatry, 36*(3), 349–356.

Lindley, S. E., Carlson, E., & Sheikh, J. (2000). Psychotic symptoms in posttraumatic stress disorder. *CNS Spectrums, 5*(9), 52–57.

Lonigan, C. J., Shannon, M. P., Taylor, C. M., Finch, A. J., & Sallec, F. R. (1994). Children exposed to disaster: II. Risk factors for the development of post-traumatic symptomatology. *Journal of the American Academy of Child and Adolescent Psychiatry, 33*(1), 94–105.

Looff, D., Grimley, P., Kuiler, F., Martin, A., & Shunfield, L. (1995). Carba-mazepine for posttraumatic stress disorder [Letter to the editor]. *Journal of the American Academy of Child and Adolescent Psychiatry, 34*(6), 703–704.

Macksoud, M. S., & Aber, J. L. (1996). The war experiences and psychosocial development of children in Lebanon. *Child Development, 67,* 70–88.

March, J. S. (1999). Assessment of pediatric posttraumatic stress disorder. In P. A. Saigh & J. D. Saigh (Eds.), *Posttraumatic stress disorder: A comprehensive text* (pp. 199–218). Boston: Allyn & Bacon.

March, J. S., Amaya-Jackson, L., Murray, M. C., & Schulte, A. (1998). Cognitive-behavioral psychotherapy for children and adolescents with posttraumatic stress disorder after a single-incident stressor. *Journal of the American Academy of Child and Adolescent Psychiatry, 37*(6), 585–593.

March, J. S., Amaya-Jackson, L., Terry, R., & Costanzo, P. (1997). Posttraumatic symptomatology in children and adolescents after an industrial fire. *Journal of the American Academy of Child and Adolescent Psychiatry, 36*(8), 1080–1088.

Martinez, P., & Richters, J. E. (1993). The NIMH community violence project: II. Children's distress symptoms associated with violence exposure. *Psychiatry, 59,* 22–35.

Matzner, F., Silva, R., Silvan, M., Chawdury, M., & Natasi, L. (1997). Preliminary test-retest reliability of the KID-SCID. In *Annual Meeting New Research Program and Abstracts* (pp. 172–173). Washington, DC: American Psychiatric Association.

McCloskey, L. A., & Walker, W. (2000). Posttraumatic stress in children exposed to family violence and single event trauma. *Journal of the American Academy of Child and Adolescent Psychiatry, 26*(5), 764–769.

McFarland, A. C. (1987). Posttraumatic phenomena in a longitudinal study of children following natural disaster. *Journal of the American Academy of Child and Adolescent Psychiatry, 26*(5), 764–769.

McLeer, S. V., Callaghan, M., Henry, D., & Wallen, J. (1994). Psychiatric disorders in sexually abused children. *Journal of the American Academy of Child and Adolescent Psychiatry, 33*(3), 313–319.

Milgram, N. A., Toubiana, Y. H., Klingman, A., Raviv, A., & Goldstein, I. (1988). Situational exposure and personal loss in children's acute and chronic stress reactions to a school bus disaster. *Journal of Traumatic Stress, 1,* 339–352.

Miller, T. W., & Veltkamp, L. J. (1988). Effects of multigenerational sexual abuse in rural America. *International Journal of Family Psychiatry, 9*(3), 259–275.

Muris, P., Merckelbach, H., Korver, P., & Meesters, C. (2000). Screening for trauma in children and adolescents: The validity of the Traumatic Stress Disorder Scale of the Screen for Child Anxiety Related Emotional Disorders. *Journal of Clinical Child Psychology, 29*(3), 406–413.

Nader, K., Kriegler, J. A., Blake, D. D., Pynoos, R. S., Newman, E., & Weathers, F. W. (1996). Clinician-Administered PTSD Scale for Children and Adolescents for *DSM-IV.* Boston: National Center for PTSD and UCLA Trauma Psychiatry Program.

Nader, K., Pynoos, R. S., Fairbanks, L., & Frederick, C. (1990). Children's posttraumatic stress disorder reactions one year after a sniper attack at their school. *American Journal of Psychiatry, 147,* 1526–1530.

Pelcovitz, D., Kaplan, S., Goldenberg, B., Mandel, F., Lehane, J., & Guarrero, J. (1994). Posttraumatic stress disorder in physically abused adolescents. *Journal of the American Academy of Child and Adolescent Psychiatry, 33*(3), 305–312.

Perry, B. D. (1994). Neurobiological sequelae of childhood trauma: Posttraumatic stress disorder in children. In M. M. Murburg (Ed.), *Catecholamine func-*

tion in Posttraumatic Stress Disorder: Emerging Concepts. Washington, DC: American Psychiatric Press.

Pine, D. C., & Cohen, J. A. (2002). Trauma in children: Risk and treatment of psychiatric sequelae. *Biological Psychiatry, 51,* 519–531.

Pitman, R. K., Orr, S. P., Altman, B., Longpre, R. E., Poire, R. E., & Macklin, M. L. (1996). Emotional processing during eye-movement desensitization and reprocessing therapy of Vietnam veterans with chronic posttraumatic stress disorder. *Comprehensive Psychiatry, 37,* 419–429.

Pynoos, R., & Eth, S. (1986). Witness to violence: The child interview. *Journal of the American Academy of Child and Adolescent Psychiatry, 25,* 306–319.

Pynoos, R. S., Frederick, C., Nader, K., Arroyo, W., Steinberg, A., Eth, S., Nunez, F., et al. (1987). Life threat and posttraumatic stress in school-age children. *Archives of General Psychiatry, 44,* 1057–1063.

Pynoos, R. S., Rodriguez, A., Steinberg, A.,Stuber, M., & Frederick, C. J. (1998). *UCLA PTSD Index for DSM-IV.* Unpublished questionnaire, UCLA. Email address: RPynoos@mednet.ucla.edu

Reinherz, H., Giaconia, R. M., Pakiz, B., Silverman, A. B., Frost, A. K., & Lefkowitz, E. S. (1993). Psychosocial risks for major depression in late adolescence: A longitudinal community study. *Journal of the American Academy of Child and Adolescent Psychiatry, 32,* 1155–1163.

Richters, J. E., & Martinez, P. (1990). *Checklist of Child Distress Symptoms: Parent report.* Washington, DC: National Institute of Mental Health.

Richters, J. E., Martinez, P., & Valla, J. P. (1990). Levonn: A cartoon-based interview for assessing children's distress symptoms. Washington, DC: National Institute of Mental Health.

Ryan, G. (1989). Victim to victimizer: Rethinking victim treatment. *Journal of Interpersonal Violence, 4*(3), 325–341.

Saigh, P. (1986). In vitro flooding in the treatment of a 6-yr-old boy's posttraumatic stress disorder. *Behaviour Research and Therapy, 24*(6), 685–688.

Saigh, P. (1988). The validity of the *DSM-III* posttraumatic stress disorder classification as applied to adolescents. *Profess School Psychol, 3*(4), 283–290.

Saigh, P. (1989a). The development and validation of the Children's Posttraumatic Stress Disorder Inventory. *International Journal of Special Education, 4,* 75–84.

Saigh, P. (1989b). The use of an in vitro flooding package in the treatment of traumatized adolescents. *Journal of Developmental and Behavioral Pediatrics, 10*(1), 17–21.

Saigh, P. A., Yule, W., & Inamdar, S. C. (1996). Imaginal flooding of traumatized children and adolescents. *Journal of School Psychology, 34,* 163–183.

Saxe, G. N., Stoddard, F. J., Markey, C., Taft, C., King, D., & King, L. (1997). *The Child Stress Reaction Checklist: A measure of ASD and PTSD in children.* Paper presented at the annual meeting of the International Society for Traumatic Stress Studies, Montreal, Canada.

Scheeringa, M. S., Peebles, C. D., Cook, C. A., & Zeanah, C. H. (2001). Toward establishing procedural, criterion, and discriminate validity for PTSD in early childhood. *Journal of the American Academy of Child and Adolescent Psychiatry, 40*(1), 52–60.

Scheeringa, M. S., Zeanah, C. H., Drell, M. J., & Larrieu, J. A. (1995). Two approaches to the diagnosis of PTSD in infancy and early childhood. *Journal of the American Academy of Child and Adolescent Psychiatry, 34,* 191–200.

Scheeringa, M. S., Zeanah, C. H., Myers, L., & Putnam, F. W. (2003). New findings on alternative criteria for PTSD in preschool children. *Journal of the American Academy of Child and Adolescent Psychiatry, 42,* 561–570.

Schwarz, E. D., & Kowalski, J. M. (1991). Posttraumatic stress disorder after a school shooting: Effects of symptom threshold selection and diagnosis by *DSM-III, DSM-III-R,* or proposed *DSM-IV. American Journal of Psychiatry, 148*(5), 592–597.

Seedat, S., Stein, D. J., Ziervogel, C., Middleton, T., Kammer, D., Emsley, R. A., Rossouw, W. (2002). Comparison of response to a selective serotonin reuptake inhibitor in children, adolescents, and adults with PTSD. *Journal of Child and Adolescent Psychopharmacology, 12,* 37–46.

Shaw, J. A., Applegate, B., Tanner, S., Perez, D., Rothe, E., Campo-Bowen, A. E., & Lahey, B. L. (1995). Psychological effect of Hurricane Andrew on an elementary school population. *Journal of the American Academy of Child and Adolescent Psychiatry, 34*(9), 1185–1192.

Singer, M. I., Anglin, T., Song, L., & Lunghofer, L. (1995). Adolescents' exposure to violence and associated symptoms of psychological trauma. *Journal of the American Medical Association, 273*(6), 477–482.

Spiegel, D. (1984). Multiple personality as a post-traumatic stress disorder. *Psychiatric Clinics of North America, 7,* 101–110.

Stallard, P., & Law, F. (1993). Screening and psychological debriefing of adolescent survivors of life threatening events. *British Journal of Psychiatry, 163,* 660–665.

Steiner, H., Garcia, I. G., & Matthews, Z. (1997). PTSD in incarcerated juvenile delinquents. *Journal of the American Academy of Child and Adolescent Psychiatry, 36,* 357–365.

Stoddard, F. J., Norman, D. K., & Murphy, M. (1989). A diagnostic outcome study of children and adolescents with severe burns. *Journal of Trauma, 29*(4), 471–477.

Stone, M. H. (1990). Abuse and abusiveness in borderline personality disorder. In P. S. Links (Ed.), *Family environment and borderline personality disorder.* Washington, DC: American Psychiatric Press.

Strasburger, L. H., Guthiel, T. G., & Brodsky, A. (1997). On wearing two hats: Role conflict in serving as both psychotherapist and expert witness. *American Journal of Psychiatry, 154*(4), 448–456.

Stuber, M. L., Nader, K., Yasuda, P., Pynoos, R. S., & Cohen, S. (1991). Stress responses after pediatric bone marrow transplantation: Preliminary results of a prospective longitudinal study. *Journal of the American Academy of Child and Adolescent Psychiatry, 30*(6), 952–957.

Sullivan, J. M., & Evans, K. (1994). Integrated treatment for the survivor of childhood trauma who is chemically dependent. *Journal of Psychoactive Drugs, 26*(4), 369–378.

Terr, L. C. (1983). Chowchilla revisited: The effect of psychic trauma four years after a school bus kidnapping. *American Journal of Psychiatry, 140,* 1543–1550.

Trowell, J., Kolvin, I., Weeramanthri, T., Sadowski, H., Berelowitz, M., Glasser, D., & Leitch, I. (2002). Psychotherapy for sexually abused girls: Psychopathological outcome findings and patterns of change. *British Journal of Psychiatry, 160,* 234–247.

Weine, S., Becker, D. F., McGlashan, T. H., Vojvoda, D., Hartman, S., & Robbins,

J. P. (1995). Adolescent survivors of "ethnic cleansing": Observations on the first year in America. *Journal of the American Academy of Child and Adolescent Psychiatry, 34*(9), 1153–1159.

Wolfe, D. A., Sas, L., & Wekerle, C. (1994). Factors associated with the development of posttraumatic stress disorder among child victims of sexual abuse. *Child Abuse and Neglect, 18,* 37–50.

Wozniak, J., Crawford, M., Biederman, J., Faraone, S., Spencer, T., Taylor, A., & Blier, H. (1999). Antecedents and complications of trauma in boys with ADHD: Findings from a longitudinal study. *Journal of the American Academy of Child and Adolescent Psychiatry, 38,* 48–55.

Yehuda, R., & McFarlane, A. C. (1995). Conflict between current knowledge about posttraumatic stress disorder and its original conceptual basis. *American Journal of Psychiatry, 152,* 1705–1713.

Yule, W., & Udwin, O. (1991). Screening child survivors for posttraumatic stress disorder: Experiences from the "Jupiter" sighting. *British Journal of Clinical Psychology, 30,* 131–138.

15

SELECTIVE MUTISM

Abbe M. Garcia, Jennifer B. Freeman,
Greta Francis, Lauren M. Miller,
& Henrietta L. Leonard

D espite having been described in the literature since 1877 (Kussmaul, 1877) and being an established diagnostic category in the current *Diagnostic and Statistical Manual of Mental Disorders: DSM-IV* (American Psychiatric Association [APA], 1994), selective mutism has not been the focus of large-scale empirical study. Rather, with a few recent notable exceptions, the literature on this relatively rare disorder is predominated by case study reports and single-case-design experiments. The evidence that emerged from these sources has led to a recent change in the prevailing view about the etiology of the disorder. Instead of focusing on more psychodynamic factors, the current literature emphasizes biologically mediated temperamental components, which point to selective mutism's relationship to anxiety disorders (Black, 1996; Black & Uhde, 1992; Dow, Sonies, Scheib, Moss, & Leonard, 1995; Leonard & Topol, 1993). In addition to reviewing the basis for this literature, this chapter provides practical guidelines for the assessment and treatment of selective mutism. To the extent possible given the state of the extant literature, the guidelines presented emphasize empirically supported methods of treatment and assessment.

PHENOMENOLOGY

In *DSM-IV*, selective mutism is grouped with the disorders usually first diagnosed in infancy, childhood, or adolescence. Selective mutism is characterized by a consistent failure to speak in one or more social situations in which speech is expected (e.g., school), despite speaking in other situations.

To fully satisfy diagnostic criteria, symptoms must persist for at least 1 month (not limited to the first month in school) and must be severe enough to interfere with educational or occupational achievement. The diagnosis of selective mutism is not appropriate in situations where there is insufficient knowledge of the language, or when the absence of speech is attributable to a communication disorder, pervasive developmental disorder, schizophrenia, or another psychotic disorder. Despite these diagnostic criteria, it is believed that the population of children with selective mutism is heterogeneous (Dow et al., 1995).

The heterogeneity of the population of children with selective mutism is also reflected in the differing opinions about its critical clinical correlates. In addition to not speaking in certain social situations, selectively mute children are also frequently described as shy, inhibited, withdrawn, anxious, and sometimes as passive aggressive, stubborn, disobedient, angry, manipulative, controlling, and oppositional. In the past, these features were considered mutually exclusive, and children were divided into two distinct groups. One group of children was thought to remain mute due to severe anxiety experienced in situations in which speech was expected, and the other group of children was thought to withhold speech in an attempt to manipulate and control others in their environment. Although it is now recognized that these clinical features are not mutually exclusive, the weight of the empirical evidence favors the anxious presentations as the most likely, with oppositional features as secondary if present at all (Black & Uhde, 1992, 1995; Dow et al., 1995; Dummit et al., 1997; Kratochwill, 1981; Leonard & Topol, 1993; Steinhausen & Juzi, 1996; Wright, Cuccaro, Leonhardt, Kendall, & Anderson, 1995). For example, Steinhausen and Juzi (1996) reported that 85% of their sample of selectively mute children were characterized as shy and 66% were described as anxious; in contrast, only 21% were described as oppositional, and only 17% were described as hyperactive. Similarly, Kumpulainen, Rasanen, Raaska, and Somppi (1998) reported that 63% of their selectively mute sample were shy, 63% were withdrawn, and 58% were described as serious by teachers, whereas only 13% were described as aggressive or hyperactive.

Dummit and colleagues (1997) examined the nature of the social avoidance displayed by their patients so that they could evaluate the hypothesis that fear of speaking could account for most, or all, of these children's social discomfort. Their results did not support this hypothesis. Rather, they found that although selectively mute children endorsed severe anxiety associated with speaking, they also endorsed mild to moderate levels of anxiety in social situations that did not require speech (e.g., writing in front of others, being the center of attention, looking people in the eyes, and eating in public). Therefore, it does not appear that the comorbidity between selective mutism and anxiety disorders, particularly social phobia, is an artifact due to overlapping symptoms in the diagnostic system.

Selectively mute children do not categorically refuse to speak in all situations, not even in all social situations. Therefore, it is important to note the situations in which this behavior is most often observed. Across studies, the pattern of situations in which the child is mute is very similar and can generally be captured along several dimensions. Being mute away from home is more likely than being mute at home. School is a very common place for this behavior to occur. Being mute with adults is more likely than with other children, and being mute with unfamiliar nonfamily members is more likely than with familiar family members (Black & Uhde, 1995; Dummit et al., 1997; Kumpulainen et al., 1998; Steinhausen & Juzi, 1996). Children whose mutism departs radically from this pattern (e.g., will not speak in any situation, or will not speak at home while speaking in other situations) may be suffering from a wholly different type of problem than the children described here.

Selective mutism has been reported in less than 1% of individuals seeking treatment, but little systematic research has been done to support this estimate (APA, 1994). Most studies find that selective mutism is slightly more prevalent in females than males, with estimates ranging from 2.6:1 to 1.5:1, females to males (Dummit et al., 1997; Kopp & Gillberg, 1997; Kristensen, 2000; Kumpulainen et al., 1998; Steinhausen & Juzi, 1996). The two most frequently cited community-based epidemiological studies reported fairly similar overall prevalence rates when equally stringent criteria were employed: 0.08% in a survey of 7-year-olds in Newcastle, England (Fundudis, Kolvin, & Garside, 1979), and 0.03% among 5- and 6-year-olds in Birmingham, England (Brown & Lloyd, 1975). However, the Brown and Lloyd study reported a much higher prevalence of 0.72% based on data obtained after only 8 weeks of school (when the children were 4–5 years of age). More recently, two studies from Scandinavia reported higher prevalence rates among slightly older populations of children: 2% (38 in 2,010) among second-graders in Finland (Kumpulainen et al., 1998), and .18% (5 in 2,793) among school-aged children (ages 7–15) in Sweden (Kopp & Gillberg, 1997).

The data for the Finnish study were collected by surveying teachers of all second-graders in the county. To confirm the diagnosis, school nurses checked the information provided by teachers against the *DSM-III-R* criteria. The authors acknowledge that the rates were closer to those reported in previous studies if only children who refused to speak to anybody at school were included (0.4%, or 8 in 2,010), or if only those children who had been referred for treatment were included (0.7%, or 16 in 2,010).

The data for the Swedish study were collected by questionnaire and follow-up interview with teachers of grades 1 through 8 in a school district in West Central Götenberg, Sweden. The five children diagnosed with selective mutism in this study ranged from 9 to 13 years of age. All five of these children had been completely silent in school since school entry, which amounted to 2 or more years for all five children. Thus, prevalence estimates range from .03% to 2%. The variability in these estimates may be a function of the age of the children sampled, differences in the application of the diagnostic criteria, or vagueness of the *DSM* criteria in terms of the degree of impairment required for this diagnosis.

DEVELOPMENTAL COURSE

Onset is often insidious, with parents reporting that the child has always been this way (Leonard & Topol, 1993). The diagnosis is frequently not made until the child enters school. Recent research provides a range for documented age of onset from 2.7 years to 4.1 years (Black & Uhde, 1995; Dummit et al., 1997; Kristensen, 2000; Steinhausen & Juzi, 1996). Typical duration is several months, but the symptoms may persist for several years (APA, 1994). Although speech inhibition may accompany social anxiety in both children and adults, it is less common to find persistent, severe selective mutism in an adult. Some authors have reasoned that this difference between child and adult presentation is attributable to the fact that adults are more able to control their environments and to avoid situations in which they are likely to be called on to speak (Black & Uhde, 1992).

DIAGNOSIS AND CLASSIFICATION

Speech inhibition can be a secondary symptom of many other psychiatric disorders, including pervasive developmental disorder, schizophrenia, and severe mental retardation. The differential diagnosis for selective mutism is broad. In addition, speech and language deficits can cause speech inhibition (Lerea & Ward, 1965), but presence of a speech and language disorder should not automatically be considered grounds to rule out the presence of selective mutism (APA, 1994). To aid in this decision, speech disturbances in pure communication disorders are generally not restricted to specific social situations, whereas in selective mutism they are, and they tend to follow the situational pattern described in the previous section of this chapter. Similarly, for the other psychiatric disorders in which speech inhibition may be a secondary symptom, speech inhibition is likely to be more pervasive across situations, or the pattern of situations in which speech is restricted is likely to differ from that reviewed above.

Several studies have looked at rates of comorbidity between selective mutism and other disorders. Three studies have reported high rates of comorbidity with anxiety disorders, including social phobia, avoidant disorder, and separation anxiety disorder—with 74% to 100% of samples with selective mutism meeting criteria for an anxiety disorder (Black & Uhde, 1995; Dummit et al., 1997; Kristensen, 2000). A high rate of affected first-degree relatives may also suggest an association between selective mutism and anxiety disorders. In one study, 70% of cases had a first-degree relative with social phobia or avoidant disorder, and 37% had a first-degree relative with selective mutism (Black & Uhde, 1995). In contrast, the rates of externalizing disorders, particularly oppositional defiant disorder, were very low; for example, 1 in 50 (Dummit et al., 1997) and 3 in 30 (Black & Uhde, 1995). However, elimination disorders appear to occur more frequently among children with selective mutism than in the general population (Kristensen, 2000; Steinhausen & Juzi, 1996).

There is mixed evidence about the association between developmental delays (particularly speech and language delays) and selective mutism. Although some studies have reported no evidence of difficulties with speech and language functioning (Black & Uhde, 1995), others have reported that rates of language disorder or delays range from 11% to 65% in this population (Dummit et al., 1997; Kristensen, 1997, 2000; Kumpulainen et al., 1998; Steinhausen & Juzi, 1996). Steinhausen and Juzi characterized the nature of the speech and language problems in their sample and reported that articulation and expressive language disorders were more common than receptive language problems or stuttering. In terms of other types of delays, rates of motor delays have been reported to range from 18% to 65% (Kristensen, 1997).

The association between selective mutism and autistic spectrum disorders is controversial because of differing interpretations of the *DSM-IV* diagnostic criteria. By *DSM-IV* criteria, selective mutism must not occur exclusively during the course of a pervasive developmental disorder (APA, 1994). Some researchers have interpreted this statement to mean that one cannot diagnose selective mutism in a child with a pervasive developmental disorder, but others have argued that, to the extent that being selectively mute can be an essential feature of a child's presentation which would not necessarily be captured by a developmental disorder (e.g., Asperger's disorder), one should be able to assign both diagnoses when warranted. On the basis of the latter belief, some research groups have examined the rates of comorbidity between selective mutism and Asperger's disorder. In one study, 7.4% of the sample with selective mutism met criteria for Asperger's disorder (Kristensen, 2000), and in another study, one of five children with selective mutism met all but one of the criteria for Asperger's disorder (Kopp & Gillberg, 1997). Some of these developmental delays may be attributable to pregnancy, labor/delivery, and neonatal complications. Steinhausen and Juzi (1996) reported that 33% of their sample had been exposed to at least one risk factor during pregnancy; 43% had complicated deliveries, and 20% had at least one complication during the neonatal period.

The relationship of early traumatic experiences to selective mutism has also been the topic of some debate. Although there is clear evidence that children may react to a traumatic situation or event in their lives by becoming mute, there is little evidence to support the claim that traumatic events are a common cause of selective mutism per se (Black & Uhde, 1995; Dummit et al., 1997; Kopp & Gillberg, 1997; Kumpulainen et al., 1998).

Some researchers have suggested that selective mutism should not continue to be a separate diagnostic category. Some of them believe that it is a symptom, or subtype, of social phobia (Anstendig, 1999; Black & Uhde, 1992, 1995; Dow et al., 1995; Dummit et al., 1997; Leonard & Topol, 1993), but others take broader views. Steinhausen and Juzi (1996) suggest that the anxious features of selectively mute children are not only indicative of social phobia but may also represent a more general personality feature, such as shyness. Alternatively, Kristensen (2000) hypothesized that, although selective mutism may be regarded as a symptom of anxiety, the cause of the anxiety may include underlying neurodevelopmental vulnerabilities that might be ignored if selectively mute children were simply lumped in with all other children with an anxiety disorder. Regardless of selective mutism's official classification in the *DSM*, conceptualizing selective mutism as being associated with anxiety should be beneficial for the treatment of these children. This point is borne out in the review of treatment outcome results later in the chapter.

ASSESSMENT

When a diagnosis of selective mutism is considered, a comprehensive evaluation is critical to rule out other explanations for the mutism, to assess comorbid factors, and to plan an individualized treatment approach. The assessment process with a selectively mute child is challenging, because in most cases selectively mute children will not speak to clinicians. Therefore, parents' reports become particularly important. However, there are still important parts of the evaluation that should be conducted directly with the child.

Parent Reports

A thorough interview with parents should assess the symptom history—in particular, onset (sudden or insidious) and patterns of mute behavior (with whom, in what situations). The selective mutism section of the Anxiety Disorders Interview Schedule for Children and Parents (ADIS-C/P; Silverman & Albano, 1996) provides a structure for asking about this information.

Patterns of behavior that are not characteristic of selective mutism, such as not talking to immediate family members, abrupt cessation of speech in one environment, or absence of speech in all settings, raise concerns about other neurological or psychiatric problems (e.g., autism, speech and language disabilities, aphasia, trauma). History should also be taken regarding developmental insults, developmental delays, neuropsychological deficits, and atypical speech and language difficulties (e.g., problems with prosody), which could be suggestive of a developmental disorder (e.g., Asperger's disorder, mental retardation), a right-hemisphere deficit, or social-emotional learning disability, rather than selective mutism. A structured diagnostic interview, such as the NIMH Diagnostic Interview Schedule for Children–Parent version 2.3 (DISC 2.3; Shaffer et al., 1996), or the Schedule for Affective Disorders and Schizophrenia for School-Age Children, Present Episode and Lifetime versions (K-SADS-PL; Kaufman et al., 1997) can be helpful in assessing for other comorbid psychiatric problems.

Also of interest is the degree to which the child is verbally and nonverbally inhibited. Some selectively mute children are shy and anxious in unfamiliar environments, whereas others will engage socially in some way even if they will not speak (e.g., nodding, smiling). Targeted questions about the child's verbal and nonverbal interactions, relationships with friends, and anxiety in social situations can be revealing. The child's social interaction outside school, such as in a restaurant or on the telephone, should also be explored. The social phobia section of the ADIS-C/P is recommended as a structured way to inquire about this information.

Academic ability should also be discussed. Because it is difficult to evaluate children with selective mutism via traditional testing, subtle learning disabilities may be overlooked. Parent and teacher comments, academic reports, and standardized testing results can all be helpful in evaluating the child's skills and determining whether further testing is indicated.

Evaluation of speech and language ability is essential; this is often coordinated with the pediatrician. Factors that might have influenced a child's language development, such as a parent with identified speech and language problems or a lack of adequate exposure to the language (as in some bilingual homes), should be considered. Inadequate or confusing language exposure may result in expressive problems, and additional practice may be necessary for the child to function at normal levels. Other questions should focus on the child's ability to communicate his or her needs, both verbally and nonverbally. Descriptions of the complexity and quality of language (e.g., mean length of utterance, range of vocabulary, use of difficult verb tenses and complicated grammar) can help in evaluation of expressive language ability. Pragmatic language abilities, such as turn-taking in conversation and understanding nonverbal communicative cues, should also be explored. Other questions might focus on the child's speech production (voice, fluency, resonance, rate, and rhythm), to identify phonological problems. Given the low probability that a child with selective mutism will speak to the clinician during the evaluation, it can also be helpful to have a parent provide an audiotape of the child speaking at home, because few of the just-mentioned attributes may be directly observable during the evaluation. If problems with any of these attributes of speech and language are suspected after the parent interview, referral to a speech and language pathologist who can more fully assess these problems is recommended.

Reviewing the child's medical history is essential, because physical problems may underlie the child's mutism. Neurological injury or delay can result in speech and language problems or social skills deficits, both of which can exacerbate speech inhibition. Hearing evaluation should also be considered (particularly if the child has a history of frequent ear infections), because hearing problems are sometimes associated with learning and language delays.

Gathering a complete family history of any psychiatric or medical diagnoses, including response to treatment, can be helpful. Family history of selective mutism, extreme shyness, or anxiety disorders (social phobia, panic disorder, obsessive-compulsive disorder) may put the child at risk for developing similar problems.

Child Reports

Although children with selective mutism are unlikely to speak to the clinician during an evaluation, meeting with the child remains a crucial part of the assessment, because it allows the clinician to directly observe the severity and nature of the child's mutism. Other forms of nonverbal communication (e.g., playing, drawing) may be used to assess anxiety or shyness in social situations. Some selectively mute children will avoid eye contact and withdraw from social situations, whereas others are more interactive and will smile, giggle, and nod answers to questions even if they will not speak. Paper-and-pencil self-report questionnaires may also be effective for assessing how engageable the child is, as well as for information about general levels of anxiety and other psychiatric symptoms (e.g., Children's Depression Inventory [CDI]; Kovacs, 1992; Multidimensional Anxiety Scale for Children [MASC]; March, 1997).

Oral and sensory motor abilities should be evaluated, with particular note to any orofacial abnormalities that might interfere with articulation. Neurological difficulties, as evidenced by drooling, grimacing, muscular asymmetry, tongue and lip weakness, abnormal gag reflex, impaired sucking or swallowing, or strong preference for a certain texture of food, can be relevant because they may impede the movements necessary for normal speech. Auditory screening, and further evaluation if indicated, should be completed to ensure that hearing difficulties are not contributing to the mutism. General auditory tests of peripheral sensitivity (using both pure-tone and speech stimuli) are usually adequate to detect problems. In addition, tympanometry and acoustic reflex testing can be used to assess middle ear function, if further assessment is required.

TREATMENT

Psychosocial Treatment: Behavioral Treatment

The empirical literature on behavioral treatment of selective mutism is very limited. A number of reviews of the treatment literature have found numerous uncontrolled case reports, a few single-case experimental designs, and only one controlled group study using a very small sample (Anstendig, 1998; Cunningham, Cataldo, Mallion, & Keyes, 1984; Labbe & Williamson, 1984). Thus, no definitive conclusions can be made about the efficacy of behavioral treatment for selective mutism at this time. Strategies that have been studied include contingency management, exposure-based techniques, and self-modeling. These treatment techniques are discussed and illustrated below.

CONTINGENCY MANAGEMENT STRATEGIES   Contingency management involves strategies based on operant learning principles. Positive and negative consequences are added or taken away to increase the frequency of speech and decrease the frequency of failing to speak. The child may be rewarded for speaking, or reinforcement may be withheld when the child does not speak. An aversive consequence may be taken away when the child speaks or added when the child does not speak. Often, shaping is used to help the child move from silence to speaking in an audible voice. For example, reinforcement first might be used to reward whispering, as a step toward audible speech. Stimulus-fading strategies also are used, with aspects of the environment in which speech occurs changed gradually to promote generalization of speech. For example, the child may be rewarded for speaking with the therapist in a treatment session and then be rewarded for speaking with the same therapist at school. Alternatively, new people might be introduced gradually into a setting where speech already occurs.

Contingency management strategies have received the most empirical attention. As reviewed by Cunningham and colleagues (1984), the six controlled single-case-design studies and one group study available in the literature all evaluated the use of reinforcement, with and without stimulus fading. The authors noted that treatment selection appeared to be related to rate of baseline speech. That is, reinforcement alone was selected more often for children with limited speech at baseline, whereas reinforcement plus stimulus fading was chosen more often for children without baseline speech.

Reinforcement has been used to establish or increase the frequency of speech. Shaping often is used to increase the length or complexity of spoken communication. Although speech is reinforced, nonverbal communication may be ignored systematically (with the goal of extinguishing the response due to lack of reinforcement) or reinforced initially as a gradual approximation of speech (as part of a shaping protocol).

The use of negative or aversive consequences is another form of contingency management. The child with selective mutism is told that he or she can avoid an aversive consequence by speaking. Negative consequences are administered, contingent on refusal or failure to speak. Strategies such as time-out (removal of positive attention and reinforcement), response cost (loss of reinforcement previously earned for speaking), punishment (e.g., after-school detention), or overcorrection (addition of unpleasant expectation, such as repeated writing of words that the child refused to speak) have been used (e.g., Griffith, Schnelle, McNees, Bissinger, & Huff, 1975; Krohn, Weckstein, & Wright, 1992; Matson, Esveldt-Dawson, & O'Donnell, 1979; Wulbert, Nyman, Snow, & Owen, 1977). The goal of these strategies is to teach the child to speak in order to avoid an aversive consequence. But reliance on aversive strategies alone to treat selective mutism has been criticized as ineffective (Crema & Kerr, 1978).

A good example of the use of contingency management was provided by Griffith and colleagues (1975). These authors conducted a multiple-baseline-across-settings design to study the use of reinforcement and response cost to treat a 6-year-old boy with selective mutism who did not speak to peers in school. Prompted and spontaneous speech directed to peers were recorded at baseline and throughout treatment. Treatment consisted of a token program in which the child earned points every time he spoke to a peer. For every 10 points earned, the child received 15 minutes of free time during a homeroom period later in the day. Treatment was conducted sequentially in 3 different settings: reading class, homeroom class, gym class.

After 3 weeks of baseline recordings, the reinforcement program was started in reading class. An increased frequency of prompted and spontaneous speech during reading class was seen over the course of the treatment phase. The treatment then was implemented in homeroom class; however, no increase in the frequency of speech was observed. Thus, a response-cost procedure was added in which the child lost 10 points if he didn't speak at least five times in class each day. Again, an increased frequency of speech was recorded. Similar to the homeroom phase, the reinforcement plan was started in gym class and then response cost was added due to lack of response to reinforcement alone. Rates of prompted and spontaneous speech increased in gym class with the combination of reinforcement and response cost. At follow-up 3 months later when the child entered second grade, gains were maintained and he was reported to be functioning well in a regular second-grade class.

Cunningham and colleagues (1984) provided a nicely done single-case design evaluating the use of contingency management (i.e., reinforcement) plus stimulus fading. These authors treated a 15-year-old boy with below-average intellectual functioning who had been selectively mute in school since age 5. He was treated on an inpatient unit. The adolescent refused to speak on the unit but communicated by gestures and written notes.

During the first phase of treatment, the adolescent was reinforced gradually for imitation of facial gestures, mouthing answers, and then whispering. The second phase of treatment consisted of a stimulus fading procedure in which new people were added into treatment sessions. These new people gradually moved closer to the adolescent and began to ask questions. The location of treatment sessions also was changed, and the criterion for reinforcement was changed from prompted speech to spontaneous speech. During the third phase of treatment, generalization was targeted by having the adolescent gather signatures from people with whom he spoke in a whisper or normal voice. The signatures were traded for reinforcers, and the criterion for reinforcement changed over time from number of signatures to number of different signatures, to increase his sphere of interactions. In the fourth and final phase of treatment, prompting, fading, and reinforcement of successive approximations were used to establish speech of a normal conversational volume.

Phase 4 was evaluated using a combination reversal design with probes on untreated baselines. Baselines included word modeling, picture naming, reading aloud, and free conversation. Results indicated that the adolescent began to use a normal voice volume on the word-modeling task once reinforcement was introduced. This appeared to generalize to other non-reinforced tasks, such as picture naming and oral reading.

The use of reinforcement alone was examined by Calhoun and Koenig (1973) in the only group study of the treatment of selective mutism. Participants were eight children in kindergarten through third grade who had been diagnosed with selective mutism due to low rates of verbal behavior in school. These students were randomly assigned to a treatment or no-treatment control condition. The treatment condition involved rewards contingent on talk directed to the teacher. Rewards were administered by the teacher and typically involved the whole class's receiving the reward. During four different baseline monitoring periods before and after treatment, all talk to adults was recorded, and the total number of words was calculated. Treatment was implemented over a 5-week period. Results indicated that children in the treatment condition showed significantly more talk to adults from baseline to posttreatment, as compared with children in the control condition. At 1-year follow-up, there was no longer a significant difference in rates of talk to adults between the two groups. However, this appears to be due to increased variability within the groups. In looking at the follow-up data, all of the children in the treated group were talking more than 50 words per monitoring period (two were in the 50-to-60 word range and two were in the 120-to-130 range). In contrast, none of the children in the control group were talking more than 40 words per monitoring period (all were in the 20-to-40 word range).

EXPOSURE-BASED STRATEGIES   Exposure-based strategies are based on classical conditioning principles. The child with selective mutism is thought to remain silent as a way of reducing or avoiding anxiety. Desensitization may be used, in which the child is taught to use an anxiety-incompatible strategy (e.g., muscle relaxation, diaphragmatic breathing, presence of a familiar and trusted adult) in response to gradually more anxiety-provoking situations. A hierarchy of situations involving the need to speak is identified and then ordered from least to most anxiety provoking. The child then works his or her way up the hierarchy in a sequential fashion. For example, the child might be cued to relax first in a mildly anxiety-provoking situation (e.g., whispering to the parent in front of the therapist) before moving to a slightly more anxiety-provoking situation (e.g., talking in an audible voice to the parent in front of the therapist).

Given that selective mutism can be related to severe anxiety, the use of exposure-based treatment has been suggested. The goal of such treatment is to pair mildly anxiety-provoking stimuli with anxiety-incompatible strategies in a gradual fashion so that the child's anxiety is reduced with repeated pairings. Typically, the presence of a familiar and trusted adult has been used as the anxiety-incompatible strategy in these treatment studies. Stimulus fading, in which a trusted adult to whom the child speaks accompanies the child into new situations, has been viewed by some as a variant of in-vivo desensitization (Cunningham et al., 1984). In addition to case reports of the use of systematic desensitization (e.g., Croghan & Craven, 1982; Rye & Ullman, 1999; Scott, 1977), a few single case designs have reported positive results for the use of stimulus fading with or without reinforcement (e.g., Cunningham et al., 1984; Sanok & Striefel, 1979; Wulbert et al., 1977).

Rye and Ullman (1999) presented a detailed case report of the use of systematic desensitization to treat a 13-year-old boy with selective mutism who had not spoken in school for about 7 years. The adolescent was described as having symptoms of anxiety related to speaking, including worry about rejection by classmates. He stayed quiet and avoided school situations in which there was a requirement to talk. His teachers eventually stopped asking him to talk. The authors noted that his silence in school had been negatively reinforced over the course of many years.

The following assessments were conducted throughout the course of treatment: self-reported anxiety during exposure tasks, frequency of speech in school, school attendance, and involvement in extracurricular activities. Treatment sessions were held over an 18-month period, and these included close collaboration with school personnel. Systematic desensitization was used, both imaginal and in vivo, and presence of the therapist served as the primary anxiety-incompatible strategy. The anxiety hierarchy contained items such as imagining speaking in school, having a therapy session on school grounds during school hours, having a teacher listen to an audiotape of the adolescent speaking, and having a conversation with a favorite teacher. Over the course of treatment sessions, baseline rates of high self-reported anxiety in response to these hierarchy items diminished and, in most cases, disappeared. Stimulus-fading procedures also were used in which new settings were introduced (started in the therapist's office and then moved to school) and new people (teachers, classmates) were brought into treatment sessions.

In addition to decreases in self-reported anxiety during treatment sessions, modest gains were made in other assessed areas. The adolescent's rate of speech in school increased to the point that he was having conversations with classmates or teachers about six times per week. Absenteeism also improved, from 23 days absent per school year prior to treatment, to 15 days absent per school year during the course of treatment, to 7 days absent per school year in the year posttreatment. The adolescent also tried out for and made a school sports team. One-year follow-up information was collected from his high school teachers, because he had graduated from junior high school. His high school teachers reported that his rate of speech was similar to that of classmates. He continued to participate in a school sport and had average attendance. The adolescent reported that he no longer felt anxious about speaking at school. Despite the absence of an experimental design, this study is an excellent illustration of a detailed and comprehensive systematic desensitization treatment of an adolescent with chronic selective mutism.

SELF-MODELING   Self-modeling is based on principles of social learning theory (i.e., observational learning). The child with selective mutism learns to demonstrate verbal behavior by watching verbal behavior displayed and reinforced. Using self-modeling, the child typically watches a videotape or listens to an audiotape of himself or herself speaking in target situations (i.e., answering a teacher's question, talking with a peer in school).

A small number of studies have evaluated the use of videotaped self-modeling to treat selective mutism (Holmbeck & Lavigne, 1992; Kehle, Owens, & Cressy, 1990; Pigott & Gonzales, 1987). One study also described the use of audiotaped self-modeling (Blum et al., 1998). The general procedure is to have the child with selective mutism videotaped while talking with a parent and then to edit the tape so that it appears as though the child is talking with the teacher. The child then views the tape and watches himself or herself modeling verbal behavior.

Pigott and Gonzales (1987) completed a multiple-baseline-across-behaviors design with a 9-year-old third-grader who had been selectively mute in school since kindergarten. Baseline data were collected by observing the child twice weekly during a reading group. Frequency counts were made of the following: number of times the child was asked a question by the teacher, number of times the child answered a question within 4 seconds in a voice loud enough for the teacher to hear, and number of times the child raised his hand to answer a question that the teacher asked of the class as a whole. Two self-modeling tapes were used, one for answering questions and another for volunteering to answer questions. Following completion of two 3-week self-modeling phases, a 3-week self-monitoring plus reinforcement phase was implemented in which the child recorded every time he volunteered to answer questions and then earned points for each day that he volunteered at least six times, with points accumulating toward a reinforcer at home (i.e., trip to amusement park).

The videotape was made while having the child raise his hand and answer questions in scenes with classmates, with his mother and brother in his line of sight but not on camera. Two short videotapes were then edited so that the child could watch himself answering questions from the teacher (Tape 1) and volunteering to answer the teacher's questions (Tape 2). On both tapes, the child also saw himself being praised by the teacher for speaking. Parents were instructed to have the child watch the tapes before school each day and to praise him for doing well on the tapes.

Interobserver reliability was calculated and found to be good. Results indicated that viewing of the self-modeling videotape for answering questions increased the child's average percentage of responding to questions from 0% during baseline to 80% following the intervention. Viewing of the self-modeling videotape for volunteering to answer questions, though it initially appeared to produce an increase in volunteering, was not effective. The child's rate of volunteering following the intervention was identical to that during baseline (0%). In contrast, the addition of self-monitoring and reinforcement for volunteering was related to an increase in volunteering from 0% at baseline to an average of 6% during the intervention. Of note, the authors also collected data from two skilled peers in order to assess the social validity of their treatment results. The treated child's rate of answering questions and volunteering approximated that of his skilled classmates.

SUMMARY   Although no definitive statements can be made regarding the efficacy of behavioral treatment for selective mutism, preliminary evidence is available for its use. The current literature suggests that contingency management, particularly reinforcement, merits systematic study and may prove to be an effective strategy. There also is some support for the use of response-cost, stimulus-fading, desensitization, and self-modeling procedures as adjuncts to reinforcement programs.

Psychosocial Treatment: Other Psychotherapeutic Modalities

Psychodynamic psychotherapy and family therapy are two other treatment modalities that have been applied to selective mutism. However, both literatures rely heavily on retrospective case study reports, which limit systematic evaluation of treatment outcome. In addition, information about the child's mutism as well as information about the specific intervention techniques employed are frequently omitted, thus making it difficult to generalize the use of these treatment modalities to other children with selective mutism.

In the largest published studies of psychodynamic psychotherapy for selective mutism, Browne, Wilson, and Laybourne (1963) and Wergeland (1979) concluded that the treatment was lengthy and the outcome poor. Therefore, there is no empiric evidence to suggest that dynamic psychotherapy is effective, and there is some evidence to suggest that it is not effective, for treatment of the primary symptoms of selective mutism.

Children with selective mutism, particularly when they are young, are embedded in a family context. Often the family's perception of the symptoms needs to be assessed. Behavioral family treatment to target family issues, or specifically to help implement the behavioral plan for the mutism, is sometimes required.

Psychopharmacological Treatment

The evidence-based treatment literature on pharmacotherapy for the treatment of selective mutism is limited at this point, although medications are frequently used and interest in this intervention is increasing. In general, a behavioral treatment plan should be initiated first. If the child does not make sufficient progress, then adjunctive medication with ongoing behavioral treatment is considered. At present, the majority of the work in the area has been single-case studies initially focusing on monoamine oxidase inhibitors, or MAOIs, and then the use of selective serotonin reuptake inhibitors, or SSRIs (Black & Uhde, 1992; Carlson, Kratochwill, & Johnston, 1999; Golwyn & Sevlie, 1999; Golwyn & Weinstock, 1990; Harvey & Milne, 1998; Thomsen, Rasmussen, & Andersson, 1999; Wright et al., 1995).

With regard to more systematic studies, there is one open treatment trial (Dummit, Klein, Tancer, Asche, & Martin, 1996) and one small, double-blind, placebo-controlled trial (Black & Uhde, 1994), both with fluoxetine. Responses of selectively mute children to pharmacologic agents for social phobia continue to raise discussions concerning the nosologic relationship of selective mutism to social phobia and other anxiety disorders. Of important note, similar treatment response does not allow conclusions about underlying mechanisms of pathophysiology or diagnoses.

There are a handful of case reports describing a positive response to either phenelzine or an SSRI. Golwyn and Sevlie (1999) reported four children, 5 to 7 years of age, who were successfully treated with phenelzine, an MAOI. Although no hypertensive or serotonin syndromes occurred in those children, it would be very unusual to use an MAOI in children, and one would certainly not start there. There are case reports of the SSRIs being successfully used in children with selective mutism. Fluoxetine, citalopram, and sertraline have all been anecdotally reported to be useful in a case (Carlson et al., 1999; Harvey & Milne, 1998; Thomsen et al., 1999). There are no reported studies using a benzodiazepine or buspirone.

Clearly, the largest literature is on the use of the SSRIs. Dummit and colleagues (1996) studied 21 children ages 5 to 14 with selective mutism, all of whom also had a comorbid anxiety disorder. Of note is that all children had had a minimum of 4 weeks of behavioral psychotherapy prior to consideration for the drug trial. Children who showed clear trends toward clinical improvement during behavioral treatment were to be excluded from participation in the fluoxetine trial, although there were none who improved in this pretreatment. This open treatment study used fluoxetine in graduated doses (range, 10 to 60 mg) for 9 weeks. (A gradual titration increase started with 1.25 mg/day for the first week, 2.5 mg/day for the second week, 5 mg/day in Week 3, and 10 mg/day in Week 4.) The mean dose at end of treatment was 28.1 mg (1.1 mg/kg of body weight per day), with two children at 60 mg, four at 40 mg, and 15 at 20 mg/day. Two children developed behavioral disinhibition and were dropped from the study. Of 21 children, 76% demonstrated clinical improvement (defined by dichotomized clinical global improvement [CGI] scores) after 9 weeks of treatment. Post hoc regression analysis showed an inverse relationship between age and overall improvement (accounting for 14% of the variance), with younger children showing better response. All measures indicated marked improvement in children's symptoms for the group, although 5 of the 21 did not reach *improved* status (CGI of 3 or less) at the end point of their treatment. The authors also noted that, even in children who showed marked treatment response, complete remission of symptoms often required more than the 9-week trial.

Black and Uhde (1994) treated 16 children with selective mutism with placebo (single blind) for 2 weeks. Fifteen placebo nonresponders were then randomly assigned to double-blind treatment with fluoxetine (targeting 0.6 mg/kg per day; $n = 6$) or continued placebo ($n = 9$) for 12 weeks.

Initial dose was 0.2 mg per kilogram per day and was titrated up to 0.6 mg per kilogram per day. The mean maximum dose of fluoxetine was 21.4 mg/day (range 12 to 27 mg/day, 0.60 to 0.62 mg/kg per day). All 15 subjects entering the double-blind assignment completed the 12 weeks. Side effects were noted to be minimal. Participants treated with fluoxetine were significantly more improved than placebo-treated participants on parent's rating of mutism change and global change. However, clinician and teacher ratings did not reveal significant differences between treatment groups, and this may be due in part to the small number of patients and the more severe baseline symptoms of the fluoxetine-treated group. Overall, the authors felt that despite some improvements, participants in both treatment groups remained very symptomatic at the end of the study. Although a small study and of short duration, this was a double-blind design and provides information for designing larger systematic studies.

Carlson and colleagues (1999) reported on five children with selective mutism who were treated with a single-case research trial with a double-blind placebo-controlled trial of sertraline in a replicated multiple-baseline-across-participants design ($n = 2$; $n = 3$) over 16 weeks. Assessment measures failed to demonstrate group changes in mutism, anxiousness, and shyness, although all individuals realized considerable improvement on some of these variables. Two (of five) participants did not meet criteria for selective mutism after 10 weeks of 100 mg of sertraline daily. A third person was asymptomatic at 20 weeks poststudy. All parents chose to continue their child on sertraline 100 mg daily at the end of the study and for an indefinite period of time. Although one cannot conclude from this study design that sertraline is effective for selective mutism, it provides several interesting leads for further research. The authors noted that the multitude of data collected from this study indicated a ladderlike nature to selective mutism, similar to hierarchical structures developed for anxious conditions such as fear of flying.

Despite the limited data on the pharmacotherapy of selective mutism, the disorder is often treated pharmacologically as if it were an anxiety disorder. Whether selective mutism is conceptualized as a childhood form of social phobia, another anxiety disorder, or an obsessive-compulsive spectrum disorder, the SSRIs would be the most likely initial agent to consider, of the different medication options. The SSRIs in general offer a more tolerable side effect profile than the tricyclic antidepressants. Phenelzine (a monoamine oxidase inhibitor), which requires dietary restrictions and concern about hypertensive crisis, would rarely, if ever, be used in children. The choice of a medication in the SSRI family would be based on systematic efficacy studies of SSRIs in adults with social anxiety (e.g., paroxetine) and the most recent controlled trial of fluvoxamine in the successful treatment of social phobia, separation anxiety, or generalized anxiety disorder in children and adolescents (Walkup et al., 2001). The largest body of safety and efficacy evidence for the use of SSRIs in children comes from the pediatric obsessive-compulsive disorder (OCD) treatment literature (March et al., 1998; Riddle et al., 2001) and depression treatment literature (Emslie et al., 1997; Keller et al., 2001).

Our clinical experience in treating children with selective mutism indicates that intervention at a young age prognosticates a better outcome. Supporting this anecdotal impression was the finding by Dummit and colleagues (1996), that improvement at Week 9 was inversely correlated with age, suggesting that it is harder to successfully treat the child who has been symptomatic for a long time (Black & Uhde, 1994; Dummit et al., 1996).

Another general clinical impression is that the more anxious and inhibited children with selective mutism tend to respond better to SSRI agents than do the less anxious children. Clearly, as the subtypes of this diagnosis are better studied, it will become clear as to whether this distinction is meaningful. The child with selective mutism may take longer to respond to pharmacotherapeutic interventions, usually 12 to 16 weeks, than children with other disorders such as anxiety, and this merits systematic study. Benzodiazepines are sometimes used for those children with high anticipatory anxiety, but in general, the symptoms in selective mutism are seen in so many situations that an SSRI is more appropriate. Benzodiazepines might be used as an augmenting agent to an SSRI, if there were specific settings for anticipatory anxiety.

In summary, we concur with others (Black & Uhde, 1994; Dummit et al., 1996) that a trial of an SSRI should be considered when the symptoms of selective mutism are of long duration or cause significant impairment, or if other treatments have been unsuccessful. Pharmacotherapy should not be used as the *only* treatment intervention for selective mutism but has been used adjunctively with the behavioral treatments. Pharmacotherapy might be utilized sooner in the treatment plan, if the child has other comorbid issues which are being targeted. Further research, specifically controlled studies with long-term outcome evaluations, are required to answer these questions, but preliminary evidence is promising.

Combined Treatments

Wright and colleagues (1995) described the successful treatment of selective mutism in a preschool-age child using a multifaceted treatment approach. The intervention included fluoxetine as well as family therapy, behavioral therapy, and play therapy. According to the authors, the components of the intervention reflect a conceptualization of selective mutism that views anxiety as a key feature but also focuses on associated features, particularly oppositional behaviors. Although this study has all of the limitations associated with a single-case design, it is included as an example of the comprehensive treatment approach that is often necessary for most children with selective mutism.

Intuitively, a combined multimodal treatment approach has clinical appeal, particularly in the treatment-refractory case or with an older child.

Unfortunately, the limited number of systematic studies of psychosocial or pharmacologic treatments leaves the field with a paucity of evidence-based intervention. Certainly, combined treatments are often required for the child with a more severe symptom picture or with multiple comorbidities.

STAGES OF TREATMENT

In an attempt to operationalize the usual practice of experts in the area, the details of common practice are provided in Figure 15.1. In general, CBT is the first-line treatment for children with selective mutism. However, treatment decisions are also based on level of functional impairment, age of the child, and any comorbidity. Medication, in combination with CBT, may sometimes be indicated in the initial treatment approach for older children (over 8 years old) with more severe selective mutism or other comorbid symptoms. Based on the studies reviewed above, partial response to pharmacotherapy alone is likely (Black & Uhde, 1994; Carlson et al., 1999), and this is one basis for the recommendation that pharmacotherapy should not be used as a single first-line treatment.

What to do with a partial response? If a partial response is achieved after an adequate trial of CBT, medication may be indicated for further resolution of symptoms. If no response is achieved after an adequate trial of CBT, medication and a change in psychotherapy approach may be indicated. If a partial response is achieved after an adequate trial of combined treatment (CBT plus medication), a change in medication, a modification of psychotherapy approach, or both may be helpful. In general, if someone were a partial or nonresponder to an SSRI, another SSRI would be tried. Alternatively, augmentation with a benzodiazepine could be tried, depending on the extent of anticipatory anxiety and the comorbidity. If no improvement is seen after an adequate trial of combined treatment, augmentation with another medication—in addition to modification of psychotherapy approach, change in medication, or both—may be considered. Particularly for medication refractory cases, clomipramine might be tried next (on the basis of extrapolations from the OCD treatment models), although there is no specific evidence that it may be more effective than an SSRI.

In terms of maintenance of treatment gains, the literature provides little guidance. The two studies with behavior therapy that reported 1-year follow-up data provide mixed evidence for the maintenance of treatment gains. One study demonstrated good maintenance of gains (Rye & Ullman, 1999), whereas the other found that the treated group no longer differed from the control group at 1-year follow up. Because the groups were small and the exact nature of the behavior therapy differed across these studies, it remains unclear to which factors the difference in maintenance of treatment effects can be attributed.

If CBT is successful, then monitoring can continue as necessary (e.g., monthly assessments for 6 months). Booster sessions may be required, if

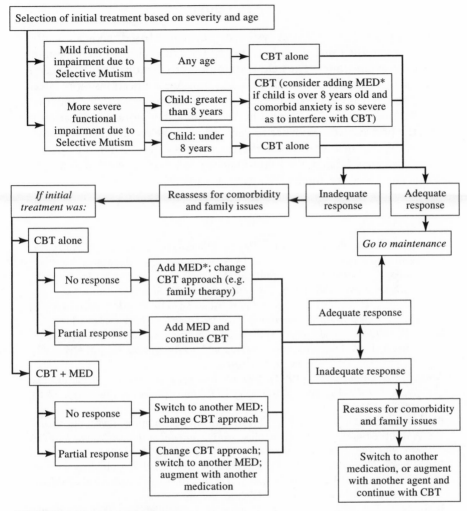

CBT* = cognitive-behavioral therapy
MED* = benzodiazepine or SSRI

Figure 15.1. Usual practices

symptoms begin to return. Patients who respond to pharmacotherapy typically are continued on the medication for 6 months after resolution of the symptoms, although this common clinical practice is based on anecdotal evidence and the premise that this time allows children to consolidate their progress and to expose themselves to the anxiety-provoking situations that previously elicited the symptoms. If symptoms have resolved for 6 months, then a slow taper of the medication can be considered, with observation for any return of the primary symptom as well as any comorbid anxiety.

452 ASSESSMENT AND TREATMENT

CONCLUSION

This disorder clearly requires systematic, evidence-based-medicine study. At this point, the usual clinical practice of the experts is the extent of practical clinical guidelines. The field is attempting to identify disorder-specific cognitive-behavioral therapy and medication. Are medications more effective than CBT; is CBT more effective than medication? Is the combination of CBT plus medications more effective than either alone? As we considered the best available evidence to date, we used the common clinical practice of experts in the area and the literature to date. After the specific treatments are validated, the field will need to address the issue of unimodal versus combined treatments in a multidisciplinary framework.

REFERENCES

American Psychiatric Association. (1994). *Diagnostic and statistical manual of mental disorders: DSM-IV* (4th ed.). Washington, DC: Author.

Anstendig, K. (1998). Selective mutism: A review of the treatment literature by modality from 1980–1996. *Psychotherapy, 35*(3), 381–391.

Anstendig, K. D. (1999). Is selective mutism an anxiety disorder? Rethinking its *DSM-IV* classification. *Journal of Anxiety Disorders, 13*(4), 417–434.

Black, B. (1996). Social anxiety and selective mutism. In L. J. Dickstein, M. B. Riba, & J. M. Oldham (Eds.), *Review of Psychiatry* (Vol. 15, pp. 469–495). Washington, DC: American Psychiatric Press.

Black, B., & Uhde, T. W. (1992). Elective mutism as a variant of social phobia. *Journal of the American Academy of Child and Adolescent Psychiatry, 31*(6), 1090–1094.

Black, B., & Uhde, T. W. (1994). Treatment of elective mutism with fluoxetine: A double-blind, placebo-controlled study. *Journal of the American Academy of Child and Adolescent Psychiatry, 33*(7), 1000–1006.

Black, B., & Uhde, T. W. (1995). Psychiatric characteristics of children with selective mutism: A pilot study. *Journal of the American Academy of Child and Adolescent Psychiatry, 34*(7), 847–856.

Blum, N. J., Kell, R. S., Starr, H. L., Lender, W. L., Bradley-Klug, K. L., Osborne, M. L., & Dowrick, P. W. (1998). Case study: Audio feedforward treatment of selective mutism. *Journal of the American Academy of Child and Adolescent Psychiatry, 37*(1), 40–43.

Brown, J. B., & Lloyd, H. (1975). A controlled study of children not speaking at school. *The Association of Workers for Maladjusted Children, 3*, 49–63.

Browne, E., Wilson, V., & Laybourne, P. C. (1963). Diagnosis and treatment of elective mutism in children. *Journal of the American Academy of Child and Adolescent Psychiatry, 2*, 605–617.

Calhoun, J., & Koenig, K. P. (1973). Classroom modification of elective mutism. *Behaviour Therapy, 4*, 700–702.

Carlson, J. S., Kratochwill, T. R., & Johnston, H. F. (1999). Sertraline treatment of 5 children diagnosed with selective mutism: A single-case research trial. *Journal of Child and Adolescent Psychopharmacology, 9*(4), 293–306.

Crema, J. E., & Kerr, J. M. (1978). Elective mutism: A child care case study. *Child Care Quarterly, 1*, 215–226.

Croghan, L. M., & Craven, R. (1982). Elective mutism: Learning from the analysis of a successful case history. *Journal of Pediatric Psychology, 7*(1), 85–93.

Cunningham, C. E., Cataldo, M. F., Mallion, C., & Keyes, J. B. (1984). A review and controlled single case evaluation of behavioral approaches to the management of elective mutism. *Child and Family Behavior Therapy, 5*(4), 25–49.

Dow, S. P., Sonies, B. C., Scheib, D., Moss, S. E., & Leonard, H. L. (1995). Practical guidelines for the assessment and treatment of selective mutism. *Journal of the American Academy of Child and Adolescent Psychiatry, 34*(7), 836–846.

Dummit, E. S., Klein, R. G., Tancer, N. K., Asche, B., & Martin, J. (1996). Fluoxetine treatment of children with selective mutism: An open trial. *Journal of the American Academy of Child and Adolescent Psychiatry, 35*(5), 615–621.

Dummit, E. S., Klein, R. G., Tancer, N. K., Asche, B., Martin, J., & Fairbanks, J. A. (1997). Systematic assessment of 50 children with selective mutism. *Journal of the American Academy of Child and Adolescent Psychiatry, 36*(5), 653–660.

Emslie, G. J., Rush, J., Weinberg, W. A., Kowatch, R. A., Hughes, C. W., Carmody, T., & Rintelmann, J. (1997). A double-blind, randomized, placebo-controlled trial of fluoxetine in children and adolescents with depression. *Archives of General Psychiatry, 54*(11), 1031–1037.

Fundudis, T., Kolvin, I., & Garside, R. (1979). *Speech retarded and deaf children: Their psychological development.* London: Academic Press.

Golwyn, D. H., & Sevlie, C. P. (1999). Phenelzine treatment of selective mutism in four prepubertal children. *Journal of Child and Adolescent Psychopharmacology, 9*(2), 109–113.

Golwyn, D. H., & Weinstock, R. C. (1990). Phenelzine treatment of elective mutism: A case report. *Journal of Clinical Psychiatry, 51*(9), 384–385.

Griffith, E. E., Schnelle, J. F., McNees, M. P., Bissinger, C., & Huff, T. M. (1975). Elective mutism in a first grader: The remediation of a complex behavioral problem. *Journal of Abnormal Child Psychology, 3*, 127–134.

Harvey, B. H., & Milne, M. (1998). Pharmacotherapy of selective mutism: Two case studies of severe entrenched mutism responsive to adjunctive treatment with fluoxetine. *South African Journal of Child and Adolescent Mental Health, 10*(1), 59–66.

Holmbeck, G., & Lavigne, J. (1992). Combining self-modeling and stimulus fading in the treatment of an electively mute child. *Psychotherapy, 29*(4), 661–667.

Kaufman, J., Birmaher, B., Brent, D. A., Rao, U., Flynn, C., Moreci, P., Williamson, D., et al. (1997). Schedule for Affective Disorders and Schizophrenia for School-Age Children–Present and Lifetime Version (K-SADS-PL): Initial reliability and validity data. *Journal of the American Academy of Child and Adolescent Psychiatry, 36*, 980–988.

Kehle, T., Owens, S., & Cressy, E. (1990). The use of self-modeling as an intervention in school psychology: A case study of an elective mute. *School Psychology Review, 19*, 115–121.

Keller, M. B., Ryan, N. D., Strober, M., Klein, R. G., Kutcher, S. P., Birmaher, B., Hagino, O. R., et al. (2001). Efficacy of paroxetine in the treatment of adolescent major depression: A randomized, controlled trial. *Journal of the American Academy of Child and Adolescent Psychiatry, 40*(7), 762–772.

Kopp, S., & Gillberg, C. (1997). Selective mutism: A population-based study: A research note. *Journal of Child Psychology and Psychiatry, 38*(2), 257–262.

Kovacs, M. (1992). *Children's Depression Inventory manual.* North Tonawanda, NY: Multi-Health Systems, Inc.

Kratochwill, T. R. (1981). *Selective mutism: Implications for research and treatment.* Hillsdale, NJ: Erlbaum.

Kristensen, H. (1997). Elective mutism—associated with developmental disorder/delay: Two case studies. *European Child and Adolescent Psychiatry, 7,* 234–239.

Kristensen, H. (2000). Selective mutism and comorbidity with developmental disorder/delay, anxiety disorder, and elimination disorder. *Journal of the American Academy of Child and Adolescent Psychiatry, 39*(2), 249–256.

Krohn, D. D., Weckstein, S. M., & Wright, H. L. (1992). A study of the effectiveness of a specific treatment for elective mutism. *Journal of the American Academy of Child and Adolescent Psychiatry, 31*(4), 711–718.

Kumpulainen, K., Rasanen, E., Raaska, H., & Somppi, V. (1998). Selective mutism among second-graders in elementary school. *European Child and Adolescent Psychiatry, 7,* 24–29.

Kussmaul, A. (1877). *Die Störungen der Sprache.* Leipzig, Germany: FCW Vogel.

Labbe, E. E., & Williamson, D. A. (1984). Behavioral treatment of elective mutism: A review of the literature. *Clinical Psychology Review, 4,* 273–292.

Leonard, H. L., & Topol, D. A. (1993). Elective mutism. In *Anxiety disorders* (Vol. 2, pp. 695–707). Philadelphia: W. B. Saunders Company.

Lerea, L., & Ward, B. (1965). Speech avoidance among children with oral-communication defects. *Journal of Psychology, 60,* 265–270.

March, J. (1997). *Multidimensional Anxiety Scale for Children.* North Tonawanda, NY: Multi-Health Systems Inc.

March, J. S., Biederman, J., Wolkow, R., Safferman, A., Mardekian, J., Cook, E. H., Cutler, N. R., et al. (1998). Sertraline in children and adolescents with obsessive-compulsive disorder: A multicenter randomized controlled trial. *Journal of the American Medical Association, 280*(20), 1752–1756.

Matson, J. L., Esveldt-Dawson, K., & O'Donnell, D. (1979). Overcorrection, modeling, and reinforcement procedures for reinstating speech in a mute boy. *Child Behavior Therapy, 1,* 363–371.

Pigott, H. E., & Gonzales, F. P. (1987). Efficacy of videotape self-monitoring in treating an electively mute child. *Journal of Clinical Child Psychology, 16*(2), 106–110.

Riddle, M. A., Reeve, E. A., Yaryura-Tobias, J. A., Yang, H. M., Claghorn, J. L., Gaffney, G., Greist, J. H., et al. (2001). Fluvoxamine for children and adolescents with obsessive-compulsive disorder: A randomized, controlled, multicenter trial. *Journal of the American Academy of Child and Adolescent Psychiatry, 40*(2), 222–229.

Rye, M. S., & Ullman, D. (1999). The successful treatment of long-term selective mutism: A case study. *Journal of Behavior Therapy and Experimental Psychiatry, 30,* 313–323.

Sanok, R., & Striefel, S. (1979). Elective mutism: Generalization of verbal responding across people and settings. *Behavior Therapy, 10,* 357–371.

Scott, E. (1977). A desensitization programme for the treatment of mutism in a 7-year-old girl: A case report. *Journal of Child Psychology and Psychiatry, 18,* 263–270.

Shaffer, D., Fisher, P., Dulcan, M. K., Davies, M., Piacentini, J., Schwab-Stone, M. E., Lahey, B. B., et al. (1996). The NIMH Diagnostic Interview Schedule for Children Version 2.3 (DISC 2.3): Description, acceptability, prevalence rates, and performance in the MECA study. *Journal of the American Academy of Child and Adolescent Psychiatry, 35,* 865–877.

Silverman, W. K., & Albano, A. M. (1996). *Anxiety Disorders Interview Schedule for DSM-IV.* San Antonio, TX: Psychological Corporation.

Steinhausen, H.-C., & Juzi, C. (1996). Elective mutism: An analysis of 100 cases. *Journal of the American Academy of Child and Adolescent Psychiatry, 35*(5), 606–614.

Thomsen, P. H., Rasmussen, G., & Andersson, C. B. (1999). Elective mutism: A 17-year-old girl treated successfully with citalopram. *Nordic Journal of Psychiatry, 53*(6), 427–429.

Walkup, J. T., Labellarte, M. J., Riddle, M. A., Pine, D. S., Greenhill, L., Klein, R., Davies, M., et al. (2001). Fluvoxamine for the treatment of anxiety disorders in children and adolescents. *New England Journal of Medicine, 344*(17), 1279–1285.

Wergeland, H. (1979). Elective mutism. *Acta Psychiatrica Scandinavica, 59,* 218–228.

Wright, H. H., Cuccaro, M. L., Leonhardt, T. V., Kendall, D. F., & Anderson, J. H. (1995). Case study: Fluoxetine in the multimodal treatment of a preschool child with selective mutism. *Journal of the American Academy of Child and Adolescent Psychiatry, 34*(7), 857–862.

Wulbert, M., Nyman, B. A., Snow, D., & Owen, Y. (1977). The efficacy of stimulus fading and contingency management in the treatment of elective mutism: A case study. *Journal of Applied Behavior Analysis, 6,* 435–441.

III

FUTURE DIRECTIONS
FOR RESEARCH
AND PRACTICE

16

ANXIETY AND
DEPRESSION
IN CHILDHOOD
Prevention and Intervention

ROBERT F. FERDINAND, PAULA M. BARRETT,
& MARK R. DADDS

The aim of the present chapter is to give an overview of existing knowledge regarding prevention of and early intervention with anxiety and depression in children and adolescents. Prevention and early intervention basically aim to identify problems at an early stage, to prevent development of problems, to promote resistance resources for at-risk subjects, and thus to reduce unnecessary suffering (Klingman, 2001). On the basis of Caplan's (1964) work on levels of prevention (primary, secondary, tertiary), Klingman identified five levels. Although Klingman's model specifically addresses posttraumatic stress disorder, it is helpful to understand principles behind prevention strategies for other internalizing disorders. With slight adjustment, the following levels of prevention may be discerned: anticipatory, primary, early secondary, intensive secondary, and tertiary prevention.

Anticipatory prevention aims at getting ready for implementation of interventions and thereby concerns the organization of the society. Whereas subsequent prevention levels directly aim at individuals who are more or less at risk, the anticipatory level aims at developing prevention protocols, organizing school programs, getting parents to attend, coordination with community mental health services, and so on. Without the anticipatory level, targeted interventions are impossible.

Primary prevention is aimed at the general population. Irrespective of individual problem levels or maladjustment, interventions are directed to all individuals of the target population, for instance, all children of a specific age, gender, or both. Depending on the target population (and the aim), interventions may involve children, teachers, or parents and may be directed via schools or families, or via other media such as television. In the case of anxiety or depression, interventions may aim to strengthen coping and problem-solving strategies that, in turn, may reduce stress in daily life and prevent the occurrence of anxiety or depressive disorders.

Secondary prevention efforts aim at intervention before a certain disorder develops. Hence, subjects at risk are identified, and the intervention is addressed. In early secondary prevention programs, individuals may receive simple advice on how to deal with the problem or where to seek help. After some time, reevaluation may take place to examine if the actions taken have had positive results. At the intensive secondary prevention level, participants receive more elaborate, treatment-based interventions, such as school programs, community programs, or a number of family therapy sessions.

Tertiary prevention aims at preventing relapse in subjects who have recovered after receiving treatment. For instance, secondary intervention may have been targeted at children who previously experienced moderate anxiety levels and who were therefore at risk for developing full-blown anxiety or depressive disorders. However, tertiary prevention is directed at preventing relapse in children who have recovered from these disorders. For instance, children who have recovered from maladjustment may need booster sessions to help them apply newly acquired problem-solving skills in daily life in the long run.

Prevention may occur at different levels simultaneously, and absolute distinctions between levels cannot be made. However, it is important to realize that an ounce of prevention may be worth a pound of cure. For instance, Dadds, Spence, Holland, Barrett, and Laurens (1997) applied a 10-week school-based cognitive-behavioral intervention, aimed at parents and children, to 7- to 14-year-olds who were selected on the basis of moderate anxiety levels. They found that, 2 years later, the intervention group showed a diagnosis rate (*DSM-IV* anxiety disorder) of 20%, compared to 39% in nontreated controls (Dadds et al., 1999). In other words, application of a targeted short intervention to children at risk may reduce the risk for later anxiety disorder. Without preventive intervention, it might be years before children at risk receive help, if they receive help at all. It is well known that a majority of problematic children do not reach mental health agencies (Verhulst & van der Ende, 1997). Besides the burden and suffering for the individuals themselves, longer duration of anxiety symptoms or disorder may result in maladaptive behavior patterns such as chronic avoidance behaviors or other adverse coping strategies. These behaviors may influence prognosis, or later therapeutic intervention, in a negative way. Hence, for a number of those who would develop full-blown anxiety disorder, a 10-week treatment protocol would probably not be enough to obtain similar results as with the same "dosage" delivered at an earlier point in time (i.e., prevention).

It is difficult to determine exactly when secondary prevention is needed. The presence of anxiety in children and adolescents should not necessarily be regarded as a sign of psychopathology or maladjustment. At some stages of development, anxiety can even be expected to occur. For instance, during infancy, the existence of separation anxiety can occur at times when the child is separated from her or his parents and may be considered age appropriate. Similarly, short-lived fears such as fear of the dark, storms, or animals can be normal phenomena, and over time, these normal fears tend to fade. However, for some children, they persist and begin to interfere with attending school, making friends, developing relationships, or day-to-day life.

Some anxious children are afraid to meet or talk to new people. Children with this difficulty may have few friends outside the family. Other children with severe anxiety may constantly worry or have concerns about school, friends, sports, or events that may or may not happen. Anxious children are often overly tense or uptight. Some may seek a lot of reassurance, and their worries may interfere with activities. Because anxious children may also be quiet, compliant, and eager to please, their difficulties may be missed.

Depression has long been thought of as an adult disorder. However, research over the past 2 decades is beginning to present a far different picture (e.g., Anderson Williams, McGee, & Silva, 1987). One Australian study (Spence, in press) found that about 2% of 13-year-old schoolchildren met the criteria for diagnosis of a depressive disorder, whereas an additional 25% showed symptoms of depression. It is common for feelings of depression to increase during middle adolescence, with approximately 3% of adolescents experiencing depression at any point in time (Clarke, Hawkins, Murphy, & Sheeber, 1993) and about 20% to 28% experiencing a depressive disorder by the time they turn 18 (Lewinsohn, Rhode, Klein, & Seeley, 1999). Rutter, Graham, and Chadwick's (1976) Isle of Wight study of a community sample also showed a marked increase in depressive symptomatology in preadolescents to middle adolescents, suggesting that depression may be part of a developmental phase, part and parcel of adolescence.

Children who experience depressive symptomatology generally have a negative view of the world, themselves, and the future. They experience disturbances of sleep, appetite, concentration, and decision making (Spence, in press). For some adolescents, suicidal ideation is also part of the depressive experience. Although it has been argued that depression is inherent to adolescent development, retrospective accounts now show that there is a strong link between adult depression and adolescent depression (Lewinsohn et al., 1999).

Controversy regarding the distinction between anxiety and depression has raged in the area of child and adolescent internalizing disorders for some time. Some researchers believe that anxiety and depression are two separate and distinct constructs, whereas others believe them to be a part of one construct that has been termed *negative affectivity* (Finch, Lipovsky, & Casat, 1989; Malcarne & Ingram, 1994; Ollendick & Yule, 1990). Although there is a strong link between anxiety and depression in childhood and adolescence (Cole, Peeke, Martin, Truglio, & Seroczynski, 1998; Kashani et al., 1987), with most support arising from strong correlations between the many common and overlapping features (Inderbitzen & Hope, 1995), there are also many distinct qualities that differentiate these disorders from one another. According to Barrett, Lowry-Webster, and Turner (1999), differences are evident with respect to age of onset, duration of illness, and associated features. Children who exhibit both anxiety and depression tend to be older than those who have only one of the disorders. In addition, when both disorders are present, anxiety tends to predate depressive symptomatology.

The tendency of anxiety disorder to predate depression has been confirmed by other studies. For instance, Woodward and Fergusson (2001) found that presence of *DSM-III-R* anxiety disorders during adolescence increases the risk for later anxiety disorder, but also for later depression. Similarly, using a genetically sensitive twin design, Silberg, Rutter, and Eaves (2001) found that genetic liability for adolescent depression in females was also associated with genetic liability for overanxious disorder and simple phobia at an earlier age (8 to 13 years). Hence, instead of waiting for depression to arise in adolescence, it may make more sense to prevent the increase, or persistence, of anxious symptoms at earlier stages of development. Given the hypothesis that increase in anxiety symptoms precedes depression, prevention of anxiety might affect the subsequent risk for depression. This strategy was followed by Dadds and colleagues (1999; 1997) in their early intervention study. Primary components of their treatment protocol—relaxation, cognitive restructuring, gradual exposure, and positive reinforcement—were based on Kendall's (1990) Coping Cat anxiety program and were aimed directly at anxiety.

Left untreated, childhood internalizing disorders (anxiety or depressive disorders) may manifest themselves later in adult clinical diagnoses. In fact, many retrospective studies (e.g., Schneider, Johnson, Hornig, Liebowitz, & Weissmann, 1992) found that internalizing disorders often appear for the first time during childhood or adolescence. Indeed, internalizing disorders such as anxiety and depression are the most commonly reported psychological problems in childhood (Barrett, Dadds, & Rapee, 1996), with estimates that about 17% to 21% of children are experiencing an anxiety disorder (Dadds et al., 1997; Kashani & Orvaschel, 1990) and about 2% to 5% of 13- to 17-year-olds in the community are experiencing depression at any given time (Anderson et al., 1987; Moor et al., 2000).

Given the high prevalence rates, the association between internalizing disorders and malfunctioning in daily life, and the tendency of internalizing disorders to persist across time, knowledge of effective prevention and early intervention strategies is critical. In adults, substantial progress has been made in the development of effective treatments for the internalizing disorders. In past decades, the efficacy of several types of psychosocial treatment—in both individual and group format—has been supported. Progress has been much slower in terms of trials assessing efficacious prevention or treatment of internalizing disorders in children and adolescents, although reported clinical and prevention trials have increased over the past 5 to 10 years, mostly because of the stabilization of the constantly changing diagnostic criteria for childhood disorders. To date, the main psychosocial treatment of choice for both anxiety and depression is cognitive-behavioral therapy.

COGNITIVE-BEHAVIORAL THERAPY

Although there are psychodynamic and behavioral treatments for childhood internalizing disorders (see Drobes & Strauss, 1993, for a review), most modern prevention programs for children and adolescents are theoretically based on cognitive-behavioral therapy (CBT). CBT-based programs help children to deal with their issues through addressing their irrational beliefs and by learning new coping skills. These coping skills are broad-based life skills that can be applied to both anxiety and depression. CBT-based approaches include a psychoeducational phase, a skills phase that includes relaxation and deep breathing, and a cognitive restructuring phase to address distorted and negative thinking that serves to maintain the problem. CBT for anxiety disorders may also include exposure and response prevention to help desensitize the child to his or her feared stimulus situations.

Although it is unclear how much the cognitive component of CBT contributes to the results in child populations, studies in adult populations (e.g., Butler, Fennell, Robson, & Gelder, 1991) have shown CBT to be superior to behavioral therapy alone. CBT-based programs have been found to be effective in the treatment of both anxiety and depression in adults and show great promise for the treatment of internalizing disorders in children. CBT-based treatments are also easily transported from an individual therapy program to a group or universal program, which increases their cost effectiveness.

CBT has long been used as an effective treatment for depression among adults, with recovery rates ranging between 65% and 85% (Clarke et al., 1992). However, its efficacy for children and adolescents has been relatively ignored. Very few articles citing clinical trials of CBT-based treatment of childhood depression exist. Those that do show mixed results. One of the reasons cited for the mixed results is that CBT is not effective with children under the age of 10 years, because they do not have the necessary cognitive resources to comprehend the cognitive component of the treatment. This is a point of contention, however (Ollendick, Grills, & King, 2001).

The current review is aimed at presenting an overview of psychosocial prevention and early intervention methods for childhood internalizing disorders. A range of options is addressed, from individual treatment and group therapy to parent and child therapy and universal preventive interventions.

Individual CBT

Several published studies over the past few years have shown support for CBT as an effective treatment for anxiety disorders, both as an individual treatment for children and with an added family component. The first clinical trial (Kendall, 1994) assessed the outcome of 47 children aged 9 to 13, who underwent 16 sessions of a CBT-based individual treatment (ICBT) for childhood anxiety. Outcome was evaluated using child, parent, and teacher reports, cognitive assessment, and behavioral observation. Compared with the wait-list group, children receiving ICBT showed improvement in coping, reported less distress, and were within the normal range on child measures and behavioral reports after treatment. Gains were maintained at a 12-month follow-up.

Using a sample of 94 anxious children, Kendall and colleagues (1997) replicated the results of Kendall's (1994) original study. After completing 16 weekly sessions, 64% of the children no longer met diagnostic criteria for their primary anxiety disorder diagnosis and demonstrated significant improvements compared with a wait list.

Barrett and colleagues (1996) added a family intervention component to the individual child treatment (CBT+FAM). The family intervention component consisted of three phases of training for the parents of anxious children: (1) skills for managing child distress and avoidance, (2) skills for managing their own anxiety, and (3) parental communication and problem-solving skills. Seventy-nine anxious children were randomly assigned to one of the two treatment conditions. At postintervention, a large proportion of the children receiving CBT (61%) and CBT+FAM (88%) were diagnosis free, compared with 30% of wait-listed children. Gains were maintained at 12 months for the children receiving CBT alone and those with the family treatment.

A 5-year follow-up (Barrett, Duffy, Dadds, & Rapee, 2001) was conducted with 52 children from Barrett et al.'s (1996) original study, and it was found that 86.5% of the children maintained their diagnosis-free status. However, the superiority of CBT plus family intervention was no longer evident, with both CBT and CBT+FAM treatments equally effective. A partial replication of these results was achieved by Howard and Kendall (1996). They conducted a multiple baseline design with six clinically anxious children aged 9 to 13 and their families, who completed 18 sessions of a CBT-based family therapy for anxiety. Substantial improvement by the families who completed the treatment program indicated that gains were maintained at 4 and 12 months posttreatment, providing further support for the effectiveness of family-based treatments of childhood anxiety.

In an attempt to assess the role of parental anxiety in the outcome of child anxiety treatment, Cobham, Dadds, and Spence (1998) added a parental anxiety management component to the individual child treatment (CBT+PAM). The 67 anxious children and a further 35 children who had at least one highly anxious parent were randomly allocated to child only treatment, or to child *and* parental anxiety treatment. In the CBT alone treatment condition, 82.4% of the child anxiety only group were diagnosis free, compared with 38.9% of the child and parent anxiety group. In the CBT+PAM condition, 80% of the child anxiety only group were diagnosis free, compared with 76.5% of child and parent anxiety. At 12 months, results for the child anxiety only group were maintained, but differential effects for the child and parent anxiety group were no longer significant. These results suggest that parental anxiety may be indicative of poorer treatment outcomes for anxious children.

Results from clinical trials assessing the efficacy of individually based CBT programs for specific types of anxiety disorders are also beginning to appear in the literature and are showing considerable promise—for example, generalized anxiety (Eisen & Silverman, 1998), social phobia (Hayward et al., 2000), and anxiety-based school refusal (King, Tonge, Heyne, & Ollendick, 2000). Individual therapy is useful when feared events or situations are unusual or embarrassing to discuss. It is also preferable when there are comorbid conditions that are not suitable for group work. Individual therapy can also provide more flexibility in terms of scheduling and content of treatment. However, individual therapy is time-consuming and costly. As a result, research has moved toward assessing the outcome of treatment of anxiety disorders in a group setting.

Group Interventions

To evaluate the therapeutic efficacy of a group CBT (GCBT) in treating anxiety disorders in children, Barrett (1998) conducted a study of 60 anxious children, aged 7 to 14 years. Children were assigned to one of three conditions, group CBT (GCBT), GCBT plus family management (GCBT+FAM), and wait-list. Children in the treatment groups underwent therapy that consisted of 12 weekly sessions. Children in both GCBT and GCBT+FAM showed significant improvement at posttreatment when compared with those in the wait-list group, but there were no statistical differences between the two active treatment groups. However, at 12 months follow-up, 84.8% of children in the GCBT were diagnosis free, compared with 64.5% of children in GCBT+FAM condition.

Silverman and colleagues (1999) also found support for the effectiveness of group CBT-based therapy. They conducted randomized clinical trials for GCBT and GCBT+FAM, comparing these with a wait-list control condition. Results showed that GCBT, and GCBT with concurrent parent sessions, were highly efficacious in producing and maintaining treatment gains. Children in GCBT showed substantial improvement on all the main outcome measures, and these gains were maintained at 3-, 6-, and 12-month follow-up.

Mendlowitz et al. (1999) assessed the effectiveness of GCBT as an intervention for anxiety, depression, and coping skills in anxious children, as well as the effect of parental involvement on treatment outcome. Sixty-two families with children aged 7 to 12 years were allocated to GCBT, GCBT plus parent intervention (GCBT+PI), or parent intervention alone (PI), and compared with a wait-list group. All treatment groups underwent 12 weekly sessions of therapy. Results showed that all treatment groups improved at posttreatment, with the CBT+PI group reporting the use of more active coping than other families and also rating their children as more improved than children from families in the other conditions.

An additional randomized clinical trial using a 10-session format was undertaken by Shortt, Barrett, and Fox (2000) to determine whether similar results could be obtained with a shorter group-CBT-based program for children (Barrett, Lowry-Webster, & Holmes, 1998). Ninety-one anxious children (aged 6 to 14 years) were randomly allocated to either a family-based CBT (FRIENDS) group or wait-list control group. (FRIENDS is an acronym referring to the therapeutic elements of this CBT program, which helps participants to remember to cope with anxiety in daily life by using several skills that are taught during the program.) Results indicated that 83% of children in the FRIENDS group were diagnosis free, compared with 18.2% of the wait-list group. Results were maintained at 12-month follow-up, with 80.5% of the children still diagnosis free.

In a pilot study conducted by Hayward and associates (2000), a CBT-based group treatment for female adolescents, who met criteria for a diagnosis of social phobia and were at risk for major depressive disorder, was examined. Thirty-five female adolescents were randomly assigned to a 16-week CBT–based group (GCBT) or wait-list control group. Preliminary results showed a significant reduction in the number of adolescents meeting the diagnostic criteria for social phobia. There were also some data suggesting that treatment of social phobia lowered the risk of relapse for major depressive disorder.

Due to the enormous cost to society of treating internalizing disorders, the mental health sector, like many other health professions, has begun to recognize the need for preventive strategies in addition to treatment. Although much of the current research into prevention of internalizing disorders has been theoretical, there have been some attempts to develop, empirically test, and report on preventive programs for both childhood anxiety and depression (Donovan & Spence, 2000).

In one of the first studies to determine the effectiveness of a preventive program for childhood anxiety, Dadds and colleagues (1997) identified 128 children at risk of anxiety disorders from a sample of 1,786 school-aged children (7 to 14 years). These children were randomly allocated to a 10-week, school-based child and family intervention group (GCBT) or wait-list control. Both groups showed improvement at postintervention; however, only the intervention group maintained improvements at 6 months. The treatment was shown to be effective as a result of the reduction in existing rates of anxiety symptomatology and prevention of the onset of new anxiety disorders at 2-year follow-up. What was especially important from this study is the notion that an anxiety program can be successfully delivered via a school-based CBT program.

Universal Interventions

It is recognized that the prevalence of anxiety disorders experienced by school-aged children is widespread. However, the National Institute of Mental Health (NIMH) has suggested that many of these children go undiagnosed and untreated (Sweeney & Rose, 2000). This is one of the major issues that arise out of targeting diagnosed or at-risk children only, as a large number of these children may inadvertently fall between the cracks. Thus, there is a push to develop more universal programs that can be applied to large numbers of children at once, especially in school-based programs. Although in its infancy, preliminary research into the effectiveness of school-based universal interventions for the prevention of anxiety and depressive symptoms in primary-school-aged children is promising.

Clarke et al. (1993), delivered one of the first school-based prevention programs. A sample of 620 Grade 9 and 10 students was randomly allocated to a three-session intervention group or wait-list control. The intervention group was targeted at reducing adolescent depressive symptomatology through education. Results of this study suggested that there was a reduction in depressive symptomatology at 3 weeks for boys but not girls, compared with a wait-list group. However, these promising results were not maintained at 3-month follow-up. Clearly, the psychoeducational component did not address all important risk factors associated with adolescent depression. A longitudinal epidemiological study of 1,500 students by Lewinsohn, Roberts, Rhodes, Seeley, Hops, and Andrews (as cited in Clarke et al., 1993) identified both low rates of pleasant events and high rates of irrational cognitions as major risk factors for onset of depression in adolescents.

In an attempt to address this issue, Clarke and associates (1993) delivered a five-session behavior-skills training intervention to 380 Grade 9 and 10 students. The intervention was aimed at increasing the number of pleasant activities experienced by children; the cognitive component (irrational cognitions) was not addressed, however. Students were randomly allocated to the treatment condition or a wait-list control condition. There were no statistically significant differences between the groups at postintervention. The two main reasons cited for the poor results of these two related studies are that the period of intervention was too short for adolescents to fully understand and integrate the psychoeducational information and that the intervention did not target irrational beliefs that are regarded as major contributors to depression for both children and adults, and the omission of this factor may have contributed to the poor results in the Clarke et al. studies.

As part of an ongoing series of clinical trials for the prevention of anxiety and depression in children, Lowry-Webster, Barrett, and Dadds (2001) randomly assigned 594 10- to 13-year-old children on a class-by-class basis to either a 10-session family group CBT program (FRIENDS) or a wait-list comparison. Results showed that children in the FRIENDS group reported fewer anxiety symptoms than wait-list children. In addition, those children who were highly anxious and completed the FRIENDS program also reported lower levels of depressive symptoms post-intervention.

To determine whether similar results could be achieved using teachers as the medium for delivering the FRIENDS program, Barrett and Turner (2002) randomly allocated 489 10- to 12-year-olds to either a psychologist-led or teacher-led preventive intervention, or to a usual care control condition with monitoring (standard curriculum) groups. The participants underwent a 12-week format of the FRIENDS program and were randomly allocated to either the psychologist-led or teacher-led program. Participants in both intervention conditions reported fewer symptoms at postintervention than those in the usual care condition. Preliminary results suggested that both psychologists and teachers are effective agents for delivering universal programs.

Results of an 8-week universal approach to treating depression in Queensland high schools initially showed great promise. The program is aimed at preventing depression in young people at risk and teaching skills to enhance general quality of life and well-being. The Problem-Solving for Life (Spence et al., 2003) program is delivered by trained teachers, within the school curriculum. Approximately 600 13-year-olds were randomly allocated to the intervention group or a monitoring control group. Adolescents in the intervention group showed a significant decline in self-reported symptoms of depression on completion of the program, compared with little change in the control group. However, these results were not maintained at 12-month follow-up.

Pragmatic Implications of Individual Versus Group CBT

Group CBT may have two important advantages over individual CBT: a better treatment environment and greater cost effectiveness. First, group therapy may provide a better treatment environment. Clients have the opportunity to practice their learning in a safe and sympathetic environment. For children, there is the added benefit of peer support and modeling from therapists. Group CBT also allows for lengthy periods of exposure, allowing for habituation of the anxiety responses to occur.

Individual CBT, on the other hand, may have the advantage that intervention is focused more clearly on the individual needs of the child. For instance, it is easier to set up individual fear hierarchies or to check difficulties with homework assignments. Also, parents may receive more attention from therapists regarding their own anxieties and parenting difficulties.

For some children, a group approach may suffice or may even be superior to individual CBT. For instance, in the case of social anxiety, children may profit from the peer interactions and practice opportunities available in the group context. However, other children may profit more from individual therapy, for instance, those who are too anxious to take part in the group process. Similarly, parents who are too anxious themselves may profit more from individual parent guidance than from group sessions with other parents, because it is impossible, or at least difficult, to discuss their own specific fears or mood states in the presence of other parents.

Level of intervention may be another factor determining success of group versus individual treatment. At the secondary level, it is more logical to use a group approach, because the aim of this type of intervention is to treat as many adolescents as possible with a small, though effective, dosage of intervention. At tertiary level, subject may have suffered from severe maladjustment that may require intensive treatment, focused as much as possible on the specific needs of a child or parent.

A second advantage above individual CBT is its presumed cost effectiveness, allowing for more efficient use of therapist time (Andrews, Crino, Hunt, Lampe, & Page, 1994). At secondary level of intervention, a group approach may be very advantageous, because it is relatively inexpensive and may yield important gains. At a tertiary or clinical level, it is not yet clear if group CBT is superior to, or even equally as cost effective as, individual therapy. Depending on the number of children treated in one session, it may require less therapist time. However, direct comparisons in a randomized fashion—regarding the outcome of group versus individual therapy in terms of psychopathological outcomes—are not available. Furthermore, the long-term cost effectiveness, for instance taking account of costs additional treatment needed after finishing manualized individual or group CBT, has not been studied.

IMPLICATIONS

Children can suffer emotionally and developmentally as a result of anxiety and depression. Anxious children tend to play less with other children, develop fewer friendships, and not to engage in organized activities such as sports teams and birthday parties. In extreme cases, anxious children may even refuse to attend school. The anxiety felt by these children results in social inhibition, whereby these children have a tendency not to develop the essential social skills necessary for normal social interactions. Anxious children often appear unhappy and report feeling sad, lonely, and shy, and they often show signs of depression (Beidel & Turner, 1998).

Similarly, children who are depressed have been shown to have impaired social, academic, and interpersonal skills. They are often sad, lonely, and isolated, with many experiencing suicidal thoughts. There is also a strong tendency for comorbidity to occur with anxiety and depression in children.

In addition, there are many similarities, such that a common approach to prevention or treatment may be possible and might serve to reduce symptomatology for both disorders.

Clinical trials of children with internalizing disorders, particularly anxiety, have shown CBT to be highly efficacious as a method of treatment. Results have consistently shown CBT to be effective in reducing symptomatology in children diagnosed with anxiety disorders or at risk for a range of anxiety disorders and depressive symptoms, compared with a wait list. In addition, these results have been found to exist whether the treatment is administered individually, in a group, or in a universally based program in, for example, school settings.

In general, CBT focused on depression may not be adequate for reducing depressive symptomatology. It is often noted, however, that the Clarke et al. (1993) studies were extremely brief in comparison to those conducted with anxious children. This length of time would have been inadequate for the children to understand the relatively complex cognitive concepts that are the basis of such CBT programs. However, a treatment that consisted of 10 or more sessions only showed somewhat greater success at short-term follow-up (e.g., Spence et al., 2003). Long-term follow-up indicated that the CBT program aimed at depression was probably not successful to prevent depression in the long run. Possibly, more intense or different approaches are needed for this purpose.

Overall, these limitations notwithstanding, CBT-based treatments appear to be highly effective for prevention of anxiety. There is reasonable support for their use as an efficacious treatment for anxiety whether treated in individual or group format, and also for the inclusion of parental or family training. Less impressive results have been found for programs that primarily focused on depression. Nevertheless, the research into prevention is in its infancy, and the results to date are impressive. It appears that a CBT-based prevention program that is universally applied within a school-like setting can lead to reduced symptomatology and diagnoses. Results even suggest that, when properly trained, teachers can administer the prevention program to the children, with equally efficacious outcomes (Barrett & Turner, 2002).

Training is a major issue when implementing prevention treatments in schools. However, there are often limited resources, such as time and teacher availability. If prevention programs require the identification of children at risk by teachers, many teachers suggest that a lack of clinical knowledge hampers their identification of these at-risk children. This could be addressed by the implementation of a clinical component aimed at educating the teachers as part of their training. Moor and colleagues (2000) developed and evaluated a training package aimed at helping teachers and school counselors to identify depressed pupils. After implementation of the training the school, staff felt more confident in their ability to recognize depressed pupils.

Although research results are promising, many questions remain unanswered. For instance, it is not clear at which age groups interventions should be aimed to obtain optimal effect with respect to prevention of anxiety or depressive disorder across the life span. From a biological point of view, prevention as early as possible might be most worthwhile, given the possible increment of biological vulnerability across time. For example, kindling processes that reflect increasing illness severity across time due to alteration in neurotransmission processes after recurrent exposure to environmental stimuli, such as life events, may be reversible if targeted as early as possible, and these may be irreversible later on (Post & Weiss, 1998; Post, Weiss, & Leverich, 1994; Weiss & Post, 1998). On the other hand, adolescents might profit more from cognitive intervention than younger children, because of their advanced cognitive abilities. More research is needed to assess associations between effectiveness of intervention and age (Ollendick & Vasey, 1999).

Other uncertainties exist regarding screening. Although knowledge exists about factors putting individuals at risk for adverse development, it is not possible to determine the prognosis of individual cases with absolute certainty. Hence, if children at risk for anxiety or depressive disorder are selected from the general population—for instance, on the basis of moderate symptom level—and treated accordingly, some children who would have done well without therapy will be treated nevertheless. Furthermore, it is not possible at present to identify children who are likely to respond to intervention in advance, so some will experience treatment failure, which may influence future help-seeking behaviors negatively. Research is needed to investigate predictors of treatment response and to find accurate signs of poor prognosis. This would enhance future screening processes for early intervention.

Besides screening issues, associations between problem characteristics (number of symptoms, level of comorbidity) and required dosage of intervention also need to be resolved. Dosage of intervention is determined by matters such as duration, frequency, and number of sessions; number of persons involved (child, parents, teacher); therapist skills; degree or extent of focusing on specific needs; and specific type of treatment ingredients. To date, ample knowledge exists about the relationship between problem characteristics and therapy dosage. Some issues are starting to be resolved— for instance, the association between parental anxiety and the need to target this anxiety to enhance treatment results in the child. However, largely, it is not known if specific types of anxiety require specific interventions (e.g., generalized anxiety disorder might especially benefit from relaxation practices). Also, despite the fact that we know that pretreatment symptom levels are predictive of treatment results to some extent (Dadds et al., 1999), it is not known if anxious children with comorbid depression or greater intensity or frequency of problems will improve with more sessions, or more parent-focused intervention, or even drug therapy. To optimally target type of intervention to individual needs, this type of issue needs to be resolved.

SUMMARY

Clinical trials to date have shown that the use of CBT in treating children with internalizing disorders such as anxiety and depression are not only efficacious but also cost effective—at secondary prevention levels—when used in a group format. The programs can be transported from an individual-based treatment to use within a school. As current findings are indicative of serious problems being experienced by many of our children, it makes sense to take on a more proactive rather than reactive approach when developing treatments for internalizing disorders in children. If under-diagnosis and undertreatment are occurring as often as described by the NIMH, then universally based treatments in schools may go a long way in addressing this issue. Future research aimed at finding the optimal match between specific interventions and individual needs is warranted.

REFERENCES

Anderson, J. C., Williams, S., McGee, R., & Silva, P. A. (1987). *DSM-III* disorders in preadolescent children: Prevalence in a large sample from the general population. *Archives of General Psychiatry, 44,* 69–76.

Andrews, G., Crino, R., Hunt, C., Lampe, L., & Page, A. (1994) *The treatment of anxiety disorders: Clinician's guide and patient manual.* Melbourne, Australia: Cambridge University Press.

Barrett, P. M. (1998). Group therapy for anxiety disorders in children. *Journal of Clinical Child Psychology, 27,* 459.

Barrett, P. M., Dadds, M. R., & Rapee, R. M. (1996). Family treatment of childhood anxiety: A controlled trial. *Journal of Consulting and Clinical Psychology, 64*(2), 333–342.

Barrett, P. M., Duffy, A. L., Dadds, M. R., & Rapee, R. M. (2001). Cognitive-behavioral treatment of anxiety disorders in children: Long-term (6-year) follow-up. *Journal of Consulting and Clinical Psychology, 69,* 135–141.

Barrett, P. M., Lowry-Webster, H., & Holmes, J. (1999). *Friends for children group leader manual* (2nd ed.). Brisbane, Australia: Australian Academic Press.

Barrett, P. M., & Turner, C. (2002). Prevention of anxiety symptoms in primary school children: Preliminary results from a universal school-based trial. *British Journal of Clinical Psychology, 40,* 399–410.

Beidel, D. C., & Turner, S. M. (1998). *Shy children, phobic adults: Nature and treatment of social phobia.* Washington, DC: American Psychological Association.

Butler, G., Fennell, M., Robson, P., & Gelder, M. (1991). Comparison of behavior therapy and cognitive behavior therapy in the treatment of generalized anxiety disorder. *Journal of Consulting and Clinical Psychology, 59*(1), 167–175.

Clarke, G. N., Hawkins, W., Murphy, M., & Sheeber, L. (1993). School-based primary prevention of depressive symptomatology in adolescents: Findings from two studies. *Journal of Adolescent Research, 8*(2), 183–204.

Clarke, G. N., Hops, H., Lewinsohn, P. M., Andrews, J., Seeley, J. R., & Williams, J. (1992). Cognitive-behavioral group treatment of adolescent depression: Prediction of outcome. *Behavior Therapy, 23,* 341–354.

Cobham, S., Dadds, M. R., & Spence, S. H. (1998). The role of parental anxiety in the treatment of childhood anxiety. *Journal of Consulting and Clinical Psychology, 66*(6), 893–905.

Cole, D. A., Peeke, L. G., Martin, J. M., Truglio, R., & Seroczynski, A. D. (1998). A longitudinal look at the relation between depression and anxiety in children and adolescents. *Journal of Consulting and Clinical Psychology, 66,* 451–460.

Dadds, M. R., Holland, D. E., Laurens, K. R., Mullins, M., Barrett, P. M., & Spence, S. H. (1999). Early intervention and prevention of anxiety disorders in children: Results at 2-year follow-up. *Journal of Consulting and Clinical Psychology, 67*(1), 145–150.

Dadds, M. R., Spence, S., Holland, D., Barrett, P. M., & Laurens, K. (1997). Prevention and early intervention for anxiety disorders: A controlled trial. *Journal of Consulting and Clinical Psychology, 65*(4), 627–635.

Donovan, C. L., & Spence, S. H. (2000). Prevention of childhood anxiety disorders. *Clinical Psychology Review, 2*(4), 509–531.

Drobes, D. J., & Strauss, C. C. (1993). Behavioural treatment of childhood anxiety disorders. *Child and Adolescent Psychiatric Clinics of North America, 2,* 779–793.

Eisen, A. R., & Silverman, W. K. (1998). Prescriptive treatment for generalized anxiety disorder in children. *Behaviour Therapy, 29*(1), 105–122.

Finch, A. J., Lipovsky, J. A., & Casat, C. D. (1989). Anxiety and depression in children and adolescents: Negative affectivity or separate constructs? In P. C. Kendall & D. Watson (Eds.), *Anxiety and depression: Distinctive and overlapping features* (pp. 171–202). New York: Academic Press.

Hayward, C., Varady, S., Albano, A. M., Thieneman, M., Henderson, L., & Schatzberg, A. F. (2000). Cognitive-behavioral group therapy for female socially phobic adolescents: Results of a pilot study. *Journal of the American Academy of Child and Adolescent Psychiatry, 39,* 721–726.

Howard, B., & Kendall, P. C. (1996). Cognitive-behavioural family therapy for anxiety disordered children: A multiple baseline evaluation. *Cognitive Therapy and Research, 20,* 423–443.

Inderbitzen, H. M., & Hope, D. A. (1995). Relationship among adolescent reports of social anxiety, anxiety and depressive symptoms. *Journal of Anxiety Disorders, 9*(5), 385–396.

Kashani, J. J., Carlson, G. A., Beck, N. C., Hoeper, E. W., Corcoran, C. M., McAllister, J. A., Fallahi, C., et al. (1987). Depression, depressive symptoms, and depressed mood among a community sample of adolescents. *American Journal of Psychiatry, 144*(7), 931–934.

Kashani, J. H., & Orvaschel, H. (1990). A community study of anxiety in children and adolescents. *American Journal of Psychiatry, 147,* 313–318.

Kendall, P. C. (1990). *Coping cat workbook.* Ardmore, PA: Workbook Publishing.

Kendall, P. C. (1994). Treating anxiety disorders in children: Results of a randomized clinical trial. *Journal of Consulting and Clinical Psychology, 62*(1), 100–110.

Kendall, P. C., Flannery-Schroeder, E., Panichelli-Mindel, S. M., Southam-Gerow, M., Henin, A., & Warman, M. (1997). Treatment of anxiety disorders in youth: A second randomized clinical trial. *Journal of Consulting and Clinical Psychology, 65,* 366–380.

King, N. J., Tonge, B. J., Heyne, D., & Ollendick, T. H. (2000). Research on the cognitive-behavioral treatment of school refusal: A review and recommendations. *Clinical Psychology Review, 20,* 495–507.

Klingman, A. (2001). Prevention of anxiety disorders: The case of posttraumatic stress disorder. In W. K. Silverman & P. D. A Treffers (Eds.), *Anxiety disorders in children and adolescents.* New York: Cambridge University Press.

Lewinsohn, P. M., Roberts, R., & Seeley, J. R. (1991). Screening for adolescent depression: A comparison of depression scales. *Journal of the American Academy of Child and Adolescent Psychiatry, 30,* 58–66.

Lowry-Webster, H. M., Barrett, P. M., & Dadds, M. R. (2000). A universal prevention trial of anxiety and depressive disorders in childhood: Preliminary data from an Australian study. *Behavior Change, 10,* 36–50.

Malcarne, V. L., & Ingram, R. E. (1994). Cognition and negative affectivity. In T. H. Ollendick & R. J. Prinz (Eds.), *Advances in clinical child psychology* (Vol. 16, pp. 141–176). New York: Plenum Press.

Mendlowitz, S. L., Manassis, K., Bradley, S., Scapillato, D., Miezitis, S., & Shaw, B. F. (1999). Cognitive-behavioral group treatments in childhood anxiety disorders: The role of parental involvement. *Journal of the American Academy of Child and Adolescent Psychiatry, 38*(10), 1223–1229.

Moor, S., Sharrock, G., Scott, J., McQueen, H., Wrate, R., Cowan J., & Blair, C. (2000). Evaluation of a teaching package designed to improve teachers' recognition of depressed pupils: A pilot study. *Journal of Adolescence, 23,* 331–342.

Ollendick, T. H., Grills, A. E., & King, N. J. (2001). Applying developmental theory to the assessment and treatment of childhood disorders: Does it make a difference? *Clinical Psychology and Psychotherapy, 8,* 304–315.

Ollendick, T. H., & Vasey, M. W. (1999). Developmental theory and the practice of clinical child psychology. *Journal of Clinical Child Psychology, 28,* 457–466.

Ollendick, T. H., & Yule, W. (1990). Depression in British and American children and its relations to anxiety and fear. *Journal of Consulting and Clinical Psychology, 58,* 126–129.

Post, R. M., & Weiss, S. R. B. (1998). Sensitization and kindling phenomena in mood, anxiety, and obsessive-compulsive disorders: The role of serotonergic mechanisms in illness progression. *Biological Psychiatry, 44*(3), 193–206.

Post, R. M., Weiss, S. R. B., & Leverich, G. S. (1994). Recurrent affective disorder: Roots in developmental neurobiology and illness progression based on changes in gene expression. *Development and Psychopathology, 6*(4), 781–813.

Rutter, M., Graham, P., & Chadwick, O. F. (1976) Adolescent turmoil: Fact or fiction? *Journal of Child Psychology and Psychiatry, 17,* 35–56.

Schneider, F. R., Johnson, J., Hornig, C. D., Liebowitz, M. R., & Weissmann, M. M. (1992). Social phobia: Comorbidity and morbidity in an epidemiological sample. *Archives of General Psychiatry, 49,* 282–289.

Shortt, A. L., Barrett, P. M., & Fox, T. (2000). A family-based cognitive behavioural group treatment for anxious children: An evaluation of the FRIENDS program. Manuscript submitted for publication.

Silberg, J. L., Rutter, M., & Eaves, L. (2001). Genetic and environmental influences on the temporal association between earlier anxiety and later depression in girls. *Biological Psychiatry, 49*(12), 1040–1049.

Silverman, W. K., Kurtines, W. M., Ginsburg, G. S., Weems, C. F., Lumpkin, P. W., & Carmichael, D. H. (1999). Treating anxiety disorders in children with group cognitive-behavioral therapy: A randomized clinical trial. *Journal of Consulting and Clinical Psychology, 67(6)*, 995–1004.

Spence, S. H., Sheffield, J. K., & Donovan, C. L. (2003). Preventing adolescent depression: An evaluation of the problem solving for life program. *Journal of Consulting and Clinical Psychology, 71(1)*, 3–13.

Sweeney, R., & Rose, V. L. (2000). Report shows childhood anxiety disorders are underdiagnosed and undertreated. *American Family Physician, 61(6)*, 1606.

Verhulst, F. C., & van der Ende, J. (1997). Factors associated with child mental health service use in the community. *Journal of the American Academy of Child and Adolescent Psychiatry, 36(7)*, 901–909.

Weiss, S. R. B., & Post, R. M. (1998). Kindling: Separate vs. shared mechanisms in affective disorders and epilepsy. *Neuropsychobiology, 38(3)*, 167–180.

Woodward, L. J., & Fergusson, D. M. (2001). Life course outcomes of young people with anxiety disorders in adolescence. *Journal of the American Academy of Child and Adolescent Psychiatry, 40(9)*, 1086–1093.

17

FROM EFFICACY
TO EFFECTIVENESS
RESEARCH
What We Have Learned
Over the Last 10 Years

ROBIN NEMEROFF, POLLY GIPSON, & PETER JENSEN

embers of the public often assume that when they take a child to a
mental health professional for treatment, the clinician will have a
broad base of knowledge from which to determine the type of treatment
that is most likely to alleviate that child's symptoms. Truly, most people
would be surprised to discover how little we know and, in the last 10 years,
how little we have learned about the effectiveness of mental health treatments for childhood anxiety problems. With this in mind, the following
chapter details the current evidence base for childhood anxiety disorder
treatments, comments on the quality of these research findings, and makes
recommendations for future research into this underexplored area.

For the purposes of this chapter, it should be noted that we have only
considered studies that incorporate a randomly assigned comparison group
into the research design, because the absence of a comparison group would
preclude our making any true conclusions about the efficacy of various treatments and whether, in fact, they are superior to a placebo condition, another treatment condition, or no treatment at all. With this criterion in mind,
we are aware of only 27 studies published since 1990 that compare the outcomes of childhood anxiety disorder treatments to the outcomes of alternative treatment conditions.

Recent publications have begun to articulate the differences between
efficacy and effectiveness research and to plot various experimental designs

that fall on the continuum between these two research models (Clarke, 1995; Hoagwood, Hibbs, Brent, & Jensen, 1995; Weisz & Jensen, 1999; Weisz, Weiss, & Donenberg, 1992). In an attempt to clarify the terms *efficacy* and *effectiveness*, Hoagwood and colleagues (1995) have described efficacy studies as "studies in which considerable control has been exercised by the investigator over sample selection . . . , over delivery of the interventions, and over conditions under which the intervention or treatment occurred" (p. 683). In contrast, they described effectiveness studies as research "in which a previously tested efficacious intervention is examined with a more heterogeneous sample within a more naturalistic setting, . . . or is provided by real-world service practitioners rather than research therapists" (p. 683). Thus, research design factors such as participant composition, degree of treatment structure, compliance with treatment structure, and selection of treatment settings are all important considerations in the existing body of research, as we consider the degree to which the study findings reported below apply to real-world treatment settings.

ANXIETY DISORDERS BROADLY DEFINED

A great deal of the research conducted in the last decade has explored the effects of specific treatments on a broad range of childhood anxiety disorders. That is, many studies have used samples that included children in a wide age range with varied and sometimes even comorbid anxiety diagnoses. In fact, there are some potential advantages to defining the target patient population so broadly, because many children have complicated presentations that are not entirely captured by a single Axis I diagnosis. Thus, looking at anxiety symptoms without strictly adhering to a specific diagnosis may provide a better gauge of a treatment's effectiveness in addressing the complex range of problems clinicians often observe in children and adolescents who are referred for treatment. On the other hand, because anxiety disorders may have vastly different presentations, studying them together might reduce our ability to identify treatments that are effective for one type of anxiety problem but not for another. As we consider recommendations for future research, it may be useful for investigators to selectively group problems that are often interrelated in the presentation of childhood anxiety, because this type of research may more accurately assess treatments for symptom clusters that frequently present in the real world. However, as long as we fail to consider the real-world correlates of our sample statistics, we run the risk of misinterpreting critical research findings.

In total, we are aware of seven controlled studies that have evaluated treatments for childhood anxiety disorders as a whole. Among these, four studies have explored the impact of cognitive-behavioral therapy (CBT) in a traditional, one-on-one setting; one study has evaluated the efficacy of CBT in a group treatment setting; and two studies have investigated the benefits of medication treatments. Separately, an eighth study evaluated the effectiveness of a psychosocial intervention in preventing the onset of full-blown anxiety disorders in children with subthreshold anxiety.

CBT for Anxiety Disorders as a Whole

To examine the effectiveness of individual CBT, Kendall (1994) conducted a controlled randomized clinical trial with 47 children between the ages of 9 and 13. Although a range of anxiety diagnoses were represented in their sample, the vast majority of the children who participated in this study carried a diagnosis of generalized anxiety disorder (64%), with the remaining children carrying a diagnosis of either social phobia (19%) or separation anxiety disorder (17%). Participants were randomly assigned to a CBT condition for 16 weeks or a wait-list condition for 8 weeks. Thereafter, the wait-list controls were assigned to a CBT condition if they maintained an anxiety disorder diagnosis.

In this study, the structure of the CBT reflected five primary treatment strategies: (1) awareness of anxious feelings and the physical correlates of anxiety, (2) identification of negative thoughts associated with anxiety-provoking situations, (3) coping strategies, (4) monitoring progress and reinforcing gains, and (5) implementing a strategic plan to manage anxious feelings. Although therapists adhered to the aforementioned principles throughout the course of the treatment, it is noteworthy that the design of this study permitted therapists to apply treatment techniques flexibly, to individualize the treatment for each subject. Treatment materials were taken from the *Coping Cat Workbook* (Kendall, 1990).

Both child and parent reports indicated that children who received CBT had a greater decrease in anxiety symptoms and a greater increase in the ability to cope with stress immediately following treatment. Moreover, all reported gains by the children treated with CBT were maintained at 1-year follow-up and at a long-term follow-up averaging 3 years posttreatment (Kendall & Southam-Gerow, 1996). However, teacher reports failed to indicate significantly more improvement in the group that received CBT.

In a subsequent study designed to test the benefits of the five cognitive-behavioral strategies just listed, Kendall and colleagues (1997) randomly assigned 94 children between the ages of 9 and 13 to either a 16-week CBT condition or a wait-list condition. Over half of the children who participated in this study were diagnosed with generalized anxiety disorder (59%), with the remaining children carrying a primary diagnosis of either separation anxiety disorder (23%) or social phobia (18%). Analyses of the psychoeducation and exposure components of the CBT treatment indicated that psychoeducation alone was not responsible for patients' improvement—instead, exposure applied after the psychoeducation component of CBT appeared to contribute to significant improvements in children's outcomes.

Aside from its contribution to our knowledge about the components of treatment that are associated with improved outcomes, this study also highlights a major problem in the area of treatment efficacy research—inconsistent findings across different evaluators and different outcome measures. Although self-reports of coping ability, frequency of anxious self-statements, and scores on one measure of chronic anxiety—the Revised Children's Manifest Anxiety Scale (RCMAS)—were improved among children who had received CBT, other measures of both chronic and temporal anxiety (the State-Trait Anxiety Inventory–Children [STAIC], STAIC A-State, STAIC A-Trait; the Fear Survey Schedule for Children–Revised [FSSC-R]) as well as a measure of depression reflected no differences between treatment groups. Although mothers' ratings of their child's depression and anxiety differed between treatment groups, fathers' ratings failed to discriminate between children who had received CBT and those who had not. Thus, this study raises important questions about the validity, reliability, and specificity of the assessment instruments used to gauge outcomes. However, the stability of outcome measures was not called into question by this study, as those measures reflecting clinical improvement immediately following CBT found similar levels of improvement at 1-year follow-up.

In a study designed to assess the benefits of augmenting traditional CBT with a family component, Barrett, Dadds, and Rapee (1996) conducted a 12-week experiment in 79 children between the ages of 7 and 14 who were diagnosed with either separation anxiety disorder (38%), generalized anxiety disorder (38%), or social phobia (24%). Participants were randomly assigned to one of three conditions: CBT, CBT with a family management component, or a wait-list condition. The CBT child treatment paralleled Kendall's (1990) *Coping Cat Workbook*, whereas the family management component focused on (a) teaching parents contingency strategies to help manage their children's behaviors, (b) strategies for dealing with their own anxiety responses and modeling adaptive responses to stressful situations, and (c) training in communication and problem-solving skills. Results at study end point indicated that children in either form of treatment were less likely to continue to meet criteria for an anxiety disorder diagnosis than children in the wait-list condition.

Although the children who received the CBT treatment with a family component were less likely to have an anxiety diagnosis than children who received the standard CBT treatment immediately following treatment (16% vs. 43%) and at 12-month follow-up (4% vs. 30%), there were no significant differences in the prevalence of anxiety disorders between the two active treatment groups at 6-month follow-up (16% vs. 29%). Additional variations in the response to the family component were noted among different demographic groups. That is, females and children ages 7 to 10 responded better to the CBT treatment when it included the family component, but no differences were reported among boys and children between the ages 11 and 14. Thus, this study raises important questions about variations in the response to family treatments over time and across different patient populations.

In a second study exploring the benefits of extending anxiety disorder treatments beyond the identified patient to include the larger family system, Cobham, Dadds, and Spence (1998) examined the outcomes of 67 anxious children between the ages of 7 and 14. In this study, children's principal diagnoses were as follows: 12% had separation anxiety disorder, 64% had generalized anxiety disorder, 18% had a simple phobia with severe functional impairment, 4% had a social phobia, and 1% had agoraphobia. Children were partitioned into two groups based on their parents' anxiety level. Subsequently, children in each parental anxiety level group were randomly assigned to either a traditional CBT treatment or a CBT treatment that also included a 4-week parental anxiety management component. The researchers found that fewer children with highly anxious parents met the diagnostic criteria for an anxiety disorder posttreatment when the parental anxiety management component was added to CBT (23% vs. 61%). In contrast, the outcomes for children whose parents were not anxious were indistinguishable between the two treatment groups (80% vs. 82%).

Although the benefits of the parental anxiety management component were maintained at 6-month follow-up, the investigators failed to find a significant difference in the prevalence of anxiety diagnoses between treatment groups at 1-year follow-up, raising questions about the potential need for additional booster sessions to maintain earlier treatment gains. In addition, clinician's global ratings of improvement failed to discriminate between the outcomes of children receiving traditional CBT and those receiving CBT plus parental anxiety management at any point, with clinician's ratings reflecting equal levels of improvement across both treatment and parental anxiety level groups.

Consistent with the Barrett et al. (1996) study described above, Cobham and colleagues (1998) also observed gender differences in children's responses to family treatment, finding significantly fewer girls with an anxiety diagnosis under the CBT plus parental anxiety management treatment condition, but no difference in the outcomes of boys across treatment conditions. Unfortunately, because this study lacked a wait-list condition, we cannot determine whether both CBT and CBT plus parental anxiety management are efficacious in reducing anxiety symptoms and increasing clinician's ratings of global improvement, or whether these effects were due to other factors such as the passage of time or rater's expectations of change. Thus, the results of this study only serve to demonstrate the short-term benefits of parental anxiety management on the outcomes of girls and children with anxious parents.

Addressing the aforementioned shortcoming in the design of the Cobham et al. (1998) study, Barrett (1998) randomly assigned 60 children between the ages of 7 and 14 who were diagnosed with either overanxious disorder (50%), separation anxiety disorder (43%), or social phobia (7%) to one of the three treatment conditions: group CBT, group CBT with an added family component, or a wait list. Although treatment was conducted in a group setting rather than in a one-to-one, individual-session format, treatment protocols paralleled those used in Barrett's earlier study (Barrett et al., 1996). Results indicated that both group CBT and group CBT with

an added family component were superior to the wait-list condition immediately following the 12-week treatments and at 1-year follow-up. That is,
the percentage of children who no longer met the criteria for an anxiety
disorder was greater in both CBT treatment groups than in the wait-list
group (65% vs. 25%). However, although children who received group CBT
were equally likely to be diagnosis free posttreatment regardless of whether
there was a family component to the treatment, children who received group
CBT with a family component were more likely to have superior outcomes
on a variety of measures including global functioning, overall anxiety, reduction of avoidant behaviors, change in family disruption by the child's
behavior, change in family's skill in dealing with child's behavior, and change
in child's ability to deal with difficult situations up to a year after treatment
(according to clinician, parent, and self-report ratings).

In sum, overall findings suggest that for some children, inclusion of a
family treatment component in CBT interventions for children with anxiety disorders may offer modest incremental advantages over child-focused
CBT alone. Because these findings were not consistently found across all
studies, however, additional studies clarifying this possible effect are needed.

Pharmacotherapy for Anxiety Disorders as a Whole

In an experiment designed to examine the efficacy of clonazepam (Klonopin)
in the treatment of child anxiety disorders, Graae, Milner, Rizzotto, and Klein
(1994) randomly assigned 15 children between the ages of 7 and 13 to an
8-week double-blind, crossover placebo controlled study, with each child
receiving 4 weeks of clonazepam (up to 2 mg/day) and 4 weeks of placebo. Whereas 14 of the 15 participants in this study had a diagnosis of
separation anxiety disorder, all but two participants had at least one
comorbid psychiatric diagnosis, ranging from attention-deficit/hyperactivity
disorder (ADHD) and oppositional defiant disorder to other anxiety diagnoses such as simple phobia, social phobia, and overanxious disorder. Although clinicians reported a greater reduction in symptoms and global
improvements in functioning during the period that children were receiving clonazepam, data analyses of treatment group differences failed to reach
statistical significance.

Unfortunately, the study conducted by Graae and colleagues (1994)
poses several problems that may affect the interpretation of the findings.
First, it is worth noting that, because of the small number of children who
participated in this study, there may have been insufficient statistical power
to discern any real differences in the outcomes of these children. Thus, the
discrepancy between the clinician's perception of change and the results of
statistical analyses may be an artifact of the small sample size of this study.
The investigators also suggest that the short duration of the clonazepam
treatment may have contributed to the lack of significant outcomes. Moreover, the complex diagnostic presentations of the children who participated
in this study may have made this a relatively difficult group of children to

treat successfully with clonazepam alone. Thus, it seems possible that, had this study been conducted with a less complex, more homogeneous sample of children, the results might have found clonazepam to be more efficacious than placebo.

Recently, the Research Unit on Pediatric Psychopharmacology (RUPP) Anxiety Study Group (2001) researched the efficacy of fluvoxamine (Luvox) in treating childhood anxiety. In this study, 128 children between the ages of 6 and 17 were randomly assigned to a double-blind, 8-week trial of either fluvoxamine or a placebo following a 3-week open trial of supportive psychotherapy that excluded any elements of CBT. Like the aforementioned medication study, participants in this study carried a variety of diagnoses including social phobia (66%), separation anxiety (59%), and generalized anxiety disorder (57%). Using a flexible dose of up to 300 mg of fluvoxamine per day, the investigators found a greater decrease in clinicians' ratings of anxiety and higher ratings of clinical response in the group receiving the medication (78% vs. 29%). Thus, the authors suggest that fluvoxamine, a medication demonstrated to be effective in the treatment of adult anxiety disorders, may be an effective treatment for childhood anxiety disorders as well. However, to date, the empirical support for pharmacotherapy interventions remains limited in comparison to the current evidence base for cognitive-behavioral interventions.

Psychosocial Intervention for Subthreshold Anxiety: A Prevention Strategy

In an attempt to prevent the onset and development of childhood anxiety disorders, Dadds, Spence, Holland, Barrett, and Laurens (1997) randomly assigned 128 children to a monitoring condition or a 10-week school-based child-and-family-focused cognitive-behavioral intervention derived from Kendall's (1990) *Coping Cat Workbook*. Participants in this study were children between the ages of 7 and 14 who had anxiety symptoms that were either subthreshold or sufficient for a *DSM-IV* anxiety diagnosis, but not severe enough to be markedly disturbing or disabling. Analyses indicated that the percentage of children meeting criteria for a full-blown anxiety disorder was diminished immediately following treatment, with no significant differences in the prevalence of anxiety disorders between treatment groups posttreatment. However, at 6-month follow-up, significant differences emerged between the two treatment conditions, with children in the intervention group demonstrating continued improvement and children in the monitoring group continuing to have a greater likelihood of meeting criteria for a *DSM-IV* diagnosis (56% vs. 27% in the intervention group). In addition, greater improvements in global functioning, anxiety symptoms, and avoidance behaviors were evidenced among children who had received the 10-week intervention both immediately following treatment and at 6-month follow-up.

It is of interest that, in a later study designed to investigate the long-term outcomes of the aforementioned intervention, Dadds and colleagues

(1999) failed to find any treatment group differences at 1-year follow-up. However, this phenomenon may be somewhat attributable to the monitoring group's exposure to an interpersonal coping skills treatment at that time. In fact, at 2-year follow-up, treatment group differences emerged once again, with children who received the CBT intervention experiencing greater clinician ratings of global functioning and having a significantly lower incidence of full-blown anxiety disorder diagnoses than at earlier assessment points (27% at 6-month follow-up, 37% at 1-year follow-up, and 20% at 2-year follow-up). Thus, this study suggests that a short-term psychosocial intervention may be efficacious in preventing the development of more severe anxiety disorders among children who have mild to moderate anxiety problems. Yet, the absence of group differences at several assessment points is curious and might be interpreted as evidence that the success of the psychosocial intervention may rest on its ability to buffer an anxious child's tendency to become more symptomatic during certain periods of time (e.g., periods of extreme stress).

OBSESSIVE-COMPULSIVE DISORDER

Obsessive-compulsive disorder (OCD) is one of the most widely researched childhood anxiety diagnoses to date. Possibly as a result of the greater body of research on this disorder, we have more empirically-supported treatments for childhood OCD than for any other anxiety disorder that manifests in childhood. Yet, even though several treatments have been demonstrated to be superior to placebo in treating OCD, it is important to remember that symptom improvement is not the same as symptom remission. Unfortunately, despite considerable improvement in the severity of OCD symptoms, an overwhelming number of children who participated in these studies continued to be relatively symptomatic . . . even after receiving these high-quality, closely monitored, empirically supported treatments.

In total, there have been five controlled research studies published since 1990—four of which explored the efficacy of pharmacologic treatments for OCD and one that compared the benefits of behavioral therapy to clomipramine. Although not a controlled study, a separate investigation explored the long-term outcomes of children who received a variety of treatments for OCD.

Pharmacotherapy for OCD

Two of the four pharmacotherapy studies for childhood OCD that have been conducted since 1990 focused on clomipramine (Anafranil) as the medication treatment of choice. As evidence of the efficacy of clomipramine in treating childhood OCD, DeVeaugh-Geiss and colleagues (1992) evaluated the treatment outcomes of 60 children and adolescents between the ages of 10 and 17 who were diagnosed with OCD and randomly assigned to an 8-week, double-blind trial of clomipramine versus placebo. Partici-

pants in the active treatment condition were administered 25 mg of clomipramine for the initial 4 days of treatment, with a gradual titration by the
end of the second week to a minimum of 75 mg/day and a maximum of
100 mg/day, depending on the participant's body weight. Results indicated
that participants' clinical improvement was greater in the clomipramine
treatment condition than that reported in the placebo condition, based on
both clinician and patient reports. An open-label extension of the clomipramine trial allowed the investigators to demonstrate that gains in the
clomipramine treatment group were maintained at 1-year follow-up. However, since there was no comparison group at 1-year follow up, we are unable to conclude definitively that clomipramine is a more effective long-term
treatment than placebo.

Following up on an earlier study (see Leonard et al., 1989) that found
clomipramine to be superior to desipramine in reducing obsessive-compulsive
symptoms in children, Leonard and colleagues (1991) conducted an
8-month double-blind study in which 26 youths who were receiving clomipramine maintenance treatment were continued on clomipramine for
3 months, randomly assigned to either a desipramine substitution or
clomipramine continuation condition for 2 months, and then reinstated
on clomipramine for another 3 months. The participants, who ranged in
age from 6 to 18, also received individual psychotherapy throughout the
course of the study. Although 6 of the 26 patients were dropped from
the study before its completion due to noncompliance, side effects, and
exacerbation of symptoms, an analysis of the remaining 20 participants
indicated that 8 of the 9 youths in the desipramine substitution group
relapsed during the 2-month medication change, whereas only 2 of the
11 patients in the clomipramine maintenance group relapsed during the
same period. Of note, however, is the fact that 7 of the 11 patients who
were maintained on clomipramine continued to exhibit significant fluc-
tuations in symptom severity throughout the course of the study, and only
3 of the 11 patients who were maintained on clomipramine experienced
a full clinical recovery from their OCD symptoms.

Additional analyses found that youths who received the desipramine
substitution had higher symptom ratings on three measures of OCD symptomatology (the NIMH Global Scale for OCD, the Comprehensive Psychopathological Rating Scale Obsessive-Compulsive subscale, and the
NIMH Obsessive-Compulsive Rating) but were not significantly different from the group that was maintained on clomipramine on two other
measures of OCD symptomatology (the Leyton Obsessional Inventory-
Child Version, Interference subscale, and the Obsessive-Compulsive Rating–Ward Scale). Separately, although youths who received the medication
substitution had higher scores on the NIMH Global Depression Scale,
they were not significantly different from the children who were maintained on clomipramine in their Hamilton Depression Rating Scale or
NIMH Global Anxiety Scale ratings. Thus, whereas the results of this study
present some evidence of clomipramine's ability to ameliorate OCD symp-

toms, it leaves unanswered questions about the effectiveness of clomipramine in remitting OCD symptoms across a number of outcome measures, possibly either due to insufficient statistical power resulting from relatively a small sample size or due to the modest effects attributable this medication treatment.

To examine the efficacy of sertraline (Zoloft) in treating children and adolescents with OCD, March and colleagues (1998b) conducted a randomized, double-blind trial of sertraline versus placebo in 178 participants between the ages of 6 and 17. Following a week-long placebo lead-in phase designed to eliminate placebo responders, children in the treatment group received 12 weeks of sertraline treatment, with doses of up to 200 mg per day. Results of the study indicated that sertraline was more efficacious than placebo in treating OCD, with benefits of the medication first emerging after 3 weeks of the treatment. Although sertraline resulted in clinically meaningful improvement for the participants of this study (42% of youths receiving sertraline versus 26% of youths receiving placebo were rated either *much improved* or *very much improved* on the Clinical Global Impression Scale [CGI]), the authors rightfully note that most patients remained in the mildly ill range on measures of OCD symptomatology at the end of this medication trial. Thus, the investigators concluded that although pharmacotherapy may be insufficient to fully support the recovery of OCD, additional promise might be found in using cognitive-behavioral techniques to enhance medication treatment outcomes. It is interesting that neither age nor diagnostic comorbidity was associated with different treatment outcomes in this study.

To examine the efficacy of fluoxetine (Prozac) in the treatment of OCD, Riddle et al. (1992) randomly assigned 14 participants between the ages of 8 and 15 to a double-blind placebo-controlled trial. The trial lasted for 20 weeks, with a crossover to either 20 mg per day of fluoxetine or placebo after 8 weeks. Although fluoxetine was associated with significantly greater improvement in OCD symptoms according to one clinician rating (Clinical Global Impression Scale-Obsessive Compulsive Disorder Scale [CGI-OCD]), no treatment group differences were evidenced on a separate clinician rating of OCD symptomatology (the Children's Yale-Brown Obsessive-Compulsive Scale [CY-BOCS]). In addition, children's self-reports of anxiety and obsessional thoughts failed to demonstrate differences between the effects of fluoxetine and placebo. Although improvement in anxiety symptoms was evidenced during both the fluoxetine and placebo phases of the treatment protocol, this study failed to provide strong evidence for the benefits of fluoxetine over those of placebo.

CBT Versus Medication for OCD

Investigating the relative efficacy of two OCD treatments, de Haan, Hoogduin, Buitelaar, and Keijsers (1998) randomly assigned 22 children between the ages of 8 and 18 to 12 weeks of either behavioral therapy or clomipramine drug therapy. If a participant failed to demonstrate a 30% reduction in symptom severity following the initial 12 weeks of treatment, an open-label extension was implemented in which the participant received a combination of both behavioral therapy and drug therapy for an additional 12 weeks. Participants in the drug therapy condition were assigned to 25 mg of clomipramine for the first week, with a gradual titration every 4 days to a maximum dosage of 3 mg per kilogram of body weight per day. In no instance did the dosage exceed 200 mg per day or the maximum tolerated by the participants. In contrast, behavioral therapy consisted of a combination of exposure and response prevention, which included some cognitive components. Results suggested that OCD symptoms, depression, and general psychopathology decreased over time in both treatment conditions. (Although this study lacked a no-treatment comparison group, it is reasonable to conclude that both treatments offer some benefits to children who suffer from OCD, because clomipramine has consistently been demonstrated to be superior to placebo in earlier studies [DeVeaugh-Geiss et. al., 1992; Leonard et al., 1991]). Additional analyses indicated that behavioral therapy was significantly more effective than clomipramine in reducing clinicians' ratings of symptom severity, although it was no more effective than clomipramine in reducing children's self-reports of the total number of symptoms they experienced. Thus, this research offers some evidence that behavioral therapy may be the preferred treatment for childhood OCD, but it provides even more compelling support for the effectiveness of combined treatment modalities . . . because more than half of the initial nonresponders showed significant improvement once they received a combination of clomipramine and behavioral therapy.

Long-Term Effectiveness of a Variety of Available Treatments for OCD

Although theirs was not a controlled study, Leonard and colleagues (1993) conducted a 2- to 7-year follow-up study of 54 children who had participated in a controlled study of clomipramine for the treatment of OCD. Because the majority of children who participated in the follow-up study had received treatments other than clomipramine after the initial clomipramine trial (96% had received alternative medications, 54% had been in individual psychotherapy that was not behavioral in nature, 33% had received behavioral therapy, and 20% had been in family therapy), this study was not able to isolate the unique long-term effects of clomipramine in treating OCD. However, this research does make an important contribution to our knowledge about the long-term effectiveness of a variety of available treatment options for childhood OCD.

Results of the initial medication study indicated that 44% of the participants no longer met criteria for OCD after 5 weeks of clomipramine treatment. Nonetheless, at assessment points 1, 2, and 3 years after they began treatment, 37% of the children still met full criteria for OCD. In addition, even the majority of children who no longer met full criteria for OCD continued to suffer from OCD symptoms and required ongoing medication treatment to stabilize their condition. Thus, among the total pool of participants, only 6% were considered to be in full remission, as they were relatively asymptomatic and were not being maintained on medication. Clearly, the results of this study point to available treatments' general ineffectiveness in fully "curing" childhood OCD. Yet, it is also important to bear in mind that participants' scores at follow-up consistently point to lower levels of anxiety, lower levels of depression, and improved global functioning than at baseline, prior to the initiation of treatment.

SEPARATION ANXIETY DISORDER AND SCHOOL REFUSAL

A total of five publications detailing the results of controlled treatment studies for separation anxiety disorder and school refusal have emerged since 1990. One article described two related medication studies, two studies explored the outcomes of CBT, and two studies investigated the benefits of augmenting CBT with medication.

Pharmacotherapy for Separation Anxiety Disorder

Bernstein, Garfinkel, and Borchardt (1990) conducted two studies to investigate the efficacy of alprazolam (Xanax) and imipramine (Tofranil) in treating separation anxiety with school refusal. The first study was an open-label trial in which 17 children between the ages of 9 and 17 were assigned to a multimodal treatment that included psychotherapy, a school reentry program, and medication. The duration of the medication treatment varied from patient to patient. Patients who were assigned to the alprazolam treatment group were given the medication two to three times each day, and the medication was increased by 0.25 mg every 3 days to attain a mean dosage of 1.43 mg daily. Alternatively, patients who were assigned to the imipramine treatment group received their medication once before going to bed, and the medication was increased by 25 mg every three days to attain a mean dosage of 135.42 mg per day. Results indicated that children in both treatment conditions showed improvement in anxiety and depression symptoms over the course of the study. Although both treatments appeared to be similarly efficacious, the lack of a no-treatment comparison group and the concurrent use of several therapeutic techniques preclude us from determining whether these effects were due to the medications, other elements of the multimodal treatment, or merely the passage of time.

In order to address the aforementioned problem, Bernstein and colleagues (2000) replicated the previous study with a double-blind comparison of alprazolam, imipramine, and a placebo condition. In this later study, 24 children and adolescents between the ages of 7 and 18 were randomly assigned to an alprazolam, imipramine, or placebo treatment condition for

8 weeks. Although initial analyses pointed to greater improvement in the medication treatment groups versus the placebo group, these treatment group differences disappeared after controlling for pretreatment differences in symptom severity.

CBT for School Refusal

King and colleagues (1998) examined the efficacy of using CBT to treat children who refused to attend school and, in many cases, carried a diagnosis of separation anxiety. In this study, 34 children between the ages of 5 and 15 were randomly assigned to either a 4-week course of CBT or a wait-list condition. The CBT treatment was primarily targeted to the child but also included parent and teacher training in child behavior management skills. Results indicated that children who received CBT had better school attendance, better coping skills, higher ratings of global functioning, and lower ratings of fear, anxiety, and depression. It is also noteworthy that these treatment group differences were evidenced across child, parent, and clinician ratings, and all differences were maintained at 3-month follow-up. However, these study findings are really not as robust as they may initially appear to be due to the failure of this study to control for the placebo effect. That is, the ratings on which the results of this study are based were produced by people who knew that the children receiving CBT were getting some form of treatment and that the children in the wait-list condition were not receiving any treatment. Thus, the raters' expectation that symptom improvement would result from treatment may have biased this study's findings in favor of CBT.

In a second study investigating the efficacy of CBT for the treatment of anxiety-based school refusal, Last, Hansen, and Franco (1998) randomly assigned 56 children and adolescents between the ages of 6 and 17 to either a CBT condition or educational-support (ES) therapy for 12 weeks. The ES treatment condition was designed as a no-treatment comparison condition, because it encompassed elements of supportive psychotherapy and psychoeducation but did not include core elements of CBT such as exposure, cognitive restructuring, and reinforcement for treatment-related gains. Thus, this research effectively addressed the concerns emerging from the aforementioned study.

The supportive therapy executed in this study was relatively structured at times, with children keeping diaries of the thoughts and feelings associated with their fears, the frequency with which they felt fearful, and the ways in which they handled their fears. However, participants in the ES condition were not taught strategies for handling their anxiety and were not reinforced for improvements in school attendance. The cognitive-behavioral treatment was based on the work done by Barlow and Beck (1994) with adult agoraphobics and consisted of two main components—systematic desensitization and cognitive restructuring. Results indicated that participants in both treatment conditions had better school attendance, higher global assessment ratings, decreases in self-reported anxiety, and a lessening of depressive symptoms. Moreover, the majority of children maintained these treatment gains at 4-week follow-up, with no difference in the maintenance of gains between treatment groups. Thus, this study suggests that CBT may be no more effective in treating school refusal than supportive therapies that incorporate a structured, psychoeducation component into the treatment format.

Due to the absence of a true no-treatment group, we cannot determine whether both treatments in this study offered equal benefits for the study participants . . . or whether the improvements experienced by these children would have occurred merely as a result of the passage of time. However, in light of King and colleagues' (1998) findings, it might be hypothesized that both of these treatments would be associated with improvements beyond that experienced by children on a waiting list. One wonders how children receiving these treatments might have faired in comparison with a group of children who received a placebo. In addition, the fact that 12 of the 28 children assigned to the CBT condition dropped out of treatment before the end of the study (compared with 3 of the 28 children assigned to the ES condition) raises concerns about the factors that may have contributed to this disproportionately high dropout rate.

Augmenting CBT With Pharmacotherapy for Separation Anxiety Disorder

In an investigation of the benefits of augmenting CBT with imipramine, Bernstein and colleagues (2000) surveyed adolescents who had been absent from school for at least 20% of school days in the last month. In order to qualify for this study, adolescents were also required to be postpubertal, between the ages of 12 and 18, and to meet criteria for a diagnosis of both major depression and at least one anxiety disorder. Sixty-three adolescents who met the selection criteria for the study and who failed to respond to a 1-week single-blind lead-in placebo phase were randomly assigned to an 8-week double-blind trial of either CBT with imipramine or CBT with placebo. The initial dosage of imipramine was based on participant's body weight and was titrated up by 3 mg per kilogram every 3 to 5 days, to a mean dose of 182 mg. CBT was based on an 8-week modification of the CBT treatment for school refusal described by Last and colleagues (1998). Results indicated that the group receiving CBT and imipramine experienced faster improvement and greater gains in school attendance. That is, after 8 weeks of treatment, adolescents who received CBT and imipramine had a 70% mean school attendance rate for the week, whereas those who received CBT with a placebo had a 28% mean school attendance rate. Although this study is promising in demonstrating the potential benefits of augmenting CBT with imipramine to increase school attendance, most measures of anxiety and depression failed to discriminate between the adolescents who received CBT with imipramine and those who received CBT with placebo.

After 4 weeks of behavioral therapy, R. G. Klein, Koplewicz, and Kanner (1992) randomly assigned 20 children with a diagnosis of separation anxiety disorder, who were between the ages of 6 and 15, to a 6-week, double-blind trial of imipramine versus placebo. It is noteworthy that only those children who did not experience significant symptom improvement following the 4-week course of behavioral therapy were entered in the subsequent imipramine trial. Thus, aside from the central hypothesis of the research, this study also offers valuable information regarding the efficacy of a short-term behavioral intervention in treating separation anxiety disorder. That is, out of 45 children who received 4 weeks of progressive, in-vivo desensitization, 20 of them continued to meet *DSM-III* criteria for separation anxiety disorder and to experience impairment significant enough to warrant their inclusion in the imipramine trial. Separately, although more than half of the children who initially presented with severe anxiety improved after the short behavioral intervention, the authors reported that most of these children continued to manifest symptoms severe enough to require additional behavioral treatment, beyond the initial 4-week period.

Among those children who failed to demonstrate significant symptom improvement following the 4-week behavioral intervention, 11 were randomized to receive 25 mg per day of imipramine for 3 days. On the 4th day, their dosage was increased to 50 mg per day, with gradual titration up to a maximum of 5 mg per kilogram per day. Throughout the medication trial, all children continued their weekly behavioral treatment sessions. Results indicated that participants' outcomes were comparable in both the imipramine and placebo treatment conditions, with mothers, children, and clinicians reporting between 40% and 60% global improvement. Thus, this study found imipramine to be no more efficacious than placebo in treating separation anxiety following a trial of behavioral therapy.

The results of this study run counter to earlier research conducted by D. F. Klein (1971, 1980), which found imipramine to be more efficacious than placebo in treating children who had school phobia with separation anxiety. In explaining this disparity, R. G. Klein and colleagues (1992) hypothesized that participants in their study may have presented with less severe pathology than the children sampled in the earlier studies, because their study did not require that children also carry a diagnosis of school phobia. Thus, it is possible that although imipramine may be beneficial for children with more complex symptom profiles, the medication may not be efficacious for the treatment of milder separation anxiety symptoms. An additional explanation for this study's failure to find a significant treatment effect for imipramine might be the small sample size. Although it is true that a sample of 20 children might have been insufficient to demonstrate statistically significant treatment group differences, R. G. Klein et al. acknowledged that their data failed to demonstrate any trends favoring imipramine over placebo. Thus, it seems highly unlikely that insufficient statistical power lies at the root of these research findings.

PHOBIC DISORDERS

To our knowledge, four controlled studies evaluating the efficacy of treatments for phobic disorders have been published since 1990. Although all of these studies explored the benefits of psychosocial interventions for phobic children, one study focused mostly on simple phobias, whereas the other three studies focused exclusively on the outcomes of children with a diagnosis of social phobia. At the present time, we are unaware of any controlled studies demonstrating the efficacy of medication in treating childhood phobias.

Psychosocial Interventions for Social Phobia

To investigate the efficacy of cognitive-behavioral group therapy for female adolescents with social phobia, Hayward and colleagues (2000) randomly assigned 35 participants to 16 weeks of either CBT or a no-treatment comparison condition. Although the investigators initially found greater improvement in phobic symptoms among the participants who received CBT, ratings of social phobia-related symptoms remained elevated in both groups posttreatment. With respect to diagnostic cutoff scores, it is noteworthy that 55% of the adolescents who received CBT met full criteria for social phobia immediately following treatment, versus 96% of the participants in the no-treatment group. However, at 1-year follow-up, treatment group differences in the incidence of social phobia failed to be significant, with 40% of the participants who received CBT and 56% of the participants who did not receive CBT continuing to meet full criteria for the disorder. Thus, although the CBT intervention appears to have produced an immediate reduction in phobic symptoms, long-term outcomes indicated that symptoms relating to social phobia may not have been significantly influenced by this short-term CBT intervention.

Drawing from an evidence-based treatment for adults with social phobia, Beidel, Turner, and Morris (2000) investigated the benefits of a multifaceted behavioral treatment for 67 children between the ages of 8 and 12 who were diagnosed with social phobia. The treatment, called social effectiveness therapy for children (SET-C), was designed to improve children's social skills and reduce their anxiety in social situations. With this in mind, SET-C consisted of child and parent psychoeducation (one session conducted with the family), social skills training (12 weekly 60-minute group sessions with four to six children), in-vivo exposure (12 weekly individual sessions lasting approximately 60 minutes), and "peer generalization" activities (during which children in the social skills training group joined in a 90-minute, weekly recreational activity with an equal number of nonanxious children for 12 weeks). Children were randomly assigned to either the SET-C treatment condition or a Testbusters control group in which children met both individually and in small groups weekly to parallel two aspects of the SET-C treatment format. Because the Testbusters program focuses on study skills and test-taking strategies, the study investigators believed that it would have face validity for socially phobic children, who often report anxiety under testing conditions. However, it is important to note that the Testbusters treatment condition did not control for the 90-minute peer generalization activities that accompanied the SET-C treatment condition.

Results of the study indicated that children who received SET-C experienced a greater reduction in social phobia symptoms than children in the Testbusters control group, according to both children's self-reports and clinician ratings. Consistent with these findings, 67% of the children who received SET-C no longer met the criteria for a diagnosis of social phobia posttreatment, in comparison with 5% of the children in the Testbusters group. Results such as these are particularly impressive in light of the fact that Social Effectiveness CBT was compared with an alternative treatment condition in this study, instead of a wait-list control. However, it is curious that other measures of emotional distress such as the STAIC failed to reflect any significant gains for the SET-C group beyond that experienced by the Testbusters comparison group. Of additional concern is the fact that observers' ratings of children's anxiety level during role-play exercises and children's self-ratings of the frequency and intensity of their distress in social situations failed to improve in either treatment group over the course of this study.

Exploring the benefits of CBT and parent involvement in the treatment of children with a primary diagnosis of social phobia, Spence, Donovan, and Brechman-Toussaint (2000) randomly assigned 50 children between the ages of 7 and 14 to either (a) a cognitive-behavioral intervention involving social skills training, cognitive restructuring, relaxation techniques, and in-vivo exposure; (b) a similar cognitive-behavioral intervention that also included parent training in modeling and reinforcing desired social skills and nonanxious behaviors; or (c) a wait-list control condition. Both treatment conditions consisted of 12 weekly sessions followed by one booster session at 3 months and a second booster session at 6 months. Sessions lasted for 1 hour and were followed by a half-hour games session, during which children were able to practice their social skills.

Results of the study indicated that children in both treatment groups experienced significantly greater improvement in anxiety and social phobia symptoms than children who were assigned to the wait-list condition. That is, in comparison with 7% of the children who were assigned to the wait-list condition, 88% of children who received CBT with parent involvement and 58% of the children who received CBT without parent involvement no longer met the criteria for a diagnosis of social phobia after the 12-week treatment period. Although no information was gathered regarding the wait-list control group at 12-month follow-up, the majority of children in both CBT groups maintained their treatment gains, with 81% of the children who received CBT with parent involvement and 53% of the children who received CBT without parent involvement continuing to be free of a diagnosis of social phobia. Although there was a trend in favor of the benefits of parent involvement, there were no statistically significant differences in the outcomes of children who received CBT with parent involvement and children who received CBT without parent involvement at any time during the course of the study.

A Comparison of Cognitive and Behavioral Techniques for the Treatment of Phobias

In an attempt to discern the relative benefits of various cognitive-behavioral techniques, Silverman and colleagues (1999) randomly assigned 81 children to a 10-week trial of either (a) graduated, in-vivo exposure with behavioral contingency management; (b) graduated, in-vivo exposure with cognitive training; or (c) educational support (ES). Unlike the two active treatment conditions, the ES condition did not involve an assigned exposure hierarchy and did not include coaching in ways to use cognitive-behavioral techniques to manage feared situations.

All three treatment conditions included both a child and family component, with weekly meetings involving 40 minutes alone with the child, 25 minutes alone with the parents, and a 15-minute meeting with both the child and parents. Participants in this study were between the ages of 6 and 16, and most of these children met the criteria for the diagnosis of a simple phobia. Results indicated that participants in all three treatment conditions experienced a reduction in phobic symptoms immediately following treatment and maintained these gains at 3-month, 6-month, and 12-month follow-up. Overall findings suggest that there were no significant differences in outcomes across treatment groups. However, the Anxiety Disorders Interview Schedule for Children (ADIS-C) and the Anxiety Disorders Interview Schedule for Parents (ADIS-P) pointed to lower posttreatment rates of diagnosis in the group that received cognitive training relative to the other two treatment conditions (12% vs. 45% and 44%).

Although the ES treatment condition was originally designed as a no-treatment comparison, the results of this study are consistent with Last and colleagues' (1998) findings that ES may be no less effective than other, more active CBT strategies. Still, it remains unclear whether all three treatments offered true benefits for these children or whether their conditions would have improved due to the passage of time or other nonspecific treatment factors. In addition, because all three experimental conditions involved parents in the treatment, it would be useful to explore the degree to which family involvement may have contributed to the improvement in child outcomes. Thus, the results of this study point to several new lines of research that are warranted to better understand the course of phobic disorders and the elements of treatment that are critical to influencing it.

GENERALIZED ANXIETY DISORDER

Since 1990, there has been only one controlled pharmacologic study investigating the efficacy of current treatments for generalized anxiety disorder in children and adolescents. Simeon and colleagues (1992) randomly assigned 30 children between the ages of 8 and 17 to receive alprazolam or placebo for 4 weeks. All children carried a *DSM-III-R* diagnosis of either overanxious disorder (70%) or avoidant disorder (30%); therefore, under the *DSM-IV* diagnostic system, most of them would be given a diagnosis of generalized anxiety disorder. The double-blind, placebo-controlled trial was preceded by a 1-week placebo lead-in phase in order to eliminate placebo responders. Depending on the participants' body weight, the initial dosage of alprazolam was either 0.25 mg per day or 0.50 mg per day, and dosage levels were increased every 2 days to reach a maximum dosage of 0.04 mg per day for every kilogram a child weighed (or, alternatively, to reach a dose sufficient to produce an optimal effect in the opinion of the clinician). Clinical global ratings appear to have favored the alprazolam treatment condition immediately following treatment, although these differences failed to reach statistical significance. In fact, although both treatment groups experienced improvement over time in ratings of anxiety, fear, withdrawal, worry, sleep, and psychosomatic problems, analyses failed to find significant outcome differences between treatment groups on 39 of the 45 assessed measures. Insufficient statistical power may have contributed to the general absence of significant findings, but it is noteworthy that across all six measures for which treatment group differences were evidenced, results favored the placebo condition over alprazolam. Thus, this study fails to provide evidence of the efficacy of alprazolam in treating GAD.

SELECTIVE MUTISM

We are aware of only one controlled study investigating the efficacy of current treatments for selective mutism; it explored the potential benefits of using pharmacotherapy to treat selective mutism. Thus, to our knowledge, we have no reliable information about the success of psychosocial interventions in remedying this difficult emotional disorder.

To evaluate the efficacy of fluoxetine in the treatment of selective mutism, Black and Uhde (1994) conducted a double-blind placebo-controlled experiment with 16 children between the ages of 5 and 16. The course of treatment consisted of two phases: Phase 1 was a single-blind, 2-week placebo trial to eliminate placebo responders, and Phase 2 ($n = 15$) was a double-blind, 12-week placebo-controlled trial. Participants assigned to the active treatment condition were administered 0.08 ml per day of fluoxetine syrup for 1 week, 0.16 ml per day for 1 week, and 0.24 ml per day for the remaining 10 weeks of treatment. Unfortunately, no statistically significant treatment differences were observed on most outcome measures, including ratings of elective mutism, anxiety, and social anxiety. However, parents of children who received fluoxetine did report a significantly greater reduction in mutism and improvement in global functioning than parents of children who received a placebo.

Despite the general lack of statistically significant findings, it is noteworthy that the average improvement among children who received fluoxetine was greater than the placebo group on 28 of the 29 outcome measures. Thus, it seems possible that greater statistical power might have uncovered treatment group differences that remain obscured by the small sample size of this study. It is also possible that the results of this study were limited by the short duration of the treatment. That is, because parent reports of children receiving fluoxetine improved considerably between Weeks 8 and 12 of treatment, it seems possible that a longer trial of fluoxetine might have produced more pronounced symptom change. Additional research into the efficacy of fluoxetine for the treatment of selective mutism is clearly warranted. Still, the limits of our ability to effectively treat selective mutism are highlighted by the fact that even children whose symptom ratings were significantly improved in Black and Uhde's (1994) study continued to be highly symptomatic posttreatment.

POSTTRAUMATIC STRESS DISORDER

To date, we are aware of only two published studies that explore the efficacy of current treatments for childhood posttraumatic stress disorder (PTSD) in comparison with a no-treatment control group. In both of these studies, cognitive-behavioral techniques were used to treat sexually abused children who were experiencing PTSD symptoms. Three recent studies have also attempted to evaluate the efficacy of psychosocial treatments for PTSD arising from single-incident stressors, using single-case experimental designs. In most cases, we have chosen not to include multiple-baseline designs in this review of the literature. However, we made an exception in our discussion of PTSD due to the relatively large sample size of these studies and the absence of other sources of empirical support for the treatment of childhood PTSD due to single-incident stressors. Still, it is important to note that the lack of a no-treatment comparison group in these studies precludes us from drawing more definitive conclusions about the efficacy of these treatment interventions.

CBT for Sexually Abused Children With PTSD Symptoms

In an attempt to evaluate the benefits of CBT in the treatment of PTSD symptoms among children with a history of sexual abuse, Deblinger, Lippmann, and Steer (1996) randomly assigned 100 children between the ages of 7 and 13 to one of the following treatment conditions: (a) 12 weekly, 45-minute CBT sessions with the child only (parents of children assigned to this treatment condition were given periodic updates on their children's progress, but no formal training was provided); (b) 12 weekly, 45-minute sessions with the nonoffending parents only, providing formal training in cognitive-behavioral strategies that could be applied to their children;

(c) 12 weekly, 80- to 90-minute CBT sessions divided between the nonoffending parents and the child; or (d) a comparison condition in which subjects were given information about PTSD and encouraged to seek therapy with other professionals in the community. Although 71% of the children met the full criteria for a diagnosis of PTSD, all of the children included in the study were experiencing at least three PTSD symptoms at the time of the study.

Results indicated that children who received direct treatment services experienced a greater reduction in PTSD symptoms. That is, the children assigned to Groups 1 and 3 were less likely to maintain a diagnosis of PTSD (16%) than the children assigned to Groups 2 and 4 (30%) following the 12 week treatment period. However, children assigned to treatment conditions in which parents received training in cognitive-behavioral techniques (Groups 2 and 3) experienced other benefits, such as reduced rates of depression (64% of the children in Groups 2 and 3 vs. 38% of the children in Groups 1 and 4 reported lower levels of depression after the 12-week treatment period), significantly fewer parent reports of behavior problems (36% in Groups 2 and 3 vs. 80% in Groups 1 and 4), and parents' perception that their parenting skills were more effective. Treatment gains across groups were maintained at 3-month, 6-month, 1-year, and 2-year follow-up (Deblinger, Steer, & Lippmann, 1999), offering strong support for the benefits of CBT interventions directed toward both children and the parents of children who are experiencing trauma-related symptoms as a result of sexual abuse.

A separate study by King and colleagues (2000) also explored the efficacy of CBT with and without parental involvement for the treatment of PTSD symptoms in children who had experienced sexual abuse. In this study, 36 sexually abused children between the ages of 5 and 17 were randomly assigned to receive either: (a) 20 weeks of individual, 50-minute CBT sessions with the child; (b) 20 weeks of individual, 50-minute CBT sessions with the child and 20 weeks of 50-minute training sessions in child behavior management and parent-child communication skills with the parent; or (c) a wait-list control condition. Of the children who participated in this study, 69% met the full criteria for a diagnosis of PTSD and, consistent with Deblinger and colleagues' (1996) study inclusion criteria, all were experiencing at least three PTSD symptoms at the onset of the study.

Results indicated that children in both CBT treatment conditions had lower rates of PTSD immediately following treatment (40% vs. 80%) and at 3-month follow-up (33% vs. 80%) than children assigned to the wait-list control condition. The benefits of the CBT interventions were also supported by significantly better outcomes on children's reports of emotional distress, parents' reports of their children's PTSD-related behaviors, and clinicians' ratings of overall functioning. However, a longer follow-up period and a comparison to an active treatment control condition would have provided a more rigorous test of the benefits of the CBT interventions. It is of interest that no significant differences were observed between the outcomes of children in the two CBT treatment groups, raising a question as to whether parent involvement truly does not contribute to improved outcomes in a group of children who are receiving individual CBT or whether the small sample size in this study might have limited the investigators' ability to discern the potential benefits of involving parents in the treatment.

Psychosocial Treatments for PTSD Resulting From Single-Incident Stressors

Using a multiple-baseline design to control for time trends and site-specific effects, March, Amaya-Jackson, Murray, and Schulte (1998a) assigned 17 children between the ages of 10 and 15 to an 18-week, manualized group CBT treatment. All children who were admitted to the study met the *DSM-IV* criteria for PTSD; and, in all cases, the syndrome was determined to have arisen from a single incident rather than a chronic, abuse-related stressor. The therapy, which was termed *multimodality trauma treatment*, consisted of several treatment modules that included psychoeducation, anxiety management, anger control, cognitive restructuring, and exposure with response prevention. Results indicated that, immediately posttreatment, 57% of the participants no longer met the *DSM-IV* criteria for PTSD; and, at 6-month follow-up, the number of children who no longer were eligible for a PTSD diagnosis grew to 86%. Significant improvement during treatment and in the 6 months following the termination of treatment was also evidenced across several measures of PTSD symptomatology and a measure of clinical global improvement.

In a study of 248 children between the ages of 6 and 12 who were experiencing high levels of PTSD symptoms 2 years after a major hurricane struck their community, Chemtob, Nakashima, Hamada, and Carlson (2002a) used a randomized, lagged-groups, multiple-baseline design to evaluate the efficacy of a 4-session, psychosocial treatment designed to help children: (a) regain a sense of safety, (b) grieve over losses and renew attachments, (c) express disaster-related anger, and (d) achieve a sense of closure regarding the disaster. Participants were randomly assigned to either an individual or a group treatment format, with both treatment modalities reflecting the aims and structure detailed above. A significant reduction in trauma-related symptoms and a lower rate of PTSD diagnoses (44% posttreatment vs. 88% pretreatment) was evidenced immediately following treatment and at 1-year follow-up, according to both children's self-reports and clinician ratings on trauma measures. No significant effects were observed for the passage of time in the absence of treatment, the type of treatment (group vs. individual), or the wave in which the treatment was administered.

In light of the fact that 44% of the children in the aforementioned study continued to meet the criteria for a diagnosis of PTSD 1 year after the completion of the 4-week psychosocial intervention described above, Chemtob, Nakashima, and Hamada (2002b) attempted to evaluate the efficacy of Eye Movement Desensitization and Reprocessing (EMDR) for this treatment-resistant group of children. Drawing from the group of children who continued to meet the criteria for a diagnosis of PTSD 1 year post-treatment and 3½ years after hurricane exposure, 32 children were randomly assigned to a lagged-groups, multiple-baseline study design in which children were assessed at fixed time intervals and received a 4-week EMDR treatment during the active phase of their group assignment. Results indicated that children experienced improvement in trauma-related symptoms, generalized anxiety, physiological symptomatology, negative affect, and worry immediately following treatment and at 1-year follow-up. In addition, 56% of these children no longer met the criteria for PTSD after receiving EMDR.

SUMMARY: TREATMENT IMPLICATIONS AND RECOMMENDATIONS FOR FUTURE RESEARCH

Unfortunately, as much as our review reflects state-of-the-art knowledge in the field, the most disappointing lesson seems to be an awareness of how little we truly know about treating childhood anxiety problems. Evidence for the efficacy of current anxiety treatments is limited by alarmingly little research with experimental designs, small sample sizes that limit the ability to discern true outcome differences, and inconsistent results across different outcome assessment measures (see Table 17.1 for a summary of research findings). And these issues do not even touch on those that limit our knowledge of the effectiveness of current treatments, such as the paucity of information about long-term outcomes and the highly complex symptom presentations that make the treatment of many children far more complicated than a single anxiety disorder diagnosis. Unfortunately, as little information as we have about the efficacy of childhood treatments, we have even less information about the *effectiveness* of these treatments in real-world settings.

Across the multiple treatments that have been researched, children often continue to be symptomatic, even if they are likely to experience some improvement in symptoms and functioning in response to evidence-based treatments. Generally speaking, the current evidence base offers reasonably consistent support for the efficacy of CBT for childhood anxiety (Barrett, 1998; Barrett et al., 1996; Kendall, 1994; Kendall et al., 1997). However, because most of these studies have compared the efficacy of CBT to wait-list control groups, an important question remains regarding the effectiveness of CBT above a no-treatment comparison condition that is blind to both recipients and raters. In addition, it remains unclear whether theory-based interventions such as CBT are any more effective than psychoeducational interventions or nonspecific supportive therapies (see results of Last et al., 1998, for example). Although there has been a recent emergence of promising new data relating to medication treatments for childhood anxiety disorders (e.g., see RUPP Anxiety Study Group, 2001), our knowledge about the efficacy of pharmacological interventions remains limited.

Research focusing on treatments for specific anxiety diagnoses may offer important guidance for clinicians. For OCD, CBT, clomipramine, and sertraline have all been shown to be efficacious treatments. Although there is limited evidence that CBT may lead to greater symptom improvement than medication treatments, the research seems to indicate that combining CBT and medication may offer the greatest benefit to children with OCD (de Haan et al., 1998; Leonard et al., 1993). CBT also seems to be the treatment of choice for children with a diagnosis of social phobia and PTSD. However, to date, evidence for the efficacy of psychosocial treatments for PTSD arising from events other than sexual abuse is limited. With this in mind, we need more research on the benefits of CBT, medication treatments, and other psychosocial treatments such as EMDR.

Unfortunately, very little may be concluded about available treatments for children who have simple phobias, generalized anxiety disorder, selective mutism, and separation anxiety disorder. Although research studies encompassing a range of anxiety disorders may lend general support for the efficacy of CBT in the treatment of separation anxiety disorder and generalized anxiety disorder (e.g., Barrett, 1998; Kendall, 1994; Kendall et al., 1997), we certainly need more information in these areas. Regardless of the diagnosis, the benefits of CBT may be enhanced by integrating family members into the treatment—particularly with younger children, girls, and children with parents who present with anxiety. Still, the benefits of family interventions with children receiving medication treatments have yet to be documented.

Additional research into treatments for childhood anxiety is clearly necessary. And as we plan future research endeavors, we should aim to make our research as applicable as possible to real-world treatment settings—but not at the sacrifice of experimental research designs. Thus, we need studies with more heterogeneous samples that evaluate the effectiveness of current treatments applied by therapists in naturalistic settings. At the same time that we are exploring new questions about which treatments effectively help which kids, it is also important to remain grounded in the basics—we need more information about the long-term outcomes associated with various treatments, we need large numbers of participants and sites so that we have sufficient statistical power to discern true outcome differences, and we need more confidence in the validity of our process and outcome assessment measures. As our knowledge about treatments for childhood anxiety increases, it would also be useful to explore the ways in which patient population differences (e.g., highly comorbid children vs. children with single diagnoses, children with internalizing vs. externalizing emotional problems, children of varying ages, and demographic group differences) may be systematically related to important child and family factors that mediate the effectiveness of various treatments.

Table 17.1. Summary of Research Findings and Methodological Shortcomings

Study	Results	Lack of Significance May Be Due to Small N	Inconsistent Results Across Measures	Inconsistent Results Across Raters	Inconsistent Results Across Time	Lack of Long-Term Follow-Up	Lack of No-Treatment Comparison Group
For a range of anxiety diagnoses:							
Barrett, 1998	CBT+FAM ≥ CBT > WL		X				
Barrett, Dadds, & Rapee, 1996	CBT+FAM ≥ CBT				X		
Cobham, Dadds, & Spence, 1998	For youths with anxious parents, CBT+PAM > CBT		X				X
Dadds, Spence, Holland, Barrett, & Laurens, 1997; Dadds et al., 1999	CBT ≥ Monitoring group		X		X		
Graae, Milner, Rizzotto, & Klein, 1994	Clonazepam = Placebo	X	X				
Kendall, 1994; Kendall & Southam-Gerow, 1996	CBT > WL			X			
Kendall et al., 1997	CBT vs. WL		X	X			
Research Unit on Pediatric Psychopharmacology (RUPP) Anxiety Study Group, 2001	Fluvoxamine > Placebo					X	
For OCD:							
de Haan, Hoogduin, Buitelaar, & Keijsers, 1998	Behavioral Tx ≥ Clomipramine		X	X			
DeVeaugh-Geiss et al., 1992	Clomipramine > Placebo						X @ LT F/U
Leonard et al., 1991	Clomipramine ≥ Desipramine	X	X				
March et al., 1998b	Sertraline > Placebo	X	X			X	
Riddle et al., 1992	Fluoxetine ≥ Placebo	X	X	X			

For separation anxiety:					
Bernstein et al., 2000	CBT + Imipramine ≥ CBT + Placebo	X			
Bernstein, Garfinkel, & Borchardt, 1990	Alprazolam = Imipramine = Placebo	X	X		
King et al., 1998	CBT > WL	X		X	
R. G. Klein, Koplewicz, & Kanner, 1992	Imipramine = Placebo	X	X	X	
Last, Hansen, & Franco, 1998	CBT = ES				X
For phobias:					
Beidel, Turner, & Morris, 2000	SET > Testbusters (active control group)	X	X		X @ LT F/U
Hayward et al., 2000	CBT ≥ WL	X		X	
Silverman et al., 1999	Exposure + BM = Exposure + CT = ES	X		X	X @ LT F/U
Spence, Donovan, & Brechman-Toussaint, 2000	CBT parent & child ≥ CBT child > WL	X			
For GAD:					
Simeon et al., 1992	Alprazolam = Placebo	X	X		
For selective mutism:					
Black & Uhde, 1994	Fluoxetine ≥ Placebo	X	X	X	
For PTSD:					
Chemtob, 2002	Post-Tx, fewer trauma symptoms				X
Chemtob, 2002	After EMDR, lower levels of anxiety and other measures of psychopathology				X
Deblinger, Lippmann, & Steer, 1996; Deblinger, Steer, & Lippmann, 1999	CBT parent & child ≥ CBT child or CBT parent alone > Community Tx	X			
King et al., 2000	CBT child = CBT parent & child > WL	X	X		X
March, Amaya-Jackson, Murray, & Schulte, 1998a	After CBT, lower rate of PTSD diagnosis	X	X		X

Note. BM = behavioral management; CBT = cognitive-behavioral therapy; EMDR = Eye Movement Desensitization and Reprocessing; ES = educational support; FAM = family anxiety management; F/U = follow-up; LT = long-term; PAM = parental anxiety management; SET = social effectiveness therapy; Tx = treatment; SET = social effectiveness therapy; WL = wait list.

In addition to research design factors such as participant composition, degree of treatment structure, compliance with treatment structure, and selection of treatment settings, it is likely that individual, organizational, and systemic factors also facilitate successful treatment outcomes in the real world or, alternatively, pose barriers to the translation of efficacious treatments into effective, available services (see Figure 17.1). These three mediators of the relationship between efficacy research and effective treatment practices have important implications for future research and children's treatment outcomes. Thus, all three of these factors need to be considered and addressed for efficacious treatments to be effectively translated to real-world settings.

Consider, for example, child and family factors such as parents' attitudes towards medications, a family's acceptance of the need for treatment, and the ease of getting the child to treatment. Clearly, without the parents' support of the treatment process, even the most efficacious therapy is likely to fail in real-world settings. On the level of provider and organizational factors, we have variables such as the training level of the clinician (who is often not trained in evidence-based treatment practices), the perceived usefulness of evidence-based treatment techniques, and size of the clinician's caseload. Unless providers are supported in their training and use of evidence-based techniques, ivory-tower treatment protocols cannot be effectively translated into available, community-based treatments. On the metalevel of systemic and societal factors, access to evidence-based services, cost of services, and lack of coordination between child agencies all continue to be barriers to the delivery of effective treatments. Future research will need to take these factors into consideration when determining whether results from efficacy studies or even many so-called effectiveness studies can be successfully applied to real-world treatment settings. Therefore, investigators may also want to incorporate some of these factors into future research designs.

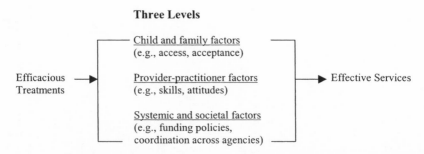

Figure 17.1. Barriers versus enhancers of delivery of effective mental health services

REFERENCES

Barlow, D. H., & Beck, J. G. (1994). The psychosocial treatment of anxiety disorders: Current status, future directions. In J. B. W. Williams & R. L. Spitzer (Eds.), *Psychotherapy research: Where are we and where should we go?* (pp. 29–69). New York: Guilford Press.

Barrett, P. M. (1998). Evaluation of cognitive-behavioral group treatments for childhood anxiety disorders. *Journal of Clinical Child Psychology, 27,* 459–468.

Barrett, P. M., Dadds, M. R., & Rapee, R. M. (1996). Family treatment of childhood anxiety: A controlled trial. *Journal of Consulting and Clinical Psychology, 64,* 333–334.

Beidel, D. C., Turner, S. M., & Morris, T. L. (2000). Behavioral treatment of childhood social phobia. *Journal of Consulting and Clinical Psychology, 68,* 1072–1080.

Bernstein, G. A., Borchardt, C. M., Perwien, A. R., Crosby, R. D., Kushner, M., Thuras, P. D., & Last, C. (2000). Imipramine plus cognitive-behavioral therapy in the treatment of school refusal. *Journal of the American Academy of Child and Adolescent Psychiatry, 39,* 276–283.

Bernstein, G. A., Garfinkel, B. D., & Borchardt, C. M. (1990). Comparative studies of pharmacotherapy for school refusal. *Journal of the American Academy of Child and Adolescent Psychiatry, 29,* 773–781.

Black, B., & Uhde, T. W. (1994). Treatment of elective mutism with fluoxetine: A double-bind, placebo controlled study. *Journal of American Academy of Child and Adolescent Psychiatry, 33,* 1000–1006.

Chemtob, C. M., Nakashima, J., & Hamada, R. S. (2002a). Psychosocial intervention for post-disaster trauma symptoms in elementary school children: A controlled community field study. *Archives of Pediatric and Adolescent Medicine, 156,* 211–216.

Chemtob, C. M., Nakashima, J., Hamada, R. S., & Carlson, J. G. (2002b). Brief treatment for elementary school children with disaster-related posttraumatic stress disorder: A field study. *Journal of Clinical Psychology, 58,* 99–112.

Clarke, G. N. (1995). Improving the transition from basic efficacy research to effectiveness studies: Methodological issues and procedures. *Journal of Consulting and Clinical Psychology, 63,* 718–725.

Cobham, V. E., Dadds, M. R., & Spence, S. H. (1998). The role of parental anxiety in the treatment of childhood anxiety. *Journal of Consulting and Clinical Psychology, 66,* 893–905.

Dadds, M. R, Spence, S. H., Holland, D. E., Barrett, P. M., & Laurens, K. R. (1997). Prevention and early intervention for anxiety disorders: A controlled trial. *Journal of Consulting and Clinical Psychology, 65,* 627–635.

Dadds, M. R., Spence, S. H., Holland, D. E., Laurens, K. R., Mullins, M., & Barrett, P. M. (1999). Early intervention and prevention of anxiety disorders in children: Results at 2-year follow-up. *Journal of Consulting and Clinical Psychology, 67,* 145–150.

Deblinger, E., Lippmann, J., & Steer, R. (1996). Sexually abused children suffering posttraumatic stress symptoms: Initial treatment outcome findings. *Child Maltreatment, 1,* 310–321.

Deblinger, E., Steer, R. A., & Lippmann, J. (1999). Two-year follow-up study of cognitive-behavioral therapy for sexually abused children suffering from posttraumatic stress symptoms. *Child Abuse and Neglect, 23,* 1371–1378.

de Haan, E., Hoogduin, K. A. L., Buitelaar, J. K., & Keijsers, G. P. J. (1998). Behavior therapy versus clomipramine for the treatment of obsessive-compulsive disorder in children and adolescents. *Journal of the American Academy of Child and Adolescent Psychiatry, 37,* 1022–1029.

DeVeaugh-Geiss, J., Moroz, G., Biederman, J., Cantwell, D., Fontaine, R., Greist, J. H., Reichler, R., et al. (1992). Clomipramine hydrochloride in childhood and adolescent obsessive-compulsive disorder: A multicenter trial. *Journal of the American Academy of Child and Adolescent Psychiatry, 31*(1), 45–49.

Graae, F., Milner, J., Rizzotto, L., & Klein, R. G. (1994). Clonazepam in childhood anxiety disorders. *Journal of the American Academy of Child and Adolescent Psychiatry, 33,* 372–376.

Hayward, C., Varady, S., Albano, A. M., Thieneman, M., Henderson, L., & Schatzberg, A. F. (2000). Cognitive-behavioral group therapy for female socially phobic adolescents: Results of a pilot study. *Journal of the American Academy of Child and Adolescent Psychiatry, 39,* 721–726.

Hoagwood, K., Hibbs, E., Brent, D., & Jensen, P. (1995). Introduction to the special section: Efficacy and effectiveness in studies of child and adolescent psychotherapy. *Journal of Consulting and Clinical Psychology, 63,* 683–687.

Kendall, P. C. (1990). *Coping cat workbook.* Ardmore, PA: Workbook Publishing.

Kendall, P. C. (1994). Treating anxiety disorders in children: Results of a randomized clinical trial. *Journal of Consulting and Clinical Psychology, 62,* 100–110.

Kendall, P. C., & Southam-Gerow, M. A. (1996). Long-term follow-up of a cognitive-behavioral therapy for anxiety-disordered youth. *Journal of Consulting and Clinical Psychology, 64*(4), 724–730.

Kendall, P.C., Flannery-Schroeder, E., Panichelli-Mindel, S. M., Southam-Gerow, M., Henin, A., & Warman, M. (1997). Therapy for youths with anxiety disorders: A second randomized clinical trial. *Journal of Consulting and Clinical Psychology, 65,* 366–380.

King, N. J., Tonge, B. J., Heyne, D., Pritchard, M., Rollings, S., Young, D., Myerson, N., & Ollendick, T. H. (1998). Cognitive-behavioral treatment of school-refusing children: A controlled evaluation. *Journal of the American Academy of Child and Adolescent Psychiatry, 37*(4), 395–403.

King, N. J., Tonge, B. J., Mullen, P., Myerson, N., Heyne, D., Rollings, S., Martin, R., & Ollendick, T. H. (2000). Treating sexually abused children with posttraumatic stress symptoms: A randomized clinical trial. *Journal of the Academy of Child and Adolescent Psychiatry, 39,* 1347–1355.

Klein, D. F. (1971). Controlled imipramine treatment of school phobia. *Archives of General Psychiatry, 25,* 204–207.

Klein, D. F. (1980). Separation anxiety in school refusal and its treatment with drugs. In L. Hersov & I. Berg (Eds.), *Out of school* (pp. 321–341). New York: Wiley.

Klein, R. G., Koplewicz, H. S., & Kanner, A. (1992). Imipramine treatment of children with separation anxiety disorder. *Journal of the American Academy of Child and Adolescent Psychiatry, 31,* 21–28.

Last, C. G., Hansen, C., & Franco, N. (1998). Cognitive-behavioral treatment of school phobia. *Journal of the American Academy of Child and Adolescent Psychiatry, 37,* 404–411.

Leonard, H. L., Swedo, S. E., Lenane, M. C., Rettew, D. C., Cheslow, D. L., Hamburger, S. D., & Rapoport, J. L. (1991). A double-blind desipramine substitution during long-term clomipramine treatment in children and adolescents with obsessive-compulsive disorder. *Archives of General Psychiatry, 48,* 922–927.

Leonard, H. L., Swedo, S. E., Lenane, M. C., Rettew, D. C., Hamburger, S. D., Bartko, J. J., & Rapoport, J. L. (1993). A 2– to 7–year follow-up study of 54 obsessive-compulsive children and adolescents. *Archives of General Psychiatry, 50,* 429–439.

Leonard, H. L., Swedo, S. E., Rapoport, J. L., Koby, E., Lenane, M. C., Cheslow, D. L., & Hamburger, S. D. (1989). Treatment of obsessive-compulsive disorder with clomipramine and desipramine in children and adolescents: A double-blind crossover comparison. *Archives of General Psychiatry, 46,* 1088–1092.

March, J. S., Amaya-Jackson, L., Murray, M. C., & Schulte, A. (1998a). Cognitive-behavioral psychotherapy for children and adolescents with posttraumatic stress disorder after a single-incident stressor. *Journal of the American Academy of Child and Adolescent Psychiatry, 37*(6), 585–593.

March, J. S., Biederman, J., Wolkow, R., Safferman, A., Mardekian, J., Cook, E. H., Cutler, N. R., et al. (1998b). Sertraline in children and adolescents with obsessive-compulsive disorder: A multicenter randomized controlled trial. *Journal of the American Medical Association, 280*(20), 1752–1756.

Research Unit on Pediatric Psychopharmacology Anxiety Study Group. (2001). Fluvoxamine for the treatment of anxiety disorders in children and adolescents. *New England Journal of Medicine, 344*(17), 1279–1285.

Riddle, M. A., Scahill, L., King, R. A., Hardin, M. T., Anderson, G. M., Ort, S. I., Smith, J. C., et al. (1992). Double-blind, crossover trial of fluoxetine and placebo in children and adolescents with obsessive-compulsive disorder. *Journal of the American Academy of Child and Adolescent Psychiatry, 31,* 1062–1069.

Silverman, W. K., Kurtines, W. M., Ginsburg, G. S., Weems, C. F., Rabian, B. & Serafini, L. T. (1999). Contingency management, self-control, and education support in the treatment of childhood phobic disorders: A randomized clinical trial. *Journal of Consulting and Clinical Psychology, 67,* 675–687.

Simeon, J. G., Ferguson, H. B., Knott, V., Roberts, N., Gauthier, B., Dubois, B. A., & Wiggins, D. (1992). Clinical, cognitive, and neurophysiological effects of alprazolam in children and adolescents with overanxious and avoidant disorders. *Journal of the American Academy of Child and Adolescent Psychiatry, 31,* 29–33.

Spence, S. H., Donovan, C., & Brechman-Toussaint, M. (2000). The treatment of childhood social phobia: The effectiveness of a social skills training-based cognitive-behavioral intervention with and without parental involvement. *Journal of Child Psychology and Psychiatry, and Allied Disciplines, 41,* 713–726.

Weisz, J. R., & Jensen, P. S. (1999). Efficacy and effectiveness of psychotherapy and pharmacotherapy with children and adolescents. *Mental Health Services Research, 1,* 125–158.

Weisz, J. R., Weiss, B., & Donenberg, G. R. (1992). The lab versus the clinic: Effects of child and adolescent psychotherapy. *American Psychologist, 47,* 1578–1585.

18

BRIDGING RESEARCH
AND PRACTICE
The Miami (United States) and
Leiden (Netherlands) Experience

WENDY K. SILVERMAN & PHILIP D. A. TREFFERS

A ll over the world, institutions for clinical child and adolescent psychology and psychiatry have developed specialized assessment and intervention research clinics for children and adolescents with anxiety disorders. The work conducted in these clinics has helped move the field forward in terms of yielding valuable knowledge about the nature of anxiety and its disorders in children and adolescents (hereafter referred to simply as *children*), and how to most effectively assess and treat these disorders.

With respect to treatment, the knowledge generated has been particularly valuable in yielding positive and strong empirical research evidence that anxiety disorders can be significantly reduced when children receive exposure-based cognitive and behavioral treatment procedures (see Silverman & Berman, 2001, for review). Despite the impressive achievements, accolades regarding the achievements often are tempered by concerns that the strategies and procedures used in research clinics are not generalizable for use in clinic settings (e.g., community mental health clinics; see Eifert, Schulte, Zvolensky, Lejuez, & Lau, 1997; Haynes, Kaholokula, & Nelson, 1999). That is, there exists a hiatus between clinical practice and clinical research (e.g., Kazdin, Siegel, & Bass, 1990; Silverman & Wallander, 1993; Weisz, Weiss, & Donenberg, 1992).

The existence of a hiatus between clinical research and clinical practice is a concern of much public health significance, because available evidence suggests that child and adolescent mental health services received in community clinics, particularly those in the United States, are *not* effective (e.g., Weiss, Catron, Harris, & Phung, 1999). In contrast, rates of positive treatment response of children with anxiety disorders have ranged from 60% to 90% in research clinics. In other words, children who receive services in nonresearch clinics generally do not fare well, especially in comparison with children who receive services in research clinics, including anxiety disorders research clinics. As a consequence, calls to bridge clinical research and practice have been published in the literature (Weisz et al., 1992), and creative ideas and suggestions have been offered about the bridging of research and practice. Many of these suggestions have focused on issues relating to rendering treatment manuals—a key feature of treatment research—more useful for clinical practice. Suggestions offered have included that treatment manuals should (a) provide sufficient detail so that specific interventions can be accurately implemented (Heimberg, 1998), (b) provide guidelines regarding when and how to switch treatments when a treatment is not working (Craighead & Craighead, 1998), and (c) emphasize the individualization of treatment by using a modular approach in which empirically derived decision rules can be applied to treatment targets as revealed by functional analyses (Eifert et al., 1997).

In general, an assumption that pervades the treatment research literature is that if nonresearch clinics begin to adapt strategies/procedures developed and evaluated in research clinics, then nonresearch clinics might begin achieving comparable treatment success rates to those achieved in research clinics.[1] This assumption needs to be established empirically, however, and such work is currently in progress (Chorpita et al., 2002; Weisz & Hawley, 1998). Even though it remains to be empirically established that the more clinic settings resemble research settings, then the greater the likelihood of positive child treatment response, myriad activities, procedures, and tasks comprise the assessments and treatments of research settings. So, even when it is empirically established that clinic settings that transport the assessments and treatments of research settings produce better outcomes than clinic settings that do not, it will require further empirical testing in research settings to determine the specific activities, procedures, and tasks that actually account for the positive changes observed (i.e., the actual mediators or mechanisms of change). Only when the mediators or mechanisms of change have been empirically established (i.e., *why* change occurs) will the field truly have the requisite knowledge regarding *what* needs to be transported to clinic settings. Despite the absence of empirical knowledge about the mediators of change in child anxiety treatment, we have some views and hypotheses about mediation. Some of the ideas expressed in this chapter regarding what should be transported are based on these views and hypotheses. The first author has recently embarked on a NIMH-funded project aimed at investigating these hypotheses about mediators of change in child anxiety treatment.

The ideas expressed in this chapter regarding what might be transported from research to clinic settings when working with children who have anxiety disorders are based on our experiences in actually doing this transportation. Specifically, Dr. Silverman, who has extensive experience in conducting randomized clinical trials in a research clinic setting, spent a sabbatical year in the Netherlands to consult with Dr. Treffers, who had the task of transforming a general child and adolescent psychiatric center into a department of an academic hospital and developing a child anxiety treatment program in that setting (described later in the chapter) that would represent a bridge between research and practice. This chapter is thus based on our actual experiences in bridging research and practice.

We begin by describing our respective clinical settings, to show the varied contexts in which we work (e.g., research-clinic setting versus clinic-research setting, psychology versus psychiatry), and some of the areas that need to be bridged. We follow this description with the historical context in which childhood anxiety disorders research clinics developed in the 1980s, because this context helps to explain the features that distinguished research clinics early on. Next, we present our conceptualization of mediators of change in child anxiety psychosocial treatments. These sections set the stage for the discussion of specific features of research clinics that we believe are most important to transport to a clinic setting such as the one we describe in the Netherlands. We conclude the chapter with a brief discussion of future directions that should be taken to help in bridging research and practice.

VARIED CONTEXTS

We work in very different contexts. Dr. Silverman is a psychology professor and a U.S. clinical child psychologist directing the Child Anxiety and Phobia Program housed in the Department of Psychology at Florida International University (FIU) in Miami. Dr. Treffers is a psychiatry professor and child and adolescent psychiatrist directing the Academic Centre for Child and Adolescent Psychiatry Curium, Leiden University Medical Center, the Netherlands.

The Child Anxiety and Phobia Program at FIU is part of the Child and Family Psychosocial Research Center under the auspices of the Department of Psychology. The anxiety program was initiated at the same time as the Center, in 1993. The Center is a research center that specializes in the development and evaluation of knowledge concerning child and family psychosocial treatment and prevention interventions. It is comprised of a number of programs and laboratories and provides multifaceted child and family interventions that include both clinic- and school-based services. A pragmatic orientation guides all the Center's clinical and research activities, as well as its efforts to bridge the gap between these activities. A pragmatic orientation grew out of the recognition that effective interventions can draw on many traditions (see Silverman & Kurtines, 1996a, 1996b, 1997). Assessment and the diagnostic workup of all children are free of charge; treatment is on a sliding fee schedule.

Within the Center, the Child Anxiety and Phobia Program (CAPP) has the distinctive mission of developing and evaluating approaches to assessment and intervention specific to the phobic and anxiety disorders of youth in a clinic setting. In striving to accomplish this mission, CAPP has focused over the years on two main objectives. The first objective has been on developing an organizational and budgetary infrastructure that will provide support for scholarly and research activities and actively pursuing the means (e.g., external funding, internal collaborative arrangement within and between disciplines, community involvement) for the conduct of psychosocial research with children and families. The second objective has been knowledge development and dissemination activities (e.g., scholarly publications in the form of journal articles, books, chapters) that contribute to the treatment of youth with phobic and anxiety disorders and the growing visibility of CAPP. Graduate students and postdoctoral fellows deliver the diagnostic assessment and treatment procedures to all children and families who present at CAPP, under Dr. Silverman's supervision. These individuals also are instrumental in helping to attain CAPP's knowledge development and dissemination objectives by developing and executing masters and doctoral theses at CAPP, also under Dr. Silverman's supervision.

The Child and Adolescent Anxiety Clinic of Curium, Leiden University Medical Center, Leiden, the Netherlands, is part of the Academic Center for Child and Adolescent Psychiatry Curium in Oegstgeest. Curium (founded in 1955), a center for child and adolescent psychiatry, comprises an outpatient clinic (22,000 operations each year), a department for day care (24 children), and a residential ward (87 beds). In addition, Curium recently developed the first specialized clinic and residential department in the world for deaf youth with severe psychiatric problems (Hindley & Van Gent, in press).

The mission of Curium is to provide inhabitants with child and adolescent psychiatric care, to train residents in child and adolescent psychiatry, to teach students of the Faculty of Medicine and the Faculty of Social Sciences of Leiden University, and to conduct research. With an eye toward research, the staff started the preparation of an outpatient Child and Adolescent Anxiety Clinic. As detailed later in the chapter, this involved a nonresearch clinic needing to adapt procedures derived from research clinics. Children who are referred to Curium are assigned to the anxiety disorders clinic on the basis of an intake screening. Assessment and treatment of children with nonanxiety disorders are done at the department. The assessment of children is mainly done by child and adolescent psychiatrists and residents (unstructured psychiatric interviews) and clinical psychologists (structured interviews and questionnaires). Psychiatrists, residents, and clinical psychologists mainly do treatment. Pharmacological therapy is reserved for psychiatrists and residents. All services are funded by medical insurance.

Similar to the CAPP at FIU, Curium's Anxiety Clinic is heavily involved in developing and evaluating approaches to assessment and intervention specific to the phobic and anxiety disorders of youth in a clinic setting. The first publications from the clinic appeared at the end of the 1990s, partly in collaboration with Dr. Silverman (e.g., Silverman, Ginsburg, & Goedhart,

1999; Silverman & Treffers, 2001; Treffers & Silverman, 2001; Van Widen-felt, Siebelink, Goedhart, & Treffers, 2002; Westenberg, Siebelink, & Treffers, 2001; Westenberg, Siebelink, Warmenhoven, & Treffers, 1999).

HISTORICAL CONTEXT

When the *Diagnostic and Statistical Manual of Mental Disorders,* third edition (*DSM-III;* American Psychiatric Association, 1980) was published, a new category of child and adolescent psychiatric disorders appeared: anxiety disorders of childhood or adolescence. Despite the increased coverage of childhood anxiety disorders in *DSM-III,* there was hardly any empirical literature to support the new classification scheme, particularly with respect to the subcategories. With regard to reliability, Rutter and Shaffer (1980) noted, "It appears extremely doubtful whether most of them would meet the second criterion of interrater reliability" (p. 383). Concerning validity, Rutter and Shaffer noted that "there is even less evidence for the nosological validity of the new syndromes" and that "little evidence could be found to justify the fine subdivisions" (p. 383). At the time, we would have further extended Rutter and Shaffer's statements about classification to treatment: With regard to the new syndromes and subsyndromes in *DSM-III,* there was no evidence about effective treatments.

What was done to help deal with these knowledge gaps? In the adult anxiety area, considerable strides in knowledge development were occurring, largely due to the establishment of adult specialty research clinics that focused on recruiting individuals with anxiety problems, forming homogenous groups of anxiety-disordered patients by using structured data-gathering procedures, and further assessing these patients by using other assessment methods (e.g., questionnaires, observations). These carefully diagnosed patients would serve as participants in randomized controlled clinical trials, similar to the trials used to evaluate the efficacy of medications, in which each would be assigned to either an experimental treatment condition (e.g., cognitive-behavioral treatment) or a control condition. Statistical comparisons between the two conditions would then be conducted to evaluate differential outcome.

In light of the success of this strategy with adult populations, it seemed reasonable to adapt a similar strategy with child populations. Hence, in the 1980s, childhood anxiety disorders specialty clinics were developed, and most focused initially on (a) developing and evaluating semistructured data-capturing instruments that would lead to reliable diagnoses of anxiety disorders in children and (b) studying these homogenous groups of children to empirically establish the external validity of the anxiety disorders categories and subcategories.

With respect to developing and evaluating semistructured data-capturing instruments (i.e., interview schedules), although there were respondent-based structured interview schedules such as the Diagnostic Interview Schedule for Children (NIMH-DISC; Shaffer, Fisher, Lucas, Dulcan, & Schwab-

Stone, 2000; Shaffer et al., 1993) and the Diagnostic Interview for Children and Adolescents (DICA; Herjanic, 1982; Reich, 2000) that were useful for epidemiological research, their coverage of anxiety disorders was light at the time, and their highly structured nature did not seem particularly useful for work with clinical samples. For this reason, Silverman and Nelles (1988) adapted the adult Anxiety Disorders Interview Schedule (Di Nardo, O'Brien, Barlow, Waddell, & Blanchard, 1983) and developed the Anxiety Disorders Interview Schedule for Children. Earlier studies on both interrater and test-retest reliability of the *DSM-III* and *DSM-III-R* anxiety diagnoses and specific symptoms using the ADIS-C/P demonstrated satisfactory to excellent levels of reliability (Silverman & Eisen, 1992; Silverman & Nelles, 1988; Silverman & Rabian, 1995). Positive support for *DSM-III-R* diagnostic reliability using the ADIS-C/P also was found in clinic samples in Australia (Rapee, Barrett, Dadds, & Evans, 1994). More recently, test-retest reliability of *DSM-IV* anxiety symptoms and diagnoses using the ADIS-C/P for *DSM-IV* (Silverman & Albano, 1996) was presented by Silverman, Saavedra, and Pina (2001). The ADIS-C has since been translated into various languages, including Spanish, Portuguese, Swedish, French, and Dutch, to allow for its use in different countries and cultures.

The accrual of large numbers of children and adolescents who present with different anxiety problems at child anxiety specialty clinics and the reliable diagnosis of these anxiety problems via semistructured and structured interviews allowed researchers in these clinics to move the external validation process forward. As proposed by researchers such as Robins and Guze (1970), Cantwell (1975), and Blashfield and Draguns (1976), different stages of the external validation process include providing evidence of distinct (a) sociodemographic factors, (b) clinical phenomenology or description, (c) psychosocial factors, (d) family genetic and family environment factors, (e) biological factors, (f) natural history, and (g) response to therapeutic interventions. In a recent review of this research, Saavedra and Silverman (2002) concluded that, overall, there seems to be converging evidence that anxiety disorders in children and adolescents have a reasonable degree of external validity. The empirical evidence is strongest when it comes to the broad category, however; the finer distinctions still require further research support.

The conclusion that the broad category of anxiety disorders in children and adolescents has a reasonable degree of external validity, but the finer distinctions have less, explains in part why most randomized clinical trials conducted in research clinics in the 1990s treated a broad spectrum of anxiety disorders (e.g., overanxious disorder, social phobia, separation anxiety disorder). Few efforts were made to develop and evaluate specific treatments for specific disorders. Additional features of the randomized clinical trials include (a) carefully selecting and identifying patient groups; (b) using manualized treatment protocols; (c) training, supervising, and monitoring therapists in the use of these protocols; and (d) assessing therapeutic targets at pretreatment, posttreatment, and follow-up.

Considerable evidence has accumulated from randomized clinical trials demonstrating that anxiety disorders in children can be reduced using individual child cognitive-behavioral therapy (Kendall, 1994; Kendall et al., 1997). There also now exists considerable empirical evidence from clinical trials that childhood anxiety disorders can be reduced when cognitive-behavioral treatments incorporate the family/parents context (e.g., Barrett, 1998; Barrett, Dadds, & Rapee, 1996; Cobham, Dadds, & Spence, 1998; Mendlowitz et al., 1999; Silverman, Kurtines, Ginsburg, Weems, Lumpkin, et al., 1999; Silverman, Kurtines, Ginsburg, Weems, Rabian, et al., 1999; Spence, Donovan, & Brechman-Toussaint, 2000), the peer group context (e.g., Barrett, 1998; Beidel, Turner, & Morris, 2000; Flannery-Schroeder & Kendall, 2000; Hayward et al., 2000; Silverman, Kurtines, Ginsburg, Weems, Lumpkin, et al., 1999; Spence et al., 2000), or both. This positive treatment evidence showing that exposure-based cognitive-behavioral treatments are efficacious using either an individual child approach or incorporating family/parents or peer group provides support (albeit indirect) for a transfer-of-control approach in treating children with anxiety disorders and provides the context in which cognitive and behavioral mediators (or both) or mechanisms of therapeutic change may work.

TRANSFER OF CONTROL

In accordance with the transfer of control (Silverman & Kurtines, 1996a, 1996b), the therapist is viewed as a consultant or collaborator who shares with or transfers to agents of child change (e.g., child, parents, peers) knowledge of behavioral and cognitive therapeutic strategies that can be used to facilitate the child's exposure to fearful or anxiety provoking situations, thereby producing positive treatment response (e.g., child anxiety reduction). The specific behavioral and cognitive therapeutic strategies that are transferred to (or used by) children, parents, or peers during therapy are hypothesized as potential mediators that lead to child anxiety reduction, in that they facilitate child exposures.

In child-focused individual cognitive-behavioral therapy (e.g., Kendall, 1994; Kendall et al., 1997), the transfer of control occurs directly from the therapist to the child himself or herself (see Figure 18.1). In this therapeutic context, a prime potential mediator is the content of child self-talk that has presumably changed (i.e., to less anxious and negative) as the therapist transfers to the child methods and procedures for changing self-talk. The less anxious and negative self-talk serves to facilitate child exposures, thereby leading to child anxiety reduction.

In peer-based group cognitive-behavioral therapy (e.g., Barrett, 1998; Beidel et al., 2000; Hayward et al., 2000; Silverman, Kurtines, Ginsburg, Weems, Lumpkin, et al., 1999), a transfer of control from therapist to child through peers occurs (see Figure 18.1). In this therapeutic context, prime potential mediators are prosocial behaviors and positive peer relationships displayed by children in the group, that have presumably changed (i.e.,

Transfer of control from therapist to child

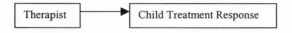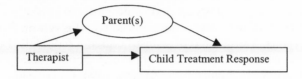

Transfer of control from therapist to parent(s) to child

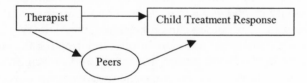

Transfer of control from therapist to peer group to child

Figure 18.1. Transfer of control

improved) as the therapist transfers—to peers in the group—methods and procedures for improving these behaviors and relationships. The use of improved child prosocial behaviors and peer relationships serves to facilitate other child group members' exposures, thereby leading to child anxiety reduction.

In family-based cognitive-behavioral therapy (Barrett et al., 1996), a transfer of control from therapist to child through parents/family members occurs (see Figure 18.1). In this therapeutic context, prime potential mediators are parenting skills and parent-child relationships that have presumably changed (i.e., improved) as the therapist transfers to parents in the family treatment the methods and procedures for improving parenting skills and parent-child relationships. The use of improved parenting skills and parent-child relationships serves to facilitate child exposures, thereby leading to child anxiety reduction.

In portions of the next section of the chapter, we show how the transfer of control approach and the cognitive and behavioral therapeutic procedures used in this approach, which are hypothesized mediators of positive child treatment response, have utility in determining features of research settings that should be transferred to or adapted in clinic settings.

TRANSPORTING/ADAPTING FEATURES OF RESEARCH SETTINGS TO CLINICAL SETTINGS

Selecting and Identifying Patient Groups

In most clinical settings, clinicians heavily rely on unstructured clinical interviews. This is notable because the literature on unstructured interviews has revealed very fundamental drawbacks—for example, the tendency to collect information selectively (McClellan & Werry, 2000). The lack of reliability and validity of unstructured clinical interviews renders it doubtful whether it is tenable to base clinical decisions exclusively on this method. In research clinics, a structured or semistructured interview is always used, because these reduce interviewer and criterion variance, thereby serving to increase diagnostic reliability (see Silverman, 1994, for review). Moreover, interview schedules can be helpful in charting comorbid disorders and determining which problems are interfering most in the daily life of the child.

It seems important to transport this type of structured/semistructured information-gathering method to clinic settings. This means that the intake of a child would involve the administration of a semistructured interview schedule. In an anxiety disorders clinic for children, the ADIS-IV-C/P (Silverman & Albano, 1996) seems to be an obvious candidate: It is the most widely used interview in childhood anxiety treatment studies. Semistructured in nature, the ADIS-IV-C/P contains specific questions that cover the diagnostic criteria for the anxiety disorders, as well as other internalizing and externalizing childhood disorders, described in the DSM-IV. The ADIS-IV-C/P also contains screening questions for other, less prevalent childhood disorders (e.g., sleep terror disorder). Additional qualities of the ADIS-IV-C/P are likely to be especially helpful to the clinician. These include questions that assist in providing a functional analysis and questions about the history of the problems and family members' reactions to the problems. All of this information contributes to case conceptualization and formulation.

In Curium, the first step in the development of an anxiety disorders clinic was the introduction of the ADIS-IV-C/P. Bart M. Siebelink and Philip Treffers translated the ADIS-IV-C/P into Dutch, in close collaboration with Dr. Silverman, and adapted it for use in the Dutch culture (Siebelink & Treffers, 2001).[2] Dr. Siebelink visited Dr. Silverman in Miami and received training from her and from CAPP staff in the use of the interview schedule. Subsequently, Siebelink trained the psychologists in Curium. Psychologists were allowed to conduct the interviews independently after matching diagnoses on five cases with a trained interviewer. Siebelink and Treffers have initiated a reliability study of the Dutch version of the interview.

There were obstacles connected with the introduction of the ADIS-IV-C/P in Curium, however. Even though it was emphasized that interview schedules can be considered as templates that guide clinicians' questioning, not as rigid, inflexible scripts (Silverman & Kurtines, 1996a), still, the introduction of a semistructured interview, conducted by a psychologist, was viewed as a "bad break" among some child and adolescent psychiatrists. Several of Curium's psychiatrists considered the introduction of the ADIS-IV-C/P as a betrayal of the unstructured psychiatric interview. The result of the interdisciplinary discussions was the decision that clinical psychologists would conduct the ADIS-IV-C/P with children and parents at the initial intake. Psychiatrists would subsequently conduct an unstructured clinical interview in the days to follow, especially focused on clarifying and elaborating on specific child problems and symptoms. Overall, in the year following the introduction of the ADIS-IV-C/P, there was a sharp decline in Curium's diagnoses of anxiety disorders not otherwise specified and dysthymia. This suggests that clinicians previously had overvalued nonspecific symptoms such as anxiety, depressed mood, and poor concentration that occur frequently in children with psychopathological conditions, just as fever and fatigue occur in many different somatic diseases (Caron & Rutter, 1991).

Using Manualized Treatment Protocols

One of the most central aspects of treatment research studies is that therapists are provided with a manual or protocol that delineates the main objectives, strategies, and procedures that are to be covered in the intervention's treatment sessions. Despite some difficulties faced in getting clinicians to use manualized treatment protocols of empirically supported treatments (for reasons we discuss shortly), we conveyed to the staff of Curium what the alternatives to empirically supported treatments are. The alternatives were expressed well by Kazdin (1999), who wrote of "empirically nonsupported treatments, nonempirically supported treatments, and . . . nonempirically nonsupported treatments" (p. 534). Helping Curium's staff to recognize these alternatives was helpful in laying the groundwork for the use of empirically supported treatments in this setting. In addition, it was conveyed to Curium's staff that manualized treatment protocols were beginning steps in working with children with anxiety disorders. We say *beginning* because we also made clear to Curium's staff the following idea conveyed by Chorpita and Donkervoet (2001): "Standardized treatments serve not so much as the panacea for the myriad of mental health difficulties facing our youth, but more likely as starting points for further innovation and development" (p. 336).

To elaborate on this point: We explained to Curium's staff that no treatment manual can ever be a substitute for sound theory/conceptualization as it relates to child anxiety disorders and the treatment of these disorders. Thus, when Dr. Silverman was on sabbatical at Curium, she gave a number of lectures and presentations to the staff that focused not so much on how to provide the treatment but on the transfer-of-control conceptualization (Silverman & Kurtines, 1996a, 1996b), especially the importance of exposure and the use of various therapeutic procedures, including behavioral and cognitive procedures, as a way to transfer control. She also emphasized that the clinical implications of the transfer of control are that there are multiple approaches (e.g., individual child therapy, parent-child therapy, peer group therapy), and there are multiple therapeutic strategies (e.g., child cognitive self-control training, parent use of positive reinforcement, peer use of positive reinforcement) that are likely to mediate positive treatment response. These clinical implications were very reassuring to the clinicians because they understood that they could be flexible and creative regarding the approaches and therapeutic strategies used in their work with children with anxiety disorders. That clinicians can be flexible in using treatment manuals without adversely affecting outcome also has been empirically demonstrated (Kendall & Chu, 2000). Thus, treatment protocols are starting points for further innovation and development (Chorpita & Donkervoet, 2001)—but one cannot innovate and develop if one lacks a conceptualization of the treatment described in the protocol.

Hence, in keeping with the transfer-of-control approach, a supplementary protocol was developed (Van Widenfelt, 2001a) in which the transfer of control from therapist to child via cognitive-behavioral therapy was supplemented with a transfer of control from therapist to parent to child. Thus, increased parental involvement via targeting parent psychopathology, parental expectations, and parent-child communication and problem solving was supplemented. Therapist- and parent-assisted in-session and out-of-session exposure exercises were conducted as described by Silverman and Kurtines (1996). Children who were not helped sufficiently by the protocol that used a therapist-to-child transfer of control would be enrolled in this supplementary protocol. This *stepped-care* model is consistent with recent recommendations in the literature: "In this approach, lower cost interventions are tried first, with more intensive and costly interventions reserved for those insufficiently helped by the initial intervention" (Haaga, 2000, p. 547).

Nevertheless, obstacles were faced in attempting to introduce any anxiety-protocolized treatment to Curium's staff. The introduction of a treatment protocol, consisting of 12 sessions, was considered as a devaluation of traditional nonprotocolized forms of therapy, be it behavioral or psychodynamic therapy. It appeared very difficult to expect experienced therapists to follow a protocol. Therefore, the staff was increased with young therapists who were prepared to execute protocolized exposure-based cognitive-behavioral treatments. Another objection to this proposal clearly had to do with interdisciplinary rivalry: Cognitive-behavioral therapy was considered an exclusively psychological treatment. Some psychiatrists pleaded for pharmacological treatment of anxiety disorders. Here, a "grand round" about the lack of empirical evidence for this form of treatment (with the exception of OCD and panic disorder) was convincing.

Training, Supervising, and Monitoring Therapists

All therapists involved in treatment research studies receive careful and intensive training in the proper administration of the interventions. Although different settings may vary in specific procedures used to train therapists, general procedures involve the following: Therapists first familiarize themselves with the treatment protocols, followed by both didactic and clinical training via extensive role-playing of the interventions' procedures. Therapists also study videotapes of interventions employed by successful therapists, and they are required to treat successfully at least one case using the particular intervention under investigation, under observation/supervision, prior to admittance as a therapist. During the treatment research studies, therapists receive weekly on-site supervision meetings to prepare for upcoming sessions and to process sessions just completed. Also during the projects, treatment sessions are videotaped, and therapists are usually aware that a proportion of these tapes will be selected for treatment-integrity checks. The latter undoubtedly serves to increase therapists' adherence to the treatment manual. In Curium, this procedure was followed as much as possible: Therapists were trained and supervised by experienced cognitive-behavioral therapists.

Assessing Therapeutic Targets

All treatment research studies involve rather extensive multisource-multimethod assessment procedures. At CAPP, for example, as in most other research clinic settings, the initial administration of the assessment measures (interviews and questionnaires) is conducted in two separate sessions within a 2-week period. During the first session, all children and parents are administered the ADIS-IV-C/P (Silverman & Albano, 1996). The interviews are administered to the children and parents in a randomly determined order. While one source is being interviewed, the other is completing a series of questionnaires, with assistance by a staff member as needed. During the second session, questionnaires that were not completed at the first session are completed, and any additional assessment procedures that are needed are administered. The assessment procedure is conducted at baseline (prior to Treatment Session 1), posttreatment, and at two follow-up points (6 and 12 months following treatment).

At CAPP, child treatment response (i.e., anxiety reduction) is assessed on two main levels. The first is a *global level* via severity and interference levels as rated by clinician, child, and parents. More specifically, each of these sources' are asked to consider, overall, how the child's anxiety symptoms interfere with respect to school (e.g., deteriorating academic performance), peer relationships (little or no social interaction), family life (e.g., leads to family disruption) and child internal distress (e.g., child is upset or distraught about symptoms). The overall impairment ratings are made using the rating scale contained in the ADIS-IV-C/P, which includes a 9-point scale ranging from 0 to 8, with adverb qualifiers underneath selected points (e.g., *no severity* to *disruption of functioning*).

The second way that child treatment response is assessed in most research clinic settings, including CAPP, is on a *specific symptom level* as rated by children and parents, using a variety of questionnaires. The most widely used questionnaires in child anxiety treatment research have been the Children's Manifest Anxiety Scale–Revised (RCMAS; Reynolds & Richmond, 1985), the Revised Fear Survey Schedule for Children (FSSC-R; Ollendick, 1983), and the Child Behavior Checklist (CBCL; Achenbach, 1991), particularly the internalizing scales. Additional measures are typically administered to assess other variables relevant toward advancing understanding regarding factors that influence child treatment response, such as levels of child depression, parental psychopathology, and so on.

In Curium, it appeared possible to introduce the assessment of the child treatment response on both the global and specific symptom levels. At the end of the treatment, all the anxiety disorders that are covered on the ADIS-IV-C/P are assessed by using both child and parent interview versions. For the purpose of an assessment on the specific symptom level at pre- and posttreatment, several additional measures were included in the battery. These included the Multidimensional Anxiety Scale for Children (MASC; March, Parker, Sullivan, Stallings, & Conners, 1997; Utens & Ferdinand, 2000), the Negative Affectivity Self-Statement Questionnaire for Children (NASSQ; Ronan, Kendall, & Rowe, 1994; Van Widenfelt & Treffers, 2000), and the Childhood Anxiety Sensitivity Index (CASI; Silverman, Fleisig, Rabian, & Peterson, 1991; Treffers, Westenberg, & Siebelink, 1998; Van Widenfelt et al., 2002).

The implementation of questionnaires in clinical work requires careful dealing with logistical issues: the staff should not be overburdened, and the same holds true for parents and children. It is a good idea to supply the clinicians as soon as possible with feedback on the data obtained on an individual child, and if possible to connect the obtained data with any existing normative data. In this way, the clinicians are helped to recognize the value in collecting these assessment data on the children for reasons beyond research. Fortunately, because Curium has a tradition of systematic collection of patient data (Treffers, Goedhart, Waltz, & Koudijs, 1990), the administration of an assessment battery to children and families was not met with much staff resistance. The staff of Curium also are well aware of the problems of the translation and cultural adaptation of instruments from the United States or the United Kingdom, realizing that culture may moderate the expression of fears (e.g., Shore & Rapport, 1998). The point of departure is thus to determine the reliability and validity of adapted instruments as critically as the psychometric data of the original instruments (Treffers, 2001; Van Widenfelt, 2001b).

FUTURE DIRECTIONS

In this chapter, we have shared our experiences in bridging research and practice with respect to a research clinic facility in Miami and a clinic research facility in Leiden. Although we believe that we have built a reasonably sound research/practice bridge, we recognize that our efforts to transport empirically based knowledge activities and procedures from CAPP in Miami to Curium in Leiden involved some constraints that were not simply due to practical/logistical issues (e.g., getting staff members to agree to use protocolized treatments), but also due to limits in current empirical knowledge. As we pointed out at the beginning of the chapter, for example, only when mediators or mechanisms of change have been empirically established (i.e., *why* change occurs) will the field truly have the requisite knowledge regarding *what* needs to be transported to clinic settings. We thus have shared in this chapter our views regarding the transfer of control and how this is a useful model that allows one to think about potential mediational candidates/variables (e.g., content of child self-talk in individual therapy, training social skills and peer relationships in peer-group therapy, training parent skills and parent-child relationships in family-based therapy) and how these candidates/variables influence notions about the specific procedures to be transported to clinic setting. As we have noted, however, these views are currently undergoing empirical testing.

Moderators of Treatment Outcome

In addition to mediation, however, there remain other unresolved issues that, until empirically resolved, will continue to deter the bridging of research and practice. For example, even when the mediators suggested by the transfer-of-control approach have been empirically established, these mediators are likely to interact in different ways with other variables (i.e., *moderators*) and the combination of these variables, such as child and parent characteristics, to influence outcome. In other words, the mediators also will likely depend on, or vary with, various moderators.

To date, with respect to child and parent background variables such as gender, ethnic, socioeconomic class, and age, with the exception of the findings of Barrett et al. (1996a) that younger children responded better to family-based treatment than individual treatment, other investigations (e.g., Berman, Weems, Silverman, & Kurtines, 2000; Treadwell, Flannery-Schroeder, & Kendall, 1995) have not found gender, ethnic, socioeconomic class, or age to moderate childhood anxiety cognitive-behavioral treatment approaches. Although child depression was found to moderate outcome in the Berman et al. (2000) study, future research is needed to examine the robustness of this finding because other studies (e.g., Kendall, Brady, & Verduin, 2001) did not evaluate the potential role of this variable.

It therefore seems very important to continue to conduct research on possible moderators of child anxiety treatment. As Kazdin (1999) has noted, however, the evaluation of moderators can be endless if one does not have a treatment theory or conceptualization of change. We view the transfer-of-control model as a useful framework for selecting relevant moderator variables, because some variables can be hypothesized as more likely to block or impede the transfer of control than others (e.g., parent psychopathology can block or interfere with the mediational role of parenting skills in family-based treatments). Those variables that block or interfere are the ones worth investigating as potential moderators. Nevertheless, a full and complete evaluation of variables as potential moderators has considerable power requirements that are rarely seen in most clinical trials, thereby increasing the difficulties in conducting research on moderators. At a minimum, though, and as an exploratory step, we recommend investigators to routinely include participant background variables such as comorbidity, medication status, parent anxiety, life events, and type of family structure/caregiver involvement in treatment as covariates in their testing of potential models.

Prescriptive Treatment

As noted by March and Curry (1998), knowledge of moderator variables is important, because such knowledge could lead to tailoring interventions that meet the specific set of circumstances for a child and his or her family. We would suggest, however, that even if particular variables are identified as moderators, it still remains an unanswered empirical question whether tailoring a treatment that meets those specific circumstances leads to a more improved outcome than a treatment that does not meet those specific circumstances.

Hence, there is a need for further research on prescriptive treatments in which children receive a given treatment (or a "prescribed" treatment) based on certain characteristics/variables. In treating generalized anxiety in children, for example, Eisen and Silverman (1993, 1998) provided preliminary evidence suggesting that a prescriptive approach can be useful. Using a multiple-baseline design across participants, Eisen and Silverman (1998) systematically prescribed specific cognitive-behavioral interventions, cognitive therapy and relaxation training, to different problematic response classes (i.e., cognitive and somatic). Participants were four overanxious children (aged 8 to 12 years) who were randomly assigned to experimental and control conditions. Experimental participants received 5 weeks of prescriptive treatment (i.e., cognitive therapy for worry symptoms, relaxation therapy for somatic symptoms). Control participants, on the other hand, first received 5 weeks of nonprescriptive treatment (i.e., relaxation therapy for worry symptoms; cognitive therapy for somatic symptoms), followed by 5 weeks of prescriptive treatment. Children with a problematic response class that was primarily cognitive responded most favorably to cognitive therapy; children with a problematic response class that was primarily somatic responded most favorably to relaxation training. If findings such as these are replicated in other research settings, then the implication would be that clinicians might consider prescribing different facets of an empirically supported treatment depending on the characteristics or needs of participants.

Varying Treatment Duration

Developing and evaluating treatment programs of specified lengths or duration (e.g., 10 weeks/sessions, 14 weeks/sessions) made a great deal of sense in the early treatment efficacy stage in childhood anxiety disorders. From a research perspective, evaluating a treatment of a specified length that was administered to all participants in an identical manner (e.g., weekly, 60 minutes) provided systematic and direct control of these important variables. From a practical perspective, evaluating a short-term, time-limited treatment program provided further evidence for the type of therapy that was particularly needed during the zeitgeist of the 1990s, in which third-party payers and HMOs had become much more financially restrictive with respect to reimbursement for medical care, in general, and mental health care, in particular.

Despite the research and practical rationale for evaluating treatments of specified lengths, the reality in most clinic settings is that therapy is rarely so specific in terms of duration. In fact, the average length of treatment received by most children and families in the mental health setting is not even as high as what is being evaluated in the efficacy trials, but instead hovers at about three to five sessions (Kazdin et al., 1990). However, there also are those children and families who stay in therapy for long periods of time, because they require support for or help with a wide of issues that crop up in their daily lives. There also are families who attend therapy on a now-and-then basis, receiving booster sessions as needed.

From a research perspective, there is a need to develop and evaluate interventions that reflect these varying lengths and patterns of therapy attendance. Although this type of research poses many methodological challenges, some of the methods and data analytic strategies procedures used by Howard, Moras, Brill, Martinovich, and Lutz (1996) in the adult psychotherapy area, and developments in other analytic areas (e.g., growth curve analyses; Duncan, Duncan, Strycker, Li, & Alpert, 1999), seem to be important tools. Once the results of such research are obtained, researchers would be in a better position to inform clinicians about the implications of varying lengths, client attendance patterns, or both on outcome, and clinicians could then adjust treatments accordingly.

Impaired But Not Diagnosed

When most children and parents present to general outpatient mental health clinics (e.g., community mental health centers, private practice), it is usually because the children are showing disturbing or severe deterioration/impairment in functioning in multiple areas, such as school, peer relationships, and family relationships; they are showing increasing signs of distress about their functioning or lack thereof; or both (Angold, Costello, Farmer, Burns, & Erkanli, 1999). Moreover, although in some cases, children's deterioration may be due entirely to anxiety and its disorders, more commonly, it is due to myriad different factors (e.g., other comorbid disorders, upsetting life events). In light of this clinical reality, we believe that treatment research's continued emphasis on DSM primary diagnoses of anxiety disorders and anxiety symptoms as the main inclusion criteria and the main outcome variables is somewhat misplaced. We believe it is important for childhood anxiety research clinics to improve their ways of assessing clinical impairment among children and to develop and evaluate interventions that are geared not just toward reducing primary anxiety diagnoses, but also toward reducing clinical impairment and associated disorders/symptoms. A refocus on children's impairment and comorbid/associated disorders/symptoms will help in future efforts to bridge research and practice.

Multidisciplinary and Transdisciplinary Collaborative Work

Which disciplines should be represented in an anxiety disorder clinic? In the United States, clinical psychologists often run child anxiety specialty clinics without the contribution of other professions. The drawback of this situation is that some medical diseases presenting as anxiety disorders, especially epilepsy (Laidlaw & Maung-Zaw, 1993; Lee, Helmers, Steingard, & DeMaso, 1997; Pegna, Perri, & Lenti, 1999), might be unrecognized. But it remains a debatable question whether it can be expected that a child psychiatrist in clinical practice would recognize these extremely rare conditions any better than an experienced clinical psychologist. Of course, it is essential that psychologists be aware of the existence of these possible conditions and know which cues are signals of an underlying medical disease. The same holds true for the presentation of anxiety disorders in the context of other psychiatric disorders (e.g., a pervasive developmental disorder, or as a prodrome of a psychotic disorder).

Another possible drawback of a monodisciplinary clinic is that some children who are referred to the clinic may be on some form of medication. Although the initial clinic trials excluded children from participating in the study if the children were on pharmacological agents (e.g., Kendall, 1994; Kendall et al., 1997; Silverman, Kurtines, Ginsburg, Weems, Lumpkin, et al., 1999; Silverman, Kurtines, Ginsburg, Weems, Rabian, et al., 1999), it now seems more common for clinical trials to include children on medications so as not to limit generalizability by excluding partial pharmacological responders. In clinic settings, a certain proportion of children also are likely to be on medications. For example, in 1995 in the United States, the number of office visits resulting in a selective serotonin reuptake inhibitor (SSRI) prescription for patients younger than 18 was about 350,000 (Jensen et al., 1999). Compared with their use in the United States, the use of SSRIs for children is more limited in Holland.

Nevertheless, it seems increasingly important for monodisciplinary clinics, particularly those in the United States, to develop some relationship with a psychiatrist who can serve, at a minimum, in a consulting role. As a consultant, the psychiatrist can help to ensure that those children who are included in the treatment (e.g., children on a selected set of anxiolytic medications such as SSRIs, buspirone, clonazepam) meet very clear requirements for a stable baseline and for no variation other than for adverse events during the course of treatment (e.g., hold constant).

We think the development of child anxiety clinics that allow for multi- and transdisciplinary collaborative work holds particular excitement, given new developments in neuropsychiatry and neurosciences: for example, neuroimaging studies suggesting a larger volume of the amygdala in children and adolescents with generalized anxiety disorder (DeBellis et al., 2000) and abnormalities in the response of the right amygdala to fear stimuli in anxious children (Thomas et al., 2001). Also, such collaboration would facilitate clinical trials that focus on the evaluation of medication usage in anxiety-disordered children (e.g., sertraline) in conjunction with, or in comparison with, psychosocial intervention.

CONCLUSION

It is our view that the bridging of research and practice is a prerequisite for the prosperous development of both research and clinical practice. Research on clinical conditions loses its goal when its attainments are not implemented in clinical practice, especially given that the rationale underlying clinical practice is to relieve the distress of children and families as much as possible. To us, "as much as possible" is via empirically supported methods.

We indicated that exposure-based cognitive-behavioral therapy is the most empirically supported intervention and that the therapy "works" using either an individual child approach, incorporating parents, the peer group, or both. We also indicated that these various approaches represent diverse pathways for a transfer of control (i.e., from therapist to child, from therapist to parent to child, from therapists to peer group to child). In addition, we discussed how a transfer-of-control model suggests potential mediators of positive child treatment response (e.g., in treatments incorporating the parent, improved parenting skills may facilitate child exposures, thereby leading to child anxiety reduction). Portions of the chapter subsequently discussed how transfer of control and its suggestive potential mediators provide suggestions about specific therapeutic procedures of exposure-based cognitive-behavioral therapy that might be transported or adapted in clinic settings. The chapter also covered other features of research settings that might be transported or adapted to clinic settings and we showed how this was done in terms of our experiences in Miami (United States) and Leiden (Netherlands).

We close with a conclusion drawn by Rush (1812/1962, p. 97) nearly two centuries ago: "Blessed science! Which thus extends its friendly empire, not only over the evils of the bodies, but those of the minds, of the children of men!"

NOTES

1. We would like to note that there are many things, in turn, that researchers need to do to render their work more applicable to the needs of clinicians. See Kazdin et al. (1990) for a discussion of this issue.

2. The Dutch version of the ADIS-IV-C/P soon became popular in the Netherlands: it was introduced in a short time in at least three Dutch centers for child and adolescent psychiatry.

REFERENCES

Achenbach, T. M. (1991). *Manual for the Child Behavior Checklist and Revised Child Behavior Profile.* Burlington: University of Vermont, Department of Psychiatry.

American Psychiatric Association. (1980). *Diagnostic and statistical manual of mental disorders* (3rd ed.). Washington, DC: Author.

Angold, A., Costello, E. J., Farmer, E. M., Burns, B. J., & Erkanli, A. (1999). Impaired but undiagnosed. *Journal of the American Academy of Child and Adolescent Psychiatry, 38,* 129–137.

Barrett, P. M. (1998). Evaluation of cognitive-behavioral group treatments for childhood anxiety disorders. *Journal of Clinical Child Psychology, 27,* 459–468.

Barrett, P. M., Dadds, M. R., & Rapee, R. M. (1996). Family treatment of childhood anxiety: A controlled trial. *Journal of Consulting and Clinical Psychology, 64,* 333–342.

Beidel, D. C., Turner, S. M., & Morris, T. L. (2000). Behavioral treatment of childhood social phobia. *Journal of Consulting and Clinical Psychology, 68,* 1072–1080.

Berman, S. L., Weems, C. F., Silverman, W. K., & Kurtines, W. M. (2000). Predictors of outcome in exposure-based cognitive and behavioral treatments for phobic and anxiety disorders in children. *Behavior Therapy, 31,* 713–731.

Blashfield, R. K., & Draguns, J. G. (1976). Toward a taxonomy of psychopathology: The purpose of psychiatric classification. *British Journal of Psychiatry, 129,* 574–583.

Cantwell, D. P. (1975). A model for the investigation of psychiatric disorders of childhood: Its application in genetic studies of the hyperkinetic syndrome. In E. J. Anthony (Ed.), *Explorations in child psychiatry* (pp. 57–59). New York: Plenum Press.

Caron, C., & Rutter, M. (1991). Comorbidity in child psychopathology: Concepts, issues and research strategies. *Journal of Child Psychology and Psychiatry and Allied Disciplines, 32,* 1063–1080.

Chorpita, B. F., & Donkervoet, J. C. (2001). Special series: Pushing the envelope of empirically based treatments for children: Introduction. *Cognitive and Behavioral Practice, 8,* 336–337.

Chorpita, B. F., Yim, L. M., Donkervoet, J. C., Arensdorf, A., Amundsen, M. J., McGee, C., Serrano, A., et al. (2002). Toward large scale implementation of empirically supported treatments for children: A review and observations by the Hawaii Empirical Basis to Services Task Force. *Clinical Psychology: Science and Practice, 9,* 165–190.

Cobham, V. E., Dadds, M. R., & Spence, S. H. (1998). The role of parental anxiety in the treatment of childhood anxiety. *Journal of Consulting and Clinical Psychology, 66,* 893–905.

Craighead, W. E., & Craighead, L. W. (1998). Manual-based treatments: Suggestions for improving their clinical utility and acceptability. *Clinical Psychology: Science and Practice, 5,* 403–407.

DeBellis, M. D., Casey, B. J., Dahl, R. E., Birmaher, B., Williamson, D. E., Thomas, K. M., Axelson, D. A., et al. (2000). A pilot study of amygdala volumes in pediatric generalized anxiety disorder. *Biological Psychiatry, 48,* 51–57.

Di Nardo, P. A., O'Brien, G. T., Barlow, D. H., Waddell, M. T., & Blanchard, E. B. (1983). Reliability of *DSM-III* anxiety disorder categories using a new structured interview. *Archives of General Psychiatry, 40,* 1070–1074.

Duncan, T., Duncan, S., Strycker, L., Li, F. & Alpert, A. (1999). *An introduction to latent variable growth curve modeling: Concepts, issues and applications.* Mahwah, NJ: Erlbaum.

Eifert, G. H., Schulte, D., Zvolensky, M. J., Lejuez, C. W., & Lau, A. W. (1997). Manualized behavior therapy: Merits and challenges. *Behavior Therapy, 28,* 499–509.

Eisen, A. R., & Silverman, W. K. (1993). Should I relax or change my thoughts? A preliminary study of the treatment of overanxious disorder in children. *Journal of Cognitive Psychotherapy, 7,* 265–280.

Eisen, A. R., & Silverman, W. K. (1998). Prescriptive treatment for generalized anxiety disorder in children. *Behavior Therapy, 29,* 105–121.

Flannery-Schroeder, E. C., & Kendall, P. C. (2000). Group versus individual cognitive behavioral treatment for youth with anxiety disorders: A randomized clinical trial. *Cognitive Therapy and Research, 24,* 251–278.

Haaga, D. (2000). Introduction to the special section on stepped care models in psychotherapy. *Journal of Consulting and Clinical Psychology, 147,* 313–318.

Haynes, S. N., Kaholokula, J. K., & Nelson, K. (1999). The idiographic application of nomothetic empirically based treatments. *Clinical Psychology: Science and Practice, 5,* 387–390.

Hayward, C., Varady, S., Albano, A. M., Thieneman, M., Henderson, L., & Schatzberg, A. F. (2000). Cognitive-behavioral group therapy for female socially phobic adolescents: Results of a pilot study. *Journal of the American Academy of Child and Adolescent Psychiatry, 39,* 721–726.

Heimberg, R. G. (1998). Manual-based treatment: An essential ingredient of clinical practice in the 21st century. *Clinical Psychology: Science and Practice, 5,* 387–390.

Herjanic, B. (1982). Development of a structured psychiatric interview for children: Agreement between child and parent on individual symptoms. *Journal of Abnormal Child Psychology, 10,* 307–324.

Hindley, P., & Van Gent, T. (2003). Psychiatric aspects of specific sensory impairments. In M. Rutter & E. Taylor (Eds.), *Child and adolescent psychiatry* (4th ed.) (pp. 842–857). Oxford, UK: Blackwell Science.

Howard, K. I., Moras, K., Brill, P. L., Martinovich, Z., & Lutz, W. (1996). Evaluation of psychotherapy: Efficacy, effectiveness, and patient progress. *American Psychologist, 51,* 1059–1064.

Jensen, P. S., Bhatara, V. S., Vitiello, B., Hoagwood, K., Feil, M., & Burke, L. (1999). Psychoactive medication prescribing practices for U.S. children: Gaps between research and clinical practice. *Journal of the American Academy of Child and Adolescent Psychiatry, 38,* 557–565.

Kazdin, A. E. (1999). Current (lack of) status of theory in child and adolescent psychotherapy research. *Journal of Clinical Child Psychology, 28,* 533–543.

Kazdin, A. E., Siegel, T. C., & Bass, D. (1990). Drawing on clinical practice to inform research on child and adolescent psychopathology: Survey of practitioners. *Professional Psychology: Research and Practice, 21,* 189–198.

Kendall, P. C. (1994). Treating anxiety disorders in children: Results of a randomized clinical trial. *Journal of Consulting and Clinical Psychology, 62,* 100–110.

Kendall, P. C., Brady, E. U., & Verduin, T. L. (2001). Comorbidity in childhood anxiety disorders and treatment outcome. *Journal of the American Academy of Child and Adolescent Psychiatry, 40,* 787–794.

Kendall, P. C., & Chu, B. C. (2000). Retrospective self-reports of therapist flexibility in a manual-based treatment for youths with anxiety disorders. *Journal of Clinical Child Psychology, 2,* 209–220.

Kendall, P. C., Flannery-Schroeder, E. C., Panichelli-Mindel, S. M., Southam-Gerow, M., Henin, A., & Warman, M. (1997). Therapy for youths with anxiety disorders: A second randomized clinical trial. *Journal of Consulting and Clinical Psychology, 65,* 366–380.

Laidlaw, J. D. D., & Maung-Zaw, K. (1993). Epilepsy mistaken for panic attacks in an adolescent girl. *British Medical Journal, 306,* 709–710.

Lee, D. O., Helmers, S. L., Steingard, R. J., & DeMaso, D. R. (1997). Seizure disorder presenting as panic disorder with agoraphobia. *Journal of the American Academy of Child and Adolescent Psychiatry, 36,* 1295–1298.

March, J. S., & Curry, J. E. (1998). Predicting the outcome of treatment. *Journal of Abnormal Child Psychology, 26,* 39–51.

March, J. S., Parker, J. D. A., Sullivan, K., Stallings, P. & Conners, K. (1997). The Multidimensional Anxiety Scale for Children (MASC): Factor structure, reliability, and validity. *Journal of the American Academy of Child and Adolescent Psychiatry, 36,* 554–565.

McClellan, J. M., & Werry, J. S. (2000). Research psychiatric diagnostic interviews for children and adolescents. *Journal of the American Academy of Child and Adolescent Psychiatry, 39,* 19–27.

Mendlowitz, S. L., Manassis, K., Bradley, S., Scapillato, D., Miezitis, S., & Shaw, B. F. (1999). Cognitive-behavioral group treatments in childhood anxiety disorders: The role of parental involvement. *Journal of the American Academy of Child and Adolescent Psychiatry, 38,* 1223–1229.

Ollendick, T. H. (1983). Reliability and validity of the Revised Fear Survey Schedule for Children (FSSC-R). *Behaviour Research and Therapy, 21,* 395–399.

Pegna, C., Perri, A., & Lenti, C. (1999). Panic disorder or temporal lobe epilepsy: A diagnostic problem in an adolescent girl. *European Child and Adolescent Psychiatry, 8,* 237–239.

Rapee, R. M., Barrett, P. M., Dadds, M. R., & Evans, L. (1994). Reliability of the *DSM-III-R* childhood anxiety disorders using structured interview: Inter-rater and parent-child agreement. *Journal of the American Academy of Child and Adolescent Psychiatry, 33,* 984–992.

Reich, W. (2000). Diagnostic Interview for Children and Adolescents (DICA). *Journal of the American Academy of Child and Adolescent Psychiatry, 39,* 59–66.

Reynolds, C. R., & Richmond, B. O. (1985). *Revised Children's Manifest Anxiety Scale.* Los Angeles: Western Psychological Services.

Robins, E., & Guze, S. B. (1970). Establishment of diagnostic validity in psychiatric illness: Its application to schizophrenia. *American Journal of Psychiatry, 126,* 983–986.

Ronan, K. E., Kendall, P. C., & Rowe, M. (1994). Negative affectivity in children: Development and validation of a self-statement questionnaire. *Cognitive Therapy and Research, 18,* 509–28.

Rush, B. (1962). *Medical inquiries and observations upon the diseases of the mind.* New York: Library of the New York Academy of Medicine/Hafner Publishing. (Original work published 1812)

Rutter, M., & Shaffer, D. (1980). *DSM-III:* A step forward or back in terms of the classification of child psychiatric disorders? *Journal of the American Academy of Child Psychiatry, 19,* 371–393.

Saavedra, L. M., & Silverman, W. K. (2002). Classification of anxiety disorders in children: What a difference two decades make. *International Review of Psychiatry, 14,* 87–100.

Shaffer, D., Fisher, P., Lucas, C. P., Dulcan, M. K., & Schwab-Stone, M. E. (2000). NIMH Diagnostic Interview Schedule for Children Version IV (NIMH DISC-IV): Description, differences from previous versions, and reliability of some common diagnoses. *Journal of the American Academy of Child and Adolescent Psychiatry, 39,* 28–38.

Shaffer, D., Schwab-Stone, M., Fisher, P. W., Cohen, P., Piacentini, J., Davies, M., Conners, C. K., et al. (1993). The Diagnostic Interview Schedule for Children–Revised version (DISC-R): Preparation, field testing, interrater reliability, and acceptability. *Journal of the American Academy of Child and Adolescent Psychiatry, 32,* 643–650.

Shore, G. N., & Rapport, M. D. (1998). The Fear Survey Schedule for Children–Revised (FSSC-HI): Ethnocultural variations in children's fearfulness. *Journal of Anxiety Disorders, 12,* 437–461.

Siebelink, B. M., & Treffers, P. D. A. (2001). *Dutch adaptation of the ADIS for DSM-IV, child version by Wendy K. Silverman and Anne Marie Albano,* Lisse, Netherlands: Swets & Zeitlinger.

Silverman, W. K. (1994). Structured diagnostic interviews. In T. H. Ollendick, N. J. King, & W. Yule (Eds.), *International handbook of phobic and anxiety disorders in children and adolescents* (pp. 293–315). New York: Plenum Press.

Silverman, W. K., & Albano, A. M. (1996). *Anxiety Disorders Interview Schedule for Children DSM-IV (Child and Parent Versions).* San Antonio, TX: Psychological Corporation.

Silverman, W. K., & Berman, S. L. (2001). Psychosocial interventions for anxiety disorders in children: Status and future directions. In W. K. Silverman & P. D. A. Treffers (Eds.), *Anxiety disorders in children and adolescents: Research, assessment and intervention* (pp. 313–334). Cambridge, UK: Cambridge University Press.

Silverman, W. K., & Eisen, A. R. (1992). Age differences in the reliability of parent and child reports of child anxious symptomatology using a structured interview. *Journal of the American Academy of Child and Adolescent Psychiatry, 31,* 117–124.

Silverman, W. K., Fleisig, W., Rabian, B., & Peterson, R. A. (1991). Childhood anxiety sensitivity index. *Journal of Clinical Child Psychology, 20,* 162–168.

Silverman, W. K., Ginsburg, G. S., & Goedhart, A. W. (1999). Factor structure of the childhood anxiety sensitivity index. *Behaviour Research and Therapy, 37,* 903–917.

Silverman, W. K., & Kurtines, W. M. (1996a). *Anxiety and phobic disorders: A pragmatic approach.* New York: Plenum Press.

Silverman, W. K., & Kurtines, W. M. (1996b). Transfer of control: A psychosocial intervention model for internalizing disorders in youth. In E. D. Hibbs & P. S. Jensen (Eds.), *Psychosocial treatments for child and adolescent disor-*

ders: Empirically based strategies for clinical practice (pp. 63–81). Washington, DC: American Psychological Association.

Silverman, W. K., & Kurtines, W. M. (1997). Theory in child psychosocial treatment research: Have it or had it? A pragmatic alternative. *Journal of Abnormal Child Psychology, 25,* 359–367.

Silverman, W. K., Kurtines, W. M., Ginsburg, G. S., Weems, C. F., Lumpkin, P. W., & Hicks-Carmichael, D. (1999). Treating anxiety disorders in children with group cognitive behavior therapy: A randomized clinical trial. *Journal of Consulting and Clinical Psychology, 67,* 995–1003.

Silverman, W. K., Kurtines, W. M., Ginsburg, G. S., Weems, C. F., Rabian, B., & Serafini, L. T. (1999). Contingency management, self-control, and education support in the treatment of childhood phobic disorders: A randomized clinical trial. *Journal of Consulting and Clinical Psychology, 67,* 675–687.

Silverman, W. K., & Nelles, W. B. (1988). The Anxiety Disorders Interview Schedule for Children. *Journal of the American Academy of Child and Adolescent Psychiatry, 27,* 772–778.

Silverman, W. K., & Rabian, B. (1995). Test-retest reliability of the *DSM-III-R* childhood anxiety disorders symptoms using the Anxiety Disorders Interview Schedule for Children. *Journal of Anxiety Disorders, 9,* 1–12.

Silverman, W. K., Saavedra, L. M., & Pina, A. A. (2001). Test-retest reliability of anxiety symptoms and disorders with the Anxiety Disorders Interview Schedule for *DSM-IV*: Child and parent versions. *Journal of the American Academy of Child and Adolescent Psychiatry, 40,* 937–944.

Silverman, W. K., & Treffers, P. D. A. (Eds.). (2001). *Anxiety disorders in children and adolescents: Research, assessment and intervention.* Cambridge, UK: Cambridge University Press.

Silverman, W. K., & Wallander, J. L. (1993). Bridging research and practice in interventions with children: An introduction to the special issue. *Clinical Psychologist, 46,* 165–168.

Spence, S. H., Donovan, C., & Brechman-Toussaint, M. (2000). The treatment of childhood social phobia: The effectiveness of a social skills training-based, cognitive behavioural intervention, with and without parental involvement. *Journal of Child Psychology and Psychiatry, and Allied Disciplines, 41,* 713–726.

Thomas, K. M., Drevets, W. C., Dahl, R. E., Ryan, N. D., Birmaher, B., Eccard, C. H., Axelson, D., et al. (2001). Amygdala response to fearful faces in anxious and depressed children. *Archives of General Psychiatry, 58,* 1057–1063.

Treadwell, K. R., Flannery-Schroeder, E. C., & Kendall, P. C. (1995). Ethnicity and gender in relation to adaptive functioning, diagnostic status, and treatment outcome in children from an anxiety clinic. *Journal of Anxiety Disorders, 9,* 373–384.

Treffers, P. D. A. (2001, July 17–21). *Interpreting cross-cultural comparisons of child assessment tools.* Paper presented at World Congress of Behavioral and Cognitive Therapies, Vancouver, Canada.

Treffers, P. D. A., Goedhart, A. W., Waltz, J. W., & Koudijs, E. (1990). The systematic collection of patient data in a centre for child and adolescent psychiatry. *British Journal of Psychiatry, 157,* 744–748.

Treffers, P. D. A., & Silverman, W. K. (2001). Anxiety and its disorders in children and youth before the twentieth century. In: W. K. Silverman & P. D. A. Treffers (Eds.), *Anxiety disorders in children and adolescents: Research, assess-*

ment and intervention (pp. 1–22). Cambridge, UK: Cambridge University Press.

Treffers, P. D. A., Westenberg, P. M., & Siebelink, P.M. (1998). *Dutch translation of the Childhood Anxiety Sensitivity Index (CASI)*. Oegstgeest, Netherlands: Academic Center for Child and Adolescent Psychiatry Curium.

Utens, E. M. W. J., & Ferdinand, R. F. (2000). *Nederlandse vertaling van de MASC: MASC-NL* [Dutch translation of the MASC]. Rotterdam, Netherlands: Department of Child and Adolescent Psychiatry, AZR-Sophia.

Van Widenfelt, B. M. (2001a). *Parent Child Treatment for Anxiety Protocol (experimental version)*. Oegstgeest, Netherlands: Academic Center for Child and Adolescent Psychiatry Curium.

Van Widenfelt, B. M. (2001b, July 17–21). *Translation and cross-cultural adaptation of child assessment tools*. Paper presented at World Congress of Behavioral and Cognitive Therapies, Vancouver, Canada.

Van Widenfelt, B. M., Siebelink, B. M., Goedhart, A. W., & Treffers, P. D. A. (2002). The Dutch Childhood Anxiety Sensitivity Index: Psychometric properties and factor structure. *Journal of Clinical Child and Adolescent Psychology, 31,* 90–100.

Van Widenfelt, B. M., & Treffers, P. D. A. (2000). *Dutch translation of the Negative Affectivity Self-Statement Questionnaire for Children (NASSQ)*. Oegstgeest, Netherlands: Academic Center for Child and Adolescent Psychiatry Curium.

Weiss, B., Catron, T., Harris, V., & Phung, T. M. (1999). The effectiveness of traditional child psychotherapy. *Journal of Consulting and Clinical Psychology, 67,* 82–94.

Weisz, J. R., & Hawley, K. M. (1998). Finding, evaluating, refining, and applying, empirically supported treatments for children and adolescents. *Journal of Clinical Child Psychology, 27,* 206–216.

Weisz, J. R., Weiss, B., & Donenberg, G. R. (1992). The lab versus the clinic: Effects of child and adolescent psychotherapy. *American Psychologist, 47,* 1578–1585.

Westenberg, P. M., Siebelink, B. M., & Treffers, P. D. A. (2001). Psychosocial developmental theory in relation to anxiety and its disorders. In W. K. Silverman & P. D. A. Treffers (Eds.), *Anxiety disorders in children and adolescents: Research, assessment and Intervention* (pp. 72–89). Cambridge, UK: Cambridge University Press.

Westenberg, P. M., Siebelink, B. M., Warmenhoven, N. J. C., & Treffers, P. D. A. (1999). Separation anxiety and overanxious disorders: Relations to age and level of psychosocial maturity. *Journal of the American Academy of Child and Adolescent Psychiatry, 38,* 1000–1007.

19

ANXIETY DISORDERS
AND ACCESS TO MENTAL
HEALTH SERVICES

HELEN L. EGGER & BARBARA J. BURNS

Although increasing attention has been paid in the last 5 years to the presentation, course, and treatment of anxiety disorders in children and adolescents (Bernstein, Borchardt, & Perwien, 1996; March, 1995), relatively little work has focused on access to mental health services by youth with anxiety disorders. Recent advances in our ability to identify and treat childhood anxiety disorders effectively, as well as our understanding of the morbidity associated with untreated anxiety disorders, highlight the importance of improving children's access to treatment.

The purpose of this chapter is to present the state of knowledge about access to mental health service use for children with anxiety disorders. We review the literature on mental health services for children and adolescents with anxiety disorders, and we present data from the Great Smoky Mountain Study (GSMS) on access to mental health care across different service sectors for children and adolescents. GSMS is a longitudinal, community study that has examined psychiatric disorders and mental health service use in rural North Carolina.

In community studies of children and adolescents, the prevalence of any anxiety diagnosis has ranged from 3% to 17% (Angold, Costello, & Erkanli, 1999; Costello & Angold, 1995). A detailed presentation of the epidemiology of anxiety disorders including rates, comorbidity, and course can be found in chapter 3 of this book, by Costello, Egger, and Angold. Anxiety disorders often co-occur with each other and with other disorders, particularly depression (Angold et al., 1999), so studies of service patterns for anxiety disorders must take into account the fact that referral patterns for comorbid conditions will be superimposed. As noted in the following review, few studies have specifically focused on mental health services for children with anxiety disorders, and none, except our recent work, have examined access to mental health services for specific anxiety disorders, taking into account the effects of comorbid disorders on service use.

MENTAL HEALTH SERVICES FOR CHILDREN AND ADOLESCENTS

Epidemiologic studies have repeatedly shown that the majority of children with psychiatric disorders do not receive treatment for their disorders (Anderson, Williams, McGee, & Silva, 1987; Burns et al., 1995; Cohen, Kasen, Brook, & Stuening, 1991; Costello & Janiszewski, 1990; Institute of Medicine, 1989; Koot & Verhulst, 1992; Leaf et al., 1996; Offord et al., 1987; U.S. Public Health Service, 1999; Verhulst & van der Ende, 1997; Zahner, Pawelkiewicz, DeFrancesco, & Adnopoz, 1992). For example, Offord and colleagues (1987) reported from the Ontario Child Health Study that, although children with psychiatric disorders were nearly four times as likely as children without psychiatric disorders to receive mental health services, only 16.1% of children between the age of 4 and 16 with a psychiatric disorder had received mental health services. In their community study of adolescents in New York State, Cohen and colleagues (1991) showed that only 33% of children 12 to 16 years old and 20% of children 17 to 20 years old with a *severe* mental disorder had consulted a mental health professional in the year prior to the interview. In the Dunedin sample, McGee and colleagues (1990) reported that only 12.5% of 15-year-olds who met criteria for a psychiatric disorder received mental health services. Data from the GSMS replicated these findings. Overall, about 16% of the children in GSMS had received some kind of mental health services in the 3 months prior to the research diagnostic interview, with only 40% of the most emotionally disturbed children having received any kind of mental health services in this same time period (Burns et al., 1995).

DIAGNOSTIC PREDICTORS OF MENTAL HEALTH SERVICE USE

A handful of studies have investigated symptom- and diagnosis-specific patterns of mental health service use. Using the Child Behavior Checklist (CBCL) as a measure of psychopathology, three studies reporting on Dutch children have suggested that internalizing symptoms were as likely as externalizing symptoms to predict mental health service use with risk ratios between 1.5 and 2 (Koot & Verhulst, 1992; Laitinen-Krispijn, van der Ende, Wierdsma, & Verhulst, 1999; Verhulst & van der Ende, 1997). Community studies using *DSM*-defined criteria for psychiatric disorders have suggested that children with behavioral disorders might be more likely than children with emotional disorders to receive mental health services. Cohen and colleagues (1991) found that the only psychiatric disorders associated with an increased likelihood of mental health services were oppositional defiant disorder, or ODD (odds ratio [OR] = 4.84; confidence interval [CI] = 2.24 to 10.46), and conduct disorder, or CD (OR = 3.74; CI = 1.57 to 8.93). Analyzing data from the NIMH Methods for the Epidemiology of Child and Adolescent Mental Disorders (MECA) study, Wu and colleagues (1999) found that disruptive disorders were significantly associated with use of mental health services but depressive disorders were not.

In Cuffe, Waller, Cuccaro, Pumariega, and Garrison's (1995) representative sample of 478 adolescents, affective disorders—a combination of depressive and anxiety disorders—showed the strongest association with treatment contact (OR = 11.25; CI = 4.53 to 27.94) compared with non-affective disorders (OR = 4.3; CI = 1.65 to 11.31). However, the results of this study were significantly limited by the use of an instrument that did not include assessments of attention deficit/hyperactivity disorder (ADHD), ODD, or substance abuse.

Very few community studies have looked specifically at anxiety disorders and mental health service use. In the Cohen et al. (1991) study, over-anxious disorder (OAD), a *DSM-III-R* disorder no longer included in *DSM-IV* and the only anxiety disorder addressed in this study, was not significantly associated with service use (OR = 1.11; CI = 0.24 to 5.10). In a study comparing treated and untreated cohorts of children, Costello and Janiszewski (1990) found that there was no statistically significant difference in the rates of anxiety disorder between the two groups. They did find a significant gender by race interaction for anxiety disorders: 57% of African American girls with an anxiety disorder compared with only 29% of the African American boys were in psychiatric treatment. There was no significant difference for white boys and girls, but treatment for anxiety disorders for white children was more common than for African American children.

The Comprehensive Community Mental Health Services for Children and Their Families Program (CMHS) collects data from 22 mental health demonstration programs serving more than 40,000 children. Its 1998 report to Congress showed that 7.8% of the children treated had a primary anxiety disorder diagnosis (Center for Mental Health Services, 1998). In contrast, 26.5% of the children were given a primary diagnosis of depression, 30% had a conduct-related diagnosis, and 13.5% an ADHD diagnosis. Although this sample did not include information on children who did not receive treatment, it does provide a picture of the relative representation of children with anxiety disorders in a large treated sample, suggesting that anxiety disorders were not a high priority in these systems of care, despite their expected rates in this population.

SERVICE SECTORS

The emerging literature on mental health service use by children and adolescents has also found that children and adolescents receive the majority of mental health services in sectors other than the specialty mental health system (Burns et al., 1995; Staghezza-Jaramillo, Bird, Gould, & Canino, 1995). For instance, in the GSMS, only one in five children receiving mental health services received care in the specialty mental health sector. Three quarters of the children receiving mental health services were seen in the education sector. For many children, this was the sole source of services (Burns et al., 1995). This predominance of education-based mental health services is typical (Cohen et al., 1991; Leaf et al., 1996; Offer, Howard, Schonert, & Ostrov, 1991; Offord et al., 1987; Staghezza-Jaramillo et al., 1995; Zahner et al., 1992).

Despite increasing reliance on managed care by pediatricians as gatekeepers to specialty services, including mental health services (Costello, Costello, et al., 1988), a number of studies have shown that pediatric primary care practitioners often do not identify children with psychiatric disorders. Only a very small percentage of the children in the GSMS received mental health services in general medical settings (Burns et al., 1995). Cohen and colleagues (1991) also found that few children with emotional or behavioral problems consulted with primary care providers about these problems. In Costello, Edelbrock, and colleagues' 1988 study of nearly 800 7- to 11-year-olds in a pediatric setting, 22% had one or more psychiatric disorder, whereas only 5% were identified as having emotional or behavioral difficulties by their pediatricians, and only 1.9% had received any mental health services during the previous year.

Burns and colleagues (1995) also found that the child welfare and juvenile justice sectors provided relatively few mental health services to children in the GSMS. Among children with a "serious emotional disturbance," defined as a psychiatric diagnosis and impairment, 16.4% received mental health services in the child welfare setting and 4.3% received services in the juvenile justice setting. Most of the children who received child welfare-based services also received services in other settings, although this was not the case for those served in the juvenile justice setting. The only data we could find on service use specifically for children with anxiety disorders in the welfare sector was from the Patterns of Care Study (POC), an ongoing longitudinal study of children age 6 through 17 involved in public service systems in San Diego County, California. This study, like the CMHS study described previously, reported on a treated population and therefore cannot provide data on children without access to services. From a sample of 425 children active in the child welfare system, 10.8% had a anxiety disorder as measured by the DISC-IV. Of these, 41.9% had received school-based services and 77.0% had received specialty mental health services (John Landsverk & Laurel Leslie, personal communication, 2001).

ANXIETY DISORDERS AND ACCESS
TO SERVICES IN THE GSMS

Our 2001 article "Anxiety Disorders and Access to Mental Health Services in a Community Sample" (Egger, Burns, Erkanli, Costello, & Angold) examined access to mental health service use across multiple service sectors for children with specific anxiety disorders in the GSMS. We included the following *DSM-IV* defined anxiety disorders: separation anxiety disorder (SAD), generalized anxiety disorder (GAD), simple phobias, social phobia, panic disorder, and posttraumatic stress disorder (PTSD). In addition, an any-anxiety-disorder variable, which required the presence of at least one of these disorders, was used in the analyses. We also controlled for the effects of other Axis I psychiatric disorders, including depression, CD, ODD, ADHD.

We considered service use in five mental health service sectors:

1. *Specialty mental health* (psychiatric hospital, psychiatric unit in a general hospital, residential treatment center, group home, partial hospitalization, therapeutic foster care, mental health center, detoxification unit, outpatient drug/alcohol clinic, case management, or private mental health professional). The majority of care was provided by public mental health centers (31.5%), private mental health providers (66.1%), or both.
2. *General medical* (medical inpatient unit, community health center, family doctor/other nonpsychiatric physician, hospital emergency room). Three-fourths of the care was provided by a pediatrician or family practitioner.
3. *Education* (guidance counselor/school psychologist, special class, or boarding school). Ninety percent of the services were provided by the school counselor.
4. *Child welfare* (social services counseling).
5. *Juvenile justice* (detention center/jail or probation officer/court counselor). Most commonly, the provider was a probation officer.

In the following section, we present data from our recent article (Egger et al., 2001) addressing these questions:

- How many children with *DSM-IV*-defined anxiety disorders received mental health services?
- In what service sector (specialty mental health, general medical, education, child welfare, juvenile justice) were children most likely to receive mental health services?
- Are the patterns of service sector use the same for children with anxiety disorders as for children with other major Axis I disorders, including depression, ODD, CD, and ADHD? If there are differences, do they exist across different service sectors?
- Are there different patterns of service sector use for specific anxiety disorders? If so, are these differences seen across the different mental health service sectors?

- Did gender, age, or ethnicity significantly affect whether children with anxiety disorders received services overall or in specific settings?
- What were the rates of psychotropic drug use for children with an anxiety disorder?

THE GSMS

The GSMS is an ongoing, longitudinal study of the development of psychiatric disorders and need for mental health services in youth living in North Carolina. The sample is a representative sample of this rural community. The details of the study design and instruments used can be found in Costello et al. (1996). About 1,400 children and their primary caretakers were separately interviewed about the child's psychiatric status and service use using the third edition of the Child and Adolescent Psychiatric Assessment (CAPA) (Angold et al., 1995), which generated *DSM-IV* diagnoses, and the Child and Adolescent Services Assessment (CASA; Burns, Angold, Magruder-Habib, Costello, & Patrick, 1992). The reference period for each of these instruments was the 3 months prior to the interview. This 3-month primary period was used rather than a longer period, because shorter recall periods are associated with more accurate recall (Angold, Erkanli, Costello, & Rutter, 1996). The data presented here are from eight annual waves of data. In all, the sample included 6,668 observations on the 1,422 subjects. The age range of the subjects was 9 to 16 years. Of the sample, 49.3% were girls. The weighted sample was comprised of 89.8% whites, 6.5% African Americans, and 3.7% Native Americans. Table 19.1 provides information about the sample characteristics of the children with anxiety disorders.

Details on the data analytic approach can be found in our article (Egger et al., 2001). The principle statistical procedure used was logistic regression with the outcomes being presence of service use in the three months preceding the interview. We used generalized estimating equations (GEE) implemented in SAS PROC GENMOD. In the first set of models, the predictors of service use were as follows:

Table 19.1. Presentation of Anxiety Disorders in the Great Smoky Mountains Study

	Prevalence	*Gender (Girls)*	*Mean Age (Years)*
Any anxiety disorder	3.0% (n = 257)	57.2%	13.0 (*SD* 2.2)
Separation anxiety disorder	1.0% (n = 107)	48.2%	10.7** (*SD* 1.4)
Generalized anxiety disorder	0.8% (n = 74)	58.7%	13.6 (*SD* 1.9)
Simple phobia	0.2% (n = 16)	55.5%	13.8 (*SD* 1.9)
Social phobia	0.5% (n = 35)	74.3%*	13.8 (*SD* 1.8)
Panic	0.2% (n = 25)	78.5%*	15.2** (*SD* 1.1)
Posttraumatic stress disorder	0.9% (n = 62)	52.7%	13.9 (*SD* 2.1)

*p < 0.05; **p < 0.001

1. Age
2. Gender
3. Race
4. An anxiety disorder
5. A depressive disorder
6. ODD
7. CD or
8. ADHD diagnosis at any or the eight waves

In the second set of models, we substituted the six specific anxiety disorders for the any-anxiety-disorder variable. Finally, we examined psychotropic medication use by children with anxiety disorders. The outcome variable was the use of one of three psychotropic medications during the 3-month primary period: antidepressants (e.g. tricyclic antidepressants, serotonin reuptake inhibitors, or atypical antidepressants such as monoamine oxidase inhibitors), stimulants (e.g. methylphenidate), or minor tranquilizers (e.g. benzodiazepines). The predictor variables were the psychiatric disorders described above.

The odds ratios represent the odds of service use for that disorder, because we controlled for the effects of the other diagnoses. Percentages reported are all weighted population estimates but do not control for the presence of other disorders. When cell sizes are given, they represent unweighted numbers of individuals in the sample.

ANXIETY DISORDERS AND OVERALL
MENTAL HEALTH SERVICE USE

Figure 19.1 show the use of mental health services across the service sectors by children with a major Axis I disorder. Children and adolescents with at least one anxiety disorder were significantly more likely than those without an anxiety disorder to have used mental health services in one of the five service sectors (OR = 2.4; 1.3, 4.3). Children with ADHD were most likely to receive some kind of mental health service (OR = 5.2; 3.2, 8.3), followed by children with CD (OR = 2.5; 1.6, 4.0), with anxiety disorders, with depression (OR = 2.0; 1.0, 4.1), and then with ODD (OR = 1.8; 1.1, 2.9).

Figures 19.2 through 19.6 show the use of mental health services, by service sector, by children with a major Axis I psychiatric disorder, including anxiety disorders. In Figure 19.2, we see that children with anxiety disorders were not more likely than children without anxiety disorders to have received services in a specialty mental health setting (OR = 1.6; 0.6, 4.0). Anxiety disorders were the only Axis I disorder not significantly associated with increased specialty mental health service use. The odds ratios for the other disorders were as follows: depression, OR = 2.7 (1.0, 7.0); CD, OR = 1.7 (1.0, 2.8); ODD, OR = 3.2 (1.7, 6.1); ADHD, OR = 2.6 (1.3, 4.9).

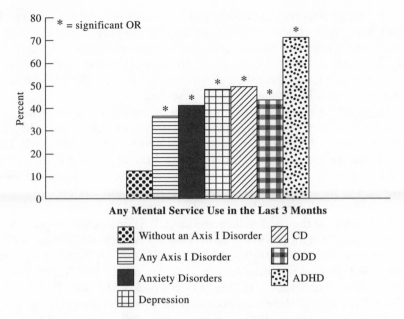

Figure 19.1. Axis I diagnoses and mental health service use

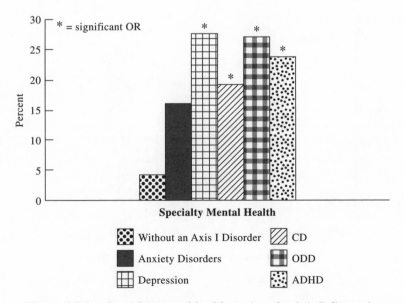

Figure 19.2. Specialty mental health services, by Axis I diagnosis

Figure 19.3 shows that children with anxiety disorders were significantly more likely than children without an anxiety disorder to receive mental health services from a pediatrician or family physician (OR = 3.0; 1.2, 7.5). Children with ADHD (OR = 5.0; 1.9, 16.8) or depression (OR = 3.8; 1.4, 9.8) were also more likely than children without these disorders to have received services in the general medical setting.

Figure 19.4 shows a different pattern of service use at schools. Children with anxiety disorders were significantly more likely than children without anxiety disorders to receive mental health services (OR = 3.0; 1.2, 7.5) in the education setting. Children with ADHD (OR = 6.5; 2.9, 14.6) and CD (OR = 2.3; 1.2, 4.6) were also more likely than those without these disorders to have received school-based mental health services.

Children with anxiety disorders were not more likely to receive mental health services in the child welfare service (CWS) or juvenile justice service (JJS) settings than those without anxiety disorders, as shown in Figures 19.5 and 19.6: CWF, OR = 2.0 [0.3, 14.2]; and JJS, OR = 0.9 [0.3, 2.3]). The only Axis I disorder significantly associated with mental health service in either of these sectors was CD (CWS, OR = 5.4 [2.5, 12.0], and JJS, OR = 4.5 [2.1, 9.7]), although there was a positive trend toward an association between ODD and services in the juvenile justice sector (OR = 2.8; 0.8, 9.8).

Although 40% of children with at least one anxiety disorder received mental health services in one of the five service sectors, this treatment rate was lower than those for all of the other Axis I disorders. The likelihood of children with any anxiety disorder receiving mental health services in any sector was similar to that for CD, and a bit higher than for depression. Yet, an examination of services by settings shows that general medical and edu-

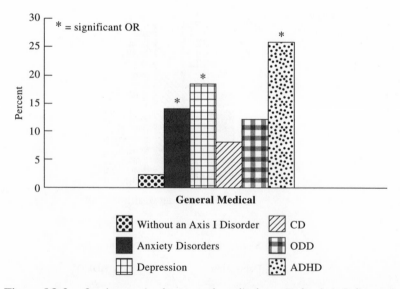

Figure 19.3. Service use in the general medical sector, by Axis I diagnosis

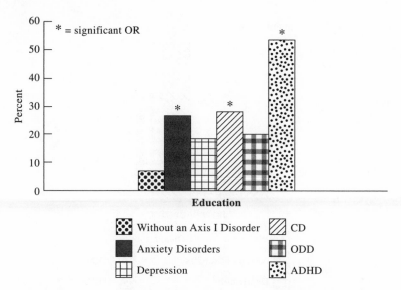

Figure 19.4. Service use in the education sector, by Axis I diagnosis

cation settings were the only two settings in which children with an anxiety disorder were more likely than children without an anxiety disorder to receive services. Children with an anxiety disorder were not more likely to receive specialty mental health services, CWS, or JJS than children without anxiety disorders.

The patterns of mental health service use differed significantly by Axis I diagnosis. The odds of a psychiatric diagnosis being associated with any mental health service use were greatest for ADHD. Yet the odds ratios for

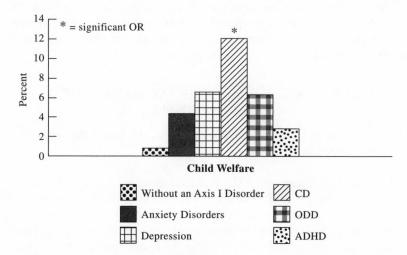

Figure 19.5. Service use in the child welfare sector, by Axis I diagnosis

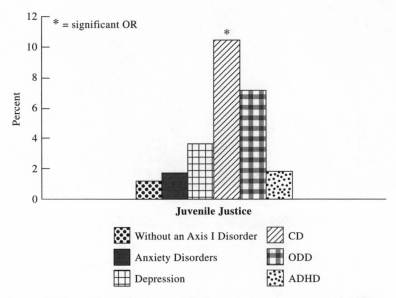

Figure 19.6.   Service use in the juvenile justice sector, by Axis I diagnosis

anxiety disorders, CD, and depression were between 2 and 2.5, and it was 1.8 for ODD. These findings do not fully support previous reports suggesting that behavioral disorders are more likely to result in mental health services than emotional disorders (Cohen et al., 1991; Wu et al., 1999). Although the relative odds of service use were roughly comparable for anxiety disorders and depression, the sector patterns differed. The specialty mental health sector was the only setting in which children with depression were more likely to receive mental health services, whereas children with anxiety disorders were served at school and by primary care practitioners. These findings call into question whether the broad affective disorders categories used for analysis of service use can effectively represent the experience of children with either diagnosis.

SPECIFIC ANXIETY DISORDERS AND MENTAL HEALTH SERVICE USE, BY SECTOR

When we examined specific anxiety disorders, we found that patterns of service use varied by diagnosis.

SAD   Overall, children with SAD were four times as likely as children without SAD to have received mental services in one of the five sectors in the 3 months prior to the interview ($OR = 4.4$; 2.0, 9.4). The two settings in which children with SAD were significantly more likely to receive mental health services were school ($OR = 5.8$; 2.4, 13.6) and specialty mental health settings ($OR = 4.2$; 2.0, 9.4). (See Figure 19.7.)

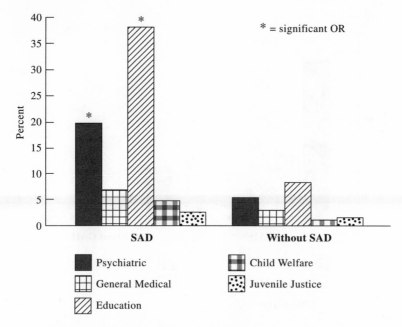

Figure 19.7.   SAD and mental health service use, by sector

GAD   GAD was not associated with an increased likelihood of mental health service use in any of the five settings. The odds ratio for service use in any setting was also not significant (*OR* = 0.6; 0.3, 1.2). (See Figure 19.8.)

Simple Phobia   Children with simple phobias were eight times as likely as children without simple phobia to have received mental health services in one of the five service sectors (*OR* = 8.3; 1.5, 45.2). Yet when we looked by sector, we found that only in the school setting were children with simple phobia more likely than children without simple phobia to receive mental health services (*OR* = 6.2; 1.0, 39.3). (See Figure 19.9.)

Social Phobia   No significant association was found between social phobia and mental health service use. The odds ratio for service in any sector was 0.6 (0.2, 1.4). (See Figure 19.10.)

Panic Disorder   Children and adolescents with panic disorder were more likely to have received mental health services in any of the five sectors than those without panic disorder (*OR* = 3.1; 1.4, 7.1). The two settings in which children with panic disorder were more likely than children without panic disorder to receive mental health services was the general medical setting (*OR* = 13.8; 2.3, 84.2) and the schools (*OR* = 3.5; 1.4, 9.0). (See Figure 19.11.)

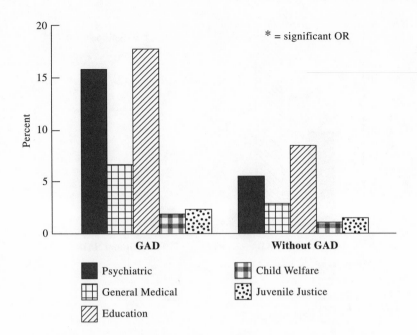

Figure 19.8. GAD and mental health service use, by sector

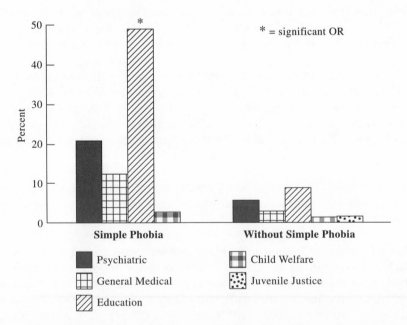

Figure 19.9. Simple phobia and mental health service use, by sector

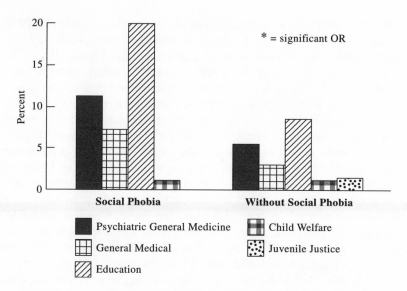

Figure 19.10. Social phobia and mental health service use, by sector

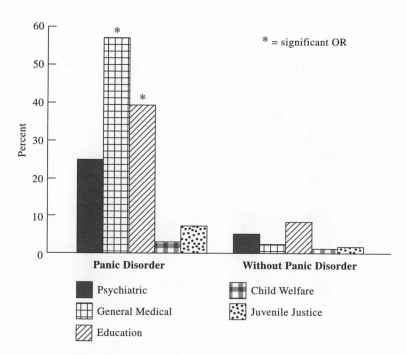

Figure 19.11. Panic disorder and mental health service use, by sector

PTSD Children with PTSD were more likely than children without PTSD to have received mental health services in a general medical setting (*OR* = 7.6; 2.2, 26.5). No other setting was significant. (See Figure 19.12.)

We found that, among the specific anxiety disorders, there was substantial heterogeneity in service access. We identified entire categories of children (those with GAD, social phobia) who were receiving little or no treatment for their disorders, except insofar as their comorbid disorders led to presentation for treatment. Only a quarter of children with GAD or social phobia had received any mental health treatment. Half of children with SAD or PTSD had received some services, whereas 60% of children with simple phobia and 80% of those with panic disorder had received some kind of mental health services. SAD was the only anxiety disorder to show an association with specialty mental health service use. Children with SAD, simple phobia, and panic disorder were significantly more likely to receive services in the education sector, yet less than half of children with these disorders received school-based mental health services.

Nearly 60% of children with panic disorder had received mental health services from their pediatricians or family physicians. The physiologic symptoms of panic, often mistaken for cardiovascular or respiratory disorders, may account for this relatively high rate of identification by nonpsychiatric physicians. Children with PTSD were also more likely to have received treatment in the general medical setting, yet only 29% of children with this disorder received services in this setting.

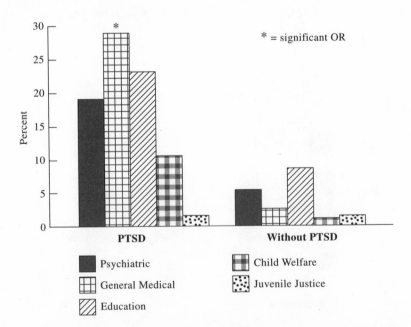

Figure 19.12. PTSD and mental health service use, by sector

AGE, RACE, AND GENDER EFFECTS

We found no significant age, gender, or race interactions for anxiety disorders overall and service use. There were no age, gender, or race effects for SAD, GAD, or social phobia. For simple phobia, girls and older children with this disorder were more likely to receive education-based mental health services than boys or younger children. A quarter (25.8%) of boys with simple phobia received education-based mental health services, compared with 74.2% of the girls with simple phobia. The only race effect found was that no Native American children with PTSD received services in the general medical setting, compared with a quarter of non–Native American children.

PSYCHOTROPIC MEDICATION AND ANXIETY DISORDERS

Fourteen percent of children with an anxiety disorder had taken stimulants, antidepressants, and minor tranquilizers within the 3 months prior to the interview. Among children with an anxiety disorder, 5.8% were taking a stimulant, 10.8% were taking an antidepressant, and 1.6% were taking a minor tranquilizer. In a multivariable model controlling for other Axis I disorders, the use of stimulants was not significantly associated with having any anxiety disorder ($OR = 0.9$; 0.3, 2.2). There was an association between having an anxiety disorder and use of an antidepressant ($OR = 5.3$; 1.5, 18.7) or a minor tranquilizer ($OR = 3.3$; 1.0, 10.6). The model for antidepressants showed that children with CD were most likely to be on antidepressants ($OR = 5.8$; 1.9, 18.1), followed by anxiety disorders, ADHD ($OR = 4.8$; 1.2, 19.7), and then depression ($OR = 4.0$; 1.0, 17.3). The only other disorder significantly associated with minor tranquilizer use was ODD ($OR = 3.5$; 1.3, 9.6). The numbers were too small to examine use of medication with specific anxiety disorders.

Our data on psychotropic medication use for children with anxiety disorders are of limited usefulness because they only report on medications used in the previous 3 months by children with a psychiatric disorder. This approach excludes from our discussion children who were on medication but whose target symptoms had resolved before the 3-month reporting period. Nonetheless, these data do provide a broadly drawn picture of medication use in this community sample. Children with an anxiety disorder were not more likely to be on stimulant medication, which suggests that clinicians were not misidentifying anxiety symptoms as ADHD symptoms, whereas children with anxiety disorders were five times more likely than children without an anxiety disorder to be taking an antidepressant and five times more likely to be on a minor tranquilizer. Comparison with other Axis I disorders showed that the relative odds of medication use were greater for children with anxiety disorders than for depression and were comparable to the conduct disorders.

LIMITATIONS OF THE GSMS DATA

Although the rates of psychopathology (Brandenburg, Friedman, & Silver, 1990) and specialty mental health service use (Bird et al., 1988; Offord et al., 1987) in our sample are similar to those in other studies, we cannot determine how generalizable these results are. The GSMS was conducted in a rural area with a well-integrated mental health services delivery system that had received support from the Robert Wood Johnson Foundation for mental health programs for children in the area. Thus, despite our findings of large unmet needs, the results may underestimate the lack of access and services provided in areas with less well developed service systems.

Although we report service utilization data, we did not examine either the type or intensity of services that children received. We know that the provision of mental health services varies within and between different sectors. Even if the services we described in our article (Egger et al., 2001) conformed to usual practice, they may not be consistent with current evidence on the efficacy or effectiveness of treatment or with current practice guidelines (Burns, Hoagwood, & Mrazek, 1999). Future analyses should take advantage of the longitudinal design of the GSMS to examine the relationship between service use and service intensity in relationship to outcomes. It would also be worthwhile to examine service use across sectors to determine pathways of systems of care in this cohort.

Despite these limitations, these data from the GSMS contribute to our understanding of access to mental health services for children with anxiety disorders. Lack of access to treatment or lack of recognition of need for treatment can lead to underutilization of mental health service. Our data suggest that we need screening programs to identify children with anxiety disorders, effective clinical services to serve children who are in need, and integration of services across sectors to help these children in the most effective and comprehensive ways possible. The lack of services provided for children with anxiety disorders in primary care settings highlights the importance of routine screening for psychiatric disorders during well-child visits and the need to educate both providers and parents about risk factors for, symptoms of, and assessment of anxiety disorders in children. Targeted screening of children whose parents themselves suffer from an anxiety disorder or other affective disorders might also serve as an effective way to increase identification. Parents and children must also be encouraged to discuss concerns about the children's emotions and behaviors and have access to information that will enable them to seek appropriate guidance. These data also suggest that better liaison between primary care and child and adolescent psychiatry is needed if these serious disorders are to be properly treated.

These data also highlight, as a number of previous studies have, the critical role of schools in identifying and treating children with psychiatric disorders. In our study, for children with any anxiety disorder, the school was one of the only settings where they were significantly more likely to receive mental health services. Yet, only 21% of the children with an anxiety disorder were treated in this setting, and little is known about the type or quality of treatment provided. School professionals, including classroom teachers, need to be taught how to recognize and refer for evaluation children with emotional and behavioral problems, including the range of anxiety disorders. Alternatively, school-based mental health services provided by mental health professionals may also improve the provision of specialty mental health services in school settings.

This chapter addresses the issue of access to services across sectors, where diagnosis and demographic characteristics are the measure of need. Additional variables (e.g. barriers to care, family characteristics) could have been addressed. Examination of the factors associated with help-seeking and service use represents the first step in mental health services research. A next research step could be to explore the outcomes of treatment provided. Future mental health services research endeavors might assess the availability of evidence-based interventions and approaches to introducing them into clinical settings. Subsequently, research could address the potential for broader dissemination when the appropriate policy and training resources are in place.

Anxiety disorders are prevalent and impairing childhood psychiatric disorders. As this book documents, there are effective psychosocial and pharmacologic assessment tools and treatments for a number of childhood anxiety disorders. The task ahead is to identify the barriers to providing care to children with anxiety disorders and to resolve them, to facilitate the identification and treatment of children with anxiety disorders.

NOTE

This project was supported by grants from the NIMH (MH-48085 and K23-MH-02016) and NIDA (DA-11301) and by Center funding from the NIMH (MH-57761).

REFERENCES

Anderson, J. C., Williams, S., McGee, R., & Silva, P. A. (1987). *DSM-III* disorders in preadolescent children: Prevalence in a large sample from the general population. *Archives of General Psychiatry, 44,* 69–76.

Angold, A., Costello, E. J., & Erkanli, A. (1999). Comorbidity. *Journal of Child Psychology and Psychiatry, 40,* 57–87.

Angold, A., Erkanli, A., Costello, E. J., & Rutter, M. (1996). Precision, reliability and accuracy in the dating of symptom onsets in child and adolescent psychopathology. *Journal of Child Psychology and Psychiatry, 37,* 657–664.

Angold, A., Prendergast, M., Cox, A., Harrington, R., Simonoff, E., & Rutter, M. (1995). The Child and Adolescent Psychiatric Assessment (CAPA). *Psychological Medicine, 25,* 739–753.

Bernstein, G. A., Borchardt, C. M., & Perwien, A. R. (1996). Anxiety disorders in children and adolescents: A review of the past 10 years. *Journal of the American Academy of Child and Adolescent Psychiatry, 35*(9), 1110–1119.

Bird, H. R., Canino, G., Rubio-Stipec, M., Gould, M. S., Ribera, J., Sesman, M., Woodbury, M., et al. (1988). Estimates of the prevalence of childhood maladjustment in a community survey in Puerto Rico. *Archives of General Psychiatry, 45,* 1120–1126.

Brandenburg, N. A., Friedman, R. M., & Silver, S. E. (1990). The epidemiology of childhood psychiatric disorders. *Journal of the American Academy of Child and Adolescent Psychiatry, 29,* 76–83.

Burns, B. J., Angold, A., Magruder-Habib, K., Costello, E. J., & Patrick, M. K. S. (1992). *The Child and Adolescent Services Assessment (CASA): Version 3.0.* Durham, NC: Duke University Medical Center.

Burns, B. J., Costello, E. J., Angold, A., Tweed, D., Stangl, D., Farmer, E. M. Z., & Erkanli, A. (1995). Children's mental health service use across service sectors. *Health Affairs, 14,* 147–159.

Burns, B. J., Hoagwood, K., & Mrazek, P. J. (1999). Effective treatment for mental disorders in children and adolescents. *Clinical Child and Family Psychology Review, 2,* 199–254.

Center for Mental Health Services, Substance Abuse and Mental Health Services Administration, U. S. Department of Health and Human Services. (1998). Annual report to Congress on the evaluation of the Comprehensive Community Mental Health Services for Children and Their Families Program: Executive summary. Atlanta, GA: Macro International.

Cohen, P., Kasen, S., Brook, J. S., & Stuening, E. L. (1991). Diagnostic predictors of treatment patterns in a cohort of adolescents. *Journal of the American Academy of Child and Adolescent Psychiatry, 30,* 989–993.

Costello, E. J., & Angold, A. (1995). Epidemiology. In J. March (Ed.), *Anxiety disorders in children and adolescents* (pp. 109–124). New York: Guilford Press.

Costello, E. J., Angold, A., Burns, B. J., Stangl, D. K., Tweed, D. L., Erkanli, A., & Worthman, C. M. (1996). The Great Smoky Mountains Study of Youth: Goals, designs, methods, and the prevalence of *DSM-III-R* disorders. *Archives of General Psychiatry, 53,* 1129–1136.

Costello, E. J., Costello, A. J., Edelbrock, C., Burns, B. J., Dulcan, M. K., Brent, D., & Janiszewski, S. (1988). Psychiatric disorders in pediatric primary care: Prevalence and risk factors. *Archives of General Psychiatry, 45,* 1107–1116.

Costello, E. J., Edelbrock, C. S., Costello, A. J., Dulcan, M. K., Burns, B. J., & Brent, D. (1988). Psychopathology in pediatric primary care: The new hidden morbidity. *Pediatrics, 82,* 415–424.

Costello, E. J., & Janiszewski, S. (1990). Who gets treated? Factors associated with referral in children with psychiatric disorders. *Acta Psychiatrica Scandinavica, 81,* 523–529.

Cuffe, S. P., Waller, J. L., Cuccaro, M. L., Pumariega, A. J., & Garrison, C. Z. (1995). Race and gender differences in the treatment of psychiatric disorders in young adolescents. *Journal of the American Academy of Child and Adolescent Psychiatry, 34,* 1536–1543.

Egger, H. L., Burns, B. J., Erkanli, A., Costello, E. J., & Angold, A. (2001). Anxiety disorders and access to mental health services in a community sample. Manuscript submitted for publication.

Institute of Medicine. (1989). *Research on children and adolescents with mental, behavioral and developmental disorders: Mobilizing a national initiative.* Washington, DC: National Academy Press.

Koot, H. M., & Verhulst, F. C. (1992). Prediction of children's referral to mental health and special education services from earlier adjustment. *Journal of Child Psychology and Psychiatry, 33*, 717–729.

Laitinen-Krispijn, S., van der Ende, J., Wierdsma, A. I., & Verhulst, F. C. (1999). Predicting adolescent mental health service use in a prospective record-linkage study. *Journal of the American Academy of Child and Adolescent Psychiatry, 38*, 1073–1092.

Leaf, P. J., Alegria, M., Cohen, P., Goodman, S. H., Horwitz, S., Hoven, C. W., Narrow, W. E., et al. (1996). Mental health service use in the community and schools: Results from the four-community MECA study. *Journal of the American Academy of Child and Adolescent Psychiatry, 35*, 889–897.

March, J. S. (1995). *Anxiety disorders in children and adolescents.* New York: Guilford Press.

McGee, R., Feehan, M., Williams, S., Partridge, F., Silva, P. A., & Kelly, J. (1990). *DSM-III* disorders in a large sample of adolescents. *Journal of the American Academy of Child and Adolescent Psychiatry, 29*, 611–619.

Offer, D., Howard, K. I., Schonert, K. A., & Ostrov, E. (1991). To whom do adolescents turn for help? Differences between disturbed and nondisturbed adolescents. *Journal of the American Academy of Child and Adolescent Psychiatry, 30*, 623–630.

Offord, D. R., Boyle, M. H., & Szatmari, P., Rae-Grant, N. I., Links, P. S., Cadman, D. T., Byles, J. A., et al. (1987). Ontario Child Health Study: II. Six-month prevalence of disorder and rates of service utilization. *Archives of General Psychiatry, 44*, 832–836.

Staghezza-Jaramillo, B., Bird, H. R., Gould, M. S., & Canino, G. (1995). Mental health service utilization among Puerto Rican children ages 4 through 16. *Journal of Child and Family Studies, 4*, 399–418.

U.S. Public Health Service. (1999). *Mental health: A report of the Surgeon General.* Washington, DC: Department of Health and Human Services.

Verhulst, F. C., & van der Ende, J. (1997). Factors associated with child mental health service use in the community. *Journal of the American Academy of Child and Adolescent Psychiatry, 36*, 901–909.

Wu, P., Hoven, C. W., Bird, H. R., Moore, R. E., Cohen, P., Alegria, M., Dulcan, M. K., et al. (1999). Depressive and disruptive disorders and mental health utilization in children and adolescents. *Journal of the American Academy of Child and Adolescent Psychiatry, 38*, 1081–1092.

Zahner, G. E. P., Pawelkiewicz, W., DeFrancesco, J. J., & Adnopoz, J. (1992). Children's mental health service needs and utilization patterns in an urban community: An epidemiology assessment. *Journal of the American Academy of Child and Adolescent Psychiatry, 31*, 951–960.

INDEX